D1443857

HOME
REHABILITATION
Guide to Clinical Practice

WENDY K. ANEMAET, MS, PT, GCS, ATC
Home Care Therapist
Board-Certified Specialist in Geriatric Physical Therapy
Miami, Florida

MICHELLE E. MOFFA-TROTTER, PT, GCS
Home Care Therapist
Board-Certified Specialist in Geriatric Physical Therapy
Clearwater, Florida

Contributions from
J MARK TROTTER, PharmD
Clinical Pharmacist Ambulatory Care
Veterans Administration Medical Center

Adjunct Faculty, Department of Pharmacy Practice
Mercer University, Southern School of Pharmacy
Macon, Georgia

with 270 illustrations

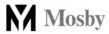

St. Louis Baltimore Boston Carlsbad Chicago Minneapolis New York Philadelphia Portland
London Milan Sydney Tokyo Toronto

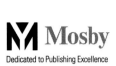
Mosby
Dedicated to Publishing Excellence

Editor-in-Chief: John Schrefer
Executive Editor: Martha Sasser
Developmental Editor: Christie M. Hart
Project Manager: Linda McKinley
Designer: Renée Duenow

Mosby, Inc.
A Harcourt Health Sciences Company
11830 Westline Industrial Drive
St. Louis, Missouri 63146

Printed in the United States of America

International Standard Book Number 0-323-00285-4

99 00 01 02 03 CA / RDC 9 8 7 6 5 4 3 2 1

About the Authors

Michelle E. Moffa-Trotter is an Honor's Scholar graduate from the University of Connecticut School of Allied Health Professions Physical Therapy Program.

Wendy K. Anemaet earned her master's degree in physical therapy at the University of Southern California.

Both authors are board-certified geriatric clinical specialists practicing in Florida. They serve as columnists and editorial consultants for ADVANCE Publications and on the editorial boards of the journals *Physical Therapy in Perspective* and *Topics in Geriatric Rehabilitation,* respectively. They lecture nationally on the topic of home rehabilitation and have written the practice-oriented text *The User Friendly Home Care Handbook.*

Preface

Home health care is one of the most rewarding and challenging settings for therapists today, allowing autonomy and flexibility as well as opportunities to provide one-on-one care and gain unique insights into patients' lives. More and more, therapists and patients are realizing the diverse benefits of home rehabilitation—of skilled therapy services provided in the environments patients use most. In turn the field of home health care has greatly expanded, allowing patients to utilize services that were previously unavailable in the home environment. Longer life spans, higher survival rates of the chronically ill, and advances in medical technology have further increased the demand for quality home health care services. As a result, home rehabilitation practice has evolved into a distinct field that requires a unique set of skills. Home health care therapists must continually hone their evaluation abilities and upgrade therapeutic program development to excel in the field. In addition, today's home rehabilitation therapists are often required to become effective and competent case managers, coordinating case and taking responsibility for the patient care plan.

Home Rehabilitation: Guide to Clinical Practice meets the multifaceted needs of today's novice and seasoned home care therapists. This portable library focuses on the necessary information required for success in home rehabilitation practice. The guide's compact size allows therapists to carry it into the home for immediate reference. The spiral binding allows it to lay flat when opened, and the wrap-around flap can be used as a built-in bookmark. The information is concise and easy to reference. Assessments offer therapists an array of tools to objectify functional status in a comprehensive range of patient populations. Standards provide a synthesis of reference information and data. Guidelines include descriptions of recommended procedures and action plans for commonly encountered conditions.

Home Rehabilitation: Guide to Clinical Practice is divided into six major parts. Part One, "The Fundamentals of Home Health Care," covers the introductory information necessary for the successful practice of home health rehabilitation. Topics include employment options, schedule maintenance, therapist equipment, infection control, personal safety, the home care team, regulatory bodies, documentation, and ethical situations. Part One orients therapists to the daily operations of home health care.

Part Two, "Pediatric Population," contains essential information that helps therapists comprehensively address the unique needs of this special population. This part includes information on environmental evaluations, developmental assessments, the special needs of neonates, and frequently encountered problems.

Additional topics include evaluation tools, milestones, and adaptive techniques for addressing the needs of children.

Part Three, "Adult Population," provides a compendium of information that can be used to meet the needs of adult home health patients. Areas covered include the home environment, affective evaluations, activities of daily living, mobility, fine motor skills, neurological disorders, integument concerns, and cardiopulmonary conditions. Functional tools, normative data, and classification guidelines fully prepare therapists for evaluating and treating adult patients in the home.

Part Four, "Emergency Situations," presents various medical scenarios that may be encountered in the home. "Warning Signs" includes the signs and symptoms and appropriate action plans for a wide range of medical conditions. "Cardiopulmonary Resuscitation Procedures" and "First Aid" provide guidelines for proper care.

Part Five, "Pharmacology," comprises pertinent medication-related information. "Medication Classification" contains a list of drugs by their generic and trade names for easy referencing and classification on medication profiles. "Medication Management" highlights key drug characteristics, including adverse reactions, that may have an impact on rehabilitation.

The appendixes contain information previously found only in agency publications. Time and time again, therapists can quickly and conveniently refer to helpful resources such as the Medicare's coverage of services guidelines, the durable medical equipment requirements, a rehabilitation abbreviation list, the ICD-9-CM common therapy diagnoses, a resource listing, and a journal and publications listing.

As the home health care field comes of age, it continues to undergo numerous changes that challenge home health care professionals. This book equips therapists with the knowledge needed for success in the rapidly evolving world of home health care.

Wendy K. Anemaet
Michelle E. Moffa-Trotter

Contents

PART FOUR *Emergency Situations, 521*

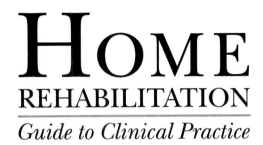

HOME
REHABILITATION
Guide to Clinical Practice

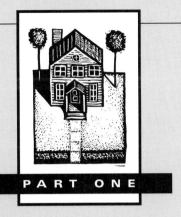

PART ONE

The Fundamentals of Home Health Care

HOME HEALTH EMPLOYMENT OPTIONS

THERAPY SCHEDULE MAINTENANCE

EQUIPMENT LISTS

INFECTION CONTROL

PERSONAL SAFETY GUIDELINES

THE HOME CARE TEAM

HOME CARE REGULATORY BODIES

HOME CARE DOCUMENTATION GUIDELINES

ETHICAL SITUATIONS IN HOME CARE

HOME HEALTH EMPLOYMENT OPTIONS

Home care therapists enjoy a wide range of employment arrangements and options not typically available to therapists in other treatment settings. A firm understanding of the employment terminology, advantages and disadvantages of staff versus independent contractor positions, and appropriate interview questions helps therapists make wise career decisions. This section provides an in-depth discussion of each topic.

Home Health Employment Options Glossary

Staff therapist status. Refers to therapists who work as employees of home health care agencies, which control the manner in which services are provided, pay their employees' taxes, define the job description, and bear the full risk for profits and losses

   Full-time staff members. Therapists who work exclusively for one agency; usually defined as such when they work a minimum number of hours or provide a minimum number of therapy visits per week

   Part-time staff members. Therapists who work outside agencies or with multiple agencies or those whose sole employment arrangements are with one agency as part-time therapists; usually defined as such when they work fewer hours or provide fewer visits than a minimum number that defines full-time status

PRN staff members. Therapists who may work in treatment settings other than home health care or with multiple agencies or whose only employment arrangement are with one agency as PRN staff therapists; usually defined as such when they accept employment on a short-term, often a fill-in, basis; *PRN* referring to the Latin phrase *pro re nata*, meaning "as needed"

Independent contractor status. Refers to therapists who control all aspects of the services they perform; handle their own taxes, build their own business reputations, contract with more than one home health care agency, and realize profits and losses

   Full-time contractors. Self-employed therapists who work solely in home care and spend at least 35 hours per week providing home care services

   Part-time contractors. Self-employed therapists who work in a variety of treatment settings, as staff therapists within agencies, or part time for one agency only; typically spend less than 35 hours per week providing home care services

Home Health Employment Settings Glossary

Home health agencies. Agencies that are usually Medicare certified and offer skilled and nonskilled home health services, such as nursing, medical social services, personal care, and rehabilitation; must supervise and control all services carefully because of strict federal guidelines; also recruit and supervise their personnel and assume liability for all care

Hospices. Providers that are usually Medicare certified and offer comprehensive, medically-directed palliative care to the terminally ill and their families; provide nursing, medical social treatment, physician care, personal care, spiritual counseling, volunteers, and rehabilitation; also must control and supervise all services carefully because of strict federal regulations; recruit and supervise their personnel and assume liability for all care

Rehabilitation contracting agencies. Providers that subcontract rehabilitation staff members to home health agencies or hospices; typically function as employers through maintenance of personnel files, handling of inservice training, and paying of employee taxes

Comparison of Staff Therapists with Independent Contractors

Variable	Staff therapists	Independent contractors
Employment status	Determined by agency	Determined by therapist
Work week	Determined by agency	Determined by therapist
Method of reimbursement	Paid per hour or per visit or included in salary	Paid per visit
Mileage reimbursement	Reimbursed fully or partially at agency's discretion	Not reimbursed
Scheduling of visits	Scheduled by agency or by therapist at agency's discretion	Scheduled by therapist
Required office time	Determined by agency	Determined by therapist
Required meeting attendance	Determined by agency	Determined by therapist
Meeting and office time reimbursement	Determined by agency; may be paid per hour or per visit or included in salary	Paid hourly reimbursement if included in work contract
Supplies	Provided by agency	Provided by therapist
Benefits	Provided by agency	Provided by therapist
Coverage for time off	Arranged by agency	Arranged by therapist

Staff Therapist Benefits

Staff therapists have access to numerous employer-sponsored benefits. Although agency benefits packages vary considerably, they may include any or all of the following items:

Insurance coverage
- Health insurance
- Dental insurance
- Disability insurance
- Life insurance

- Professional liability insurance
- Worker's compensation protection

Paid time off
- Vacation days
- Holidays
- Sick days
- Family leave

Spending accounts
- Dependent care
- Medical care

Incentive plans
- Productivity bonuses
- Quality-care bonuses
- Out-of-territory bonuses
- On-call bonuses

Investment options
- Retirement plans
- Stock option plans

Professional reimbursements
- Professional association dues
- Continuing education

Supplies
- Personal protective equipment
- Therapy evaluation equipment
- Therapy treatment equipment

Telecommunications
- Beepers
- Mobile phones
- Voice-mail systems
- Computerized documentation systems

Transportation reimbursements
- Mileage reimbursement
- Automobile provision

Guidelines for Independent Contractor Therapists

Federal and state governments and the Internal Revenue Service use various tests to determine the true nature of employment arrangements. Home care therapists working as independent contractors must prove that they function as true self-employed therapists, not agency employees. This section provides a home health care adaptation of the IRS Revenue Ruling 87-41, which provides guidance concerning 20 common law factors that individuals must consider to determine whether they are viewed as self employed or employees of a company. The guidelines allow independent therapists to self-evaluate the strengths and weaknesses of the status. Independent contractors should strive to meet a majority of the following test requirements to validate their self-employed status:*

Determination of Therapist Status

1. **Instructions.** Home care therapists who must follow agency instructions about the ways in which they provide services usually are considered agency employees because they must follow the same agency rules as staff therapists.

2. **Training.** Home care therapists who undergo training and orientation within agencies usually are considered agency employees because self-employed therapists should not require nurturing and training; instead, they should come to agencies fully able and ready to render home therapy services.

3. **Integration.** The closer an independent contractor works with an agency, the more likely that therapist is considered an agency employee. Integration is one test that independent contractor therapists fail because the provision of rehabilitation services in the home by an independent contractor overlaps with those provided by an agency.

4. **Services rendered personally.** Therapists required by agencies to provide services personally and prohibited within work contracts from independent use of therapist assistants and supplying their own vacation coverage usually are considered agency employees because agencies exert and maintain control over them.

5. **Hiring, supervising, and paying of assistants.** Home care therapists who supervise staff therapist assistants usually are considered agency employees because they do not control the hiring, paying, and firing of these assistants.

6. **Continuing relationship.** Home care therapists who contract with one agency for many years, particularly if the employment arrangements are exclusive, usually are considered agency employees because these therapists maintain continuing relationships with employers just as staff therapists do.

7. **Set work hours.** Home care therapists who must follow agency directives about availability usually are considered agency employees because they do not have the freedom to plan their own work days or weeks.

8. **Requirements for full-time work.** Home care therapists who are not free to reject or accept visits and are subject to agency-established minimum or maximum hours (or minimum or maximum visits per week) usually are considered agency employees because they do not exert full control over their business.

---

*Independent contractor therapists need not meet all 20 tests to prove self-employment status.

Box—cont'd

9. **Work performed on agency premises.** Home care therapists who routinely spend time in agencies for such things as documentation or photocopying usually are considered agency employees because they do not maintain their own place of business.

10. **Order or sequence set.** Home care therapists who must follow agency directives about visit scheduling usually are considered agency employees because they do not set their own work schedules.

11. **Oral or written reports.** Home care therapists who must complete such things as open medical record reviews usually are considered agency employees because agencies frequently require that staff therapists complete such regular reports.

12. **Payment by hour, week, or month.** Home care therapists who accept payments that are not based on a per-visit basis usually are considered agency employees because they are not paid "by the job."

13. **Business or traveling expenses.** Home care therapists who accept mileage payments, telecommunications stipends, or other types of reimbursements usually are considered agency employees because they do not cover their own business overhead.

14. **Tools and materials.** Home care therapists who accept agency supplies, such as personal protective equipment, goniometers, and cuff weights, usually are considered agency employees because they do not cover the costs of their own therapy supplies.

15. **Significant investment.** Home care therapists who accrue few business deductions usually are considered agency employees. Independent contractors by definition have significant investments in their businesses.

16. **Realization of profit or loss.** Home care therapists who accept reimbursements for canceled, refused, or missed visits usually are considered agency employees because agencies protect their employees from the burden of realizing business losses.

17. **Work performed for more than one company at a time.** Home care therapists who work exclusively for one agency usually are considered employees of the agency. Varied and substantial client bases are hallmarks of independent contractors.

18. **Services available to the general public.** Home care therapists who use agency business cards, identification badges, office space, and listed telephone numbers usually are considered agency employees because such therapists have their names in the general public only in association with an agency.

19. **Right to discharge.** Home care therapists who enter work contracts that allow agencies to discharge them usually are considered agency employees because independent contractor work contracts should delineate specific notice requirements for termination.

20. **Right to terminate.** Home care therapists who enter work contracts that allow for termination of the relationship with agencies at any time without an incurrence of liability usually are considered agency employees because such agreements suggest "at-will" relationships under which no particular notice or termination requirements exist.

Employment Interview Guidelines
Staff Therapists

Agency:
Interviewer:

Caseload

What is the expected caseload?	
What is the average caseload?	
May I see the therapy census for the past 2 months?	
Are evaluations counted as more than one visit?	
If my caseload drops, must I perform office time?	
Is office time considered part of the normal caseload?	
Are meetings considered part of the normal caseload?	
Will I be paid overtime for extra office time or meetings?	
Will I perform admissions?	
Are admissions counted as one or two visits?	
Will I be guaranteed 40 hours per week?	
What are some commonly seen diagnoses?	
What age groups do the agency's patients represent?	
What are the agency's major payer sources?	

Job Specifics

May I keep a copy of the job description?	
Who schedules visits?	
Will I work 5 days per week?	
Is on-call time required? If so, how often?	
Will I supervise home health aides?	
Will I supervise therapist assistants?	
May I follow the patients I evaluate?	
How long is orientation in the agency and the field?	
Who provides the orientation?	

How will I be reimbursed for orientation?	
Who owns the agency?	
What is the chain of command?	
Who will be my direct supervisor?	
What is the agency's level of JCAHO or CHAP accreditation?	
When was the last JCAHO or CHAP survey?	
When was the last state survey?	
What problem areas did the surveyors find?	
Does the agency have a performance improvement program in effect?	
What are the therapy performance improvement indicators?	
When are case conferences held?	
How often are the required meetings?	
How long are those meetings?	
How does the agency determine mileage reimbursements?	
What is the dress code?	
When is paperwork due?	
Is a drop box provided?	
What areas will my territory include?	

Benefits

What will be my salary, hourly rate, or per-visit rate?	
How much is the mileage reimbursement?	
What is the reimbursement for required meetings?	
Is on-call time available? If so, at what rate?	
How often will I be paid?	
Does the agency offer direct deposit?	
May I work overtime? If so, at what rate?	

Modified from Anemaet WK, Moffa-Trotter ME: *The user friendly home care handbook,* McLean, Va, 1997, LEARN Publications. *JCAHO,* Joint Commission on the Accreditation of Healthcare Organizations; *CHAP,* Community Health Accreditation Program.

Box—cont'd

Benefits—cont'd	
Is overtime required?	
Will I be required to work holidays?	
Does the agency have a holiday pay differential?	
How are visits handled during holiday weeks?	
Does the agency have a weekend differential?	
May I take time off without pay?	
How often does the agency award pay increases?	
How much was the last pay increase? When was it?	
Does the agency offer health insurance?	
Does the agency offer dental insurance?	
Does the agency offer life insurance?	
Does the agency offer disability insurance?	
Does the agency offer malpractice insurance?	

Benefits—cont'd	
How much are the copayment amounts for these insurance plans?	
Does the agency offer retirement plans?	
What are the agency's incentive plans?	
Does the agency offer a sign-on bonus?	
How much paid time off will I receive?	
Does the agency provide a beeper?	
Does the agency provide a mobile phone?	
Does the agency provide voice mail?	
Does the agency reimburse toll costs?	
Does the agency reimburse pay phone costs?	
Does the agency reimburse mobile phone costs?	
Does the agency reimburse professional organization dues?	
Do employees use dictation or computers for notes?	
Does the agency provide a company vehicle?	

Independent Contractor Therapists

Agency:	
Interviewer:	

Caseload	
How many visits are available per week?	
May I see the therapy census for the past 2 months?	
How many staff therapists do you employ?	
How many contractor therapists do you use?	
What percentage of patients are seen by staff versus contractor therapists?	
Who decides which therapists see which patients?	
Are therapists reimbursed for time spent in meetings?	

Caseload—cont'd	
What are some commonly seen diagnoses?	
What age groups do the agency's patients represent?	
What are the agency's major payer sources?	
Will I perform admissions?	

Job Specifics	
Who schedules visits?	
Is on-call time available? If so, at what rate?	
May I follow the patients I evaluate?	

Modified from Anemaet WK, Moffa-Trotter ME: *The user friendly home care handbook,* McLean, Va, 1997, LEARN Publications.

Continued

Box—cont'd

Job Specifics—cont'd	
Who provides the orientation?	
How much will I be reimbursed for orientation?	
Who owns the agency?	
What is the chain of command?	
Who is my agency contact person?	
What is the agency's level of JCAHO or CHAP accreditation?	
When was the last JCAHO or CHAP survey?	
When was the last state survey?	
What problem areas did these surveyors find?	
Does the agency have a performance improvement program in effect?	
What are the therapy performance improvement indicators?	
How often are staff meetings?	

Job Specifics—cont'd	
How long are staff meetings?	
When are case conferences held?	
How often is paperwork due?	
Does the agency have a drop box?	
What is the agency's territory?	

Benefits	
What is the rate for contractors?	
How often will I be paid?	
How much is the reimbursement for meetings?	
What is the rate for evaluations?	
What is the rate for admissions?	
What is the partial-visit rate for refusals or cancellations?	
Does the agency offer direct deposit?	
Does the agency use computerized documentation?	

Modified from Anemaet WK, Moffa-Trotter ME: *The user friendly home care handbook,* McLean, Va, 1997, LEARN Publications. *JCAHO,* Joint Commission on the Accreditation of Healthcare Organizations; *CHAP,* Community Health Accreditation Program.

THERAPY SCHEDULE MAINTENANCE

Some therapists are born organized and have their days scheduled down to the minute. Others, however, consider their days well organized when they remember to set their alarm clocks and grab their lunches before scooting out their front doors. Many others fall somewhere between these two extremes. Home care therapists must establish some level of organization in each of two areas—the scheduling of initial visits and the maintenance of weekly therapy schedules.

Initial Visit Scheduling

Inpatient facilities, such as acute-care hospitals, rehabilitation centers, and long-term care units, and outpatient facilities usually do not require that therapists schedule initial visits. Generally, office managers perform this duty; in many inpatient settings patients are accessible at all times, which makes formal scheduling unnecessary. However, because home care dictates that therapists visit their patients, not the other way around, scheduling is part of all home care therapists' jobs. Therefore therapists must possess a clear understanding of the information they must gather from agencies and patients to effectively and efficiently schedule visits.

Information Gathering

Necessary information	Possible sources	Necessary information	Possible sources
Demographics	Intake sheet	Weight-bearing status	Physician
Name	Clinical supervisor	(if applicable)	Intake sheet
Address	Case manager		Clinical supervisor
Phone number			Case manager
Diagnosis	Physician	Protocol (if applicable)	Physician
	Intake sheet		Intake sheet
	Clinical supervisor		Clinical supervisor
	Case manager		Case manager
Home rehabilitation	Clinical supervisor	Reason for therapy	Physician
admission date	Case manager	referral	Intake sheet
Physician's order for	Physician		Clinical supervisor
therapy	Intake sheet		Case manager
	Clinical supervisor	Case manager's name	Intake sheet
	Case manager	and phone number	Clinical supervisor
Physician's name and	Intake sheet	Other services in the	Intake sheet
phone number	Clinical supervisor	home (besides therapy)	Clinical supervisor
	Case manager		Case manager
Relevant medical history	Patient or caregiver	Conflicting	Patient or caregiver
	Intake sheet	appointments	
	Clinical supervisor	Patient	
	Case manager	preference	
Present medical condition	Patient or caregiver	or choice	
	Intake sheet	Physician	
	Clinical supervisor	Other disciplines	
	Case manager	Dialysis	
Mental status	Intake sheet	Chemotherapy:	
	Clinical supervisor	Directions to home	Patient or caregiver
	Case manager		Case manager
Name of caregiver	Patient or caregiver		Clinical supervisor
	Intake sheet	Pets in home	Patient or caregiver
	Clinical supervisor		Case manager
	Case manager	Meal times	Patient or caregiver
Primary language	Patient or caregiver	Parking availability or	Patient or caregiver
	Intake sheet	restrictions	Case manager
	Clinical supervisor	Security	Patient or caregiver
	Case manager		Case manager

Weekly Schedule Maintenance

Whether they use commercially produced schedule books or sheets of scrap paper, therapists must develop some organized method of maintaining visit days and times. Although this scheduling format may differ from therapist to therapist, the information remains essentially constant. Efficient therapists minimize missed visits and down time through effective organization and maintenance of weekly therapy schedules.

Weekly Schedule Formats

Type	Examples	Advantages	Disadvantages
Commercially produced schedule books	Daytimer Week-at-a-glance	Professional look Organization	Design not specific for home rehabilitation
Schedule pads	Figure 1-1	Low cost Design specific for home rehabilitation	Mail-order availability only
Schedule card systems	Figure 1-2	Low cost Ability to tailor to specific needs	Time-consuming creation
Schedule papers	Figure 1-3	Very low cost	Lack of organization Ease of misplacement

Hints for Weekly Schedule Maintenance

- Record patients' addresses and phone numbers in one location for easy reference on initial visit.
- Schedule more visits early in the week to allow time to reschedule missed visits and make room for new patients.
- Schedule admissions and evaluations at the end of the day to minimize the effects of longer-than-anticipated visits.
- Allow at least 1 hour for evaluations and 2 hours for admissions.
- When working for several agencies, highlight the names of patients with each agency in a particular color to make billing easier.
- Record all time spent in the agency and in meetings.
- Develop a shorthand coding system to justify missed visits.
- Develop a coding system for recertification dates and progress report due dates.
- Tally the number of visits and amount of mileage for the end of each day and week.
- Record all mileage for reimbursement and tax purposes.
- Record all toll fees for reimbursement and tax purposes.
- Retain weekly therapy schedules for tax purposes.

EQUIPMENT LISTS

Effective, efficient home care requires that therapists prepare themselves for unique health care settings—patients' homes. A large part of that preparation involves the gathering of necessary equipment. Agencies provide a number of necessary items, but therapists are responsible for supplying many others. Administrative equipment helps therapists organize paperwork and communicate with other members of the home care team. Evaluative equipment aids therapists in effectively quantifying and objectifying their findings. Treatment equipment lends therapists options to assist patients in achieving goals and helps make treatment sessions interesting for patients.

SCHEDULE FOR WEEK ENDING _____12/11_____

🕐	Sunday	Monday	Tuesday	Wednesday	Thursday	Friday	Saturday
7:30 AM							
7:45 AM							
8:00 AM		Allan Alibaba	Alibaba, A	Alibaba, A	Alibaba, A	Alibaba, A	
8:15 AM							
8:30 AM							
8:45 AM							
9:00 AM		Nicholas Bell	Bell, N	Case conference	Bell, N (D)		
9:15 AM							
9:30 AM						PI meeting	
9:45 AM							
10:00 AM		Sue Lee (E)			Lee, S		
10:15 AM		1234 1st St.		↓		↓	
10:30 AM		555-9876	Joy Skertz (S)				
10:45 AM		s/p THR					
11:00 AM				Rubins, B (I)			
11:15 AM							
11:30 AM		Barb Rubins					
11:45 AM							
12:00 PM			Mark James	James, M	DeVogel, J	James, M (RV)	
12:15 PM							
12:30 PM		Josie DeVogel					
12:45 PM							
1:00 PM			Joanne Diaz (E)		Diaz, J		
1:15 PM			5678 2nd Ave.				
1:30 PM			555-5432				
1:45 PM			S/P CVA				
2:00 PM		Payman Maghsoudi		Maghsoudi, P	Rob Ferrar (CM)	Maghsoudi, P (R)	
2:15 PM							
2:30 PM			Shalini Lal (E)				
2:45 PM			91011 3rd Terr.				
3:00 PM		Aviendha Taardad	555-1098	Lal, S	Taardad, A	Lal, S	
3:15 PM		(P)	Gait abnormality				
3:30 PM							
3:45 PM							
4:00 PM			Bob Edwards			Edwards, B (D)	
4:15 PM							
4:30 PM							
4:45 PM							
5:00 PM							
5:15 PM							
5:30 PM							
5:45 PM							
6:00 PM							
6:15 PM							
6:30 PM							
6:45 PM							
7:00 PM							
7:15 PM							
7:30 PM							
TOTAL MILES		61	81	47	74	54	
TOTAL VISITS		6	7	4	7	4	

(E) Evaluation	(S) Supervisory visit	(P) Missed visit—physician visit	(CM) Case management visit	TOTAL WEEK MILES	317
(D) Discharge visit	(I) Missed visit—patient ill	(R) Missed visit—patient refused	(RV) Reassessment visit	TOTAL WEEK VISITS	28

FIGURE 1-1 Schedule pad. *PI*, Performance improvement; *CVA*, cerebrovascular accident; *s/p*, status post; *THR*, total hip relacement. (Modified from Anemaet WK, Moffa-Trotter ME: *Pads with pizzazz*, Miami, 1998, Self.)

12/5 – 12/11

	Sun	Mon	Tues	Wed	Thurs	Fri	Sat
8:00		Allan Alibaba	Alibaba, A	Alibaba, A	Alibaba, A △	Alibaba, A	
9:00		Nicholas Bell	Bell, N	Case Conference	Bell, N ⊗	PI meeting	
10:00		Sue Lee ● 1234 1st St. 555-9876 s/p THR	Joy Skertz ○	↓	Lee, S	↓	
11:00		Barb Rubins		Rubins, B ✳			
12:00		Josie DeVogel	Mark James	James, M	DeVogel, J	James, M	
1:00			Joanne Diaz ● 5678 2nd Ave. 555-5432 S/P CVA		Diaz, J		
2:00		Payman Maghsoudi	Shalani Lal ● 91011 3rd Terr. 555-1098 Gait abnormality	Maghsoudi, P	Rob Ferrar ■	Maghsoudi, P	
3:00		Avienda Taardad ✳		Lal, S	Taardad, A	Lal, S	
4:00			Bob Edwards			Edwards, B ⊗	
Patients / Miles		6 / 61	7 / 81	4 / 47	7 / 74	4 / 54	

TOTAL PATIENTS 28
TOTAL MILES 317

Key
- ● Evaluation
- ⊗ Discharge
- ○ Supervisory visit
- ■ Case management visit
- ✳ Missed visit
- △ Progress note due

FIGURE 1-2 Schedule card. *PI,* Performance improvement; *CVA,* cerebrovascular accident; *s/p,* status post; *THR,* total hip relacement.

Mon	Tues	Wed	Thurs	Fri
Allan Alibaba	Alibaba, A	Alibaba, A	Alibaba, A	Alibaba, A
Nicholas Bell	Bell, N	Case	Bell, N d/c	PI meeting
		conference		
Sue Lee	Joy Skertz		Lee, S	
1234 1st St.				
555-9876				
s/p THR				
Barb Rubins		Rubins, B ill		
Josie DeVogel	Mark James	James, M	DeVogel, J	James, M
	Joanne Diaz		Diaz, J	
	5678 2nd Ave.			
	555-5432			
	s/p CVA			
Payman Maghsoudi		Maghsoudi, P	Rob Ferrar	Maghsoudi, P
				Refused
	Shalini Lal			
	91011 3rd Terr.			
Avienda Taardad	555-1098	Lal, S	Taardad, A	Lal, S
MD visit	Gait abnormality			
	Bob Edwards			Edwards, B d/c

FIGURE 1-3 Schedule paper. *PI*, Performance improvement; *CVA*, cerebrovascular accident; *s/p*, status post; *THR*, total hip replacement; *D/C*, discharge; *MD*, physician.

General equipment assists therapists in compliance with Occupational Safety and Health Administration (OSHA) and Joint Commission on the Accreditation of Healthcare Organizations (JCAHO) guidelines for infection control and safety. Each type of equipment is important to the building of a successful home care career.

Administrative Equipment

Equipment	Purpose
Appointment book	Organizes daily and weekly schedules
Beeper	Facilitates contact between agencies and other team members
Black pens	Promote clear photocopies and faxes
Mobile phone	Provides immediate access to agencies, physicians, payers, and patients
Clipboards	Serve as firm writing surfaces for documentation
Expandable files	Organize agency forms and handouts for patients
Folders	Organize information and daily notes
Highlighters	Emphasize important information on handouts for patients
Maps	Assist in location of patients' homes
Multiple copies of paperwork	Minimize unplanned trips to agencies

Modified from Anemaet WK, Moffa-Trotter ME: *The user friendly home care handbook*, McLean, Va, 1997, LEARN Publications.

Evaluative Equipment

Equipment	Purpose
Goniometer	Measures joint range of motion
Handheld dynamometer	Measures strength
Reflex hammer	Assesses deep tendon reflexes
Ruler	Measures incisions, wounds, and functional reaches
Sensation testing tools	Assess sensory status
Sphygmomanometer	Measures blood pressure and screens for deep vein thromboses
Stethoscope	Assists in blood pressure measurement and auscultation
Tape measure	Quantifies girth, extremity and incision length, and spinal range of motion
Thermometer	Measures body temperature and temperature of whirlpool
Watch	Quantifies vital signs and visit and travel times; also necessary for some functional tools

Modified from Anemaet WK, Moffa-Trotter ME: *The user friendly home care handbook,* McLean, Va, 1997, LEARN Publications.

Treatment Equipment

Equipment	Purpose
Adaptive devices	Facilitate performance of ADL
Assistive devices	Facilitate performance of gait and ADL
Bandage scissors	Cut dressings for easy removal
Cuff weights	Provide resistance for exercises
	Serve as tools for inhibition techniques
Debridement kits	Allow for removal of necrotic tissue
Dressings	Enhance wound closure
Electrical stimulation units	Facilitate edema reduction and muscle activation and recruitment
	Enhance wound closure
Exercise tubings	Provide resistance for exercises
Hand dexterity tools	Facilitate fine motor control and coordination
Platforms or steps	Provide tools for stair training during inclement weather
	Facilitate balance reactions
	Promote lower-extremity strengthening
Splinting materials	Help therapists fabricate splints
Sterile fields	Provide clean barriers for wound care
Therapy balls	Facilitate balance training, reaction times, strengthening, and coordination
Transcutaneous electrical nerve stimulation units	Provide pain management
Ultrasound units	Facilitate heating of deep tissues and edema reduction

Modified from Anemaet WK, Moffa-Trotter ME: *The user friendly home care handbook,* McLean, Va, 1997, LEARN Publications. *ADL,* Activities of daily living.

General Equipment

Equipment	Purpose
Barriers	Minimize risk of contact between "clean" items and potentially infectious microorganisms
Coolers	Keep drinks and snacks cool throughout the day
Cardiopulmonary resuscitation shields	Provide barriers to minimize transmission of infectious disease during mouth-to-mouth resuscitation
Equipment cleansers	Clean equipment in accordance with OSHA guidelines
Gait belts	Assist therapists in the maintenance of balance with gait and transfers
	Minimize the risk that therapists or patients may sustain injuries during gait and transfer training
Gloves	Minimize the risk of hand contact with potentially infectious microorganisms
Gowns	Minimize the risk of skin contact with potentially infectious microorganisms
Hand cleansers	Minimize the risks of viral and bacterial spread
Masks	Minimize the risk of contact with airborne microorganisms
Personal defense equipment	Prepares therapists for dangerous situations
Safety glasses or eye shields	Minimize the risk of contact between the eyes and potentially infectious microorganisms
Spill kits	Minimize the risk of contact between the skin and potentially infectious liquids during cleanup
Therapy bag	Facilitates transportation of necessary therapy equipment from the vehicle to the patients' homes

Modified from Anemaet WK, Moffa-Trotter ME: *The user friendly home care handbook,* McLean, Va, 1997, LEARN Publications.

INFECTION CONTROL

Home care therapists come in contact with dangerous bacteria and viruses every day when they treat and care for patients. This contact places them at risk for contracting a variety of illnesses and diseases and makes them potential carriers of these microorganisms. Therapists can spread diseases to agencies and patients' homes. Therefore therapists must adhere to certain infection-control procedures, including universal precautions, tuberculosis precautions, proper handling of biomedical waste and sharp items, hand washing, proper use of barriers, proper bag techniques, and proper procedures for equipment cleanup.

Infection Control Glossary

Acquired immunodeficiency syndrome. An immune system syndrome caused by the human immunodeficiency virus; characterized by opportunistic infections

Barriers. Materials that prevent items from coming into direct contact with patients' environments; used for items therapists must bring to and from patients' homes

Biomedical waste. Material that presents a risk of infection to humans

Body fluids. Blood; blood products; semen; vaginal secretions; fluid in the uterus of a pregnant woman; fluid surrounding the brain, spine, heart, or joints; fluid in the chest or abdomen; or other fluids that may contain blood, such as saliva

Bloodborne pathogens. Pathogenic microorganisms found in human blood that can cause disease in humans

"Clean." The absence or reasonably anticipated absence of infectious materials on items or surfaces

Contaminated. The presence or reasonably anticipated presence of potentially infectious materials on items or surfaces

Hepatitis B. Inflammation of the liver caused by a DNA virus; usually transmitted by contact with infected blood or blood derivatives

Hepatitis C. Inflammation of the liver caused by an RNA virus; usually transmitted by contact with infected blood or blood derivatives

Human immunodeficiency virus. The virus that causes AIDS

Occupational Safety and Health Administration. Federal agency that oversees and implements standards and guidelines for safety and health on the job or in the workplace

Personal protective equipment. Barriers worn or used to avoid contact with potentially infectious materials

Sharps. Objects that can puncture, lacerate, or in some other way penetrate the skin

Sterile. The absence of all microbial life, including highly resistant bacterial endospores

Tuberculosis. An infectious disease of the respiratory system caused by airborne pathogens

Universal precautions. An approach to infection control that treats all human blood and body fluids as if they carry HIV, HBV, and other bloodborne pathogens

Universal Precautions

Universal precautions are part of an approach to infection control established by OSHA; all health care workers must follow this approach. Simply put, universal precautions mean that the blood and bodily fluids of every individual must be treated as infectious. This assumption minimizes the risk that bloodborne pathogens—bacteria, viruses, and other microorganisms carried in the bloodstream or other bodily fluids—may be spread. Universal precautions encompass the first line of defense in infection control.

Universal Precautions for Home Care Therapists

- Wash hands before and after every visit.
- Maintain a "clean" working area in homes and place all equipment in that "clean" area.
- Use personal protective equipment when appropriate.
- Cover cuts, scrapes, rashes, and hangnails.
- Dispose of sharps in appropriate containers.
- Replace barriers and personal protective equipment when items appear visibly contaminated.
- Wear gloves when wiping up spills.
- Clean spilled blood or bodily fluids with spill kit.

- Dispose of biomedical waste in appropriate containers.
- Do not eat or drink in areas where bloodborne pathogens may be present.
- Clean equipment after use and when visibly contaminated.

Appropriate Use of Personal Protective Equipment

Type of equipment	Indication for use
Cardiopulmonary resuscitation mask	Mouth-to-mouth resuscitation
Gloves	Contact with blood, bodily fluids, mucous membranes, or broken skin
Gown	Potential bodily exposure to blood or bodily fluids
Mask	Possible splash, spray, or splatter of blood or bodily fluids that may reach the nose or mouth
	Contagious respiratory diagnoses, such as TB
Safety glasses or eye shields	Possible splash, spray, or splatter of blood or bodily fluids that may reach the eyes
Spill kit	Cleanup of potentially infectious liquids

TB, tuberculosis.

Tuberculosis

TB is a disease of the respiratory system caused by airborne pathogens. When an individual infected with TB talks, coughs, or sneezes, the disease is transmitted to others. Signs of active TB include a persistent cough that lasts 3 weeks or more, weakness, fever, weight loss, night sweats, chest pain during coughs, and coughing up of blood. Because TB is highly infectious, therapists must follow strict precautions to avoid contracting or spreading the disease.

Precautions for Home Care Therapists

- Identify patients who may have active TB as quickly as possible.
- Isolate patients with active TB.
- Wear approved respirators when in contact with individuals who have active TB. (Simple face masks do not provide adequate protection.)
- Encourage patients to cover their mouths when coughing or sneezing.

Biomedical Waste

Materials that present risks of infection to individuals are considered biomedical waste. Because of these risks, therapists must handle and dispose of such waste in a special manner. Home care therapists follow certain measures to ensure the proper handling of biomedical waste in patients' homes.

Handling of Biomedical Waste in the Home

- Always wear gloves when handling biomedical waste.
- Place all contaminated waste (except sharps) in leak-proof containers or bags in patients' homes.

- Place all leak-proof containers or bags with contaminated waste in red biomedical waste bags in reusable, rigid, puncture-resistant, leak-resistant containers in the nonpassenger section of the vehicle.
- Seal and label the filled red bags immediately.
- Write the agency's name and address and the date that you used and sealed the bag outside the red bag.
- Make sure that the outside of the red bag clearly displays the international biological hazard symbol (Figure 1-4) and the words *biomedical waste, biohazardous waste, biohazardous infectious waste,* or *infectious substance.*
- Store sealed and labeled red bags in the agency's biomedical storage area until a biomedical disposal company can remove them.

Sharps

Sharps are objects that can puncture, lacerate, or in some other way penetrate skin; they include needles, syringes, scalpels, and scissors. Therapists must handle these items as biomedical waste; however they cannot simply place sharps in red bags like other such waste. To effectively implement infection control programs, home care therapists must understand the procedure for the proper handling of sharps.

Handling of Sharps in the Home

- Wear gloves at all times when handling sharps.
- Dispose of sharps immediately after use.
- Place sharps in rigid, leak-resistant, puncture-resistant containers.
- Do not force anything into sharps containers.
- Do not reach inside sharps containers.
- Make sure that containers clearly display the international biological hazard symbol (see Figure 1-4).
- Seal sharps containers when they are two-thirds full.
- Label each sealed sharps container with the agency's name and address and the date the container was used.
- Place sharps containers in the nonpassenger area of the vehicle during transport.
- Keep sharps containers in upright positions at all times.
- Store sealed and labeled sharps containers in the agency's biomedical storage area until a biomedical disposal company can remove them.

FIGURE 1-4 The international biological hazard symbol.

Hand Washing

Hand washing is an important line of defense against the spread of infections. Soap, water, and vigorous rubbing help remove germs and reduce the risk that therapists may spread potentially infectious microorganisms. Therapists should wash their hands before and after each visit; after the removal of personal protective equipment; after bathroom use, coughing, sneezing, or eating; and after their hands become visibly contaminated.

Hand Washing Technique

1. Use bathroom sinks for hand washing. Avoid kitchen sinks to prevent contamination of or from food-preparation areas.
2. Place barriers between the counter surfaces and soap containers.
3. Push clothing sleeves above the elbows and remove jewelry before washing.
4. Do not allow clothing to touch the sink or water to splash on clothing.
5. Use paper towels to turn on the faucets.
6. Avoid hot water, which can dry and irritate skin.
7. Hold the hands with the fingertips down and wet them completely from above the wrists.
8. Use liquid soap instead of bar soap, which contains microorganisms.
9. Use antimicrobial soap before treating patients with known infections and patients at increased risk for infections.
10. Rub the hands together under flowing water for at least 15 seconds.
11. Clean under the nails by rubbing the fingertips against the palms.
12. Rinse the hands from above the wrists to the fingertips.
13. Pat the hands dry with clean, disposable paper towels.
14. Use paper towels to turn off the faucets.
15. Dispose of paper towels in patients' homes.

Barriers

Home care therapists carry their offices with them as they travel from home to home. Each home has different microorganisms, some potentially infectious. To minimize the risks of spreading infectious bacteria and viruses from one home to the next, therapists utilize barriers. Barriers are materials that prevent items therapists bring into homes and intend to remove from making direct contact with patients' environments. Commercially produced disposable fields, gowns or aprons; paper towels; and newspapers are all acceptable barriers. Each visit, therapists bring new barriers into homes and leave them, properly disposed, in each home. By using barriers correctly, therapists help prevent cross-contamination between patients.

Barrier Use in the Home

- Bring new barriers with each visit.
- Place barriers beneath bags and clipboards.
- Place barriers beneath hand soap brought into the home.
- Keep equipment that has not touched patients on barriers to prevent contamination.

- If kneeling or sitting in patients' homes, place barriers on those surfaces.
- Place all equipment items used with patients on barriers after cleaning them.
- Dispose of barriers before leaving patients' homes.

Bags

Therapists require the use of numerous items and pieces of equipment during treatment sessions. Because they cannot feasibly carry everything in their hands and pockets, many therapists utilize home health bags. These bags and the items contained within go into foreign environments (patients' homes) and may spread potentially infectious microorganisms. Therefore therapists must follow proper methods for the handling of home care bags and their contents to maximize infection control.

Bag Technique

1. Store multiple barriers, soap, and paper towels in the outside pocket of the bag.
2. Place the bag on a barrier on arrival at patients' homes.
3. Remove hand washing equipment and place it on a barrier at the sink.
4. Wash the hands before entering the "clean" inside area of the bag.
5. Remove necessary items and pieces of equipment from the bag and place them on a barrier until they are needed.
6. Remove cleaning materials needed for equipment and place them on a barrier for later use.
7. Close the bag when all the necessary items are removed.
8. Wash the hands before reentering the "clean" inside area of the bag if contact with patients occurred.
9. Clean used items and equipment before returning them to the "clean" inside area of the bag.
10. Return all clean items to the bag before leaving patients' homes.
11. Dispose of barriers in patients' homes.
12. Store the bag in a "clean" area of the vehicle.

Equipment Cleaning

Therapists use various pieces of equipment in the course of their days. When therapists use these items with numerous patients, the items can spread infectious microorganisms. Therefore therapists must possess a complete understanding of equipment-cleaning procedures, including knowledge of when to clean the equipment and what materials to use.

Cleaning of Evaluative Equipment

Equipment item	Frequency of cleansing	Cleansing agent	Appropriate barrier	Special instructions	Replacement instructions
Dynamometer	After each patient use	Disinfectant spray or wipes Alcohol pads 1:10 bleach solution	For handheld instruments: Disposable gloves For multijoint instruments: Plastic wrap Paper towel Wax paper Medical barrier Newspaper	Lubricate the spring mechanism with mineral oil.	Replace if instrument leaks or needle fluctuates.
Goniometer	After each patient use	Disinfectant spray or wipes Alcohol pads 1:10 bleach solution	Plastic wrap	Use a barrier only if the instrument makes contact with the patient's skin.	Replace if instrument becomes warped or damaged.
Neurological testing equipment	After each patient use	Disinfectant spray or wipes Alcohol pads 1:10 bleach solution	None (may impede accuracy of patient response)	Consider purchasing disposable sharp or dull testing equipment to prevent patient-to-patient contact.	Replace if equipment becomes warped or damaged.
Sphygmomanometer	After each patient use	Bladder meter with alcohol pads or a 1:10 bleach solution Cuff with disinfectant spray or wipes	Plastic wrap Paper towel Wax paper Medical barrier Newspaper	Wash or dry-clean cuffs with Velcro in the closed position. Calibrate once per year.	Replace if instrument leaks, does not inflate fully, or demonstrates needle fluctuation.
Stethoscope	After each patient use	Disinfectant spray or wipes Alcohol pads 1:10 bleach solution	None (may impede accuracy)	Clean diaphragm before and after each patient use.	Replace if hard, crystalline substance is palpable inside tubing.

Modified from Anemaet WK, Moffa-Trotter ME: *The user friendly home care handbook*, McLean, Va, 1997, LEARN Publications.

Cleaning of Treatment Equipment

Equipment item	Frequency of cleansing	Cleansing agent	Appropriate barrier	Special instructions	Replacement instructions
Assistive devices	After each patient use	Disinfectant spray or wipes Alcohol pads 1:10 bleach solution	Gloves (may impede performance)	Lubricate adjustable legs with petroleum jelly.	Replace if rubber tips or grips are worn or torn.
Cuff weight or dumbbell	After each patient use	Disinfectant spray or wipes Alcohol pads 1:10 bleach solution	Paper towel Plastic wrap Wax paper Medical barrier Newspaper Gloves	Use barrier only if cuff weight makes contact with patient's skin.	Replace if the item has an irreparable puncture or tear.
Gait belt	Once per month unless belt is soiled with bodily fluid	1:10 bleach solution Warm, soapy water	Paper towel Plastic wrap Wax paper Medical barrier Newspaper	Use barrier only if gait belt makes contact with patient's skin.	Replace if belt is heavily soiled or damaged or if clasp no longer works.
Exercise band or tubing	Never (not to be shared among patients; may degrade bands or tubing)	N/A	None	Give exercise band or tubing to patient to keep.	Replace if band or tubing splits or breaks.
Therapy ball	After each patient use	Warm, soapy water	Gloves (may impede performance)	Keep underinflated during transport in high elevations or warm climates because of risk of expansion.	Replace if ball has irreparable puncture or tear.

Modified from Anemaet WK, Moffa-Trotter ME: *The user friendly home care handbook*, McLean, Va, 1997, LEARN Publications.
N/A, Not applicable.

Cleaning of Modalities

Equipment item	Frequency of cleansing	Cleansing agent	Appropriate barrier	Special instructions	Replacement instructions
Cold pack	After each patient use	Warm, soapy water	Towel	Instruct patient to purchase cold pack to minimize patient-to-patient contact.	Replace if pack is punctured or torn.
Hot pack	After each patient use	Warm, soapy water	Towel	Instruct patient to purchase hot pack to minimize patient-to-patient contact.	Replace if pack is punctured or torn.
Electrical stimulation unit	After each patient use	Warm, soapy water	None	Instruct patient to obtain electrodes to minimize patient-to-patient contact.	Replace when unit no longer operates properly.
Transcutaneous electrical nerve stimulation unit	After each patient use	Warm, soapy water	None	Instruct patient to obtain electrodes to minimize patient-to-patient contact.	Replace when unit no longer operates properly.
Ultrasound unit	After each patient use	Warm, soapy water	None	Keep a calibration schedule with the unit to ensure that calibration is as manufacturer suggests.	Replace when unit no longer operates properly.

Modified from Anemaet WK, Moffa-Trotter ME: *The user friendly home care handbook*, McLean, Va, 1997, LEARN Publications.

Fundamentals of Home Health Care

PERSONAL SAFETY GUIDELINES

In hospitals, outpatient clinics, and extended-care settings, administrators enact rules and policies about procedures and conduct for patients to ensure the safety of staff members. These policies address issues such as drug abuse, weapons, and acceptable business conduct. In contrast, home health care agencies have limited control over actual treatment settings because care takes place in the home. Home care therapists must maximize their safety accordingly by following key guidelines.

Personal Safety Guidelines in the Community

Appearance and Communication
- Wear a name badge that identifies the home health care agency.
- Call patients in advance with approximate visit times.
- Clarify directions if necessary.
- Request that patients or caregivers secure menacing pets before visits.
- Back, do not run, from dogs.
- Walk around cows, pigs, and other farm animals to avoid frightening them.
- Keep change for phone calls in shoes or pockets.
- Lock purses in the vehicle's trunk or glove compartment.
- Consider carrying a mobile phone.

Driving
- Keep the vehicle in good working order, with sufficient fuel for the day.
- Store blankets, snacks, and fluids in the vehicle for emergencies.
- If the vehicle breaks down, turn on the emergency flashers and wait, with the doors locked, for the police.

Driving—cont'd
- Decline rides from strangers.
- Keep the vehicle doors locked and all the windows rolled up.
- Avoid parking in alleys or deserted side streets.

Walking
- Keep the therapy bag or equipment handy when exiting the vehicle.
- Keep one arm free at all times.
- Walk directly to visits in a professional, businesslike manner.
- Cross to the other side of the street when passing groups of strangers.
- Carry the vehicle keys in hand when leaving patients' homes.

Visiting
- Use common walkways in buildings.
- Avoid isolated stairs or entrances.
- Knock on doors before entering homes.
- Make joint visits with other staff members if relatives or neighbors pose safety problems.
- Request escort services or consider working in teams in high-crime areas.

Modified from Rice R: *The manual of home health nursing procedures,* St Louis, 1994, Mosby.

Personal Safety Guidelines in the Inner City

Safety Checklist

- Note any histories of violence, drug abuse, or mental illness before visits.
- Schedule visits as early in the day as possible.
- Secure purses and wallets in the locked vehicle trunk or glove compartment.
- Obtain accurate and exact directions.
- Alert patients or caregivers of approximate visit times.
- Check with the housing project building captains before visits.
- Drive with the windows up or rolled down no lower than the level of the earlobe and the doors locked.
- Remove personal belongings from the vehicle's interior.
- Park in well-lighted, accessible, safe areas for night visits.
- Check the surroundings (location, activities of strangers, building condition) before exiting the vehicle.
- Remain in the vehicle if feeling uneasy and contact the agency supervisor for directions.
- Remain alert at all times.
- Use escort services for high-risk areas.
- Remain calm, speak softly, and leave as quickly as possible in potentially threatening crisis situations. Do not panic.
- Keep therapy supplies out of sight while in the vehicle or patients' homes.

Security Tips

- Avoid lengthy or heavy conversations with family members or neighbors, no matter how pleasant they appear.
- Walk around crowded sidewalks and streets so that crowds do not block escape routes.
- Avoid being intimidated or provoked into confrontation.
- Do not attempt to break up domestic arguments.
- Notify patients of immediate departure when witnessing drug use and call the supervisor immediately.
- Leave unsafe areas immediately and notify the agency.

Security Tips—cont'd

- Maintain strong eye contact with everyone and always assess buildings, elevators, strangers, and body language for safety risks.

Agency protocol

1. Therapists should report immediately to the agency supervisor and security supervisor any suspicion of drug or violent activity.
2. The security supervisor then determines whether to share the safety information with other supervisors and staff members.
3. If an incident jeopardizes the safety of any staff member, that individual should report the specifics of the occurrence to the agency immediately.
4. Incidents involving drug arrests, weapons, or threats of violence result in the suspension of home care services for patients involved until the agency can ensure the safety of all its staff members.
5. The security supervisor then notifies all supervisors about the suspension of services to ensure that scheduled staff visits stop and staff members are not at risk.
6. The security supervisor dispatches an escort to any staff member not informed by telephone of the suspension in services.
7. The security supervisor, urban director, supervisor providing services, and staff members involved in the incident should attend an immediate meeting to determine the status of future home rehabilitation services.
8. If services resume, patients or caregivers must sign written contracts enhancing the safety of staff members.
9. The security supervisor accompanies staff members when they present such contracts to patients or caregivers.
10. The written contract outlines under what conditions the agency provides services and notifies patients of discharge if a contract violation occurs.
11. The agency places a copy of the signed contract in the permanent record and distributes copies to all supervisors, who share the contract with all staff members involved.

Modified from Nadwairski JA: Inner-city safety for home care providers, *J Nurs Adm* 22(9):42-47, 1992.

Personal Safety Equipment Glossary*

Vehicle antitheft devices. Devices, ranging from The Club to automated car alarms, that deter criminals from quick and discreet access to vehicles

***Call police* signs.** Light-reflective, large signs that alert passersby to the need for assistance

Flashlights. Portable light sources used during evening visits to illuminate surroundings and facilitate assessment and awareness of the area

Mobile phones. Portable telecommunications devices that allow instant access to assistance in dangerous situations

Nonlethal sprays. Handheld spray canisters that emit tear gas to stun potential assailants and allow those in danger to escape quickly

Roadside service membership. Paid service that offers 24-hour assistance for breakdowns, vehicle lockouts, and battery jumps

Sirens. Beeper-sized devices activated with pins so that removal of a pin triggers a loud, piercing sound to startle assailants and attract attention

Whistles. Safety devices that surprise assailants with loud, shrill, attention-attracting noises

THE HOME CARE TEAM

Home care therapists no longer can work in isolation. Therapists must maximize their communication with the home care team to help enhance efficiency, streamline duties, and promote quality, cost-effective care. Knowing the members who comprise the home care team is a necessary first step in the understanding of proper delegation and referral.

Home Care Team Glossary

Audiologists. Health care professionals with at least 6-year college degrees who evaluate and treat patients with hearing losses resulting from injury or disease; provide hearing-aid or assistive-listening system selection, fitting, and training

Case managers. Nurses and therapists who assess, plan, implement, coordinate, monitor, and evaluate home rehabilitation options and services to promote quality, cost-effective solutions; typically supervise home health aides, oversee total care plans, and perform admissions

Certified nursing assistants. Health care providers who undergo at least 90-hour training programs and demonstrate proficiency on certification exams; work under the supervision of nurses or therapists and help patients with bathing, personal care, catheter care, ambulation, exercises, meal preparation, and light housekeeping

Certified registered rehabilitation nurses. Health care professionals with at least 4-year college degrees in nursing and 1 year of experience in rehabilitation who demonstrate proficiency on competency exams; diagnose and treat the re-

---

*Anemaet WK, Moffa-Trotter ME: *Home care reality handout*, Chevy Chase, Md, 1998, GREAT Seminars.

sponses of patients and groups to actual or potential health problems that stem from altered functional abilities and altered lifestyles; provide comfort, therapy, and adaptive techniques and promote healthy adjustments

Companions. Individuals who provide companionship, comfort, and respite for patients who, for medical or safety reasons, cannot be left alone

Dietitians. Health care professionals with at least 4-year college degrees in dietetics who possess the credentials to evaluate and treat individuals who require dietary guidance to properly manage illnesses or disabilities; help develop nutritional plans and provide dietary counseling

Dietary technicians. Health care providers with 2-year college degrees who help assess the nutritional states of patients and the development, implementation, and review of nutritional care plans

Enterostomal therapy nurses. Health care professionals with at least 4-year college degrees in nursing who have undergone 4-week enterostomal therapy nursing education programs and provide acute and rehabilitative care for patients with select gastrointestinal, genitourinary, or integumentary system disorders; also provide direct care services for patients with abdominal stomas, wounds, fistulas, drains, pressure ulcers, and incontinence

Home health aides. Health care providers who complete 75-hour training programs and demonstrate proficiency on competency evaluations; work under the supervision of nurses or therapists; help patients with bathing, personal care, catheter care, ambulation, exercises, meal preparation, and light housekeeping

Homemakers. Individuals who perform environmental services, such as light household and homemaking duties, for patients who require assistance

Home medical equipment suppliers. Individuals who deliver medical equipment and fit it to patients; also help instruct patients in the proper uses of such devices

Licensed practical nurses. Licensed health care professionals with 2-year college degrees in practical nursing who work under the supervision of registered nurses

Licensed vocational nurses. Licensed health care professionals who undergo at least 1-year education programs in vocational nursing and work under the supervision of registered nurses

Medical social workers. Health care professionals with at least 6-year college degrees in social work who use their skills to help patients address health problems, disabilities, social conflicts, and mental illnesses; provide counseling, crisis intervention, community resource planning, and financial resource referrals

Medical social worker assistants. Health care providers with at least 4-year college degrees in social work, sociology, or psychology who work under the supervision of medical social workers

Occupational therapists. Certified health care professionals with at least 4-year college degrees in occupational therapy who evaluate and treat patients with limitations resulting from physical illnesses, injuries, dysfunctional conditions, cognitive impairments, mental illnesses, developmental disabilities, learning disabilities, psychosocial conditions, or adverse environmental conditions; also help maintain health and prevent dysfunction; provide functional training, physical agent modalities, environmental adaptations, and design, application, and training in assistive technology devices, orthotic devices, and prosthetic devices

Occupational therapist assistants. Certified health care providers with 2-year college degrees who work under the supervision of occupational therapists and provide high-quality occupational therapy services

Personal care attendants. Health care providers who demonstrate proficiency on competency exams and work under the supervision of nurses or therapists; assist patients with activities of daily living (ADL) and light housekeeping

Pharmacists. Licensed health care professionals with at least 5-year college degrees in pharmacy who improve quality of life through definite, medication-related therapeutical outcomes; prepare and dispense medications, identify and address medication-related problems, counsel, clinically monitor, and develop and implement pharmaceutical care plans

Physical therapists. Licensed health care professionals with at least 4-year college degrees in physical therapy who evaluate and treat patients with impairments, functional limitations, disabilities, or changes in physical function resulting from injury, disease, or other causes; also provide prevention and wellness services; therapeutical exercises; functional training; manual therapy techniques; medical equipment prescription, fabrication, and application; airway clearance techniques; wound management; and electrotherapeutical, physical agent, and mechanical modalities

Physical therapist assistants. Health care providers with 2-year college degrees who work under the supervision of physical therapists and provide delegated therapy procedures and related tasks to patients with health problems resulting from injury or disease

Physicians. Licensed health care professionals with at least 8-year college degrees in medicine who evaluate, treat, and refer patients with health problems to home health care agencies and therapists and oversee their plans of care

Psychiatric-mental health clinical nurse specialists. Licensed health care professionals with at least 6-year college degrees in nursing who assess, diagnose, and treat psychiatric disorders and potential mental health problems; perform all interventions that psychiatric nurses perform and sometimes prescribe medications

Psychiatric nurses. Licensed health care professionals with at least 4-year college degrees in nursing who assess mental health needs; develop diagnoses; and plan, implement, and evaluate nursing care; provide coping strategies, prevention interventions, management of therapeutical environments, administration and monitoring of psychobiological regimens, psychoeducation, crisis intervention, and counseling

Registered nurses. Licensed health care professionals with at least 4-year college degrees in nursing who identify and treat human responses to actual or potential health problems; perform services that include assessment; comfort care; and treatments, such as wound care, medication administration, venipuncture, colostomy care, diabetic care, disimpaction, catheter care, and teaching and training activities

Rehabilitation aides. Home health aides who possess advanced rehabilitation training* and work under the supervision of nurses or therapists; provide range-of-motion exercises, mobility assistance, positioning, personal care, and ostomy care for individuals with complex rehabilitation needs

---

*Advanced training is not mandatory for such aides. However, most aides do pursue further training.

Respiratory therapists. Health care providers with at least 2-year college degrees in respiratory therapy who evaluate and treat patients with breathing disorders; operate and maintain breathing equipment, administer medications, perform respiratory activities, maintain artificial airways, and operate smoking-cessation programs

Respiratory technicians. Health care providers with at least 1 year of respiratory therapy study who work under the supervision of respiratory therapists or physicians

Restorative aides. Home health aides who possess advanced rehabilitation training* and work under the supervision of nurses or therapists; perform services that include range-of-motion exercises, mobility assistance, positioning, personal care, and ostomy care for patients with complex rehabilitation needs

Restorative nurses. Health care professionals with at least 2-year college degrees in nursing who possess advanced rehabilitation training;* provide teaching and training on bowel and bladder programs, mobility, ADL, and assistive and adaptive equipment use and care

Sitters. Individuals who provide companionship and comfort to patients who, for medical or safety reasons, cannot be left alone; fill in when regular caregivers require respite

Speech-language pathologists. Health care professionals with at least 6-year college degrees in speech-language pathology who evaluate and treat patients with speech and language disorders resulting from injury or disease; help patients with speech-voice-language communication tasks, speech-voice production techniques, dysphagia treatments, language and speech articulation disorder procedures, aural treatments, and cognitive training

Speech-language pathologist assistants. Health care providers with at least on-the-job training who perform delegated tasks as prescribed, directed, and supervised by speech-language pathologists

Spiritual counselors. Individuals with theological backgrounds who provide patients with ministry services, including counseling, crisis intervention, and spiritual support

Volunteers. Nonpaid individuals who provide a variety of services, such as companionship, transportation, personal care, and counseling, for patients who require such assistance

HOME CARE REGULATORY BODIES

Home care regulatory bodies establish guidelines for the home health industry. Each regulatory body has its own focal point (for example, safety of the work environment or provision of quality care) and an array of survey and audit tools to assess agency compliance with the body's specific regulations. Therapists must possess a working knowledge of the existing regulatory bodies to ensure that their documentation and clinical practices meet the minimum regulatory standards of care.

---

*Advanced training is not mandatory. However, most restorative aides and nurses do pursue further training.

Breakdown of Regulatory Bodies

- **Agency administration.** Agency administrations organize, manage, and administer agency resources to attain and maintain the highest practical functional capacity for plans of care. Agency regulations are found in policy and procedure manuals that contain in-house rules for provision of home health services. Policies and procedures should be no less stringent than those mandated by the Health Care Financing Administration (HCFA), OSHA, state law, and accrediting organizations (if applicable). Penalties for noncompliance with agency policies and procedures range from disciplinary action to termination of employment.

- **Community Health Accreditation Program (CHAP).** CHAP is an accrediting organization that assesses home health care agencies' compliance with CHAP-developed standards for quality care. Registered nurses with 6-year college degrees and at least 5 years of experience in home health upper management visit agencies and conduct this voluntary survey process. They audit the agency's adherence to CHAP standards through home visits, telephone surveys, staff interviews, medical records reviews, and personnel file audits. CHAP awards accreditation to agencies based on the level of compliance with CHAP standards. Noncompliance with CHAP standards results in loss of accreditation or nonaccreditation.

- **Health Care Financing Administration (HCFA).** HCFA is a federal agency within the Department of Health and Human Services that administers the Medicare, Medicaid, and Child Health Insurance programs. In particular, HCFA manages and operates the Medicare program, establishes provider reimbursement policies, conducts research, and assesses the quality of health care services. The regulations concerning Medicare services are in two publications—the Conditions of Participation for Home Health Agencies, which establishes guidelines that Medicare-certified agencies must follow, and the Health Insurance Manual-11, which contains the federal guidelines for the rendering of home health services, including coverage of services, homebound requirements, and billing procedures. Penalties for noncompliance with the Conditions of Participation include agency exclusion from the Medicare program. Penalties for noncompliance with Health Insurance Manual-11 guidelines include denial of claims or charges of fraud, which can result in fines or criminal prosecution.

- **Joint Commission on the Accreditation of Healthcare Organizations.** JCAHO is an accrediting organization that assesses home health care agencies' compliance with JCAHO-developed standards for quality care. Registered nurses with at least 5 years of experience in home health care conduct this voluntary survey process. They audit adherence to JCAHO standards through visits, staff interviews, medical records reviews, and personnel file audits. JCAHO awards each agency a specific level of accreditation that agrees with that agency's level of compliance with JCAHO standards. Noncompliance with JCAHO standards results in loss of accreditation or nonaccreditation.

- **Occupational Safety and Health Administration.** OSHA is a federal agency within the United States Department of Labor that sets standards for workplace safety. OSHA works with state partners, inspectors, discrimination investigators, engineers, physicians, educators, standards writers, and support personnel to establish protective standards, enforce those standards, and educate employers and employees about safe work practices. Specific standards relevant to home care include the OSHA Standard on Occupational Exposure to Bloodborne Pathogens, OSHA Tuberculosis Requirements, and OSHA Infection Control Requirements. Penalties for noncompliance with OSHA standards include monetary fines.

- **Professional organizations.** The American Occupational Therapy Association and the American Physical Therapy Association are the professional organizations for occupational and physical therapists and assistants in the United States. Published documents, such as the respective codes of ethics and guidelines for the use of support personnel, provide standards of care for each profession. The American Occupational Therapy Association's Community Home Health Special Interest Group provides *Guidelines for Occupational Therapy in the Home,* which offers recommendations for the practice of occupational therapy in home health care. The American Physical Therapy Association's Community Home Health Section provides *Guidelines for the Provision of Physical Therapy Services in the Home,* which lists the minimum performance criteria for the administration of physical therapy in the home. Noncompliance with either organization's guidelines results in disciplinary action from the respective professional organization.
- **Regional home health intermediaries.** The intermediaries are contractors for HCFA who perform specific functions regarding Medicare. Examples of such functions include home health agency cost report audits, provider payments, productivity investment programs, benefits integrity programs, bill payments, medical claims and utilization reviews, claims reconsideration and hearings, and Medicare secondary payer reviews. Essentially, the intermediaries determine agency compliance with Health Insurance Manual-11 guidelines. Penalties for noncompliance include claims denials and referrals to the antifraud department.
- **State boards of therapy practice.** Most states regulate therapy services through practice acts for licensed therapists. Therapy practice acts detail state-specific regulations for such things as the scope of therapy services, minimum standards of care, disciplinary guidelines, and license eligibility requirements. Penalties for noncompliance with these acts include fines, practice restrictions, license revocations, and criminal prosecutions.
- **State health departments.** Most states set specific regulations that agencies must follow to become licensed home health care providers. State surveyors assess compliance with these laws. Penalties for noncompliance with state regulations include fines and home health license revocations.
- **State survey agencies.** These agencies ensure that home health agencies meet minimum health and safety requirements as established in the HCFA's Conditions of Participation for Home Health Agencies. Surveyors review Medicare certification application forms and perform on-site agency visits. Penalties for noncompliance with the conditions include revocation of Medicare certification or noncertification.
- **Third-party payers.** Third-party payers are non–HCFA-administered insurance providers that manage and operate insurance programs, establish provider reimbursement policies, and assess the quality of health care services. The regulations concerning third-party payer benefits are found in the payer's service benefit plan manual. Penalties for noncompliance with third-party payer guidelines include agency exclusion from the insurance program and denial of claims.

HOME CARE DOCUMENTATION GUIDELINES

In all therapy settings documentation provides valuable information about patients' courses of care. Documentation provides basic qualitative information about treatments and outcomes, both of which are used in claims determination and internal performance improvement measurement. At more advanced levels, documentation provides data for researchers and legal evidence to support liability claims. Therapists must follow proper home rehabilitation documentation guidelines to ensure adherence with minimum standards of care.

Documentation *Do's* and *Dont's*

Home Care Specific *Do's*

Use agency-approved abbreviation lists. These abbreviation lists keep documentation consistent among team members and eliminate the confusion created by cryptic symbols during chart audits and claims reviews. In addition, approved lists help ensure the same abbreviation does not stand for more than one task or term.

Determine therapy diagnoses. Therapists generally treat only those patients with acceptable therapy problems or diagnoses, which generally involve the musculoskeletal, neurological, or respiratory systems.

Include all pertinent diagnoses. Pertinent diagnoses are those that affect patients' predicted responses to therapy treatments. By including pertinent diagnoses, such as chronic obstructive pulmonary disease, rheumatoid arthritis, or prostate cancer, therapists can help substantiate longer-than-normal periods of care.

Detail pain. To reflect the skill in pain management, therapists must document pain carefully by including a description of the location, intensity, duration, and type of pain patients experience.

Justify homebound status. Therapists should summarize why patients require home therapy versus outpatient therapy. A description of homebound status should include the functional limitations or medical contraindications that preclude patients from leaving the home without assistance.

Demonstrate discharge planning on the first visit. Discharge planning should begin on the first visit, when the therapist develops the

Home Care Specific *Do's—cont'd*

Demonstrate discharge planning on the first visit.—cont'd therapy plan. Therapists then should record patients' responses to the plan to demonstrate involvement in the planning process.

Document why patients or caregivers cannot be taught. Because of dementia, severe aphasia, blindness, or sensory impairments, many patients cannot learn to perform various aspects of care themselves. For instance, blind patients cannot inspect their skin or apply ice or heat modalities safely. Patients with dementia may never attain independence in a home program because of recall deficits. By explaining why patients cannot learn such things, therapists help justify the necessity of their skilled interventions to perform normally unskilled procedures.

Explain why patients or caregivers require repeated instruction. To justify reinstruction of education topics for patients, such as home exercises or the use of assistive devices, therapists must document how patients perform specific tasks unsafely or ineffectively.

Document instruction in the proper use and care of medical equipment. JCAHO requires complete education for patients in the proper use, care, and maintenance of medical equipment. Because therapists are best suited to evaluate, fit, and train patients with assistive devices, prosthetics, orthoses, and adaptive or other medical equipment, they also are well qualified to instruct patients in the proper use and care of those devices.

Modified from Anemaet WK, Moffa-Trotter ME: *The user friendly home care handbook,* McLean, Va, 1997, LEARN Publications.

Box—cont'd

Home Care Specific *Do's—cont'd*

Record all education of patients. Because teaching is a skilled intervention, therapists should summarize education for patients and caregivers during each visit. In cases of noncompliance, therapists must document complete education of patients about the purpose of therapy and the deleterious effects of noncompliance with therapy. This step minimizes the therapist's liability in cases of abandonment, when discharge occurs as a result of noncompliance and subsequent lack of progress.

Document patients' responses to each treatment. Medicare and JCAHO request that therapists document patients' verbal or observed physical responses to each treatment. Noting the successful carryover of education topics or a normalized gait pattern after specific gait training are two examples of the ways therapists may document such responses.

Summarize the skill involved in each treatment. To justify reimbursement, therapists must show why specific treatment interventions require their oversight to ensure safety and effectiveness.

Write patients' names on all documentation and handouts. To expedite accurate filing of clinical notes, home exercises, and team communications, therapists should record patients' names and case numbers on all pages submitted for inclusion in the medical record.

Include license numbers after therapist signatures. The therapist's license number validates that a qualified therapist rendered the treatment. The number also helps expedite intermediary review and claims determination.

Record all interdisciplinary communication. Discussions with other team members about patients—whether at formal case conferences, via telephone, or outside patients' front doors—must be included in medical records. This written communication shows coordinated and complementary care and fulfills JCAHO expectations for interdisciplinary communication.

Reassess patients every 2 weeks. Objective reassessments demonstrate in measurable terms the gains patients have

Home Care Specific *Do's—cont'd*

Reassess patients every 2 weeks.—cont'd made, the effectiveness of therapy interventions, and the need for therapy program updates or adjustments. Most importantly, reassessments help justify the services and prove that patients made material progress in reasonable periods of time.

Perform documentation soon after visits. Charting during treatments or shortly after visits improves the accuracy of the documentation.

Home Care Specific Dont's

Do not chart arbitrary numbers. Anyone can estimate an individual's strength or range of motion. Therapists must measure and document accurately the exact numbers obtained through objective testing (for example, expressing range of motion in actual degrees, not percentages).

Do not use unnecessary phrases. To streamline documentation, therapists should include only informative and relevant statements in notes or reports. Comments such as "patient tolerated treatment well" or "patient is without any new complaints" do not give team members or reviewers any substantial information about the impact of therapy on patients' functional statuses.

Do not document out-of-house trips except those that are medically related. Although federal guidelines allow patients to leave their homes for nonmedical purposes, such as occasional visits to the barber or church, documentation of these outings may call into question patients' homebound statuses. If therapists do document such outings, however, they should provide details about the assistance that patients require to complete the trips and any adverse reactions to affirm their homebound statuses.

Do not record excessive gait distances. Neither intermediary, state, nor federal guidelines define excessive gait distances. Therefore therapists must use common sense when documenting such numbers. During the initial evaluation therapists should document the farthest distances patients must walk to function in their homes or exit their homes in emergencies. Therapists then can gait-train "safely" up to those distances. Once patients can ambulate up to the

Continued

Box—cont'd

Home Care Specific *Dont's*—cont'd

Do not record excessive gait distances.—cont'd
established threshold, therapists should quantify gait as either household or environmental and stop documenting distance altogether, emphasizing instead those aspects that necessitate skilled therapy intervention (for example, gait pattern normalization or assistance and specific training required).

Do not note increased weights, distances, and repetitions as the only measures of progress. Although increased gait distances and higher weight tolerance with exercise may indicate improved function, therapists must demonstrate progress clearly in functional areas, such as mobility, safety, and ADL, rather than relying on parameters that simply reflect improved tolerance.

Do not leave poor progress unexplained. All patients experience periods of plateau and contrasting bad weeks. Therapists should cite the reasons for periods in which progress is

Home Care Specific *Dont's*—cont'd

Do not leave poor progress unexplained.—cont'd
slowed for some patients. A statement that one patient experienced an arthritic exacerbation, a cold, or unstable blood glucose levels may help explain poor progress.

Do not settle disputes in documentation. Therapists should limit documentation to observations and patients' statements. "Rash" statements that may conflict with the documentation of other team members, such as "patient no longer needs home health aides," should be discussed in team conferences, not in clinical therapy notes.

Do not change frequency of visits or treatment interventions without a physician's order. In home care, physicians establish and manage plans of care. Therefore any changes, such as the addition of new interventions or the permanent decrease in the frequency of therapy sessions, must be approved by and signed by a physician.

Modified from Anemaet WK, Moffa-Trotter ME: *The user friendly home care handbook,* McLean, Va, 1997, LEARN Publications.

Federal Standards for the Definition of Skilled Therapy Services*

Therapy interventions must be skilled for intermediaries to reimburse therapists for their services. Federal regulations state that therapy services are skilled if therapists meet one or more of the following conditions:

1. **Services are inherently complex.** Complex therapy interventions require performance by or supervision of therapists to ensure safety and effectiveness. Examples of such sufficiently complex interventions include joint mobilization, electrical stimulation, and neuromuscular facilitation.

2. **Services necessitate case management.** Case management is the development, implementation, management, and evaluation of care plans; it is a skilled intervention often performed by nursing professionals. At times, however, therapists also serve as case managers. For instance, certain conditions—cerebrovascular accidents and total hip replacements, to name a few—warrant the skills of therapists in the management of care plans to ensure that patients' needs are met, medical safety is ensured, and recovery occurs. Therapists also undertake case management when patients demonstrate identified dangers,

---

*Modified from Anemaet WK, Moffa-Trotter ME: *The user friendly home care handbook,* McLean, Va, 1997, LEARN Publications.

such as a high probability of relapse or a secondary complication, which necessitate periodical reevaluation and management of care plans.

3. **Services cannot be performed by laypersons.** If laypersons, such as caregivers, can perform given interventions or services, the interventions or services are not considered skilled. If therapists document continual interventions provided with unchanging levels of assistance and patients' functional statuses do not change from treatment to treatment, a caregiver may be able to provide such services. Therapists must demonstrate the skill carefully by documenting the type and amount of assistance provided to ensure that patients can perform the activities safely and effectively.

4. **Patients demonstrate medical complications.** Normally unskilled services may be considered skilled if patients experience medical complications and require the skills of therapists to perform or supervise the tasks. Examples of unskilled services that may be considered skilled if medical complications exist include range-of-motion exercises in patients who have unhealed fractures or the application of simple modalities for patients with vision impairments or those who cannot examine their skin reliably.

5. **Services are reasonable and necessary.** Services also must be both reasonable and necessary to be considered skilled.

Federal Standards for the Definition of Reasonable and Necessary Services*

1. **The type and amount of services are consistent with the diagnosis.** The interventions and activities provided during therapy treatments must be consistent with the nature and severity of patients' illnesses or injuries and medical needs. For example, therapists reasonably may address cognitive training in patients who have experienced recent strokes and who demonstrate cognitive deficits. In contrast, therapists may not perform cognitive training reasonably on patients with shoulder fractures because cognitive impairment typically does not result from such a diagnosis.

   In addition, the frequency and duration of services must be reasonable and necessary. A stroke survivor who is moderately to totally dependent for all ADL, transfers, and mobility may warrant intensive daily rehabilitation. Conversely, daily therapy for a stroke survivor who is only minimally dependent for ADL and mobility is probably not reasonable and necessary.

2. **The services are specific and effective treatments for the diagnosis.** The therapy interventions must be considered, under accepted standards of medical practice, specific and effective treatments for the diagnosis. For example, ultrasound is an appropriate modality for such uses as tissue warming because it increases circulation at a cellular level. Intermediaries would not consider ultrasound reasonable and necessary if therapists used it on patients' heads to improve cognition through increased cerebral blood circulation; studies do not support such a theory.

---

*Modified from Anemaet WK, Moffa-Trotter ME: *The user friendly home care handbook,* McLean, Va, 1997, LEARN Publications.

3. **Patients' conditions are expected to improve.** Reasonable and necessary services are accompanied by an expectation that patients' conditions may improve materially in a reasonable, generally predictable period of time. During therapy patients must demonstrate gains consequential to independent function. Note, however, that only the expectation of improvement is necessary; unforeseen circumstances, such as hospitalizations, poor compliance, and relapses, may compromise the ability of patients to achieve those goals without affecting the reasonable and necessary status of services.

4. **Patients require maintenance programs.** The instruction, periodical reassessment, and advancement of safe and effective maintenance programs are reasonable and necessary therapy services. These maintenance programs must address specific patients' deficits. General exercises to promote overall fitness or flexibility, activities to provide diversion or general motivation, repetitive exercises to improve gait, or exercises to maintain strength and endurance ordinarily are not skilled because any layperson can perform such activities independently.

5. **Patients or caregivers require education and training.** Education and training of patients and caregivers about techniques, exercises, and precautions related to therapy diagnosis must be reasonable and necessary. Examples of education include durable medical equipment training, home programs, and energy-conservation strategies.

Home Care Documentation Formats

Although agency forms may dictate the layout and contents of home therapy documentation, therapists still may benefit from studying alternative formats. Learning new methods for documentation allows therapists to incorporate key aspects in their own charts. For example, the data-driven format of focus charting may provide an easy-to-follow template for critical pathway documentation forms that home health care agencies use. This process improves the objectivity, clarity, and reflection of functional outcomes associated with good documentation.

Focus Charting
Three steps in focus charting

Step	Definition	Items for inclusion
D	Data	Signs and symptoms
		Patient's complaints
		Observed status
A	Action	Completed therapy interventions
R	Response	Verbal responses to treatment
		Physical responses to treatment

Modified from Lampe SS: Focus charting: streamlining documentation, *Nurs Manage* 16(7):43, 1985.

Sample focus charting form

Focus of Treatment	DAR Format
	D
	A
	R
	D
	A
	R

DAR, Data, action, response.

Functional Outcome Report (FOR) Format
Six steps in FOR documentation

Step	Clinical reasoning	FOR documentation
1	Establish patient's needs.	Report reason for referral.
2	Analyze patient's performance.	Identify and report functional limitations.
3	Identify clinician's impression.	Establish physical therapy assessments.
4	Postulate relationships between impairment and performance.	Identify therapy problems.
5	Predict functional outcome.	List functional outcome goals.
6	Devise treatment strategy.	Present treatment plan and rationale.

Modified from Stewart DL, Abeln SH: *Documenting functional outcomes in physical therapy,* St Louis, 1993, Mosby.
FOR, Functional outcome report.

Sample FOR form

Reason for Referral

Functional limitations	
Activity	*Current performance status*

Physical Therapy Assessment

Therapy Problems

Functional outcome goals		
Activity	*Target performance status*	*Due date*

Treatment Plan with Rationale

Modified from Stewart DL, Abeln SH: *Documenting functional outcomes in physical therapy,* St Louis, 1993, Mosby.

Problem Focus Progress Format
Four steps in focus progress documentation

Step	Definition	Items for inclusion
1	Problem	Area of dependence or difficulty
2	Progress	Objective status of patient
		Assessment of progress
3	Program	Completed treatment interventions
4	Plan	Description of treatment planned for next visit
		Discharge plans

Sample focus progress form

Problem	Progress	Program	Plan

From Pedretti L: *Occupational therapy: practice skills for physical dysfunction,* ed 4, St Louis, 1996, Mosby.

SOAP Format
Four steps in SOAP documentation

Step	Definition	Items for inclusion
S (subjective information)	Patient's or caregiver's statements, preferably quoted, relevant to the therapy plan of care or the current patient's condition	Medical history Psychosocial history Prior level of function Chief problem Pain Paresthesias Personal therapy goal Patient's response
O (objective findings)	Therapist's delineation of the objective patient's status and completed treatment interventions	General appearance Mental status Vital signs Gross motor function Fine motor function ADL/IADL status Posture Neurological status Respiratory status Cardiovascular status Integumentary status Home assessment Completed treatment interventions
A (assessment)	Summary of or justification for patient's problems, progress toward goals, and rehabilitation potential	Problem list Therapy goals Rehabilitation potential Justification for therapy Summary of patient's progress Reasons for problems encountered
P (plan)	Description of treatment plan for next visit or discharge plan	Therapy frequency Therapy duration Planned treatment interventions Treatment progression plan Discharge plan

Modified from Weed LL: *Medical records, medical education, and patient care: the problem-oriented record as a basic tool,* Chicago, 1971, Year Book.
ADL, Activities of daily living; *IADL,* instrumental activities of daily living.

Sample SOAP form

Subjective information
Objective findings
Assessment
Plan

ETHICAL SITUATIONS IN HOME CARE

Home care therapists make decisions daily about their delivery of care and service and their interactions with patients, caregivers, and other home care team members. As a result of this decision-making role, therapists encounter situations in which their values conflict with regulations or with the values of others. In these instances therapists must rely on their own systems of ethics, the internal beliefs that guide their actions. Each therapist develops a system of beliefs over time as a result of life experiences. In addition, each therapist develops ways in which to deal with ethical situations. Therefore therapists must recognize ethical situations in home rehabilitation and develop effective strategies to resolve them before they become dilemmas.

Commonly Encountered Ethical Situations

Type of situation	Examples
Patient related	Patient attachment (for example, patient without potential for improvement not agreeing to discharge of therapy services)
	Poor compliance (for example, patient with potential for improvement not following therapy plan)
	Patient not homebound (for example, patient who doesn't meet requirements for homebound status receiving services meant for homebound patients)
Co-worker related	Improper use of a home health aide
	"Correction" of previous documentation
	Inappropriate physician order
Regulation related	Abandonment of patient
	Billing for nonskilled visits
	Inappropriate supervision of assistants (for example, therapist appointing tasks that assistant is not qualified or trained to perform)

Levels of Ethical Reasoning

Level	Motivation	Foundation for decision
Primary	Avoid punishment	Fear of retribution
Secondary	Obtain compensation	Expectation of reward
Tertiary	Give in to peer pressure	Attempt to "fit in"
Quaternary	Fulfill moral obligation	Belief in a higher standard

Guidelines for the Resolution of Ethical Situations

1. Identify the situation.
2. Establish how and why the situation occurred.
3. Determine the type of ethical situation and the possible implications it presents.
4. Clarify the understanding of the situation.
5. Gather as much relevant information as possible.
6. Outline the possible solutions.
7. Distinguish the advantages and disadvantages of each solution and establish the level of ethical reasoning involved in each.
8. Select a strategy to resolve the situation.
9. Implement the chosen plan.
10. Evaluate the effectiveness of the strategy.

Case Illustrations

The following scenarios illustrate possible applications of the aforementioned guidelines applied to potential ethical situations:

Potential Abandonment

1. Identify the situation.
   - A physical therapist has been working with Ms. Pereira, a moderately confused but cooperative patient, 3 times per week for 2 weeks to help her improve her gait strength, balance, and safety, all of which deteriorated after a lengthy hospitalization and stay in a skilled-nursing facility. When supervising her home exercise program, her family members, although motivated, still require verbal cues for two of the six exercises she must perform.

     Before her hospitalization, Ms. Pereira could walk without an assistive device; however, she required standby assistance because her dementia causes her to wander. Currently, she walks with a small-based quad cane and minimal assistance for loss of balance, which she experiences every 30 feet. Her Tinetti Assessment Tool score is 17/28, placing her at a high risk for falls (see Part Three). Ms. Pereira belongs to a Medicare health maintenance organization (HMO) that authorized six physical therapy visits and denied requests for additional treatment, stating that Ms. Pereira resides with family members who helped her before the hospitalization and can help her again.

2. Establish how and why the situation occurred.
   - The HMO case manager was not aware of the differences between the assistance Ms. Pereira requires now (minimal assistance for loss of balance) and the assistance she required before her hospitalization (standby assistance for cognitive reasons).
   - Ms. Pereira's family members did not know the limitations of her insurance.
   - The HMO case manager was not aware of Ms. Pereira's need for physical therapy.
   - The physical therapist did not explain to the HMO case manager Ms. Pereira's need for physical therapy.
3. Determine the type of ethical situation and the possible implications it presents.
   - This is a regulation-related ethical situation, which may evolve into claims of abandonment of a patient if the therapist discharges Ms. Pereira because her HMO no longer authorizes treatment.
4. Clarify the understanding of the situation.
   - Ms. Pereira requires more skilled physical therapy than the authorized six visits to regain the level of function she enjoyed before her hospitalization and to decrease her risk of falling.
   - Ms. Pereira has the potential to achieve her former level of function; however, she cannot become completely independent because of her dementia.
   - The HMO refuses to pay for additional physical therapy visits.
   - If the physical therapist discharges Ms. Pereira with the knowledge that she may benefit from further skilled physical therapy, family members may claim that the therapist abandoned Ms. Pereira.
5. Gather as much relevant information as possible.
   - Obtain the HMO's service coverage requirements.
   - Determine Ms. Pereira's former level of function.
   - Ascertain Ms. Pereira's current level of function.
   - Provide documentation stating that family members cannot supervise Ms. Pereira's home exercise program effectively.
   - Locate research-based evidence that explains Ms. Pereira's increased risk of falling based on her Tinetti score and the potential ramifications of this risk.
   - Obtain a physician's statement that Ms. Pereira needs more physical therapy.
6. Outline the possible solutions.
   - Discharge Ms. Pereira because she does not have insurance coverage.
   - Notify the HMO case manager of Ms. Pereira's potential for improved function, high risk for falls, potential for serious injury, and associated medical costs.
   - Request that a physician explain to the HMO case manager the need for additional physical therapy.
   - Encourage family members to request from the HMO more physical therapy.
   - Offer family members the option of private pay therapy, incorporating a sliding-fee scale and alternative payment options if finances present a problem.
   - Continue providing physical therapy services pro bono.
7. Distinguish the advantages and disadvantages of each solution and establish the level of ethical reasoning involved in each.

Solution	Advantages	Disadvantages
Discharge Ms. Pereira because of a lack of insurance coverage.	Agency does not lose money. Premature discharge appears the fault of the HMO.	Ms. Pereira does not receive necessary skilled physical therapy. Therapist risks claims of abandonment.
Notify HMO.	Case manager is fully informed of the situation. Therapist gains an opportunity to discuss Ms. Pereira's situation fully.	Notification is time consuming.
Ask physician to notify HMO.	HMO case manager may put more stock in physician's assessment. Therapist and HMO share the risk of abandonment because physician agrees that Ms. Pereira needs more physical therapy.	Physician's involvement in an HMO may foster reluctance. Physician may not take the necessary time.
Ask family members to notify HMO.	HMO is pressured to allow more physical therapy to prevent the loss of customer satisfaction. Family members take active roles in the search for authorization.	HMO case manager may resent therapist's request that family members call.
Offer private-pay therapy services.	Ms. Pereira continues to receive physical therapy treatment. Family members take responsibility for situation.	Family members may not be able to afford private therapy.
Continue therapy pro bono.	Ms. Pereira receives necessary skilled therapy. Family members cannot claim that therapist abandoned Ms. Pereira.	Therapist and agency are not reimbursed. Most agencies cannot afford to do this routinely.

HMO, Health maintenance organization.

- The previously mentioned solutions involve a combination of the following levels of ethical reasoning:
  a. Primary—avoidance of nonreimbursement
  b. Secondary—expectation of reimbursement from either the HMO or family members
  c. Quaternary—fulfillment of a moral obligation through enactment of the necessary steps to provide physical therapy services for Ms. Pereira
8. Select a strategy to resolve the situation (in this case one that involves several steps).
   - The physical therapist contacts the HMO case manager and discusses Ms. Pereira's situation.
   - The physical therapist notifies the physician of the situation and requests that the physician contact the HMO case manager.
   - The physical therapist encourages family members to notify the HMO that Ms. Pereira has not achieved her former level of function and needs physical therapy to do so.
   - The agency offers the family members the option of private therapy services if the HMO does not authorize additional therapy.

9. Implement the chosen plan.
   - After discussing Ms. Pereira's situation with the physical therapist, the case manager still denies authorization.
   - The physician phones the HMO and is told that Ms. Pereira exhausted her physical therapy benefits for this illness.
   - The family members are reluctant to call the HMO, stating that the task is part of the agency's job.
   - Family members pay for four more physical therapy sessions, after which Ms. Pereira can walk with a small-based quad cane without losing her balance. In addition, the family can supervise her home exercise program independently.
   - Family members refuse to pay for more physical therapy services, which would allow Ms. Pereira to walk without the use of an assistive device and further decrease her risk of falling. They state that Ms. Pereira needs the services to regain her former level of function but do not want to pay for those services. Family members agree that Ms. Pereira has reached an acceptable functional level.
   - Ms. Pereira is discharged from physical therapy because her family members will not pay for more services.
10. Evaluate the effectiveness of the strategy.
   - The physical therapist clearly documented the need for further physical therapy, Ms. Pereira's risk for falls, and all education provided to family members.
   - The agency, HMO, and physician shared the risk of abandonment claims.
   - The decision to discharge Ms. Pereira was not unilateral on the agency's part but was a shared decision between the agency and the family members, who decided that Ms. Pereira did not need physical therapy services if they had to pay.
   - Ms. Pereira regained some function but did not achieve the level she enjoyed before her hospitalization.

Patient Not Homebound

1. Identify the situation.
   - A physical therapist has been treating Mr. Afonso, who was active and independent in the community without an assistive device before he suffered a mild cerebrovascular accident. He requires verbal cues for four of his six home exercises and ambulates with a front-wheeled walker and minimal assistance because of inadequate foot clearance, which results in loss of balance. He also requires minimal assistance during sit-to-stand transfers from a chair of average height and scores 14/28 on the Tinetti Assessment Tool (see Part Three). In addition, Mr. Afonso receives home health aide services and skilled nursing services twice a week.

     The therapist arrives at Mr. Afonso's for the scheduled appointment and cannot reach him after repeated knocks on the door and phone calls. After notifying the office, the therapist later reaches Mr. Afonso and discovers that he went out for lunch with several friends. Further conversation reveals that he routinely leaves his home and drives, accompanied by a friend.

2. Establish how and why the situation occurred.
   - Mr. Afonso was not aware of the Medicare homebound requirement.
   - The agency or physical therapist did not explain adequately to Mr. Afonso the requirements for homebound status.

- The agency or physical therapist did not assess Mr. Afonso's homebound status accurately.
3. Determine the type of ethical situation and the possible implications it presents.
   - This is a regulation-related ethical situation, which may evolve into an ethical situation related to a co-worker if another team member is aware of Mr. Afonso's true status and chooses to overlook it.
4. Clarify the understanding of the situation.
   - Mr. Afonso requires skilled physical therapy to become independent with transfers, to attain gait without an assistive device, to perform his home exercise program, and to decrease his risk of falling.
   - Mr. Afonso is not homebound because he leaves the home frequently for nonmedical reasons.
   - Physical therapy services cannot continue under Medicare's home health benefit (Medicare Part A).
   - Home health aide and skilled nursing services cannot continue under Medicare's home health benefit (Medicare Part A).
5. Gather as much relevant information as possible.
   - Obtain Medicare's coverage of homebound services requirement.
   - Determine Mr. Afonso's current functional status.
   - Ascertain Mr. Afonso's former level of function.
   - Document Mr. Afonso's progress to date with physical therapy.
6. Outline the possible solutions.
   - Continue providing home health physical therapy services to Mr. Afonso and bill under Medicare Part A.
   - Discharge Mr. Afonso from physical therapy services.
   - Refer Mr. Afonso to outpatient physical therapy.
   - Provide outpatient physical therapy to Mr. Afonso in his home and bill under Medicare Part B.
7. Distinguish the advantages and disadvantages of each solution and establish the level of ethical reasoning involved in each.

Solution	Advantages	Disadvantages
Continue providing services under Medicare Part A.	Mr. Afonso continues to receive needed physical therapy services. Home health aide and nurse need not discharge Mr. Afonso	Therapist's actions constitute Medicare fraud.
Discharge Mr. Afonso from physical therapy.	Therapist does not bill Medicare for services to a patient who is not homebound.	Mr. Afonso does not receive needed skilled physical therapy services.
Refer Mr. Afonso to outpatient physical therapy.	Mr. Afonso receives needed physical therapy services. Mr. Afonso increases his socialization Mr. Afonso can interact with other patients with similar impairments.	Mr. Afonso may not have transportation. Mr. Afonso may choose not to visit an outpatient facility. The home health aide and nurse must discharge Mr. Afonso.

Continued

Table—cont'd

Solution	Advantages	Disadvantages
Continue providing services under Medicare Part B.	Mr. Afonso continues to receive needed physical therapy services. The therapist provides services in the home and can tailor them to Mr. Afonso's needs. Solution adheres to Medicare's guidelines for billing for physical therapy services to a nonhomebound patient in the home.	Mr. Afonso must use supplemental insurance or pay the copayment privately. Billing system is different for the agency, which is accustomed to billing Medicare Part A only. The home health aide and nurse must discharge Mr. Afonso.

The aforementioned solutions involve a combination of the following levels of ethical reasoning:

a. Primary—avoidance of Medicare fraud

b. Secondary—maintenance of Mr. Afonso on services to retain higher census (the total number of patients to which an agency provides services)

c. Tertiary—continuance of services under Medicare Part A because other physical therapists do it or because the home health aide or nurse does not want to discharge Mr. Afonso

d. Quaternary—a moral obligation to inform Medicare that Mr. Afonso is no longer homebound and provide therapy services under Medicare Part B, either in the home or in an outpatient facility

8. Select a strategy to resolve the situation.
   - Refer Mr. Afonso to outpatient physical therapy services.

9. Implement the chosen plan.
   - The therapist notifies the agency that Mr. Afonso is no longer homebound.
   - The therapist notifies the physician that the home health physical therapy services must end and Mr. Afonso will be referred to an outpatient facility.
   - The therapist notifies Mr. Afonso that he cannot receive home health services because he no longer meets the requirements for Medicare Part A home rehabilitation services and instructs him to call an outpatient facility and schedule an appointment. Medical social services also provides Mr. Afonso a list of community homemaker services.
   - All home health services (physical therapy, home health aide, and skilled nursing) are discharged.

10. Evaluate the effectiveness of the strategy.
   - Mr. Afonso continues to receive physical therapy services. Several friends take turns driving him to his appointments.
   - Mr. Afonso arranges for assistance in the home through Neighborly Senior Services and his church.
   - Mr. Afonso is not violating Medicare homebound regulations.

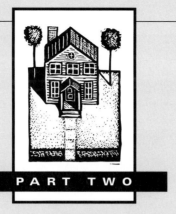

PART TWO

Pediatric Population

PEDIATRIC ENVIRONMENTAL EVALUATION

PEDIATRIC DEVELOPMENTAL EVALUATION

SPECIAL CONSIDERATIONS FOR PRETERM NEWBORNS AND INFANTS

FREQUENTLY ENCOUNTERED PEDIATRIC PROBLEMS

PEDIATRIC ENVIRONMENTAL EVALUATION

Psychologists, geneticists, and even the general public long have debated the nature vs. nurture question. Are children's development affected more by their genetic compositions or their surroundings? Although no one individual can answer these questions with certainty, little doubt exists that both components play vital roles. Therapists cannot alter their patients' genetic compositions; however, they can facilitate changes to patients' surroundings. Therapists positively affect pediatric patient development by assessing patients' homes and caregivers and then implementing measures to ensure that homes are accessible and safe.

Home Assessments

Home Observation and Measurement of the Environment Inventory

The Home Observation and Measurement of the Environment (HOME) Inventory is an observation tool therapists can use in the home to assess parent-child interactions. Three scales exist, each based on age—infants and toddlers, preschoolers, and elementary school children. Each scale is divided into subscales that outline a number of observed items or behaviors. Scoring the HOME Inventory involves tallying the number of observations on each subscale.

HOME Inventory for Families of Infants and Toddlers

Bettye M. Caldwell and Robert H. Bradley

Family name _____ Visitor _____ Date _____

Address _____ Phone _____

Child's name _____ Birthdate _____ Age _____ Sex _____

Parent or caregiver present _____ Relationship to child _____

Family composition _____
(individuals living in household, including sex and age of children)

| Family ethnicity _____ | Language spoken _____ | Maternal education _____ | Paternal education _____ |

| Mother employed? _____ | Type of work when employed _____ | Father employed? _____ | Type of work when employed _____ |

Current child care arrangements _____

Summary of past year's arrangement _____

Other individuals present _____

Comments _____

_____

Summary

Subscale	Score	Lowest fourth	Middle half	Upper fourth
I. Responsiveness		0-6	7-9	10-11
II. Acceptance		0-4	5-6	7-8
III. Organization		0-3	4-5	6
IV. Learning materials		0-4	5-7	8-9
V. Involvement		0-2	3-4	5-6
VI. Variety		0-1	2-3	4-5
Total score		0-25	26-36	37-45

Modified from Caldwell BM, Bradley RH: *Manual of home observation for measurement of the environment,* ed 2, Fayetteville, Ark, 1984, The University of Arkansas Press.

HOME Inventory for Families of Infants and Toddlers—cont'd

Place a plus (+) or minus (−) in the box alongside each item if the behavior is observed during the visit or if the parent (or primary caregiver) reports that the conditions or events are characteristic of the home environment. Count the number of plus signs and enter the subtotals and the total in the spaces provided.

I. Responsiveness

1. Parent spontaneously vocalizes to child at least twice.
2. Parent responds verbally to child's vocalizations or verbalizations.
3. Parent tells child name of object or individual during visit.
4. Parent's speech is distinct, clear, and audible.
5. Parent initiates verbal interchanges with therapist.
6. Parent converses freely and easily with therapist.
7. Parent permits child to engage in "messy" play.
8. Parent spontaneously praises child at least twice.
9. Parent's voice conveys positive feelings toward child.
10. Parent caresses or kisses child at least once.
11. Parent responds positively to praise of child that visitor offers.

II. Acceptance

12. Parent does not shout at child.
13. Parent does not express overt annoyance with or hostility toward child.
14. Parent neither slaps nor spanks child during visit.
15. Parent reports no more than one instance of physical punishment during the past week.
16. Parent does not scold or criticize child during visit.
17. Parent interferes with or restricts child fewer than three times during visit.

II. Acceptance—cont'd

18. At least 10 books are present and visible.
19. Family owns a pet.

III. Organization

20. Child care is provided by one of three regular substitutes.
21. Child is taken to grocery store at least once a week.
22. Child gets out of house at least four times a week.
23. Child is taken regularly to doctor's office or clinic.
24. Child has a special place for toys and treasures.
25. Child's play environment is safe.

IV. Learning Materials

26. Child uses muscle-activity toys or equipment.
27. Child uses push or pull toy.
28. Child uses stroller or walker, kiddie car, scooter, or tricycle.
29. Parent provides toys with which child can play during visit.
30. Child uses cuddly toy or role-playing toys.
31. Child uses learning facilitators, such as a mobile, table and chair, high chair, or playpen.
32. Child uses simple eye-hand coordination toys.
33. Child uses complex eye-hand coordination toys.
34. Child uses toys for literature and music.

Continued

HOME *Inventory for Families of Infants and Toddlers—cont'd*

V. Involvement

35. Parent keeps child in visual range and looks at child often.

36. Parent talks to child while performing household work.

37. Parent consciously encourages developmental advancements.

38. Parent invests maturing toys with value via personal attention.

39. Parent structures child's play periods.

40. Parent provides toys that challenge child to develop new skills.

VI. Variety

41. Father provides some care daily.

42. Parent reads stories to child at least three times weekly.

43. Child eats at least one meal a day with mother and father.

44. Family visits relatives or receives visits once per month or so.

45. Child owns three or more books.

	I	II	III	IV	V	VI	Total
Totals							

Modified from Caldwell BM, Bradley RH: *Manual of home observation for measurement of the environment,* ed 2, Fayetteville, Ark, 1984, The University of Arkansas Press.

HOME Inventory for Families of Preschoolers (Ages 3 to 6)

Bettye M. Caldwell and Robert H. Bradley

Family name _____ Date _____ Visitor _____

Child's name _____ Birthdate _____ Age _____ Sex _____

Parent or caregiver present _____ Relationship to child _____

Family composistion _____
(individuals living in household, including sex and age of children)

Family ethnicity _____   Language spoken _____   Maternal education _____   Paternal education _____

Mother employed? _____   Type of work when employed _____   Father employed? _____   Type of work when employed _____

Address _____   Phone number _____

Current child care arrangements _____

Summary of past year's arrangement _____

Other individuals present _____

Comments _____

Summary

Subscale	Score	Percentile range*		
		Lowest fourth	Middle half	Upper fourth
I. Learning stimulation		0-2	3-9	10-11
II. Language stimulation		0-4	5-6	7
III. Physical environment		0-3	4-6	7
IV. Warmth and affection		0-3	4-5	6-7
V. Academic stimulation		0-2	3-4	5
VI. Modeling		0-1	2-3	4-5
VII. Variety in experience		0-4	5-7	8-9
VIII. Acceptance		0-2	3	4
Total score		0-29	30-45	46-55

Modified from Caldwell BM, Bradley RH: Manual of home observation for measurement of the environment, ed 2, Fayetteville, Ark, 1984, The University of Arkansas Press.

*For rapid profiling of a family, place an X in the percentile range box that corresponds to the raw score.

Continued

HOME Inventory for Families of Preschoolers (Ages 3 to 6)—cont'd

Place a plus (+) or minus (−) in the box alongside each item if the behavior is observed during the visit or if the parent (or primary caregiver) reports that the conditions or events are characteristic of the home environment. Count the number of plus signs and enter the subtotals and the total in the spaces provided.

I. Learning Stimulation

1. Child has toys that teach color, size, shape.
2. Child has three or more puzzles.
3. Child has record player and at least five children's records.
4. Child has toys permitting free expression.
5. Child has toys or games requiring refined movements.
6. Child has toys or games that help teach numbers.
7. Child has at least 10 children's books.
8. At least 10 books are visible in the home.
9. Family buys and reads a daily newspaper.
10. Family subscribes to at least one magazine.
11. Child is encouraged to learn shapes.

Subtotal

II. Language Stimulation

12. Child has toys that help teach animal names.
13. Child is encouraged to learn the alphabet.
14. Parent teaches child simple verbal manners (for example, please, thank you).

II. Language Stimulation—cont'd

15. Parent uses correct grammar and pronunciation.
16. Parent encourages child to talk and takes time to listen.
17. Parent's voice conveys positive feeling to child.
18. Child is permitted choice in breakfast or lunch menu.

Subtotal

III. Physical Environment

19. Home appears safe.
20. Outside play environment appears safe.
21. Interior of home is not dark or perceptually monotonous.
22. Neighborhood is aesthetically pleasing.
23. Home has 100 square feet of living space per individual in it.
24. Rooms are not overcrowded with furniture.
25. Home is reasonably clean and minimally cluttered.

Subtotal

IV. Warmth and Affection

26. Parent holds child close 10 to 15 minutes per day.
27. Parent converses with child at least twice during visit.

Modified from Caldwell BM, Bradley RH: Manual of home observation for measurement of the environment, ed 2, Fayetteville, Ark, 1984, The University of Arkansas Press.

HOME Inventory for Families of Preschoolers (Ages 3 to 6)—cont'd

IV. Warmth and Affection—cont'd

28. Parent answers child's questions or requests verbally.

29. Parent usually responds verbally to child's speech.

30. Parent praises child's qualities twice during visit.

31. Parent caresses, kisses, or cuddles child during visit.

32. Parent helps child demonstrate some achievement during visit.

Subtotal

V. Academic Stimulation

33. Child is encouraged to learn colors.

34. Child is encouraged to learn patterned speech such as songs.

35. Child is encouraged to learn spatial relationships.

36. Child is encouraged to learn numbers.

37. Child is encouraged to learn to read a few words.

Subtotal

VI. Modeling

38. Some delay of food gratification is expected.

39. Television is used judiciously.

40. Parent introduces child to visitor.

41. Child can express negative feelings without reprisal.

42. Child can hit parent without harsh reprisal.

Subtotal

VII. Variety in Experience

43. Child has real or toy musical instrument.

44. Child is taken on outing by family member at least every other week.

45. Child has been on trip of more than 50 miles during last year.

46. Child has been taken to a museum during past year.

47. Parent encourages child to put away toys without help.

48. Parent uses complex sentence structure and vocabulary.

49. Child's artwork is displayed some place in home.

50. Child eats at least one meal per day with mother and father.

51. Parent lets child choose some foods or brands at grocery store.

Subtotal

VIII. Acceptance

52. Parent does not scold or disparage child more than once.

53. Parent does not use physical restraint during visit.

54. Parent neither slaps nor spanks child during visit.

55. Parent reports no more than one instance of physical punishment during the past week.

Subtotal

HOME Inventory for Families of Elementary Schoolchildren

Bettye M. Caldwell and Robert H. Bradley

Family name _____ Date _____ Visitor _____

Child's name _____ Birthdate _____ Age _____ Sex _____

Parent or caregiver present _____ Relationship to child _____

Family composition _____
(individuals living in household, including sex and age of children)

Family
ethnicity_____

Language
spoken _____

Maternal
education _____

Paternal
education _____

Mother
employed?_____

Type of work
when employed _____

Father
employed? _____

Type of work
when employed _____

Address _____ How long? _____ Phone _____

Current child-care arrangements _____

Summary of past year's arrangement _____

Other individuals present _____

Summary

	Score
I. Emotional and verbal responsiveness	
II. Encouragement of maturity	
III. Emotional climate	
IV. Growth-fostering materials and experiences	
V. Provision for active stimulation	
VI. Family participation in developmentally stimulating experiences	
VII. Paternal involvement	
VIII. Aspects of physical environment	

Modified from Caldwell BM, Bradley RH: *Manual of home observation for measurement of the environment,* ed 2, Fayetteville, Ark, 1984, The University of Arkansas Press.

HOME Inventory for Families of Elementary Schoolchildren—cont'd

Place a plus (+) or minus (−) in the box alongside each item if the behavior is observed during the visit or if the parent (or primary caregiver) reports that the conditions or events are characteristic of the home environment. Count the number of plus signs and enter the subtotals and the total in the spaces provided.

I. Emotional and Verbal Responsiveness

1. Family has fairly regular and predictable daily schedule for child (for example, meals, daycare, bedtime, television, and homework).

2. Parent sometimes yields to child's fears or rituals (e.g., allows nightlight, accompanies child to new experiences).

3. Child has been praised at least twice during past week for doing something.

4. Child is encouraged to read independently.

5. Parent encourages child to contribute to conversation during visit.

6. Parent shows some positive emotional responses to therapist's praise of child.

7. Parent responds to child's questions during visit.

8. Parent uses complete sentence structure and some long words in conversation.

9. When speaking of or to the child, parent's voice conveys positive feelings.

10. Parent initiates verbal interchanges with therapist, asks questions, and makes spontaneous comments.

Subtotal

II. Encouragement of Maturity

11. Family requires child to carry out certain self-care routines (for example, make bed, clean room, clean up after spills, bathe self). (A plus sign requires three out of four).

II. Encouragement of Maturity—cont'd

12. Family requires child to keep living and play area reasonably clean and straight.

13. Child puts outdoor clothing, dirty clothes, and night clothes in special places.

14. Parent sets limits for child and generally enforces them (e.g., curfew, homework before television, or other regulations that fit family pattern).

15. Parent introduces visitor to child.

16. Parent consistently establishes or applies family rules.

17. Parent does not violate rules of common courtesy.

Subtotal

III. Emotional Climate

18. Parent has not lost temper with child more than once during previous week.

19. Parent reports no more than one instance of physical punishment occurred during past month.

20. Child can express negative feelings toward parents without harsh reprisals.

21. Parent has not cried or been visibly upset in child's presence more than once during past week.

22. Child has a special place in which to keep possessions.

23. Parent talks to child during visit beyond correction and introduction.

Continued

HOME Inventory for Families of Elementary Schoolchildren—cont'd

III. Emotional Climate—cont'd

24. Parent uses some term of endearment or some diminutive for child's name when talking about child twice during visit.

25. Parent does not express overannoyance with or hostility toward child (e.g., complaining, describing child as "bad," saying child won't mind).

Subtotal

IV. Growth-fostering Materials and Experiences

26. Child has unlimited access to record player or radio.

27. Child has unlimited access to musical instrument (e.g., piano, drum, ukelele, guitar).

28. Child has unlimited access to at least 10 appropriate books.

29. Parent buys and reads a newspaper daily.

30. Child has unlimited access to desk or other suitable place for reading or studying.

31. Family has a dictionary and encourages child to use it.

32. Child has visited a friend unaccompanied in the past week.

33. House has at least two pictures or other types of artwork on the walls.

Subtotal

V. Provision for Active Stimulation

34. Family has a television, and it is used judiciously, not left on continuously. (No television requires an automatic minus sign; any scheduling scores plus sign.)

35. Family encourages child to develop or sustain hobbies.

36. Child is regularly included in family's recreational hobby.

37. Family provides lessons to organizational membership to support child's talents (e.g., YMCA membership or gymnastic lessons).

38. Child has ready access to at least two pieces of playground equipment in the immediate vicinity of the home.

39. Child has access to a library card, and family arranges for child to go to library once per month.

40. Family member has taken child or arranged for child to go to a scientific, historical, or art museum within past year.

41. Family member has taken child or arranged for child to take a trip on a plane, train, or bus within past year.

Subtotal

VI. Family Participation in Developmentally Stimulating Experiences

42. Family visits or receives visits from relatives or friends at least once every other week.

Modified from Caldwell BM, Bradley RH: *Manual of home observation for measurement of the environment*, ed 2, Fayetteville, Ark, 1984, The University of Arkansas Press.

HOME Inventory for Families of Elementary Schoolchildren—cont'd

VI. Family Participation in Developmentally Stimulating Experiences—cont'd

43. Child has accompanied parent on family business venture 3 or 4 times within past year (e.g., to garage, clothing shop, or appliance repair shop).

44. Family member has taken child or arranged for child to attend some type of live musical or theatre performance.

45. Family member has taken child or arranged for child to go on a trip of more than 50 miles from home (50-mile radial distance, not total distance).

46. Parent discusses television programs with child.

47. Parent helps child achieve motor skills (for example, ride a two-wheel bicycle, roller skate, ice skate, or play ball).

Subtotal

VII. Paternal Involvement

48. Father (or father substitute) regularly engages in outdoor recreation with child.

49. Child sees and spends time with father or father figure 4 days per week.

50. Child eats at least one meal per day on most days with mother and father (or mother and father figures). (One-parent families rate an automatic minus sign.)

VII. Paternal Involvement—cont'd

51. Child has remained with this primary family group for all of his life aside from 2 or 3 week vacations, illnesses of mother, visits of grandmother, or other unexpected events. (A plus sign requires no changes in mother's, father's, grandmother's or grandfather's presence since birth).

Subtotal

VIII. Aspects of Physical Environment

52. Child's room has picture or wall decoration appealing to children.

53. Home's interior is not dark or perceptually monotonous.

54. In terms of available floor space, the rooms are not overcrowded with furniture.

55. All visible rooms in the home are reasonably clean and minimally cluttered.

56. At least 100 square feet of living space exists per individual in the home.

57. Home is not overly noisy with sounds such as television, shouts of children, or a radio.

58. Home has no potentially dangerous structural or health defects (e.g., plaster coming down from ceiling, stairway with boards missing, or rodents).

59. Child's outside play environment appears safe and free of hazards. (No outside play area requires an automatic minus sign).

Subtotal

Pediatric Population

Home Screening Questionnaire

The Home Screening Questionnaire assesses the home environments of at-risk children through use of separate forms for two different age groups—0 to 3 years and 3 to 6 years. The questionnaire was designed as a simple, economical, and brief test, requiring only 5 minutes to complete. Its purpose is to determine whether a particular home environment meets the cognitive needs of a certain child.

---

*Home Screening Questionnaire**
Ages 0 to 3 Years

Child's Name _____ Birthdate _____ Age _____

Parents' Names _____ Phone _____

Address _____ Date _____

Please answer *all* the following questions about the ways in which your child spends time and some of your family's activities. On some questions, you may want to check more than one choice.

For office use only	
_____	1. How often do you and your child see relatives?
	_____ Never
	_____ At least once per year
	_____ At least 6 times per year
	_____ At least once per month
	_____ At least once per week
_____	2. Do you subscribe to any magazines?
	Yes No
	If yes, what kind?
	_____ Home and family magazines
	_____ News magazines
	_____ Children's magazines
	_____ Other
_____	3. About how many hours each day does your child spend in a playpen, jumpchair, infant swing, or infant seat?
	_____ None
	_____ Up to 1 hour
	_____ 1 to 3 hours
	_____ More than 3 hours

For office use only	
_____	4. Does your child have a toybox or other special place where to store toys?
	Yes No
_____	5. How many children's books does your child own?
	_____ 0—too young
	_____ 1 or 2
	_____ 5 to 9
	_____ 10 or more
_____	6. How many books do you own?
	_____ 0 to 9
	_____ 10 to 20
	_____ More than 20
	Where do you keep them?
	_____ In boxes
	_____ On a bookcase
	_____ Other _____

From William K Frankenburg, 1981, 1988, WK Frankenburg.
*For more information on using this form, call 1-800-419-4729.

Home Screening Questionnaire
Ages 0 to 3 Years—cont'd

For office use only	

7. How often does someone take your child into a grocery store?
_____ Hardly ever
_____ At least once per month
_____ At least twice per month
_____ At least once per week

8. How many different babysitters or day-care centers have you used in the past 3 months?

_____

9. Do you have any pets?
Yes   No

10. About how many times in the past week did you have to spank or slap your child to get him or her to mind?

_____

11. How old was your child when you began talking to him or her?
_____ 0 to 3 months
_____ 3 to 9 months
_____ 9 to 15 months
_____ When he or she was old enough to understand

12. How do you feel that your child behaves most of the time?
_____ Smiles and acts pleasant
_____ Prefers to be by himself or herself
_____ Responds readily to affection
_____ Gets angry when he or she does not get his or her way
_____ Is often cranky

13. Do you talk to your child as you are doing the housework?
Yes   No   Too Young

*Home Screening Questionnaire**
Ages 3 to 6 Years

Child's Name _____ Birthdate _____ Age _____

Parents' Names _____ Phone _____

Address _____ Date _____

Please answer *all* the following questions about the ways in which your child spends time and some of your family's activities. On some questions, you may want to check more than one choice.

For office use only		**For office use only**	
_____	1. a) Do you get any magazines in the mail? 　　Yes　　No 　b) If yes, what kind? 　　_____ Home and family magazines 　　_____ News magazines 　　_____ Children's magazines 　　_____ Other	_____	4. How many books do you own besides children's books? 　_____ 0 to 9 　_____ 10 to 20 　_____ More than 20
		_____	5. How often does someone take your child into a grocery store? 　_____ Hardly ever 　_____ At least once per month 　_____ At least twice per month 　_____ At least once per week
_____	2. Does your child have a toy box or other special place to store toys? 　Yes　　No		
_____	3. How many children's books does your family own? 　_____ 0 to 2 　_____ 3 to 9 　_____ 10 or more	_____	6. About how many times in the past week did you have to spank your child? 　_____
		_____	7. Do you have a television? 　Yes　　No About how many hours is the television on each day? 　_____

From William K Frankenburg, 1981, 1988, WK Frankenburg.
*For more information on using this form, call 1-800-419-4729.

Home Screening Questionnaire
Ages 3 to 6 Years—cont'd

For office use only

8. How often does your child have stories read to him or her?
   _____ Hardly ever
   _____ At least once per week
   _____ At least 3 times per week
   _____ At least 5 times per week

9. Do you ever sing to your child when he or she is nearby?
   Yes   No

10. Does you child put away toys by himself or herself most of the time?
    Yes   No

11. Is your child allowed to walk or ride a tricycle by himself or herself to the house of a friend or relative?
    Yes   No

For office use only

12. What do you do with your child's artwork?
    _____ Let the child keep it
    _____ Put it away
    _____ Hang it somewhere in the home
    _____ Throw it away shortly after looking at it

13. In the space below, write what you might say if your child said, "Look at that big truck."

14. What do you usually do when a friend is visiting you in your home and your child has nothing to do?
    _____ Suggest something for your child to do
    _____ Offer your child a toy
    _____ Give your child a cookie or something to eat
    _____ Put your child to bed for a nap
    _____ Play with your child

Family and Caregiver Assessments
Family Screening

The Family American Pediatric Gross Assessment Record (APGAR) is a screening questionnaire that assesses satisfaction with the functional state of the family. It scores family members' answers to questions about five areas of family dynamics—adaptation, partnership, growth, affection, and resolve—by assigning a 0 for answers of "hardly ever," 1 for "some of the time," or 2 for "almost always." Scores of 7 to 10 represent functional families, whereas scores of 4 to 6 suggest moderate dysfunction and 0 to 3 denote severe dysfunction. No special training is required to administer the questionnaire.

The family APGAR scale

The following questions have been designed to help us better understand you and your family. You should feel free to ask questions about any item in the questionnaire.

Please use the comment space should you need to provide additional information or discuss the way the question applies to your family. Please try to answer all questions.

The word *family* describes the individual(s) with whom you usually live. If you live alone, consider family members as those with whom you now have the strongest emotional ties.

	For each question, check only one box		
	Almost always	**Some of the time**	**Hardly ever**
I am satisfied that I can turn to my family for help when something is troubling me. Comments:	☐	☐	☐
I am satisfied with the way my family talks over things with me and shares problems with me. Comments:	☐	☐	☐
I am satisfied that my family accepts and supports my wishes to take on new activities or directions. Comments:	☐	☐	☐
I am satisfied with the way my family expresses affection and responds to my emotions, such as anger, sorrow, and love. Comments:	☐	☐	☐
I am satisfied with the way my family and I share time together. Comments:	☐	☐	☐

Modified from Smilkstein G: The family Apgar: a proposal for a family function test and its use by physicians, *J Fam Pract* 6(6):1232-1235, 1978.

Coping for Parents

The Coping Health Inventory for Parents is a self-report checklist of 45 coping behaviors parents use to weather the hardships associated with management of a family life that includes a seriously ill child. Each behavior is scored on a 4-point scale, with 0 assigned to answers of "not helpful," 1 to "minimally helpful," 2 to "moderately helpful," and 3 to "extremely helpful."

Coping health inventory for parents

Purpose

The Coping Health Inventory for Parents was developed to record the behaviors that parents find helpful and those they do not find helpful in the management of family life when one or more family members is ill for a brief period or has a medical condition that calls for continued medical care. *Coping* is defined as personal or collective (with other individuals or programs) efforts to manage the hardships associated with health problems in the family.

Directions

- To complete this inventory, please read the list of coping behaviors one at a time.
- For each coping behavior you used, please record how helpful it is:
  - 3 = Extremely helpful
  - 2 = Moderately helpful
  - 1 = Minimally helpful
  - 0 = Not helpful
- For each coping behavior you do not use, please record your reason.
  - Chose not to use it
  - Not possible

Please begin; read and record your decision for each coping behavior.

Coping behaviors	Extremely helpful	Moderately helpful	Minimally helpful	Not helpful	I do not cope this way because:	
					Chose not to	Not possible
1. Talking over personal feelings and concerns with spouse	3	2	1	0	☐	☐
2. Engaging in relationships and friendships that help me feel important and appreciated	3	2	1	0	☐	☐
3. Trusting my spouse (or former spouse) to help support me and my child(ren)	3	2	1	0	☐	☐
4. Sleeping	3	2	1	0	☐	☐
5. Talking with medical staff (nurses, social workers) when visiting the medical center	3	2	1	0	☐	☐
6. Believing that my child(ren) will get better	3	2	1	0	☐	☐
7. Working (outside employment)	3	2	1	0	☐	☐

Modified from McCubbin HI and others: The coping health inventory for parents (CHIP). In McCubbin HI, Thompson AI, McCubbin MA: *Family assessment: resiliency, coping, and adaptation—inventories for research and practice,* Madison, Wis, 1996, University of Wisconsin.

Continued

Table—cont'd

Coping behaviors	Extremely helpful	Moderately helpful	Minimally helpful	Not helpful	I do not cope this way because:	
					Chose not to	Not possible
8. Showing that I am strong	3	2	1	0	☐	☐
9. Purchasing gifts for myself or other family members	3	2	1	0	☐	☐
10. Talking with other individuals or parents in my same situation	3	2	1	0	☐	☐
11. Taking good care of all medical equipment at home	3	2	1	0	☐	☐
12. Eating	3	2	1	0	☐	☐
13. Ensuring that other members of the family help with chores and tasks at home	3	2	1	0	☐	☐
14. Getting away by myself	3	2	1	0	☐	☐
15. Talking with the doctor about my concerns regarding my sick child(ren)	3	2	1	0	☐	☐
16. Believing that the medical center or hospital has my family's best interest in mind	3	2	1	0	☐	☐
17. Building close relationships with other individuals	3	2	1	0	☐	☐
18. Believing in God	3	2	1	0	☐	☐
19. Developing myself as a person	3	2	1	0	☐	☐
20. Talking with other parents in the same type of situation and learning about their experiences	3	2	1	0	☐	☐
21. Doing things together as a family (involving all members of the family)	3	2	1	0	☐	☐
22. Investing time and energy in my job	3	2	1	0	☐	☐
23. Believing that my child is getting the best medical care possible	3	2	1	0	☐	☐
24. Entertaining friends in our home	3	2	1	0	☐	☐
25. Reading about how other individuals in my situation handle things	3	2	1	0	☐	☐
26. Doing things with family relatives	3	2	1	0	☐	☐
27. Becoming more self reliant and independent	3	2	1	0	☐	☐

Modified from McCubbin HI and others: The coping health inventory for parents (CHIP). In McCubbin HI, Thompson AI, McCubbin MA: *Family assessment: resiliency, coping, and adaptation—inventories for research and practice,* Madison, Wis, 1996, University of Wisconsin.

Table—cont'd

Coping behaviors	Extremely helpful	Moderately helpful	Minimally helpful	Not helpful	I do not cope this way because:	
					Chose not to	Not possible
28. Telling myself that I have many things for which to be thankful	3	2	1	0	☐	☐
29. Concentrating on hobbies (for example, art, music, or jogging)	3	2	1	0	☐	☐
30. Explaining the family situation to friends and neighbors so they will understand	3	2	1	0	☐	☐
31. Encouraging child(ren) with medical condition to be more independent	3	2	1	0	☐	☐
32. Keeping myself in shape and well groomed	3	2	1	0	☐	☐
33. Becoming involved in social activities (for example, parties) with friends	3	2	1	0	☐	☐
34. Going out with my spouse on a regular basis	3	2	1	0	☐	☐
35. Being sure prescribed medical treatments for child(ren) are carried out at home each day	3	2	1	0	☐	☐
36. Building a closer relationship with my spouse	3	2	1	0	☐	☐
37. Allowing myself to get angry	3	2	1	0	☐	☐
38. Investing myself in my child(ren)	3	2	1	0	☐	☐
39. Talking to someone (not professional counselor or doctor) about my feelings	3	2	1	0	☐	☐
40. Reading more about the medical problem that concerns me	3	2	1	0	☐	☐
41. Trying to maintain family stability	3	2	1	0	☐	☐
42. Being able to get away from the home care tasks and responsibilities for some relief	3	2	1	0	☐	☐
43. Ensuring that my child with the medical condition is seen at the clinic or hospital on a regular basis	3	2	1	0	☐	☐
44. Believing that things will always work out	3	2	1	0	☐	☐
45. Doing things with my children	3	2	1	0	☐	☐

Toy Guidelines

Play and play activities have roles in child development, and toys are important components of play. However, for infants and children with impairments, special considerations and adaptations are necessary for the safe and effective use of toys and the enhancement of development.

Suggestions for Play Adaptations

Children who may need adaptations	Adaptations (not age-specific)
Children with sensory impairments	
Auditory	Colorful toys
	Large facial expressions (smiles)
	Tactile toys, such as terrycloth, velour
	Water play
	Gestures and signs
	Toys with lights, vibrating switches
	FM amplifier, hearing aids
	Speakers for extra volume on computers
	Positioning changes so that child can see activity
Visual	Toys with sound (rattle)
	Singing
	Music boxes
	Enlarged pictures or print
	Tactile toys, such as terrycloth, velour
	Vibrating switches
	Computer programs with large print
	Computer voice output
	Scanner to read to data to computer
	Braille
Children with motor impairments	Toys hung near child's hands and feet (overhead bar, chair)
	Wrist or ankle fasteners for rattles
	Squeaky toys from pet store that squeak easily (may not be safe for use in mouth)
	Toys adapted for easy grasping (sew-on fabric flap, bottle with divided trunk that can be grasped by smaller hands)

Modified from Ratliffe KT: *Clinical pediatric physical therapy,* St Louis, 1998, Mosby.

Table—cont'd

Children who may need adaptations	Adaptations (not age-specific)
Children with motor impairments—cont'd	Large crayons, puzzles with large pieces
	Positioning for optimal use of hands or feet (head and trunk supported in midline)
	Positioning devices (corner seat, infant seat, adapted stroller, custom molded seat, stander, mobile stander)
	Toys adapted to give auditory feedback if touched or swiped, even without grasping
	Toys adapted for switch use
	Clamp or glue toys that do not move (to lap tray, table, chair, high chair, stroller, floor)
	Built-up seat, back, handlebars on ride-on toys and tricycles
	Switch access for computer
	Weight bases on toys
	Electric toys or equipment adapted for switch operation (electric car, electric train, battery-operated toys, bubble generator, toy house with lights, tape recorder, fan, blender)
	Equipment to facilitate difficult movements (wedge for rolling, scooter board or floor cart for moving on floor, special seat for swing)
	Equipment to facilitate access to playground equipment (positioning device for sandbox, seat for swing, seat or cart for playhouse, vest for slide)
Children with cognitive impairments	Simplified rules for games
	Peer buddies for support
	Simple, clear instructions
	Simplified role that allows child to participate in activity

Pediatric Population

Appropriate Toys and Motivational Strategies for Children

Age range	Appropriate toys	Motivational strategies
Young infants (newborn-6 mo)	Rattles	Smile.
	Plastic keys	Coo.
	Stuffed animals	Tickle.
	Mobiles	Play pat-a-cake.
	Busy boxes	Play "This little piggy went to market."
	Bubbles	Hold toys for which newborn or infant
	Pinwheels	can reach.
	Black and white, color pictures	

Modified from Ratliffe KT: *Clinical pediatric physical therapy,* St Louis, 1998, Mosby.   *Continued*

Table—cont'd

Age range	Appropriate toys	Motivational strategies
Older infants (6-12 mo)	Music boxes Busy boxes Stackable or nesting toys, blocks Push toys Ride-on toys Infant books (cloth, cardboard) Puzzles with large pieces Stuffed animals Teethers Mirrors	Work through caregiver (teaching caregiver how to perform activity with child). Use interesting toys. Follow infant's lead until relationship is established, then shape behavior toward desired therapy goals.
Toddlers (1-3 yr)	Balls Dolls Toy animals Ride-on toys, tricycles Toddler slides Plastic baseballs, golf balls, basketballs Farm sets Playhouses with furniture Pretend food Grocery carts Push or pull toys Shape-sorter toys Simple puzzles Books, crayons Toy telephones Computers Age-appropriate software	Present interesting toys. Set up interesting environments. Include family members in therapy. Allow toddler to explore beyond boundaries of therapy setting. Use the body as therapy tool to climb on, under, across. Read books. Use familiar routines.
Preschoolers (3-5 yr)	Crayons Books Puzzles Play-dough Music tapes, tape recorders Building toys (blocks) Dress-up clothes Legos Groups of related toy figures Puppets Dolls Rocks, sticks, boards Pillows, blankets Action figures	Initiate gross motor play. Rough-house with child. Allow child to explore environment. Use peer support through closely planned group activities. Use simple, imaginative games. Create art projects child can take home, follow child's lead. Involve family members or classmates in therapy sessions.

Modified from Ratliffe KT: *Clinical pediatric physical therapy,* St Louis, 1998, Mosby.

Table—cont'd

Age range	Appropriate toys	Motivational strategies
Preschoolers (3-5 yr)—cont'd	Doctor's kits Art supplies Children's athletic equipment (plastic bats, lightweight balls, portable nets) Marbles Computers with software	
Young school-aged children (5-8 yr)	Same as for preschoolers, plus board games Playground equipment Bicycles Athletic equipment (balls, nets, bats, goals) Dolls and action figures Beads to string Knitting materials Pasting, tracing, drawing materials Magic sets Trading cards Checkers Dominoes Make-up Water play equipment	Play imaginative games (e.g., pirates, ballet dancers, gymnastics, baseball). Draw family members into therapy sessions. Give child sense of accomplishment (help child complete project to take home or learn specific skill that child can demonstrate to family members). Incorporate child's goals into therapy goals. Use chart to document progress. Use small toys, objects as rewards.
Older school-aged children (8-12 yr)	Art supplies Board games Tape recorders (music) Exercise equipment (stationary bike, rowing machine, kinetic exercise equipment, pulleys, weights) Athletic equipment Model kits Puzzles Collections (stamps, marbles, dolls, cars, angels) Computers with software	Initiate competition between child and self, therapy provider, family member, peers. Document progress on chart using stars or stickers. Discover child's goals and incorporate them into therapy. Give child sense of success (make goals small enough that immediate progress is visible). Find out what motivates child (ask child, family members, peers).
Adolescents (12-18 yr)	Same as above	Develop system of rewards and consequences for home programs or progress that is attainable and meaningful. Use chart to document goals and progress.

Toy Safety Guidelines

Selection

- Select toys that suit the skills, abilities, and interests of children.
- Select toys that are safe for the specific child; look for label that indicates the intended age group. Toys that are safe for one age may not be safe for another.

  For infants, toddlers, and all children who still place objects into the mouth, avoid toys with small parts that may pose fatal choking or aspiration hazards. Toys in this category are usually labeled: "Not recommended for children under 3 years."

  For infants avoid toys with strings or cords that are 7 inches or longer because they may cause strangulation.

  For all children under 8 years, avoid electric toys with heating elements.

  For children under 5 years, avoid arrows or darts.
- Check for safety labels, such as "flame retardant" or "flame resistant."
- Select toys durable enough to survive rough play; look for sturdy construction, such as tightly secured small parts.
- Look for toys with smooth, rounded edges. Avoid toys with sharp edges that can cut or that have sharp points. Points on the inside of the toy can puncture the child if the toy is broken.
- Avoid toys with shooting or throwing objects that can injure eyes.

  Avoid toys into which other missiles, such as sticks or pebbles, may be used as substitutes for the intended projectiles.

  Ensure that any arrows or darts have blunt tips and are manufactured from resilient materials; ensure that tips are securely attached.

Selection—cont'd

- Ensure that materials in toys are nontoxic.
- Avoid toys that make loud noises that may damage a child's hearing.

  Check to determine whether squeaking toys are too loud when held close to the ear.

  If selecting caps for cap guns, look for the label required by federal law to be on boxes or packages of caps: "Warning—Do not fire closer than 1 foot to the ear. Do not use indoors."
- Ensure that arrows or darts have soft tips, rubber suction cups, or other protective tips. Ensure that tips are secure.
- If selecting a toy gun, ensure that the barrel or the entire gun is brightly colored to avoid being mistaken as a real gun.
- Check toy instructions for clarity. They should be clear to an adult and, when appropriate, to a child.

Supervision

- Maintain a safe play environment.

  Remove and discard plastic wrappings on toys immediately: they can suffocate a child.

  Remove large toys, bumper pads, and boxes from playpens; an adventuresome child can use such items to climb or fall out.
- Set "ground rules" for play.
- Supervise young children closely during play.
- Teach children how to use toys properly and safely.
- Instruct older children to keep their toys away from younger brothers, sisters, and friends.
- Keep children who are playing with riding toys away from stairs, hills, traffic, and swimming pools.

Modified from Wong D: *Wong and Whaley's clinical manual of pediatric nursing*, ed 4, St Louis, 1996, Mosby.

Box—cont'd

Supervision—cont'd

- Establish and enforce rules regarding protective gear.

  Insist that children wear helmets when using bicycles, skateboards, or in-line skates.

  Insist that children wear gloves and wrist, elbow, and knee pads when using skateboards or in-line skates.

- Instruct children on electrical safety.

  Teach children the proper way to unplug an electrical toy—pulling on the plug, not the cord.

  Teach children to beware of electrical appliances and electrically operated playthings; children frequently are unfamiliar with the hazards of electricity and water.

- Teach children the safe use of utensils that under certain circumstances can cause injury, such as scissors, knives, needles, heating elements, loops, long strings, or cords.

Maintenance

- Inspect old and new toys regularly for breakage, loose parts, and other potential hazards.

  Look for jagged or sharp edges or broken parts that may constitute choking hazards.

  Check movable parts to ensure that they are attached securely to toys; sometimes pieces that are safe when attached to the toy become dangerous when detached.

  Examine all outdoor toys regularly for rust and weak or sharp parts that can become dangerous to a child.

  Check electrical cords and plugs for cracked or fraying parts.

Maintenance—cont'd

- Maintain toys in good repair, without signs of possible hazards, such as sharp edges, splinters, weak seams, or rust.

  Make repairs immediately, or discard the toys out of reach of children.

  Sand sharp wooden toys or splintered surfaces smooth.

  Use only nontoxic paint to repaint toys, toy boxes, or children's furniture.

Storage

- Provide a safe place for children to store toys.
- Select a toy chest or toy box that is ventilated, is free of self-locking devices that can trap a child inside, and has a lid designed not to pinch a child's fingers or fall on a child's head.
- If containers other than toy chests are used for storage purposes, fit them with spring-loaded support devices if they have hinged lids to avoid entrapment and suffocation.
- Teach children to store toys safely to prevent accidental injury from stepping, tripping, or falling on a toy.
- Playthings meant for older children and adults should be stowed away safely on high shelves, in locked closets, or in other areas unavailable to younger children.

Pediatric Population

Toys for Tots

Age range	Abilities	Appropriate toys
Birth-3 mo	Follows sounds and objects Responds to voices Enjoys simple patterns with high contrasts	Mobiles Rattles Squeeze toys Musical toys
3-6 mo	Bats, kicks, grasps (but does not let go of grasp) Brings most things to mouth	Crib gyms Unbreakable mirrors Simple picture books Soft toys Items of varying textures
6-9 mo	Mouths, grasps and releases, hands toy back and forth Sits and creeps	Activity boxes Simple stacking toys Soft blocks Containers
9-12 mo	Manipulates objects and "finds" hidden toys Enjoys increased mobility	Balls Wheeled toys Stacking or nesting toys Containers
12-18 mo	Crawls and walks Imitates others Demonstrates increased fine-motor coordination	Dolls Stuffed animals Reality-based toys Pull toys Simple puzzles Sorting toys
18-24 mo	Walks Mimics others Engages in imaginative play	Ride-on toys Push and pull toys Dolls Clay Finger paints Large crayons Simple musical instruments

Modified from Wingate C: Let's play! *Am Baby* 5:10, 1998.

Types and Examples of Age-Specific Play Activities

Category (characteristic age)	Description	Properties of activities	Representative toys and activities
Exploratory play (0-2 yr)	Play and recreational experiences through which child develops body scheme, sensory integrative and motor skills, and concepts of sensory characteristics and actions of human and nonhuman objects	Material and objects: Child's own body Significant others Environmental textures Infant toys with distinct sensory characteristics and actions Everyday household objects Human relationships: Strongest relationships occurring through play among child and parents	Auditory toys (rattles, play piano), balls (all sizes and textures), bells, blocks, busy boxes, containers and nesting toys, dolls and stuffed animals, hammers and pegs, imitative hand-body games, inflatables, language games with parents, mirrors, mobiles, pop-up toys, pots and pans, rolling and crawling and cruising activities, sand and water toys and activities, brightly colored scarves, scooter boards, scribbling with crayons, See 'N' Say, sensory play with parents, shape boxes, empty spice bottles, squeeze toys, teething toys, textured surfaces, one-to three-piece puzzles
Symbolic play (2-4 yr)	Play and recreational experiences through which child formulates, tests, classifies, and refines ideas, feelings, and combined actions Category associated with the development of language Objects given importance according to the child's ability to symbolize, control, change, and master	Materials and objects: Gross-motor play equipment Simple construction toys Simple art materials Toys for fantasy, imaginative play Human relationships: Play with peers beginning with parallel imitation and developing into cooperative interaction	Balance-rocker boards, blocks, beads, blowing bubbles, cars, trucks, trains, chalk and blackboard activities, clay, modeling dough, colorforms, construction kits, crayons, paints, paper, dolls and stuffed animals, dollhouses, dramatic songs, "dress up" materials, fingerpaints, hand puppets, household play items, inflatables, magnets, miniature figures, musical instruments, nesting toys, play tunnel, put-together toys, puzzles, records, rocking horses, rolling in the grass, sand and water toys, sewing cards, simple story books, slides, space stations, stacking toys, swings, toy telephones, tricycle riding

Continued

Modified from Pratt PN, Allen AS: *Occupational therapy for children*, ed 2, St Louis, 1989, Mosby.

Pediatric Population

Table—cont'd

Category (characteristic age)	Description	Properties of activities	Representative toys and activities
Creative play (4-7 yr)	Play and recreational experiences through which the child refines sensory, motor, cognitive, and social skills; explores combinations of actions on multiple objects; and develops interests and competencies that promote performance of school-related and work-related activities	Materials and objects: Arts and crafts Complex construction toys Dramatic play materials Household activities, such as cooking, simple woodwork, pet care, and gardening Human relationships: Play beginning in cooperative peer groups with gradual emergence of competitive atmosphere, peer validation of play products becoming increasingly important Parents assisting and validating in the absence of peers	Baking cookies, stringing beads, bicycle riding, craft kits, cutting and pasting, finger painting, gardening, origami, painting, paperdolls, play houses, simple weaving (placemats and pot holders), simple woodworking, stencils

Games (7-12 yr)	Materials and objects:	Board games, card games, checkers, clubs, collections, computer games, field days (races and tug-of-war), hangman, jacks, marbles, jump rope, organized outdoor games, ping pong, roller skating and ice skating, school plays, performances, scooter board races, team sports, trading cards
Play and recreational experiences that have distinct rules and involve skill development and social interaction in a competitive atmosphere	Arts and crafts	
	Complex construction toys	
	Dramatic play materials	
	Household activities, such as cooking, simple woodwork, pet care, and gardening	
Actions and results of actions being compared against those of peers	Human relationships:	
	Play beginning in cooperative peer groups with gradual emergence of competitive atmosphere, peer validation of play products becomes increasingly important	
	Parents assisting and validating in the absence of peers	

Modified from Pratt PN, Allen AS: *Occupational therapy for children*, ed 2, St Louis, 1989, Mosby.

Pediatric Population

Gross Motor Activities

Activity	Adaptations	Purposes
Pass the beanbag	Imitate manner that beanbag is passed (for example, under one leg, behind back). Sit on floor or therapy balls. Use only right or left hand. Play "hot potato." Individual holding beanbag when music stops is loser.	Grasp and release Crossing midline of body Motor planning Sitting balance Body scheme Right-left discrimination
Animal walk	Use for relay races or "Mother may I." Include in obstacle course. Walk along rope or line on floor. Perform walk blindfolded.	Motor planning Bilateral integration Body scheme
Cross the river: Step on "stepping stones" to "cross the river" (walk across room) without "getting feet wet" (missing stepping stone and putting foot on floor).	Use carpet squares, cardboard pieces, tape marks, and so on for stepping stones. Jump or hop on squares. Color code for right and left. Vary placement of squares. Step on rope laid across floor. Walk across by stepping in shoe boxes.	Motor planning Crossing midline of body Balance Bilateral integration Right-left discrimination
Obstacle course: Arrange course of objects to go over, under, around, through, between, and so on.	Arrange under chair or table. Step in boxes. Roll on carpet or mat. Step between rows of blocks. Jump over boxes. Crawl around desk.	Motor planning Body scheme Bilateral integration Tactile input Sequencing
Hopscotch	Use jumps instead of hops. Reduce size or number of squares. Use beanbag as marker.	Motor planning Equilibrium Sequencing Bilateral integration
Hit the target: Throw beanbag or ball in box or trash can or use Velcro dartboard.	Throw from different positions—all fours, prone, and so on. Sit on therapy balls. Throw with both hands simultaneously. Cross body's midline when throwing. Throw while swinging. Throw with right or left hand on command.	Motor planning Eye-hand coordination Crossing midline of body Sitting balance Right-left discrimination

Modified from Pratt PN, Allen AS: *Occupational therapy for children,* ed 2, St Louis, 1989, Mosby.

In-Hand Manipulation Treatment Activities

Preparation Activities

General tactile awareness activities
1. Using crazy foam
2. Using shaving cream
3. Applying hand lotion
4. Finger painting

Activities involving proprioceptive input
1. Weight bearing—wheelbarrow, activities on a small ball
2. Pushing heavy objects (e.g., boxes, chairs, benches)
3. Pulling (tug-of-war)
4. Pressing different parts of the hand into clay
5. Pushing fingers into clay or therapy putty
6. Pushing shapes out of perforated cardboard
7. Tearing packages or boxes open
8. Playing clapping games

Activities involving regulation of pressure
1. Tearing edges off computer paper
2. Rolling clay into a ball
3. Squeezing water from a sponge or washcloth
4. Pushing snaps together

Activities involving tactile discrimination
1. Performing finger games and songs
2. Playing finger-identification games
3. Discriminating stabilized objects
4. Discriminating stabilized shapes
5. Writing on the body and identifying the shape, letter, or object drawn
6. Discriminating textures

Specific In-Hand Manipulation Activities

Translation: fingers to palm
1. Removing coin from a change purse
2. Hiding a penny in the hand (magic trick)
3. Crumpling paper
4. Picking up and bringing small piece of food into the palm

Translation: fingers to palm with stabilization
1. Removing two or more coins from a change purse, one at a time
2. Taking two or more chips off a magnetic wand, one at a time

Specific In-Hand Manipulation Activities—cont'd

Translation: fingers to palm with stabilization—cont'd
3. Picking up pegs or paper clips one at a time and holding two or more in the hand at one time
4. Picking up several utensils one at a time and holding two or more in the hand at one time

Translation: palm to fingers
1. Moving a penny from palm to fingers
2. Moving a chip to fingers to put on a magnetic wand
3. Moving an object to put it into a container
4. Moving a food item to put it in mouth

Translation: palm to fingers with stabilization
1. Holding several chips to put on a wand, one at a time
2. Handling money to put into a bank or soda machine
3. Putting one utensil down while holding several
4. Holding several game pieces (chips, pegs, markers)

Shift
1. Turning pages in a book
2. Picking up sheets of paper, tissue paper, or dollar bills
3. Separating playing cards
4. Stringing beads (shifting string and bead as string goes through the bead)
5. Shifting a crayon, pencil, or pen for coloring or writing
6. Shifting paper in nonpreferred hand while cutting
7. Playing with tinkertoys (long, thin pieces)
8. Moving a cookie while eating
9. Adjusting a spoon, fork, or knife for appropriate use
10. Rubbing pain, dirt, or tape off pad of a finger

Shift with stabilization
1. Holding a pen and pushing the cap off with the same hand
2. Holding chips while flipping one from the fingers

Modified from Case-Smith J, Allen AS, Pratt PN, editors: *Occupational therapy for children*, ed 3, St Louis, 1996, Mosby.

Pediatric Population

Continued

Box—cont'd

Specific In-Hand Manipulation Activities—cont'd

Shift with stabilization—cont'd

3. Holding fabric in the hand while attempting to button or snap
4. Holding a key ring with keys in hand, shifting one for placement in a lock

Simple or complex rotation (depending on object orientation)

1. Removing or fitting a small jar lid
2. Removing or fitting bolts from nuts
3. Rotating a crayon or pencil—tip oriented ulnarly (simple rotation)
4. Rotating a crayon or pencil—tip oriented radially (complex rotation)
5. Removing a crayon from the box and preparing it for coloring
6. Rotating a pen or marker to put on the top
7. Rotating toy people to put them in chairs, a bus, or a boat

Specific In-Hand Manipulation Activities—cont'd

Simple or complex rotation (depending on object orientation)—cont'd

8. Rotating a puzzle piece for placement in board
9. Feeling objects or shapes to identify them
10. Handling construction-toy pieces
11. Turning cubes that have pictures on all six sides
12. Constructing twisted shapes with pipe cleaners
13. Rotating a toothbrush or eating utensils during use

Simple or complex rotation with stabilization

1. Handling parts of a small-shape container while rotating the shape to put it into the container
2. Holding a key ring with keys, rotating correct one for placement in lock

Modified from Case-Smith J, Allen AS, Pratt PN, editors: *Occupational therapy for children,* ed 3, St Louis, 1996, Mosby.

Adaptations

Development requires interaction with the environment. Children with impairments have numerous barriers to such interactions. Therapists assist in overcoming these barriers by developing structural changes, providing assistive devices (Figure 2-1), and modifying tasks (Figures 2-2 through 2-4).

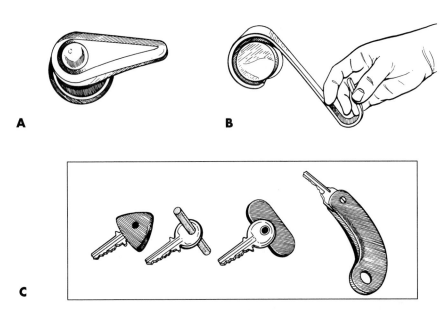

A

B

C

FIGURE 2-1 Adaptive devices for opening doors. A, Rubber knob extension that snaps onto doorknobs. **B,** Portable doorknob turner. **C,** Key adaptations that increase leverage to facilitate turning. (From Pratt PN, Allen AS: *Occupational therapy for children,* ed 2, St Louis, 1989, Mosby.)

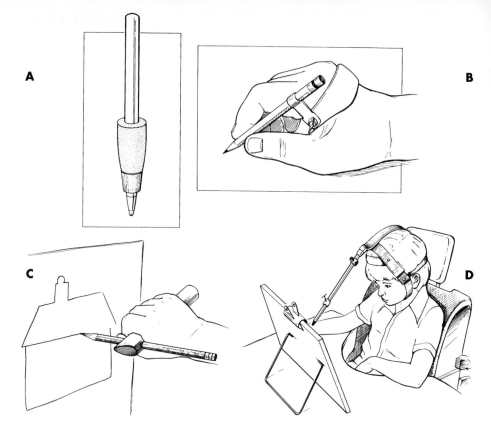

FIGURE 2-2 Adapted writing tools. A, Foam cylinder that increases grasp surface area. **B,** Adaptation used to encourage tripod-type grasp. **C,** Adaptive device that accommodates various grasp and wrist positions. **D,** Headwand with felt-tip pen attached used to mark in a workbook that is clipped to a slanted board. (From Case-Smith J et al: *Occupational therapy for children,* ed 3, St Louis, 1996, Mosby.)

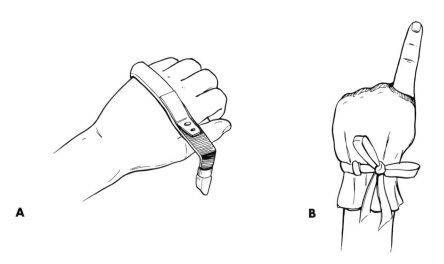

FIGURE 2-3 Adapted keyboard access tools. A, Angled pointer that accommodates forearm and palmar grasp positions. **B,** Mitten for isolating one finger. (From Pratt PN, Allen AS: *Occupational therapy for children,* ed 2, St Louis, 1989, Mosby.)

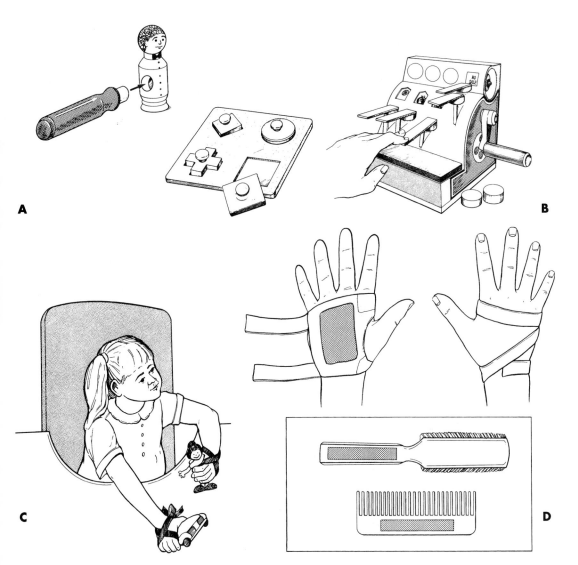

FIGURE 2-4 Adaptations for play. A, Handles and knobs increase grasping ability. **B,** Lever extensions permit operation of toy with less force and control. **C,** Straps allow individuals who cannot grasp objects to play with toys. **D,** Velcro mitts allow individuals who have no grasping ability to hold objects. (From Case-Smith J et al: *Occupational therapy for children,* ed 3, St Louis, 1996, Mosby.)

Environmental Adaptations for Homes with Limited Accessibility

Architectural barriers	Structural changes	Possible assistive devices	Task modifications
Entrances and exits	Hand rails Hand stairs Ramps Built-up terrains to door height Stair lifts In-home elevators Increased door widths (33-36 in minimum) Step-back hinges Rehinged doors that open in or out Pocket doors Folding doors Electric door openers	Strapping or loops on door handles Lever handles Portable door knobs Built-up key holders Combination locks Environmental control units	Use different entrances. Remove inside doors. Use curtains for privacy. Use hips or wheelchairs to open doors.
Bathrooms	Enlarged rooms Low-mounted sinks Open spaces under cabinets Shower seats Changed placements of tub faucets Ramped shower stalls Toilet bidets Linen closet shelves with no doors	Safety rails Seat reducers Raised commode seats Wheelchair commodes Steps placed in front of commodes Insulated pipes Single-lever faucets Tub seats Hydraulic lifts Toilet paper tongs Toilet paper mountings Angled mirrors Wall-mounted hairdryers with switches Wheelchair shower chairs	Place free-standing commodes in secluded areas. Use urinals. Empty leg bags into litter containers. Use bed baths. Use sponge baths. Use liquid soap. Place soap on a string. Use shampoo pumps. Use dry shampoo.

Modified from Case-Smith J, Allen AS, Pratt PN, editors: *Occupational therapy for children*, ed 3, St Louis, 1996, Mosby.

Table—cont'd

Architectural barriers	Structural changes	Possible assistive devices	Task modifications
Bedrooms	Bedrooms on first floor Enlarged spaces Enlarged closet doors Low closet poles Closet storage systems with shelves Built-in bookshelves at low and medium heights Holes cut in work surfaces for holding of objects and electrical cords Built-in dressers or dressers bolted to the walls Special glides for wall drawers	Leg extenders Bed rails Firm mattresses Straps or rope ladders Mounted shoe racks Environmental control units or switches for television, radio, and light access Enlarged or added loops on drawer handles Positioning devices Adaptive chairs	Place beds on floor. Keep most used clothes in accessible drawers. Use shelves instead of dresser drawers for clothes. Store toys in shoe bags.
Kitchens	Enlarged spaces Lowered countertops Lowered cabinets Sinks without cabinets under them Built-in range tops Sliding drawers and organizers in cabinets Wall-mounted ovens side by side Dishwashers mounted higher Front-opening washers	Adapted utensils Automated learning devices for appliances turned on by switches Adapted seats Wheelchair lap trays Barstools	Keep most frequently used items in low cupboards. Hang bowls and pans on wall instead of in cabinet. Eat on wheelchair lap trays instead of tables. Store water in insulated bottles with pumps on tables. Keep items used most frequently on accessible surfaces. Use stools for washing dishes.

Pediatric Population

Useful Adaptations For Living Areas

Living area	Adaptation
Kitchen	Make access to countertop via bar stool, standing frame, or prone stander.
	Place frequently used utensils and food in low cupboards to improve access.
	Perform food preparation or clean-up while seated at table if countertop is inaccessible.
	Avoid stacking heavy bowls and pans.
	Use time- and energy-saving devices, such as microwave ovens with large touch controls, food processors, electric mixers, and blenders.
	Use other adapted kitchen aids and utensils.
Dining room	Use adapted chairs for posture control and proper seat height.
	Use a wheelchair lap tray as an eating surface.
Variable areas	Use push-button telephones, mounted on walls at relatively low heights for access and stability.
	Use special telephone functions, such as automatic dialing, speaker phone, or receiver amplification available through the special services division of the local telephone company.
	Use environmental control switches, remote units, or systems for lights and appliances.
	Avoid thick pile carpet or throw rugs to optimize mobility.

Modified from Pratt PN, Allen AS: *Occupational therapy for children,* ed 2, St Louis, 1989, Mosby.

Support of Function through Adaptive Aids

Function	Adaptive aid
Arm movement	**Suspension sling.** A device to support the upper extremity in which cuffs fit under the elbow and wrist and are spring-suspended from overhead bars; assisted motions including shoulder horizontal abduction and adduction, shoulder external and internal rotation, shoulder abduction, and elbow flexion and extension
	Mobile arm support. A frictionless arm support that uses the concept of the inclined plane in which a trough supports the forearm and connects to a series of movable bars with adjustable stops and the unit fastens to a wheelchair with brackets; provides movement in space and helps weak shoulder and elbow muscles to position the hand
	Gooseneck spoon. A spoon that is mounted to a gooseneck holder that is clamped to the table edge; provides resistance through the motions of scooping and bringing food on the spoon to the mouth; can help inhibit extraneous movement and athetosis
Wrist support	**Cock-up splint.** A simple splint that extends from the distal palmar crease, supports the wrist, and ends two-thirds up the distance of the forearm; stabilizes and positions the wrist to provide mechanical advantage fingers need in prehension and grasp
Grasp	**Universal cuff (utensil holder).** A cuff that fits around the palm, has a pocket for the insertion of handles of utensils, and can be used when grasp is not possible
	Built-up handle. An enlarged handle that facilitates grasp
	Modified handle for cup or glass. A projection on the utensil that accommodates a child's grasping pattern; must maintain low center of gravity when weakness is present
Reach	**Curved handle.** A handle adjusted to form an angle so that a child can reach body parts
	Extended handle. An elongated handle that provides reach; becomes less stable with length and weight
	Sandwich holder. A plastic holder with a rubber band that grips the sandwich; inserted in universal cuff
Supination	**Swivel spoon.** Spoon with swivel mechanism that levels the bowl when wrist or finger motion is not present
Stabilization of equipment or food	**Nonslip mat.** A nonslip plastic material that holds plates and glasses steady
	Plate guard. A rim that clips onto a plate; provides a "wall" against which the child scoops food with a fork or spoon
	Scoop dish. A plate molded low in front and high in back to facilitate scooping of food
One-handed feeding	**Rocker knife.** A knife with a curved blade; cuts with rocking motion provided by one hand; other aids including the plate guard and nonslip mat
Self-feeding	**Electric or battery feeder.** An expensive device that enables self-feeding without use of the arms; requires a single motion to control switches; must be set up by caregiver

Pediatric Population

Modified from Pratt PN, Allen AS: *Occupational therapy for children*, ed 2, St Louis, 1989, Mosby.

Stabilization Materials and Applications

Materials	Applications
Tape	Material that is generally a temporary solution; can be applied quickly as need arises; is inexpensive and readily available in households, schools, and therapy units; duct tape being very sturdy, with good holding power; masking and cellophane tapes being less sturdy but widely used
Nonslip, pressure-sensitive matting	Material that can be ordered through therapy supply catalogs in rolls or pads; becoming available to the public in kitchen stores; minimizes slipping and sliding of objects with large bases that are placed on it; can be glued to small objects in small pieces to aid stabilization; relies on friction between materials for stabilization
Suction cup holders	Devices that are widely available in both stores and through therapy supply catalogs; single-faced suction cups being generally permanently applied to a toy or object; double-faced suction cups being set up where suction is needed between the object and work surface
C-clamps	Devices that are readily available and suitable for the securing of flat objects to lap trays, table edges, and other surfaces
Tacking putty	Product that is sold for the sticking of posters onto walls; useful for the holding of lightweight objects on tables, lap trays, angle boards, and walls
Pressure-sensitive hook and loop tapes	Tapes that can be glued to the base of toys and other objects and to play or work surfaces for stabilization; soft loop tape being used on areas that come into contact with child's skin or clothing
Wing nuts and bolts	Items that often can bolt toys and other objects to a table surface through holes drilled through the object and holding surface; stabilizes objects more permanently
Magnets	Devices that can be affixed to toys and aid stabilization in metallic surfaces, such as refrigerator doors, metal tables, and magnetic play boards
L-brackets	Hardware-store items that are particularly effective for the stabilization of items in an upright plane; holes being drilled in both the work or play surface and the toy or other object to correspond with the L-bracket holes; objects then being secured with nuts and bolts
Soldering clamps	Small clamps that are mounted to free-standing bases that are weighted or suction-cupped or that use clamps for stability; best used to hold small items for intricate play, hobbies, or work
Elastic or webbing straps	Materials that can be attached to toys to tie them down or to play or work surfaces to secure flat objects

Modified from Case-Smith J, Allen AS, Pratt PN, editors: *Occupational therapy for children,* ed 3, St Louis, 1996, Mosby.

Computer and Typewriter Keyboard Adaptations

Adaptation	Applications
Key latch	Device that locks the "shift" and "control" keys to allow simultaneous activation of another key; for children who are able to use only one finger, a headwand, or mouth-stick
Keyguard	Device that improves accuracy when the child has difficulty hitting one key at a time; acts as a guide for finger placement and resting surface for the hand; typical errors that indicate the need for a keyguard including frequent hitting of the keys next to desired letters or unintentional activation of other keys with other fingers or parts of the hand because of uncontrolled motion; most commercial keyguards being equipped with a latching feature for the "control" and "shift" keys
Special placement of the keyboard	Adaptation for one-handed typists and children who have difficulty crossing the midline; placement of the keyboard being offset toward the dominant hand; placing the keyboard on an inclined surface possibly facilitating key selection
Arm support systems	Wrist rests or arm supports that can be secured in front of the keyboard when motor weakness or extraneous movements are present; may be continuous with the front of the keyboard or raised; effective for increases in speed, accuracy, and endurance; overhead slings and mobile arm supports being alternative adaptations
Disabling of the repeat function	Modifications in software and hardware designed to prevent children with slow reactions or poorly moderated downward pressure from activating repeat functions through sustained pressure on keys; contact special services divisions of computer manufacturers for assistance

Modified from Pratt PN, Allen AS: *Occupational therapy for children,* ed 2, St Louis, 1989, Mosby.

Positioning Guidelines

Positioning patients is an important part of home rehabilitation for any population, but especially for children. Many infants and children lack the ability to position themselves for play and activities of daily living and cannot provide adequate pressure relief. Home care therapists educate patients and caregivers on the role of positioning and provide instructions for specific positioning techniques (Figure 2-5).

Pediatric Population

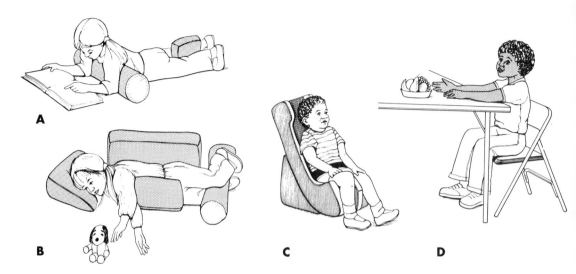

FIGURE 2-5 Adapted positioning for improved function. A, Prone position. **B,** Sidelying position. **C,** Grading sitting balance in partial recliner. **D,** Increasing postural stability by elevating working surface. (From Pratt PN, Allen AS: *Occupational therapy for children*, ed 2, St Louis, 1989, Mosby.)

Medical and Developmental Considerations

Medical factors	Developmental factors
Prone	
Advantages	
Improved oxygenation and ventilation (despite increased total "work" of breathing) in infants with and without ventilatory support[1,8,16,18,23]	Facilitates development of flexor tone
	Facilitates hand-to-mouth pattern for self-calming
Better gastric emptying than in supine or on left side (unless feedings pool regardless)[25]	Facilitates active neck extension and head raising
Less reflux, especially if head of bed is elevated 30°[3,19,20]	Improves coping with extrauterine environment (if sleep more, cry less)[4]
Decreased risk of aspiration[11]	May decrease persistent head turning to the right and skull asymmetry

Modified from Case-Smith J, Allen AS, Pratt PN, editors: *Occupational therapy for children*, ed 3, St Louis, 1996, Mosby.

[1]Alastair AH, Ross KR, Russell G: The effect of posture on ventilation and lung mechanics in preterm and light-for-date infants, *Pediatrics* 64:429, 1979.

[3]Blumenthal I, Lealman GT: Effect of posture on gastroesophageal reflux in the newborn, *Arch Dis Child* 57(7):555, 1982.

[4]Bottos M, Stafani D: Postural and motor care of the premature baby, *Dev Med Child Neurol* 24:706, 1982 (letter).

[8]Fox M, Molesky M: The effects of prone and supine positioning on arterial oxygen pressure, *Neonat Network* 25, 1990.

[11]Hewitt V: Effect of posture on the presence of fat in tracheal aspirate in neonates, *Aust Paediatr J* 12:267, 1976.

[16]Martin RJ and others: Effect of supine and prone positions on arterial oxygen tension in the preterm infant, *Pediatrics* 63(4):528, 1979.

[18]Mendoza J, Roberts J, Cook L: Postural effects on pulmonary function and heart rate of preterm infants with lung disease, *J Pediatr* 118:445, 1991.

[19]Meyers WF, Herbst JJ: Effectiveness of position therapy for gastroesophageal reflux, Pediatrics 69(6):768, 1982.

[20]Orenstein S, Whitington P, Orenstein D: The infant seat as treatment for gastroesophageal reflux, *N Engl J Med* 309:760, 1983.

[23]Wagaman MJ and others: Improved oxygenation and lung compliance with prone positioning of neonates, *J Pediatr* 94(5):787, 1979.

[25]Yu VYH: Effect of body position on gastric emptying in the neonate, *Arch Dis Child* 50:500, 1975.

Table—cont'd

Medical factors	Developmental factors

Prone—cont'd
Advantages—cont'd

More sleep and less crying when term and preterm infants are prone rather than supine[4,6]

Less energy expenditure when prone rather than supine[17]

Less sleep apnea in prone than in supine in term infants[12]

Best position to expose diaper rash to air or heat lamp

Disadvantages

Access for medical care more difficult

Possible self-extubation with agitated or active infant

| | Makes visual exploration more difficult for baby |
| | Makes face-to-face social contact more difficult |

Supine
Advantages

Easier access to infant for medical care (in hammock)

Increase in sleep time for preterm infants (versus "flat" supine)[5]

Facilitates easier visual exploration by infant

May facilitate midline position in supine in hammock

Ensures easier positioning of head in midline (than in prone)

Disadvantages

Decreased arterial oxygen tension, lung compliance, and tidal volume than in prone[1,16,23]

More reflux than in prone at any time or than in upright sitting if infant is awake[19,20]

Greater risk of aspiration than in prone or right sidelying[11]

More sleep and less crying for term and preterm infants in supine than prone[4,6]

Possible decrease in respiration in supine in hammock if infant had decreased lung compliance (respiratory distress syndrome)[5]

Greater energy expenditure in supine than prone[17]

Encourages extension rather than flexion (increased muscle tone with hyperextension of head, neck, and shoulders)[2]

Encourages external rotation positional deformities of arms and legs (with later delayed hands-to-midline or out-toeing gait)

[2]Anderson J, Auster-Liebhaber J: Developmental therapy in the neonatal intensive care unit, *Phys Occup Ther Pediatr* 4:89, 1984.

[5]Bottos M and others: The effect of a containing position in a hammock versus the supine position on the cutaneous oxygen level in premature and term babies, *Early Hum Dev* 11:265, 1985.

[6]Brackbill Y, Douthitt T, West H: Psycholphysiologic effects in the neonate of prone versus supine placement, *J Pediatr* 82:82, 1973.

[12]Hoshimoto T and others: Postural effects on behavioral states of newborn infants: a sleep polygraph study, *Brain Dev* 5:286, 1983.

[17]Masterson J, Zucker C, Schulze K: Prone and supine positioning effects on energy expenditure and behavior of low birth weight neonates, *Pediatrics* 80(5):689, 1987.

Continued

Pediatric Population

Medical factors	Developmental factors

Sidelying

Advantages

Better gastric emptying when lying on right side than in supine or left side lying (about same as prone)[25]	Encourages midline orientation of head and extremities
Better oxygenation for infant with unilateral lung disease, with good lung positioned uppermost[10]	Counteracts external rotation of limbs, promotes flexion and extremity adduction
	Facilitates hand-to-mouth pattern for self-calming
	Facilitates hand-to-hand activity

Disadvantages

Decreased gastric emptying when lying on left side than in prone or right sidelying[25]	May be difficult to maintain flexed position with irritable or hypertonic extended infant

Sitting

Advantages

Alternative position (for variety and skin integrity)	Is an alerting posture (upright)
	Encourages infant visual exploration
	Encourages social interaction
	May allow use of swing for older neonatal intensive care unit infants
	May help temporarily "break up" (relax) high tone

Disadvantages

Increased frequency and duration of reflux for infant seat elevated 60°[20]	May be difficult to properly position infant without slumping or slouching of head and trunk[22]
Increased heart rate and mean arterial pressure in preterm infants in more upright position (90°)[22]	
Possible decrease in oxygen saturation in some preterm infants in semireclined position[24]	

Head Position and Midline Position

Advantages

Decrease intracranial pressure and intraventricular hemorrhage when head in midline[9]	May improve head shape with head in midline
Possible reduction in intracranial pressure when head of bed elevated 30°[9]	Reduces asymmetry and encourages development of flexion
	May reduce head flattening with use of waterbeds and water pillows[7,13,15,21]

Disadvantages

Creation of pressure sores if too long on firm surface	May be difficult in prone

Modified from Case-Smith J, Allen AS, Pratt PN, editors: *Occupational therapy for children*, ed 3, St Louis, 1996, Mosby.

[7]Fay MJ: The positive effects of positioning, *Neonat Network* 8:23, 1988.

[9]Goldberg RN and others: The effect of head position on intracranial pressure in the neonate, *Crit Care Med* 11(6):428, 1983.

[10]Heaf D and others: Postural effects of gas exchange in infants, *N Engl J Med* 308:1505, 1983.

[13]Kramer LI, Pierpont ME: Rocking waterbeds and auditory stimuli to enhance growth of preterm infants, *J Pediatr* 88(2):297, 1976.

[14]Mansell A, Bryan C, Levison H: Airway closure in children, *J Appl Physiol* 33:711, 1972.

[15]Marsden DJ: Reduction of head flattening in preterm infants, *Dev Med Child Neurol* 22:507, 1980.

[21]Schwirian P, Eesley T, Cuellar L: Use of water pillows in reducing head shape distortion in preterm infants, *Res Nurs Health* 9:203, 1986.

[22]Smith P, Turner B: The physiologic effects of positioning premature infants in car seats, *Neonat Network* 9:11, 1990.

[24]Willet L and others: Risk of hypoventilation in premature infants in car seats, *J Pediatr* 109:245, 1986.

Ideal Positioning

	Supine	Prone	Sidelying	Sitting
Pelvis and hips	Pelvis in line with trunk Hips in 30°-90° flexion Neutral rotation of pelvis Hips symmetrically abducted 10°-20°	Pelvis in line with trunk Hips in extension Neutral rotation Hips symmetrically abducted 10°-20°	Pelvis in line with trunk Hips in flexion Neutral rotation of pelvis Hips in 10°-20° abduction	Pelvis in line with trunk Hips at 90° flexion Neutral rotation of pelvis Hips symmetrically abducted 10°-20°
Trunk	Straight trunk Shoulders in line with hips Neutral rotation of trunk	Straight trunk Shoulders in line with hips Neutral rotation	Straight trunk Shoulders in line with hips Slight sidebending OK	Straight trunk Shoulders over hips Trunk not rotated
Head and neck	Head in neutral position Head facing forward Slight cervical flexion	Head in neutral position Head facing to one side Slight cervical flexion	Head in neutral position Head facing forward Slight cervical flexion	Head in neutral position Head facing forward Head evenly on shoulders
Shoulders and arms	Arms fully supported Arms forward of trunk Forearms resting on trunk or pillow	Arms fully supported Arms forward of trunk Flexion at shoulder Flexion at elbows	Both arms supported Lower arm forward Arms not lying on point of shoulder Lower arm neutral rotation Upper arm internally rotated 0°-40°	Arms fully supported Elbows in flexion Shoulders internally rotated 0°-40°
Legs and feet	Knees supported in flexion Feet held at 90°	Knees extended Feet supported at 90°	Knees in flexion Feet positioned at 90° Pillow between knees	Knees at 90° Ankles at 90° Feet fully supported Thighs fully supported

Pediatric Population

Modified from Ratliffe KT: *Clinical pediatric physical therapy*, St Louis, 1998, Mosby.

Functional Positions and Possible Adaptations for Children with Severe Disabilities

Activity, positioning devices	Functional goal	Possible postural problems	Possible adaptations
Activity Sleeping in supine position **Devices** Crib Bassinet Blanket Adult arms or lap Bed Mat	The infant or child maintains a neutral alignment of the head and trunk with age-appropriate flexion of the extremities while sleeping in supine position.	Infant or child with low postural tone: • Cannot keep head in midline • Demonstrates excessive passive extension in arms and legs Infant or child with high postural tone: • Exhibits strong influence of ATNR, causing head to turn to side and trunk to arch • Demonstrates asymmetry in posture caused by ATNR	Purchase or make a U-shaped towel roll to put around the head (works better for infants and small children). If the towel roll gets pushed out of position, attach to a flat surface on which body can lie on to anchor the device. Make a double-wedged pillow that guides the infant's or child's head to midline. Use towel rolls to encircle an infant's body, or sandbags, bolsters, or stuffed animals supporting the arms and legs of a child in a symmetrical flexed position.
Activity Playing with toy truck in prone position **Devices** Crib Blanket Adult lap Adult body Mat Carpeted floor Scooter board Bolster	Infant or child moves toy truck at least 3 in across floor, using arm to propel.	Infant or child with low postural tone: • Cannot lift head and upper trunk • Cannot lift arms to reach • Holds arms and legs in excessive passive extension Infant or child with high postural tone: • Exhibits strong influence of STNR, causing difficulty extending arm when head is extended • Cannot maintain head in midline to look at toy • Makes jerky and poorly graded movements • Cannot extend arm when head is in midline	Use small roll, pillow, or wedge under the chest so that the head is not forced into hyperextension when prone and the arms to fall into flexion. Support both arms at the elbow to prevent asymmetries of trunk and head position. Purchase lateral trunk pads to provide extra stability and allow arm movement. Use gravity to help with head control. Recline the device if it has posterior head support. Create base to allow variations of recline. Create posterior head support by building a padded solid seat insert or a custom foam insert

Activity			
Activity Going to the beach with family **Devices** Car seat Infant seat Beach chair Lawn chair Bath seat or ring Jog stroller	Infant or child plays with sand toys while sitting on the sand at the beach.	Infant or child with low postural tone: • Sits with rounded trunk, unable to lift head to see or interact • Cannot lift arms to reach • Holds arms and legs in excessive passive extension • Cannot grasp or lift toy Infant or child with high postural tone: • Tends to arch and move out of sitting position • Cannot maintain head in midline to look at toys or friends • Makes jerky and poorly graded movements • Cannot extend arm when head is in midline	Use a plastic-molded lawn chair with a high back. Either bury the legs so that the chair seat is on or below the level of the sand or cut off the legs. Use a pelvic belt or strap in the lawn chair to hold the pelvis in place. Make a wedge to hold the head in slight flexion to decrease the effects of extension pattern of movement. Cut out a cardboard box to use as a table for toys. Dig out the sand so that sand can support legs, knees, hips, and ankles can be supported at 90° or appropriate angles. Build up lateral trunk supports that can be placed in lawn or beach chair. Towel rolls or foam blocks work well. Use a wide strap that can be pulled through cutout slots in the back of the seating device for trunk support.

Continued

Modified from Ratliffe KT: *Clinical pediatric physical therapy*, St Louis, 1998, Mosby.
ATNR, Asymmetrical tonic neck reflex; *STNR*, symmetrical tonic neck reflex.

Pediatric Population

Table—cont'd

Activity, positioning devices	Functional goal	Possible postural problems	Possible adaptations
Activity Playing with toys while standing at a coffee table	Infant or child plays with toys while standing at the coffee table for 5 min.	Infant or child with low postural tone: • Cannot bear full weight through legs • Cannot free arms to play with toys • Demonstrates poor foot and leg position in standing • Experiences difficulty holding head upright for extended periods of play Infant or child with high postural tone: • Stands on toes with poor lower-extremity alignment • Demonstrates poor balance in standing • Makes jerky and poorly graded movements • Experiences difficulty using arms while standing	Manually support the infant or child's head. Use a soft, thick, foam collar supporting occiput and chin, which rests on the chest to allow free breathing while supporting the head upright. Provide graded posterior support either by using an adult's body or a sturdy chair. Use orthotics to facilitate lower-extremity alignment in standing. Place furniture next to infant or child to help with balance. Use a stander with support at feet, knees, hips, and trunk, as needed, for stability.
Devices Infant walker Low table Playpen Stander Ring walker Pickup walker Rolling walker			

Modified from Ratliffe KT: *Clinical pediatric physical therapy,* St Louis, 1998, Mosby.

Buying, Adapting, or Fabricating Positioning Equipment

	Benefits	Difficulties	Situations in which method used
Commercially available equipment	Is durable Supported by vendor for defects or problems Has been thought about carefully by many design professionals May be purchased by medical insurance or other third-party funding agency	Is expensive Is heavy Is imposing May be more complicated than needed Usually takes a long time to obtain if waiting for funding	Can get medical insurance coverage Need the special features built into device Do not have time to adapt or fabricate device Do not have skills to adapt or fabricate device
Adapted equipment	May be able to complete sooner than can buy commercially made equipment Can customize to specific needs and desires Can use equipment and materials on hand Promotes team building in design and adaptation	Takes time to make Takes creativity to design May be difficult to obtain materials May be less durable than commercially made equipment	Own equipment that can be adapted Possess skills to do adaptation Have materials and time to do adaptation Need device quickly
Fabricated equipment	Can customize to specific needs and desires May be able to get completed in timely manner May be less expensive than commercially available equipment Promotes team building in design and adaptation	Takes time to make Takes creativity to design May need specific skills, such as sewing, carpentry, or metal work May have difficulty finding materials or resources to fabricate May be less durable	Possess skills and resources to fabricate equipment Do not have money to buy equipment Need device quickly Need equipment not available commercially

Modified from Ratliffe KT: *Clinical pediatric physical therapy,* St Louis, 1998, Mosby.

Childproofing Guidelines

Performing pediatric comprehensive environmental assessments involves instructing parents or caregivers about appropriate childproofing strategies to ensure the safety of children in and around the home. Measures vary based on a child's level of development and physical capabilities. The goal of home rehabilitation is to allow maximal exploration of the environment for optimal development with minimal hazards.

Child Safety Home Checklist

Fire, Electricity, Burns

☐ Guards in front of or around heating appliances, fireplaces, or furnaces (including floor furnace)*

☐ Electrical wires hidden or far from reach*

☐ Frayed or broken wires absent, sockets not overloaded

☐ Plastic guards or caps over electrical outlets, furniture in front of outlets*

☐ Hanging tablecloths far from reach and away from open fires*

☐ Smoke detectors tested and operating properly

☐ Kitchen matches stored far from child's reach*

☐ Large, deep ashtrays (if used) throughout house

☐ Small stoves, heaters, and other hot objects (cigarettes, candles, coffee pots, slow cookers) placed where they cannot be tipped over or reached by children

☐ Hot water heater set at 49 degrees Celsius (120 degrees Fahrenheit) or lower

☐ Pot handles turned toward back of stove, center of table

☐ Loose clothing not worn near stove

☐ Cooking or eating hot foods or liquids far from child standing nearby or sitting in lap

☐ All small appliances, such as iron, turned off, disconnected, and placed out of reach when not in use

☐ Cool, not hot, mist vaporizer used

☐ Fire extinguisher available on each floor and checked periodically

☐ Electrical fuse box and gas outlet accessible

☐ Family escape plan in case of a fire practiced periodically, fire escape ladder available on upper-level floors

☐ Telephone number of fire or rescue squad and address of home with nearest cross street posted near phone

Suffocation and Aspiration

☐ Small objects stored far from child's reach*

☐ Toys inspected for small removable parts or long strings*

☐ Hanging crib toys and mobiles placed far from reach

☐ Plastic bags stored far from child's reach, large plastic garment bags discarded after tied in knots*

☐ Mattress or pillow not covered with plastic or other material that could be harmful to child*

☐ Crib designed according to federal regulations and with snug-fitting mattress*†

☐ Crib positioned far from other furniture or windows*

☐ Portable playpen gates up at all times while in use

☐ Accordion-style playpen gates not used*

☐ Bathroom doors kept closed and toilet seats down*

☐ Faucets turned off firmly*

☐ Pool fenced with locked gate

☐ Poolside equipped with proper safety tools

☐ Electric garage door openers stored safely and garage door equipped with sensor to rise when door strikes object

☐ Doors of ovens, trunks, dishwashers, refrigerators, and front-loading clothes washers and dryers kept closed*

☐ Unused appliances, such as refrigerators, securely closed with locks or doors removed*

☐ Food served in small noncylindric pieces*

☐ Toy chests not equipped with lids or with lids that securely lock in open position*

☐ Buckets and wading pools kept empty when not in use*

☐ Clothesline above head level

☐ At least one member of household trained in basic life support, including first aid for choking†

Modified from Wong D: *Wong and Whaley's clinical manual of pediatric nursing,* ed 4, St Louis, 1996, Mosby.

*Safety measures are specific for homes with young children. All safety measures should be implemented in homes where children reside and visit frequently, such as those of grandparents or babysitters.

†Federal regulations are available from U.S. Consumer Product Safety Commission: (800) 638-CPSC.

‡For home care instructions for infant cardiopulmonary resuscitation and infant child choking, see Part IV, "Emergency Situations."

Box—cont'd

Poisoning

- [ ] Toxic substances, including batteries, placed on high shelves, preferably in locked cabinets
- [ ] Toxic plants hung or placed far from reach*
- [ ] Excess quantities of cleaning fluids, paints, pesticides, drugs, and other toxic substances not stored in home
- [ ] Used containers of poisonous substances discarded where child cannot obtain access
- [ ] Telephone number of local poison control center and address of home with nearest cross street posted near phone
- [ ] Syrup of ipecac in home and containing two doses per child
- [ ] Medicines clearly labeled in childproof containers and stored far from reach
- [ ] Household cleaners, disinfectants, and insecticides kept in their original containers, separate from food and far from reach
- [ ] Smoking in areas far from children

Falls

- [ ] Nonskid mats, strips, or surfaces in tubs and showers
- [ ] Exits, halls, and passageways in rooms kept clear of toys, furniture, boxes, or other items that can obstruct them
- [ ] Stairs and halls well lighted and switches at both tops and bottoms
- [ ] Sturdy handrails for all steps and stairways
- [ ] Stairways free of clutter

Falls—cont'd

- [ ] Treads, risers, and carpeting in good repair
- [ ] Glass doors and walls marked with decals
- [ ] Safety glass used in doors, windows, and walls
- [ ] Gates on top and bottom of staircases and elevated areas, such as porches and fire escapes*
- [ ] Guardrails on upstairs windows with locks that limit height of window opening and access to areas such as fire escapes*
- [ ] Crib side rails raised to full height, mattress lowered as child grows*
- [ ] Restraints used in high chairs, walkers, or other baby furniture, walkers not used near stairs*
- [ ] Scatter rugs secured in place or equipped with nonskid backing
- [ ] Walks, patios, and driveways in good repair

Bodily Injury

- [ ] Knives, power tools, and unloaded firearms stored safety or placed in locked cabinet
- [ ] Garden tools returned to storage racks after use
- [ ] Pets properly restrained and immunized for rabies
- [ ] Swings, slides, and other outdoor play equipment kept in safe conditions
- [ ] Yard free of broken glass, nail-studded boards, other litter
- [ ] Cement birdbaths placed where child cannot tip them*

Injury Prevention During Infancy

Birth to 4 months

Major developmental accomplishments

May be propelled forward or backward
  by involuntary relexes (crawling reflex) or
  make jerking movements because of
  startle reflex

May roll over
Demonstrates increasing eye-hand
  coordination and voluntary grasp reflex

Injury prevention

Aspiration

Begin practicing safeguarding early (see 4-7
  months), even though danger to this age
  group is not great.
Never shake baby powder directly on infant;
  place powder in hand and then on infant's
  skin; store container closed and out of
  infant's reach.
Hold infant for feeding; do not prop bottle.
Know emergency procedures for choking.*
Use pacifier with one-piece construction and a
  loop handle.

Suffocation and Drowning

Keep all plastic bags stored out of infant's
  reach; discard large plastic garment bags
  after tying them in knots.
Do not cover mattress with plastic.
Use a firm mattress and loose blankets but no
  pillows.
Ensure that crib design follows federal
  government regulations and mattress fits
  snugly.
Position crib far from other furniture and
  radiators.
Avoid sleeping in bed with infant.
Do not tie pacifier on string around infant's neck.
Remove bibs at bedtime.
Never leave infant alone in bath.
Do not leave infant younger than 12 months
  alone on adult or youth mattress.

Falls

Always raise crib rails.
Never leave infant on raised, unguarded
  surface.
When in doubt as to where to place infant, use
  floor.

Falls—cont'd

Restrain child in infant seat and never leave
  child unattended while seat is resting on
  raised surface.
Avoid using high chair until child can sit well
  with support.

Poisoning

Begin practicing safeguards early (see 4-7 months),
  even though danger to this group is not great.

Burns

Install smoke detectors in home.
Use caution when warming formula in
  microwave oven; always check temperature
  of liquid before feeding.
Check bathwater.
Do not pour hot liquids when infant is nearby.
Beware of cigarette ashes that may fall on infant.
Do not leave infant in sun for more than a few
  minutes; keep exposed areas covered.
Wash flame-retardant clothes according to label
  directions.
Use cool-mist vaporizers.
Do not leave child in parked car.
Check surface heat of car restraint before
  placing child in seat.

Motor-Vehicle Injuries

Transport infant in federally approved, rear-
  facing car seat.*
Do not place infant on seat or in lap.
Do not place child in carriage or stroller behind
  parked car.

Body Damage

Avoid sharp, jagged objects.
Keep diaper pins closed and far from infant.

Modified from Wong D: *Wong and Whaley's clinical manual of pediatric nursing*, ed 4, St Louis, Mosby.
*Because a considerable risk of major and minor injury and even death exists from the use of walkers and because no clear benefit is obtained from their use, the American Academy of Pediatrics recommends a ban on the manufacture and sale of mobile infant walkers in the United States. The particular risk of walkers in households with stairs is falls. (American Academy of Pediatrics, Committee on Injury and Poison Prevention: Injuries associated with infant walkers, *Pediatrics* 95(5):778-780, 1995.)

4 to 7 months

Major developmental accomplishments

Rolls over

Sits momentarily

Grasps and manipulates small objects

Resecures dropped objects

Demonstrates well-developed eye-hand coordination

Can focus on and locate very small objects

Mouths prominently

Can push up on hands and knees

Crawls backward

Injury prevention

Aspiration

Keep buttons, beads, syringe caps, and other small objects from infant's reach.

Keep floor free of small objects.

Do not feed infant hard candy, nuts, food with pits or seeds, or whole or circular pieces of hot dogs.

Exercise caution when giving teething biscuits because large chunks may be broken off and aspirated.

Do not feed infant while infant is lying down.

Inspect toys for removable parts.

Keep baby powder far from reach.

Avoid storing large quantities of cleaning fluids, paints, pesticides, and other toxic substances.

Discard used containers of poisonous substances.

Do not store toxic substances in food containers.

Suffocation

Keep uninflated balloons far from reach.

Remove all crib toys that are strung across crib or playpen when infant begins to push up on hands or knees or is 5 months old.

Falls

Restrain infant in high chair.

Keep crib rails raised to full height.

Poisoning

Ensure that paint for furniture or toys does not contain lead.

Place toxic substances on high shelves or in locked cabinets.

Hang plants or place on high surfaces rather than on floors.

Discard used button-sized batteries; store new batteries in safe areas.

Know telephone number of local poison control center (usually listed in front of telephone directory).

Burns

Keep faucets far from reach.

Place hot objects (cigarettes, candles, incense) on high surfaces.

Limit exposure to sun; apply sunscreen.

Motor-Vehicle Injuries

See birth to 4 months.

Body Damage

Provide toys that are smooth and rounded, preferably made of wood or plastic.

Avoid long, pointed objects as toys.

Avoid toys that are excessively loud.

Keep sharp objects far from infant's reach.

Pediatric Population

Continued

Table—cont'd

8 to 12 months
Major developmental accomplishments

Crawls, creeps
Stands while holding onto furniture
Stands alone
Cruises around furniture
Walks
Climbs
Pulls on objects

Throws objects
Can pick up small objects and use pincer grasp
Explores by putting objects in mouth
Dislikes being restrained
Explores farther from parent
Demonstrates increasing understanding of
    simple commands and phrases

Injury prevention

Aspiration

Keep lint and small objects off floor and
    furniture and far from reach of infant.
Take care in feeding solid table food to ensure
    that very small pieces are given.
Do not use beanbag toys or allow infant to play
    with dried beans.
See also 4 to 7 months.

Suffocation and Drowning

Keep doors of ovens, dishwashers, refrigerators,
    coolers, and front-loading clothes washers
    and dryers closed at all times.
If storing an unused appliance, such as a
    refrigerator, remove the door.
Supervise contact with inflated balloons;
    immediately discard popped balloons and
    keep uninflated balloons far from reach.
Fence swimming pools.
Always supervise infant when near sources of
    water, such as cleaning buckets, drainage
    areas, and toilets.
Keep bathroom doors closed.
Eliminate unnecessary pools of water.
Keep one hand on infant at all times in tub.

Motor-Vehicle Injuries

See birth to 4 months.

Falls

Fence stairways at tops and bottoms if infant has
    access to either end.
Dress infant in safe shoes and clothing (soles
    that do not "catch" on floor, tied shoelaces,
    pant legs that do not touch floor).
Avoid walkers, especially near stairs.*
Ensure that furniture is sturdy enough for infant
    to pull self to standing position and cruise.

Poisoning

Administer medications as drugs, not candy.
Do not administer medications unless so
    prescribed by practitioner.
Replace medications and poisons immediately
    after use; replace caps properly if child-
    protector cap is used.
Keep syrup of ipecac in home; use only if advised.

Burns

Place guards in front of or around any heating
    appliance, fireplace, or furnace.
Keep electrical wires hidden or far from reach.
Place plastic guards over electrical outlets; place
    furniture in front of outlets.
Keep hanging tablecloths far from reach
    (because infant may pull down hot liquids or
    heavy or sharp objects).

Modified from Wong D: *Wong and Whaley's clinical manual of pediatric nursing,* ed 4, St Louis, Mosby.
*Because a considerable risk of major and minor injury and even death exists from the use of walkers and because no clear benefit is obtained from their use, the American Academy of Pediatrics recommends a ban on the manufacture and sale of mobile infant walkers in the United States. The particular risk of walkers in households with stairs is falls. (American Academy of Pediatrics, Committee on Injury and Poison Prevention: Injuries associated with infant walkers, *Pediatrics* 95(5):778-780, 1995.)

Injury Prevention During Early Childhood

Developmental abilities related to risk of injury	Injury prevention
Walks, runs, climbs Can open doors and gates Can ride tricycle Can throw ball and other objects	**Motor-Vehicle Injuries** Use federally approved car restraint; if restraint is not available, use lap belt. Supervise child during outside play. Do not allow child to play on curb or behind parked car. Do not permit child to play in pile of leaves, snow, or large cardboard container in area of heavy traffic. Supervise tricycle riding. Lock fences and doors if not directly supervising child. Teach child to obey the following pedestrian safety rules: Obey traffic regulations; walk only at crosswalks and when traffic signals indicate it is safe to cross. Stand back a step from curb until time to cross. Look left, right, and left again and check for turning cars before crossing street. Use sidewalks; when no sidewalk exists, walk on left side, facing traffic. Wear light colors at night and attach fluorescent material to clothing.
Can explore if left unsupervised Demonstrates great curiosity Is helpless in water and unaware of its danger; has no idea of significance of water's depth	**Drowning** Supervise closely when near source of water, including bucket. Keep all bathroom doors and lids on toilets closed. Build fence around swimming pool and lock gate. Teach swimming and water safety (not a substitute for protection).
Can reach heights by climbing, stretching, standing on toes, and using objects as ladders Pulls objects Explores holes and openings Can open drawers and closets Unaware of potential sources of heat or fire Plays with mechanical objects	**Burns** Turn pot handles toward back of stove. Place electric appliances, such as coffee makers, frying pans, and popcorn machines, toward back of counter. Place guardrails in front of radiators, fireplaces, or other heating elements. Store matches and cigarette lighters in locked or inaccessible areas; discard carefully. Place burning candles, incense, hot foods, ashes, embers, and cigarettes far from reach. Do not let tablecloth hang within child's reach. Do not let electric cord from iron or other appliance hang within child's reach. Cover electrical outlets with protective devices. Keep electrical wires hidden or far from reach.

Pediatric Population

Modified from Wong D: *Wang and Whaley's clinical manual of pediatric nursing,* ed 4, St Louis, 1996, Mosby.

Continued

Table—cont'd

Developmental abilities related to risk of injury	Injury prevention
	Burns—cont'd
	Do not allow child to play with electrical appliance, wires, or lighters.
	Stress danger of open flames; teach meaning of word *hot*.
	Always check bathwater temperature; adjust hot-water heater temperature to 120°F or lower; do not allow children to play with faucets.
	Apply a sunscreen with a protection factor of 15 or higher when child is exposed to sunlight.
Explores by putting objects in mouth	**Poisoning**
Can open drawers, closets, and most containers	Place all potentially toxic agents in a locked cabinet or far from reach (including plants).
Climbs	Replace medications and poisons immediately; replace child-resistant caps properly.
Cannot read warning labels	Refer to medications as drugs, not candy.
Does not know safe dose or amount	Do not store large surpluses of toxic agents.
	Promptly discard empty poison containers; never reuse to store a food item or other poison.
	Teach child not to play in trash containers.
	Never remove labels from containers of toxic substances.
	Keep syrup of ipecac in home; use only if advised.
	Know number and location of nearest poison control center (usually listed in front of telephone directory).
Can open doors and some windows	**Falls**
Goes up and down stairs	Keep screens in windows, nail securely, and use guardrails.
Demonstrates unrefined depth perception	Place gates at tops and bottoms of stairways.
	Keep doors locked or use child-resistant doorknob covers at entries to stairs, high porches, or other elevated areas, such as laundry chutes.
	Remove unsecured or scatter rugs.
	Apply nonskid mat in bathtub or shower.
	Keep crib rails fully raised and mattress at lowest level.
	Place carpeting under crib and in bathroom.
	Keep large toys and bumper pads from crib or playpen (can be used as "stairs" to climb out), then move to youth bed when child can crawl out of crib.
	Avoid using walkers, especially near stairs.
	Dress in safe clothing (soles that do not "catch" on floor, tied shoelaces, pant legs that do not hang on floor).

Modified from Wong D: *Wong and Whaley's clinical manual of pediatric nursing,* ed 4, St Louis, Mosby.

Table—cont'd

Developmental abilities related to risk of injury	Injury prevention
	Falls—cont'd Keep child restrained in vehicles; never leave unattended in shopping cart or stroller. Supervise at playgrounds; select play areas with soft ground cover and safe equipment.
Puts things in mouth May swallow hard or nonedible pieces of food	**Choking and Suffocation** Avoid large, round chunks of meat, such as whole hot dogs; slice lengthwise into short pieces. Avoid fruit with pits, fish with bones, dried beans, hard candy, chewing gum, nuts, popcorn, grapes, and marshmallows. Choose large, sturdy toys without sharp edges or small removable parts. Discard old refrigerators, ovens, and other appliances; if storing old appliances, remove doors. Keep automatic garage door transmitter in inaccessible place. Select safe toy boxes or chests without heavy, hinged lids.
Still demonstrates clumsiness in many skills Is easily distracted from tasks Unaware of potential danger from strangers or other individuals	**Body Damage** Avoid sharp or pointed objects, such as knives, scissors, or toothpicks, especially when walking or running. Do not allow lollipops or similar objects in mouth when walking or running. Teach safety precautions (carrying fork or scissors with pointed end away from face). Store all dangerous tools, garden equipment, and firearms in locked cabinets. Be alert to danger of animals, including household pets. Use safety glass and decals on large glassed areas, such as sliding glass doors. Teach name, address, and phone number and to ask for help from appropriate individuals (cashiers, security guards, police) if lost; keep identification on child (sewn in clothes or inside shoe). Avoid personalized clothing in public places. Teach child never to go with stranger. Teach child to tell parents if anyone makes child feel uncomfortable in any way. Always listen to child's concerns regarding others' behavior. Teach child to say "no" when confronted with uncomfortable situations.

Pediatric Population

Injury Prevention During School-Age Years

Developmental abilities related to risk of injury	Injury prevention
Is increasingly involved in activities outside home Is excited by speed and motion Is easily distracted by environment Can listen to reason	**Motor-Vehicle Injuries** Educate child regarding proper use of seat belts while passenger in vehicle. Maintain discipline while passenger in vehicle; keep arms inside and do not lean against doors or interfere with driver. Emphasize safe pedestrian behavior. Insist on wearing safety apparel (helmet) where applicable, such as riding bicycle, motorcycle, moped, and all-terrain vehicles.
Is apt to overdo things May work hard to perfect skill Has cautious, but not fearful, gross-motor actions Likes swimming	**Drowning** Teach child to swim. Teach basic rules of water safety. Select safe and supervised places to swim. Check sufficient water depth before diving. Swim with companion. Use approved flotation device in water or boats. Become advocate for legislation requiring fencing around pools. Learn cardiopulmonary resuscitation.
Demonstrates increasing independence Is adventuresome Enjoys trying new things	**Burns** Instruct child in behavior in areas involving contact with potential burn hazards (gasoline, matches, bonfires or barbecues, lighter fluid, firecrackers, cigarette lighters, cooking utensils, chemistry sets); avoid climbing or flying kites around high-tension wires. Instruct child in proper behavior in the event of fire (fire drills at home, school). Teach child safe cooking (use low heat; avoid frying; be careful of steam burns, scalds, or exploding foods, especially from microwaving).
Adheres to group rules May be influenced easily by peers Exhibits strong allegiance to friends	**Poisoning** Educate child regarding hazards of taking nonprescription drugs and chemicals, including aspirin and alcohol. Teach child to say "no" if offered illegal or dangerous drugs or alcohol. Keep potentially dangerous products in properly labeled receptacles, preferably out of reach.

Modified from Wong DL: *Wong and Whaley's clinical manual of pediatric nursing*, ed 4, St Louis, 1996, Mosby.

Table—cont'd

Developmental abilities related to risk of injury	Injury prevention
Has increased physical skills Needs strenuous physical activity Is interested in acquiring new skills and perfecting attained skills Is daring and adventurous, especially with peers Frequently plays in hazardous places Demonstrates confidence that often exceeds physical capacity Desires group loyalty and has strong need for friends' approval Attempts hazardous feats Accompanies friends to potentially hazardous facilities Delights in physical activity Is likely to overdo things Grows taller faster than grows muscles or achieves coordination	**Body Damage** Help provide facilities for supervised activities. Encourage play in safe places. Keep firearms safely locked up except during adult supervision. Teach proper care of, use of, and respect for potentially dangerous devices (power tools, firecrackers, and so on). Teach children not to tease or surprise dogs, invade their territories, take dogs' toys, or interfere with dogs' feeding. Stress eye, ear, or mouth protection when using potentially hazardous objects or devices or when engaged in potentially hazardous sports. Teach safety regarding use of corrective devices (glasses); monitor duration of wear of contact lenses to prevent corneal damage. Stress careful selection, use, and maintenance of sports and recreation equipment, such as skateboards and in-line skates. Emphasize proper conditioning, safe practices, and use of safety equipment for sports or recreational activities. Caution against engaging in hazardous sports such as those involving trampolines. Use safety glass and decals on large glassed areas, such as sliding-glass doors. Teach name, address, and phone number and to ask for help from appropriate individuals (cashiers, security guards, police) if lost; have identification on child (sewn in clothes or inside shoe). Avoid personalized clothing in public places. Teach child never to go with a stranger. Teach child to tell parents if anyone makes child feel uncomfortable in any way. Always listen to child's concerns regarding others' behavior. Teach child to say "no" when confronted with uncomfortable situations.

Injury Prevention During Adolescence

Developmental abilities related to risk of injury	Injury prevention

Need independence and freedom

Test independence

Permitted to drive a motor vehicle (age varying)

Inclined to take risks

Feel indestructible

Need to discharge energy, often at expense of logical thinking and other control mechanisms

Demonstrate strong need for peer approval

May attempt hazardous feats

Experience peak incidence for practice and participation in sports

May have access to more complex tools, objects, and locations

Can assume responsibility for own actions

Motor- and Nonmotor-Vehicle Injuries

Pedestrian

Emphasize and encourage safe pedestrian behavior.

Passenger

Promote appropriate behavior while riding in motor vehicle.

Driver

Provide competent driver education; encourage judicious use of vehicle; discourage drag racing and "playing chicken"; maintain vehicle in proper condition (brakes, tires).

Teach and promote safety and maintenance of two-wheeled vehicles.

Promote and encourage wearing of safety apparel, such as helmet or long trousers.

Reinforce dangers of drugs, including alcohol, when operating motor vehicle.

Drowning

Teach nonswimmers to swim.

Teach basic rules of water safety, including judicious selection of place to swim, sufficient water depth for diving, and swimming with companion.

Burns

Reinforce proper behavior in areas involving contact with burn hazards (gasoline, electric wires, fires).

Provide advice regarding excessive exposure to natural or artificial sunlight (ultraviolet burn).

Discourage smoking.

Encourage use of sunscreen.

Poisoning

Educate in hazards of drug use, including alcohol.

Falls

Teach and encourage general safety measures in all activities.

Body Damage

Promote acquisition of proper instruction in sports and use of sports equipment.

Instruct in safe use of and respect for firearms and other potentially dangerous devices (power tools, firecrackers).

Provide and encourage use of protective equipment when using potentially hazardous devices.

Promote access to or provision of safe sports and recreational facilities.

Be alert for signs of depression (potential suicide).

Discourage use or availability of hazardous sports equipment (trampoline, surfboards).

Provide instructions regarding proper use of corrective devices, such as glasses, contact lenses, and hearing aids.

Encourage and foster judicious application of safety principles and prevention.

Modified from Wong D: *Wong and Whaley's clinical manual of pediatric nursing,* ed 4, St Louis, 1996, Mosby.

PEDIATRIC DEVELOPMENTAL EVALUATION

Throughout the first years of life, a plethora of changes occur. Home care therapists use a variety of tools to determine whether patients are progressing normally. These tools range from developmental screens to comprehensive developmental assessments. For effective implementation of such tools, therapists must understand the proper use of each tool and when and for whom each device may be used appropriately. In addition, therapists also must possess clear understandings of the reflexes and reactions that drive child development.

Commonly Used Evaluation Tools

Evaluation tool	Age range	Key features	Reference
Neonatal Behavioral Assessment Scale	3 days-4 wk	Assesses interactive behavior, infant competence, and neurological status; effective predictor of future neurological problems; good tool for teaching of parents about infant behaviors	Brazelton TB: *Clinics in developmental medicine,* no. 50, Philadelphia, 1973, JB Lippincott.
Neurological Evaluation of the Newborn and Infant	Birth-12 mo	Measures reflexes and muscle tone and provides range of motion expectations	Amiel-Tison C, Grenier A: *Current problems in pediatrics,* vol. III, no. 1, Chicago, 1976, Year Book.
Movement Assessment of Infants	Birth-12 mo	Assesses muscle tone, reflexes, automatic reactions, and purposeful movement	Chandler LS, Swanson MW, Andrews MS: *Movement assessment of infants,* Rolling Bay, Wis, 1980, Infant Movement Research.
Alberta Infant Motor Scale	Birth-walking age	Identifies the components of motor development; differentiates atypical development and small increments that may be attributed to maturation or intervention	Piper MC and others: *Motor assessment of the developing infant,* Philadelphia, 1993, WB Saunders.
Milani-Comparetti Motor Development Screening Test	Birth-2 yr	Measures functional movement and related reflex and automatic responses; demonstrates age-appropriate responses through profile	Tremblath J, Kliewer D, Brauce W: Omaha, 1977, Nebraska Medical Center.

Modified from Ratliffe KT: *Clinical pediatric physical therapy,* St Louis, 1998, Mosby.

Continued

Evaluation tool	Age range	Key features	Reference
Hawaii Developmental Charts (formerly Hawaii Early Learning Profile)	Birth-3 yr	Graphically demonstrates approximate age ranges in motor, cognitive, language, self-help and social skills; intended for use in planning intervention programs, documenting progress, and monitoring achievement of individual objectives	Furuno S and others: *Hawaii developmental charts*, Tucson, 1993, Therapy Skill Builders.
Revised Gesell and Amatruda Developmental Neurological Exam	1 mo-5 yr	Provides developmental quotient in four areas—motor, adaptive, language, and personal-social	Knobloch H, Pasamanick B: *Developmental diagnosis*, ed 3, Philadelphia, 1974, JB Lippincott.
Bayley Scales of Infant Development II	Birth-42 mo	Includes mental scale, motor scale, and behavioral record; scored as developmental index; includes data on special populations (prematurity, Down syndrome, HIV, developmental delays)	Bayley N: *Bayley scales of infant development*, San Antonio, 1993, Harcourt Brace.
Denver Developmental Screening Test	2 wk-6 yr	Measures four domains—personal-social, fine motor adaptive, language, and gross motor; screens children for delays and determines need for further evaluation	Frankenburg WK, Dodds J: *Denver developmental screening test*, Denver, 1990, Archer Petal.
Peabody Developmental Motor Scales	Birth-83 mo	Includes gross and fine-motor scales; gives standard scores and age-equivalent scores; identifies emerging skills; may be used on children who do not understand verbal language	Folio M, Fewell R: *Peabody developmental motor scales*, Allen, Tex, 1983, DLM Teaching Resources.
The Pediatric Evaluation of Disability Inventory	6 mo-7½ yr	Assesses functional skills; designed for rehabilitation use; includes self-care, mobility, and social skills; scores based on function, amount of assistance required, and need for equipment or modification	Haley SM and others: *The pediatric evaluation of disability inventory*, Boston, 1989, New England Medical Center.

Modified from Ratliffe KT: *Clinical pediatric physical therapy,* St Louis, 1998, Mosby.
HIV, Human immunodeficiency virus.

Evaluation tool	Age range	Key features	Reference
Miller Assessment for Preschoolers	2 yr, 9 mo- 5 yr, 8 mo	Identifies children with mild to moderate delays; combines sensory-motor and cognitive domains; uses developmental approach; does not provide age-equivalent scores	Miller LJ: *The foundation of knowledge in development,* San Antonio, 1982, The Psychological Corporation.
Tufts Assessment of Motor Performance-Pediatric Clinical Version	3 yr and above	Measures functional and motor performance skills to monitor child's response to treatment and to determine if treatment goals were met; includes measurements of proficiency of skill and time to complete skill	Haley SM, Inacio CA, Mann NR: *Tufts assessment of motor performance-pediatric clinical version,* Boston, 1989, Tufts New England Medical Center.
Bruininks-Oseretsky Test of Motor Performance	4½-14½ yr	Assesses gross and fine-motor function for educational and therapeutic placement decisions; gives scores as age equivalents	Bruininks RH: *Bruininks-Oseretsky test of motor performance,* Circle Pines, Minn, 1978, American Guidance Service.
Purdue Perceptual Motor Survey	6-10 yr	Identifies children lacking perceptual motor abilities needed to acquire academic skills; includes balance and postural flexibility, body image and differentiation, perceptual-motor match, ocular control, and visual achievement forms	Roach EG, Kephart NC: *The Purdue perceptual motor survey,* Columbus, Ohio, 1966, Merrill.
Test of Motor Impairment	5-13 yr	Detects motor dysfunction problems indicative of possible neurological dysfunction; is divided into five areas—balance, upper-limb coordination, whole-body coordination, manual dexterity, and simultaneous movement	Stott DH, Moyes FA, Henderson FA: *Test of motor impairment,* Guelph, Ontario, 1972, Brook Educational.

Pediatric Population

Common Pediatric Evaluation Tools

Alberta Infant Motor Scales (AIMS)

Piper MC, Darrah, J (1994)
Motor assessment of the developing infant
WB Saunders
Philadelphia, PA 19106

Battelle Developmental Inventory

Newborg J and others (1988)
Riverside Publishing
8420 West Bryn Mawr Avenue
Chicago, IL 60631
(800) 767-8378

Bayley Scales of Infant Development, Ed 2

Bayley N (1994)
The Psychological Corporation
555 Academic Court
San Antonio, TX 78204
(210) 299-1061

Beery Developmental Test of Visual Motor Integration (Rev #3)

Beery KE (1989)
Modern Curriculum Press
13900 Prospect Road
Cleveland, OH 44136
(216) 572-0690

Brigance Diagnostic Inventories

Brigance AH (1978)
Curriculum Associates
5 Esquire Road, North
Billerica, MA 01862

Bruininks-Oseretsky Test of Motor Proficiency

Bruininks R (1978)
American Guidance Service
4201 Woodland Road
Circle Pines, MN 55014
(612) 786-4343

Coping Inventory

Zeitlin S (1991)
Scholastic Testing Service
Bensenville, IL 60106-8056

DeGangi-Berk Test of Sensory Integration

Berk RA, DeGangi GA (1983)
Western Psychological Services
1203 Wilshire Boulevard
Los Angeles, CA 90025-1251
(310) 478-2061

Denver Developmental Screening Test (Rev)

Frankenburg W and others (1990)
Ladoca Publishing Foundation
University of Colorado
Denver, CO 80216

Developmental Programming for Infants and Young Children

Schafer DS, Moersch MS (1981)
The University of Michigan Press
Ann Arbor, MI 48106
(313) 764-4392

Developmental Test of Visual Perception, Ed 2

(previously called the *Marianne Frostig Developmental Test of Visual Perception*)
Hammill DD, Pearson NA, Voress JK (1993)
Pro Ed
8700 Shoal Creek Boulevard
Austin TX 78757-6897
(512) 451-3246

Early Coping Inventory

Zeitlin S, Williamson GG, Szczepanski M (1988)
Scholastic Testing Service
Bensenville, IL 60106-8056

Early Intervention Developmental Profile

Rogers SJ and others (1981)
University of Michigan Press
Ann Arbor, MI 48106
(313) 764-4392

Modified from Case-Smith J, Allen AS, Pratt PN: *Occupational therapy for children*, ed 3, St Louis, 1996, Mosby.

Box—cont'd

Erhardt Developmental Prehension Assessment

Erhardt RP (1982)
Therapy Skill Builders
3830 East Bellevue
P.O. Box 42050-TS4
Tucson, AZ 85733
(602) 323-7500

Erhardt Developmental Vision Assessment

Erhardt RP (1988)
Therapy Skill Builders
3830 East Bellevue
P.O. Box 42050-TS4
Tucson, AZ 85733
(602) 323-7500

The First STEP

Miller LJ (1993)
The Psychological Corporation
555 Academic Court
San Antonio, TX 78204
(210) 299-1061

Gesell Preschool Test

Ames LB and others (1980)
Programs for Education, Inc.
P.O. Box 167
Rosemont, NJ 08556
(609) 397-2214

Gross Motor Function Measure (GMFM)

Russell D and others (1989)
Gross Motor Measures Group
c/o Dianne Russell
Building 74, Room 29
Station 9
Hamilton, Ontario
Canada L8N 3Z5

Hawaii Early Learning Profile (HELP)

Furuno S and others (1984)
Vort Corporation
P.O. Box 60123
Palo Alto, CA 94306
(415) 322-8282

Home Observation and Measurement of the Environment (HOME)

Caldwell B (1984)
Center for Early Development and Education
University of Arkansas
Little Rock, AR 77204

In-Hand Manipulation Test (Research Ed Only)

Exner CE
Occupational Therapy Department
Towson State University
Towson, MD 21204

Miller Assessment for Preschoolers (MAP)

Miller LJ (1982)
The Psychological Corporation
555 Academic Court
San Antonio, TX 78204
(210) 299-1061

Motor-Free Visual Perception Test (MVPT)

Colarusso RP, Hammill DD (1983)
Academic Therapy Publications
20 Commercial Boulevard
Novato, CA 94947-6191
(800) 422-7249

Movement Assessment of Infants (MAI)

Chandler LS, Andrews, MS, Swanson MW (1980)
P.O. Box 4631
Rolling Bay, WA 98061

Pediatric Population

Continued

Peabody Developmental Motor Scales

Folio R, Fewell R (1983)
Riverside Publishing
8420 West Bryn Mawr Avenue
Chicago, IL 60631
(800) 767-8378
(800) 323-9540

Pediatric Evaluation of Disability Inventory (PEDI)

Haley SM and others (1992)
PEDI Research Group
Department of Rehabilitation Medicine
New England Medical Center Hospital, #75K/R
750 Washington Street
Boston, MA 02111-1901
(617) 956-5031

Pediatric Examination of Educational Readiness

Levine MD, Schneider EA
Educators Publishing Service, Inc.
75 Moulton Street
Cambridge, MA 02238-9101

Pediatric Extended Examination at Three

Blackman JA, Levine MD, Markowitz M
Educators Publishing Service, Inc.
75 Moulton Street
Cambridge, MA 02238-9101

Quick Neurological Screening Test (QNST)

Mutti M, Sterling HM, Spalding NV (1978)
Academic Therapy Publications
20 Commercial Boulevard
Novato, CA 94949
(415) 883-3314

Sensory Integration and Praxis Tests (SIPT)

Ayres AJ and staff (1989)
Western Psychological Services
1203 Wilshire Boulevard
Los Angeles, CA 90025-1251
(310) 478-2061

Test of Infant Motor Performance (TIMP)

Cambell SK and others (1993)
Development of the Test of Infant Motor
    Performance
In Granger CV, Gresham GE, editors: *New
    Developments in Functional Assessment*
WB Saunders
Philadelphia, PA 19106

Test of Sensory Functions in Infants (TSFI)

DeGangi GA, Greenspan SI (1989)
Western Psychological Services
1203 Wilshire Boulevard
Los Angeles, CA 90025-1251
(310) 478-2061

Test of Visual-Perceptual Skills (Nonmotor)

Gardner MF (1982)
Psychological and Educational Publications, Inc.
1477 Rollins Road
Burlingame, CA 94010-2316
(800) 523-5775

Test of Visual-Motor Skills (TVMS)

Gardner MF (1986)
Psychological and Educational Publications, Inc.
1477 Rollins Road
Burlingame, CA 94010-2316
(800) 523-5775

Toddler and Infant Motor Evaluation (TIME)

Miller LJ, Roid GH (1994)
Therapy Skill Builders
3830 East Bellevue
P.O. Box 42050
Tucson, AZ 85733
(602) 323-7500

Transdisciplinary Play-Based Assessment

Linder TW (1993)
Paul H. Brookes Publishing
P.O. Box 10624
Baltimore, MD 21285-0624
(800) 638-3775

Modified from Case-Smith J, Allen AS, Pratt PN: *Occupational therapy for children*, ed 3, St Louis, 1996, Mosby.

Developmental Assessments
System Screening

The Apgar Scoring System is a screen of the cardiac, neurological, and respiratory systems of newborns. It is computed at 1 minute and 5 minutes after birth through scoring of heart rate, respiratory effort, muscle tone, reflex irritability, and color on a scale of 0 to 2. The sum of these parts forms the Apgar score; totals closer to 10 (the maximum score) represent the healthiest newborns. Lower scores may indicate newborns with higher potentials for future functional problems, but the Apgar Scoring System is not always an accurate prognostic indicator. Most newborns score lower at minute 1 than at minute 5.

Apgar scoring system

	Sign				
	Heart rate (beats/min)	Respiratory effort	Muscle tone	Reflex irritability	Color
Score 0	Absent	Absent	Flaccid	No response	Blue, pale
Score 1	Slow (less than 100)	Slow, irregular; hypoventilation	Slightly active (some flexion)	Cry; some motion	Pink body; blue hands and feet
Score 2	Good (more than 100)	Good (lusty cry)	Active, well flexed	Vigorous cry	Completely pink

Total score	Condition
0-3	Severe distress
4-6	Moderate difficulty
7-10	Absence of stress

Modified from Apgar V and others: Evaluation of the newborn infant, *JAMA* 168:1988, 1958.

Function in Newborns

One of the most frequently used tools in the assessment of neurological and interactive function in newborns is the Brazelton Neonatal Behavioral Assessment Scale. The scale is composed of 20 elicited responses and 28 interactive items that provide information useful in the detection of neurological problems, teaching of parents and caregivers, and determining of the skills of interaction. Using a 9-point scale, therapists score items based on the newborn's best performance; the method effectively highlights subtle differences among different newborns. The therapist then scores the newborn's responses on a 4-point ordinal scale; approximately 80% of newborns receive scores of 2.

Pediatric Population

Brazelton Scale Scoring Form

Name _____ Sex _____ Date of birth _____

Examiner _____ Place of examination _____

Date _____ Birth weight _____ Current weight _____ Height _____

Head circumference _____ Time examined _____ Time last fed _____

Type of delivery _____ Length of labor _____ Apgar score _____

Abnormalities of labor _____

Initial State: Observe 2 Minutes

1	2	3	4	5	6
deep	light	drowsy	alert	active	crying

Predominant States: Mark Two

1	2	3	4	5	6

Elicited Responses

	0 None	1 Low	2 Med	3 High	Asymmetric
Plantar grasp	☐	☐	☐	☐	☐
Hand grasp	☐	☐	☐	☐	☐
Ankle clonus	☐	☐	☐	☐	☐
Babinski reflex	☐	☐	☐	☐	☐
Standing	☐	☐	☐	☐	☐
Automatic walking	☐	☐	☐	☐	☐
Placing	☐	☐	☐	☐	☐
Incurvation	☐	☐	☐	☐	☐
Crawling	☐	☐	☐	☐	☐
Glabellar reflex	☐	☐	☐	☐	☐
Tonic deviation of head and eyes	☐	☐	☐	☐	☐
Nystagmus	☐	☐	☐	☐	☐
Tonic neck reflex	☐	☐	☐	☐	☐
Moro reflex	☐	☐	☐	☐	☐
Rooting (intensity)	☐	☐	☐	☐	☐
Sucking (intensity)	☐	☐	☐	☐	☐
Passive movement RUE	☐	☐	☐	☐	☐
Passive movement LUE	☐	☐	☐	☐	☐
Passive movement RLE	☐	☐	☐	☐	☐
Passive movement LLE	☐	☐	☐	☐	☐

Modified from Brazelton TB: *Neonatal behavioral assessment scale,* Philadelphia, 1973, JB Lippincott.
RUE, Right upper extremity; *LUE,* left upper extremity; *RLE,* right lower extremity; *LLE,* left lower extremity.

Brazelton Scale Scoring Form—cont'd

Behavior

	9	8	7	6	5	4	3	2	1	Comments
Habituation										
Response decrement to light	☐	☐	☐	☐	☐	☐	☐	☐	☐	_____
Response decrement to rattle	☐	☐	☐	☐	☐	☐	☐	☐	☐	_____
Response decrement to bell	☐	☐	☐	☐	☐	☐	☐	☐	☐	_____
Response decrement to foot probe	☐	☐	☐	☐	☐	☐	☐	☐	☐	_____
Social-interactive responses										
Animate visual response	☐	☐	☐	☐	☐	☐	☐	☐	☐	_____
Inanimate visual response	☐	☐	☐	☐	☐	☐	☐	☐	☐	_____
Animate auditory response	☐	☐	☐	☐	☐	☐	☐	☐	☐	_____
Inanimate auditory response	☐	☐	☐	☐	☐	☐	☐	☐	☐	_____
Animate visual and auditory responses	☐	☐	☐	☐	☐	☐	☐	☐	☐	_____
Inanimate visual and auditory responses	☐	☐	☐	☐	☐	☐	☐	☐	☐	_____
Alertness	☐	☐	☐	☐	☐	☐	☐	☐	☐	_____
Motor system										
General tone	☐	☐	☐	☐	☐	☐	☐	☐	☐	_____
Motor maturity	☐	☐	☐	☐	☐	☐	☐	☐	☐	_____
Pull-to-sit ability	☐	☐	☐	☐	☐	☐	☐	☐	☐	_____
Defense mechanisms	☐	☐	☐	☐	☐	☐	☐	☐	☐	_____
Activity level	☐	☐	☐	☐	☐	☐	☐	☐	☐	_____
State organization										
Peak of excitement	☐	☐	☐	☐	☐	☐	☐	☐	☐	_____
Rapidity of buildup	☐	☐	☐	☐	☐	☐	☐	☐	☐	_____
Irritability	☐	☐	☐	☐	☐	☐	☐	☐	☐	_____
Lability of states of being	☐	☐	☐	☐	☐	☐	☐	☐	☐	_____
State regulation										
Cuddliness	☐	☐	☐	☐	☐	☐	☐	☐	☐	_____
Consolability	☐	☐	☐	☐	☐	☐	☐	☐	☐	_____
Self-quieting ability	☐	☐	☐	☐	☐	☐	☐	☐	☐	_____
Hand-to-mouth movement	☐	☐	☐	☐	☐	☐	☐	☐	☐	_____
Autonomic system										
Tremulousness	☐	☐	☐	☐	☐	☐	☐	☐	☐	_____
Startles	☐	☐	☐	☐	☐	☐	☐	☐	☐	_____
Lability of skin color	☐	☐	☐	☐	☐	☐	☐	☐	☐	_____
Smiles	☐	☐	☐	☐	☐	☐	☐	☐	☐	_____

Pediatric Population

Continued

Brazelton Scale Scoring Form—cont'd

Summary:

Strengths

Concerns

Recommendations

Modified from Brazelton TB: *Neonatal behavioral assessment scale*, Philadelphia, 1973, JB Lippincott.

Developmental Ratings from Birth to 6 Years

Another widely used developmental screen is the Denver Developmental Screening Test (see pp. 121-122), which rates development from birth to 6 years in four areas—gross motor, language, fine motor adaptive, and personal-social. Its purpose is not diagnostic, and the test does not establish developmental levels; instead it screens for abnormalities or delays in development.

Movement, Postural Reactions, and Primitive Reflexes

The Milani-Comparetti Motor Development Screening Test (see p. 123) measures functional movement, the emergence of postural reactions, and the integration of primitive reflexes in infants from birth to 2 years. Therapists use this test to obtain graphic records of neuromotor development.

Sensorimotor Performance

Norton's Basic Motor Evaluation (see pp. 124-133) is an observation-based tool that assesses the quality of sensorimotor performance in the contexts of both purposeful and reflexive movements. Children of any age may be evaluated. Tests are scored on a scale of 0-4; the higher the score, the more normal the child's sensorimotor function.

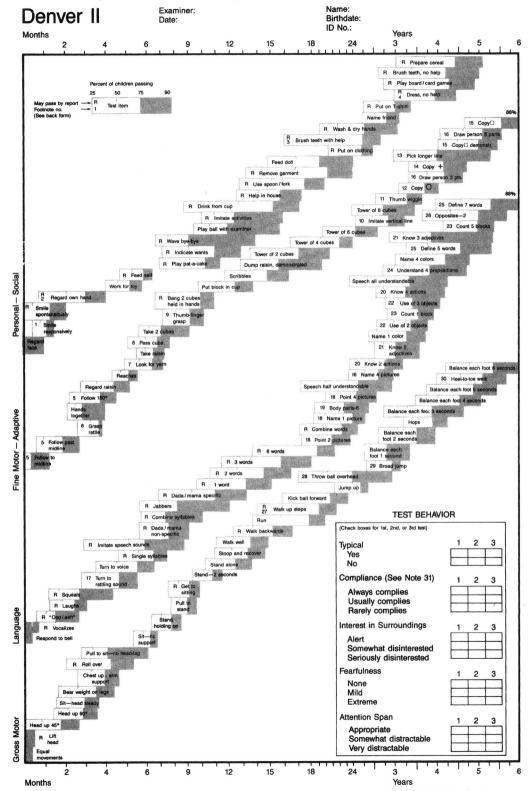

Denver II

Denver Developmental Screening Test

Examiner:
Date:

Name:
Birthdate:
ID No.:

From William K Frankenburg and JB Dodds, 1981, 1988, WK Frankenburg and JB Dodds; 1978, WK Frankenburg.
*For more information on using this form, call 1-800-419-4729.

Continued

DIRECTIONS FOR ADMINISTRATION

1. Try to get child to smile by smiling, talking, or waving. Do not touch child.
2. Child must stare at hand several seconds.
3. Parent may help guide toothbrush and put toothpaste on brush.
4. Child does not have to be able to tie shoes or button/zip in the back.
5. Move yarn slowly in an arc from one side to the other, about 8 inches above child's face.
6. Pass if child grasps rattle when it is touched to the backs or tips of fingers.
7. Pass if child tries to see where yarn went. Yarn should be dropped quickly from sight from tester's hand without arm movement.
8. Child must transfer cube from hand to hand without help of body, mouth, or table.
9. Pass if child picks up raisin with any part of thumb and finger.
10. Line can vary only 30 degrees or less from tester's line.
11. Make a fist with thumb pointing upward and wiggle only the thumb. Pass if child imitates and does not move any fingers other than the thumb.

12. Pass any enclosed form. Fail continuous round motions.

13. Which line is longer (not bigger)? Turn paper upside down and repeat. (Pass 3 of 3 or 5 of 6.)

14. Pass any lines crossing near midpoint.

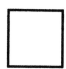
15. Have child copy first. If failed, demonstrate.

When giving items 12, 14, and 15, do not name the forms. Do not demonstrate 12 and 14.

16. When scoring, each pair (2 arms, 2 legs, etc.) counts as one part.
17. Place one cube in cup and shake gently near child's ear but out of sight. Repeat for other ear.
18. Point to picture and have child name it. (No credit is given for sounds only.)
    If less than 4 pictures are named correctly, have child point to picture as each is named by tester.

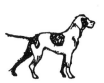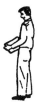

19. Using doll, tell child: Show me the nose, eyes, ears, mouth, hands, feet, tummy, hair. Pass 6 of 8.
20. Using pictures, ask child: Which one flies?... says meow?... talks?... barks?... gallops? Pass 2 of 5, 4 of 5.
21. Ask child: What do you do when you are cold?... tired?... hungry? Pass 2 of 3, 3 of 3.
22. Ask child: What do you do with a cup? What is a chair used for? What is a pencil used for? Action words must be included in answers.
23. Pass if child correctly places *and* says how many blocks are on paper. (1, 5).
24. Tell child: Put block **on** table, **under** table, **in front of** me, **behind** me. Pass 4 of 4. (Do not help child by pointing, moving head or eyes.)
25. Ask child: What is a ball?... lake?... desk?... house?... banana?... curtain?... fence?... ceiling? Pass if defined in terms of **use, shape, what it is made of, or general category** (such as banana is fruit, not just yellow). Pass 5 of 8, 7 of 8.
26. Ask child: If a horse is big, a mouse is __? If fire is hot, ice is __? If the sun shines during the day, the moon shines during the __? Pass 2 of 3.
27. Child may use wall or rail only, not person. Child may not crawl.
28. Child must throw ball overhand 3 feet to within arm's reach of tester.
29. Child must perform standing broad jump over width of test sheet ($8\frac{1}{2}$ inches).
30. Tell child to walk forward, ∞➝ heel within 1 inch of toe. Tester may demonstrate. Child must walk 4 consecutive steps.
31. In the second year, half of normal children are noncompliant.

OBSERVATIONS:

From William K Frankenburg and JB Dodds, 1981, 1988, WK Frankenburg and JB Dodds; 1978, WK Frankenburg.
*For more information on using this form, call 1-800-419-4729.

Milani-Comparetti Motor Development Screening Test

NAME

RECORD NO.

	YR	MO	DAY
TEST DATE	____	____	____
BIRTH DATE	____	____	____
AGE	____	____	____

GE IN MONTHS: 1 2 3 4 5 6 7 8 9 10 11 12 15 18 21 24

- Body lying supine — lifts
- Hand grasp
- Foot grasp
- Supine equil.
- Body pulled up from supine
- Sitting — L3
- Sitting equil.
- Sideway parachute
- Backward parachute
- Body held vertical
- Head righting
- Downwards parachute
- Standing — supporting reactions / astasia / takes weight
- Standing equil.
- Locomotion — automatic stepping / roll P→S / roll S→P / GI crawling / crawls / cruising / walks / high/medium/no guard / recip. mvts. / runs
- Landau
- Forward parachute
- Body lying prone
- Prone equil.
- All fours — forearms / hands / 4 pt / kneeling / plantigrade standing
- All fours equil.
- Sym T.N.
- Body derotative
- Standing up from supine — with rotation and support / without support
- Body rotative — rotates out of sitting / rotates into sitting
- Asym. T.N.
- Moro

MONTHS: 1 2 3 4 5 6 7 8 9 10 11 12 15 18 21 24

TESTER: _____ *Record General Observations on Back of Score Form

Pediatric Population

From Milani-Comparetti A, Gidoni: Routine developmental examination in normal and retarded children, *Dev Med Child Neurol* 9:635, 1967.

ASSESSMENT CHART: MINIMAL CEREBRAL DYSFUNCTION
Movement and posture with inborn reactions

Name _____ Bd. _____ Patient's clinic _____

0—Cannot assume test posture even after demonstration
1—Can assume an approximate test posture after demonstration
2—Can assume test posture in an awkward manner on command
3—Can assume and sustain test posture in a near normal manner on command
    (note abnormal details)
4—Normal

Examiner:

DA	Test movements and postures	

Supine
6-7 months
	1. Rolls completely over
	   a. To right
	   b. To left	

4-10 months	2. Pulls hips and knees to chest fully flexed, arms crossed, palms on shoulders, fingers extended	

4 months	3. With hips, knees fully flexed
	   a. Extend right leg
	   b. Extend left leg	

5-7 months	4. Head in midline, arms at sides, raise head:
	   a. Influence on arms
	   b. Influence on legs	

36-60 months (3-5 years)	5. Pulls up to sit, support on forearms, then by extending elbows	

Prone
 	
4-6 months
+ 24 months
	6. Extends arms beside head, legs abducted
	   a. Raises head in midline
	   b. Supinates forearms
	     (palms toward ceiling)	

+ 24 months	7. Brings arms down beside body; extends arms, palms down	
3-6 months + 36 months	8. a. Flexes right knee, hips extend b. Flexes left knee, hips extend	

Modified from Norton Y: Minimal cerebral dysfunction—part II: modified treatment and evaluation of movement, *AJOT* 26(4):193-195, 1972.

ASSESSMENT CHART: MINIMAL CEREBRAL DYSFUNCTION—cont'd
Movement and posture with inborn reactions

Examiner:		
DA	**Test movements and postures**	
3 months	9. a. Supports trunk on forearms; upper trunk extended, face vertical b. Flexes knees	
5 months 8 months 6 months	10. a. Supports trunk on hands; elbows and hips extended, face vertical b. Flexes neck c. Extends neck d. Balances	
8 months +9–11 months	11. Moves from prone to sit a. All fours push back b. Transitional between quadrupedal and adult method: (1) Side sit right (2) Side sit left	
Sitting erect 8 months 10 months 10 months	12. Sits with soles of feet together, hips flexed and externally rotated to at least 45° a. Round sit b. Pushes laterally: (1) Right (2) Left c. Balance extended, flexes legs	
8 months 10 months 10 months	13. Extends knees, abducts legs, pushes forward and backward a. Hips 60°-70° b. Hips 90°-100° c. Hips 110°-120°	
+ 15 months	14. Hangs legs over edge of platform a. Extends right knee b. Extends left knee	

Continued

		Examiner:
DA	**Test movements and postures**	

Kneeling and crawling
7 months
 	
8 months
	15. Gets into four-point kneel and rocks (back straight)
	  a. Weight on knees
	  b. Weight on hands
	    (1) Neck extends
	    (2) Neck flexes
	  c. Crawls	

9 months
36 months
	16. Moves to kneel-stand; head in midposition, arms at side, hips fully extended
	  a. Pushes: (1) Forward
	          (2) Backward	

10 months	17. Moves to half-kneel
	  a. Weight on right knee
	  b. Weight on left knee	

Squat 21 months	18. Squats; heels down, toes not clawed, knees pointing in same direction as toes, hips fully flexed, head in line with trunk, arms forward	
Standing and components of walking +15 months	19. Stands up; correct alignment, feet separated 6 inches	

36 months	20. Bears weight on one leg
	  a. Shifts weight over right leg: _____ seconds
	  b. Shifts weight over left leg: _____ seconds	

+24 months
 	
36 months
	21. Walks (adult method)
	  a. Forward
	  b. Backward
	  c. Stairs: alternates feet
	    (1) Up
	    (2) Down	

Modified from Norton Y: Minimal cerebral dysfunction—part II: modified treatment and evaluation of movement, *AJOT* 26(4):193-195, 1972.

+ − = Present or absent inborn reactions
IR = Inborn reactions
* = Equilibrium reactions = learned reactions
M&P = Movements and posture
( ) = Retarding influences
STNR = Symmetrical tonic neck reflex
DA = Age at which normal responses, movement, and behavior develop in these positions because of presence or absence of certain basic reflexes and reactions

Test				Retest			
Inborn reactions	+	−	Date	Remarks: M&P	IR +	−	Date	Remarks: M&P
(Neck righting)	+	−			+	−		
Head on body								
(Body on body)			R				R	
Body on head								
Labyrinthine			L				L	
(Tonic neck)								
Associated reactions								
(Tonic labyrinthine)								
(Crossed extension)			R				R	
(Tonic labyrinthine)								
(Tonic neck)			L				L	
(Tonic) labyrinthine			a				a	
Associated reactions +								
STNR			b				b	
(Tonic) labyrinthine								
Head on body								
Head on body								
(Tonic) labyrinthine			a				a	
Landau on floor								
(Tonic neck)			b				b	
(Neck righting)								
(Tonic neck)								
(Tonic labyrinthine)								
(Amphibian)			R				R	
			L				L	
Labyrinthine			a				a	
Optical righting								
Body on head			b				b	

Pediatric Population

Continued

ASSESSMENT CHART: MINIMAL CEREBRAL DYSFUNCTION—cont'd
Movement and posture with inborn reactions

Test					Retest		
Inborn reactions			**Date**	**Remarks: M&P**	**IR**	**Date**	**Remarks: M&P**
Labyrinthine Optical (STNR) Equilibrium			a				a
			b				b
			c				c
			d				d
Labyrinthine Optical Head on body Body on head (Amphibian) Equilibrium			a				a
			R				R
			L				L
Labyrinthine Optical Protective extension of arms Equilibrium			a				a
			R				R
			L				L
			c				c
Labyrinthine Optical Protective extension of arms Equilibrium			a				a
			b				b
			c				c
Labyrinthine (Adductor reflex)			R				R
			L				L
Labyrinthine Optical (STNR) (Asymmetrical TNR) Equilibrium			Rock				Rock
			Knees				Knees
			(1) (2)				(1) (2)
			Crawl				Crawl

Modified from Norton Y: Minimal cerebral dysfunction—part II: modified treatment and evaluation of movement, *AJOT* 26(4):193-195, 1972.

ASSESSMENT CHART: MINIMAL CEREBRAL DYSFUNCTION—cont'd
Movement and posture with inborn reactions

Inborn reactions			Date	Remarks: M&P	IR	Date	Remarks: M&P
Test					**Retest**		
Labyrinthine			F			F	
Optical							
Protective extension of arms			B			B	
Equilibrium							
Labyrinthine			R			R	
Optical							
Equilibrium			L			L	
Labyrinthine							
Equilibrium							
Labyrinthine							
Optical							
Equilibrium							
Labyrinthine			R			R	
Optical							
Equilibrium			L			L	
Positive			a			a	
Negative			b			b	
Support							
Equilibrium			c			c	
			(1)			(1)	
			(2)			(2)	

Continued

HEAD IN MIDLINE FOR POSITIONS

Tests: supine

Test 1
Purpose: To test the level of and ability to roll completely over in both directions
Instructions: "Roll to your tummy and keep rolling to your back again. Now do it on the other side. Lie on your back."
Note: Stiffness; lack of trunk-pelvis separation (body on body righting); hyperextended neck in backward roll; rolling at angle.
Normal: Head, hip, top knee slightly flexed in turning over to side

Test 2 (from position of Test 1)
Purpose: To test for freedom from hypertonicity and lack of associated movement in the supine position
Instructions: "Pull your knees close up to your chest. Bend your elbows and cross your arms. Put your hands on your shoulders. Raise up your elbows. Rest your arms."
Note: Finger clawing; downward pull of scapular depressors preventing elbows from remaining away from the body (children with this difficulty seeming to have trouble writing); feet neither inverted nor dorsiflexed

Test 3 (from position of Test 2)
Purpose: To test for lower-extremity differentiation or identify hypertonicity preventing that differentiation
Instructions: "Put your arms beside your body. Straighten that leg (right). Bend that same knee (right) and straighten the other leg (left). Relax!"
Note: Internal rotation of either leg; adduction of either thigh; feet inverted, plantar flexed; extension of opposite leg when other extends; back arched; body asymmetrical

Test 4 (from position of Test 3)
Purpose: To test ability to raise head from the supporting surface without affecting extremities
Instructions: "Raise just your head. Put it back down. Now relax."
Note: Inability of head to differentiate from rest of body; symmetrical tonic neck reflex causing arms to flex and tone to increase in the legs; feet inverted

Test 5 (from position of Test 4)
Purpose: To test the ability and method of moving from supine to sit
Instructions: "Sit up, please. Now lie down."
Note: Adult method, 5-year level: symmetry of movement, head forward, bilateral elbow flexion to extension, hips flexing; versus pathological process of hypertonicity in back and lower extremities preventing hip flexion as back raises off support; transitional method: + 10-month level: from prone to side sit; infant method, 8-month level: from quadriped position to sit

Tests: prone

Test 6
Purpose: To test freedom from hypertonicity in prone position
Instructions: "Get onto your tummy. Straighten your arms beside your head. Raise it. Turn the palms of your hands toward the ceiling. Straighten your fingers. Put your head down."
Note: Shoulders and hips: tightness in upper or lower extremities; inversion of feet; inability to supinate (after + 24 months); inability to straighten fingers (asymmetry); hypertonic upper extremity and trunk flexors, adductors of upper extremity and trunk shoulder girdle depressors, and pronators affecting ability to write in cursive; heavy

Modified from Norton Y: Minimal cerebral dysfunction—part II: modified treatment and evaluation of movement, *AJOT* 26(4):193-195, 1972.

Note—cont'd

head: tonic labyrinthine abnormality; lower extremity tightness affecting the degree of upper extremity freedom of movement

Test 7 (from position of Test 6)
Purpose: To further test freedom of shoulders and arms from flexor hypertonus in prone
Instructions: "Bring your arms down straight beside your body. Put the palms of your hands on the mat. Now relax."
Note: Freedom of head movement; influence of head position on tone of extremities (asymmetrical tonic neck reflex) affecting ability in fine skill and possibly figure ground; balance during movement and upright positions; feet adducted, inverted

Test 8 (from position of Test 7)
Purpose: To test selective control of hips and knees
Instructions: "Bend your right knee. Put it down and bend your left knee. Now relax."
Note: 90-degree knee flexion with completely extended hips sometime after 36 months; hip raising, toppling of leg in inward or outward direction, foot inversion; tightness at hips and knees affecting balance during movement and in upright positions; amphibian reactions of forward flexion capable of being a retarding influence for hip extension but a precursor for crawl

Test 9 (from position of Test 8)
Purpose: To test postural control in spinal extension and with knee flexion
Instructions: "Pull up onto your elbows. Bend both knees. Now straighten your knees."
Note: Inability to place arms at a 90-degree flexion, with slight abduction, forearms straight, hands opened: hypertonicity of adductors, flexors of arms, forearms, and

Note—cont'd

fingers; toppling to either side; hip flexion with knee flexion; control in this position needed to crawl and the beginning use of hands with balance

Test 10 (from position of Test 9)
Purpose: To test the ability to support weight on extended arms, regardless of the position of the head
Instructions: "Straighten your elbows. Put your weight on your opened hands. Now bend your neck. Raise your head, (pushing laterally for balance). Now get onto your tummy."
Note: Inability to carry weight on extended elbows, perform finger extension with neck flexion, or bend elbows with neck extension; leg thrust with neck flexion, (due to symmetrical tonic neck reflex); hip internal rotation and foot inversion; lack of equilibrium reactions

Test 11 (from position of Test 10)
Purpose: To test the ability and method of getting from prone to sit
Instructions: "Sit up, please. Now bring your legs in front."
Note: Symmetry in getting up if the infant method in the quadrupedal position is used; preferred side that the child turns toward if the transitional method is chosen, or whether the child pushes up to the knees, sits, swings the legs over and forward

Tests: sitting erect

Test 12 (from position of Test 11)
Purpose: To test the ability to round sit and the development of lateral protective extension and balance reactions
Instructions: "Sit up tall. Put the soles of your feet together. Relax your arms." (Push the child gently and laterally at each shoulder to observe balance and protective extension of the supporting

Continued

Instructions—cont'd
   arm with abduction of the opposite arm, and balance reactions as the therapist alternately flexes and extends the legs.) "Now put your legs out straight."
Note: Inability to balance; presence or absence of protective extension of arms and the side of the absence; straight (normal) back versus the need for head-forward flexion compensation to prevent backward tipping; lack of adequate hip flexion and external rotation of the legs

Test 13 (from position of Test 12)
Purpose: To test balance reactions and protective extension of the arms in long sit
Instructions: "Separate your legs. Sit up tall and let your arms go limp." (Push child forward then backward.) "Now sit at the edge of the platform."
Note: Inability to balance or lack of protective extension of the limbs (elbows extended) when pushed forward or backward; inadequate amount of hip flexion in forward, straight position; internal rotation of thighs; foot inversion

Test 14 (from position of Test 13)
Purpose: To test the ability to extend one leg without associated reactions in the other
Instructions: "Sit up tall. Raise that (right) leg and straighten your knee. Relax, raise and straighten the other (left) knee. Rest. Now get onto your hands and knees."
Note: Any adduction or internal rotation of the other leg when either (first) leg extends; foot inversions

Tests: kneeling and crawling

Test 15 (from position of Test 14)
Purpose: To test weight bearing, balance, and control in four-point position on open hands, regardless of the position of the head

Instructions: "Rock backward. Rock forward (3 times). Raise your head. Lower your head. Crawl. Now raise up onto your knees."
Note: Lordosis; flexion of elbows when the neck flexes with thrust of lower extremities (symmetrical tonic neck reflex); extension of the elbows only if the neck extends (symmetrical tonic neck reflex); extension of one arm only when the head turns toward that arm (asymmetrical tonic neck reflex); raising of knees off the supporting surface in moving onto extended elbows (symmetrical tonic neck reflex); inversion of feet and asymmetry in crawling

Test 16 (from position of Test 15)
Purpose: To test for anteroposterior control of pelvis, trunk, and thighs during movement
Instructions: "Straighten your trunk and hips." (Push forward, backward.) "Remain in that position."
Note: Inability to regain balance without difficulty from forward or backward push; lack of or inadequate protective extension of arms; feet inverted; hips flexed; back lordosed

Test 17 (from position of Test 16)
Purpose: To test the control of hip rotation and the effect on the lower extremities and balance
Instructions: "Raise the left leg, bend the knee, and put your foot down flat. Change legs. Squat."
Note: Inadequate flexion of hip or knee; angle of forward leg (more than 90 degrees); thigh adducted; balance unstable; toes constantly clawed; heel off ground; lower leg of supporting leg occasionally raised off support and that foot inverted and the hip of the supporting leg inadequately extended

Modified from Norton Y: Minimal cerebral dysfunction—part II: modified treatment and evaluation of movement, *AJOT* 26(4):193-195, 1972.

Tests: squat

Test 18 (from position of Test 17)
Purpose: To test control of hypertonicity throughout the body
Instructions: "Squat. Separate your knees. Put your heels down on the floor. Bring your arms forward. Shift weight sideways. Now stand up."
Note: Inability to put heels down on the floor; constant clawing of toes; tendency to topple backward or sideways in movement; pain behind the knees or in the buttocks or calf of the leg

Tests: standing, components of walking

Test 19 (from position of Test 18)
Purpose: To test for normal distribution of tone in standing
Instructions: "Stand up tall. Separate your feet so far (about 6 inches). Remain in that position."
Note: Inability to extend hips adequately; excessive lordosis, geno recurvatum; unequal weight distribution: shoulders of unequal height, spine curved laterally, feet inverted; balance tenuous

Test 20 (from position of Test 19)
Purpose: To test the time ability (in seconds) to support the body over one leg
Instructions: "Shift your weight onto the (right) leg and hold it as long as you can. Do it on the other leg. Now stand on both legs."
Note: Time (recorded) in seconds that steady balance can be maintained on either leg; flexed leg having inadequate hip extension; thigh being internally

Note—cont'd
rotated and adducted; foot inverted; difficulty in weight shift

Test 21 (from position of Test 20)
Purpose: To test heel strike and dorsiflexion in forward movement; adult approach: hip extension in backward walk; freedom of upper extremity in stair climb
Instructions: "Walk forward to (specifying point) and stop. Walk backward to me and stop. Climb the stairs."
Note: Internal rotation of the thigh, hip-knee flexion, foot inversion; a lack of reciprocal arm movement with rigid spine; forward walk: alignment of hips, knees, and ankles; dorsiflexion of forward foot on heel strike; rear leg outwardly rotated at hip; roll off from head of first metatarsal; slight rotation of trunk; arms swinging freely and alternating with leg movements (right arm with left leg in normal postural control); backward walk: alignment of hip, knee, ankle, or forward leg; back leg extended, outwardly rotated at hip; hip extended, knee flexed so that back foot touches first metatarsal and leg somewhat laterally for support; feet not inverted in normal postural control; climbing stairs (without bannister): alternate flexed hip, knee, ankle dorsiflexion; weight firmly on lower stair; pulling up onto forward extending leg; back leg flexed at knee, hip extended, and thigh abducted; standing leg: leg, foot aligned, arms free in normal postural control; no internally rotated thigh, adducted forward leg, or inverted feet (for children at least 4 years)

Developmental Reflexes and Reactions

Primitive reflexes are innate responses or movements elicited by particular stimuli. As children mature, the reflexes are integrated to allow normal development. As these primitive reflexes disappear, developmental reactions emerge. Therapists must understand when children should have these reflexes and reactions and the consequences for children who are missing them.

Developmental Reactions and Reflexes Glossary

Reactions

Amphibian. Lifting of the pelvis on one side in a prone position producing arm and leg flexion on the same side

Associated. An action (e.g., squeezing a ball) that produces mirroring on the opposite side or increased muscle tone in other parts of the body

Body righting. Restoration or maintenance of normal postural relationships of the head, trunk, and extremities during activity

Equilibrium. Automatic, compensatory movements that adapt the body to changes in the center of gravity and in the position of the extremities in relation to the trunk

Head righting. Restoration of normal position of the head in space

Landau response. Extension of the head producing lower-extremity and spinal extension and flexion of the head producing lower-extremity and spinal flexion when the head is held in the prone position in space at the thorax

Protective extension. Sudden loss of balance producing immediate upper extremity extension, finger abduction, and finger extension

Reflexes

Asymmetrical tonic neck reflex (ATNR). Passive head rotation in the supine position producing extension of the arm and leg on the face side and flexion of the arm and leg on the back of the head side

Babinski Stroking of the lateral sole of the foot from the heel to the ball of the foot producing splaying of the toes and dorsiflexion of the hallux

Crossed extension. Firm pressure on the ball of the foot or noxious stimulus of the extended leg producing extension and adduction of the opposite leg

Flexor withdrawal. Noxious stimuli applied to the bottom of the foot producing uncontrolled flexion of the lower extremity

Gag. Stimulation of the posterior pharynx producing a gag response

Galant. Sweeping of the paravertebral area between the twelfth rib and the iliac crest with fingernail in the prone position producing trunk curvature to the same side

Glabellar. Brisk tapping of the bridge of the nose producing eye closure

Moro's. Dropping of the head from a semiflexed position producing upper-extremity abduction and extension followed by upper-extremity flexion and adduction, lower-extremity extension and adduction, and crying

Palmar grasp. Pressure on the palmar surface of the hand producing full finger flexion

Placing. Top of the foot touching a hard object and producing lifting of the leg

Plantar grasp. Pressure on the ball of the foot producing toe flexion

Positive support. Bouncing on the soles of the feet producing increased lower-extremity extension tone and partial weight bearing

Rooting. Touching beside the mouth producing head turning to that side and sucking

Startle. Loud noise producing upper-extremity abduction and extension followed by upper-extremity flexion and adduction

Stepping. Sole of the foot touching a hard surface and producing reciprocal flexion and extension of the leg

Sucking. Stimulation of the oral area producing sucking movements

Symmetrical tonic neck reflex (STNR). Neck flexion in the quadruped position producing upper-extremity flexion and lower-extremity extension

Tonic labyrinthine. Change in position of the head or body in space producing extension of the extremities in the supine position and flexion of the extremities in the prone position

Traction. Pulling on the upper extremities and producing neck flexion, elbow flexion, and attempts at pull to sit

Newborn and Infant Reflexes and their Possible Adverse Effects

Primitive reflex	Possible negative effect on movement with abnormal persistence of reflex
Asymmetrical Tonic Neck Reflex (ATNR)	Interferes with the following:
Stimulus: head position, turned to one side	• Feeding
Response: arm and leg on face side extended, arm and leg on scalp side flexed, spine curved with convexity toward face side	• Visual tracking
	• Midline hand use
Normal age of response: birth to 6 mo	• Bilateral hand use
	• Rolling
	• Development of crawling
	Can lead to skeletal deformities (for example, scoliosis, hip subluxation, hip dislocation)
Symmetrical Tonic Neck Reflex (STNR)	Interferes with the following:
Stimulus: head position, flexion or extension	• Ability to prop on arms in prone position
Response: when head in flexion, arms flexed and legs extended; when head in extension, arms extended and legs flexed	• Attaining and maintaining of hands-and-knees position
	• Reciprocal crawling
Normal age of response: 6-8 mo	• Sitting balance when looking around
	• Use of hands when looking at object in hands in sitting position
Tonic Labyrinthine Reflex (TLR)	Interferes with the following:
Stimulus: position of labyrinth in inner ear; reflected in head position	• Ability to initiate rolling
Response: in supine position, body and extremities held in extension; in prone position, body and extremities held in flexion	• Ability to prop on elbows with extended hips in prone position
	• Ability to flex trunk and hips to come to sitting position from supine position
Normal age of response: birth to 6 mo	Often causes full body extension, which interferes with balance in sitting or standing

Modified from Ratliffe KT: *Clinical pediatric physical therapy,* St Louis, 1998, Mosby.

Continued

Pediatric Population

Primitive reflex	Possible negative effect on movement with abnormal persistence of reflex
Galant Reflex Stimulus: touch to skin along spine from shoulder to hip Response: lateral flexion of trunk to side of stimulus Normal age of response: 30 wk of gestation to 2 mo	Interferes with development of sitting balance Can lead to scoliosis
Palmar Grasp Reflex Stimulus: pressure in palm on ulner side of hand Response: flexion of fingers causing strong grip Normal age of response: birth to 4 mo	Interferes with the following: • Ability to grasp and release objects voluntarily • Weight bearing on open hand for propping; crawling; protective responses
Plantar Grasp Reflex Stimulus: pressure to base of toes Response: toe flexion Normal age of response: 28 wk of gestation to 9 mo	Interferes with the following: • Ability to stand with feet flat on surface • Balance reactions and weight shifting in standing
Rooting Reflex Stimulus: touch on cheek Response: turning of head to same side with mouth open Normal age of response: 28 wk of gestation to 3 mo	Interferes with the following: • Oral motor development • Development of midline control of head • Optical righting, visual tracking, and social interaction
Moro Reflex Stimulus: head dropping into extension suddenly for a few inches Response: arms abducting with fingers open, then crossing trunk into adduction; crying Normal age of response: 28 wk of gestation to 5 mo	Interferes with the following: • Balance reactions in sitting • Protective responses in sitting • Eye-hand coordination; visual tracking
Startle Reflex Stimulus: loud, sudden noise Response: similar to Moro response but elbows flexed and hands closed Normal age of response: 28 wk of gestation to 5 mo	Interferes with the following: • Sitting balance • Protective responses in sitting • Eye-hand coordination; visual tracking • Social interaction; attention
Positive Support Reflex Stimulus: weight placed on balls of feet when upright Response: stiffening of legs and trunk into extension Normal age of response: 35 wk of gestation to 2 mo	Interferes with the following: • Standing and walking • Balance reactions and weight shift in standing Can lead to contractures of ankles into plantar flexion
Walking (Stepping) Reflex Stimulus: supported upright position with soles of feet on firm surface Response: reciprocal flexion and extension of legs Normal age of response: 38 wk of gestation to 2 mo	Interferes with the following: • Standing and walking • Balance reactions and weight shifting in standing • Development of smooth, coordinated reciprocal movements of lower extremities

Modified from Ratliffe KT: *Clinical pediatric physical therapy,* St Louis, 1998, Mosby.

Reflexes and Developmental Reactions of Children

Developmental reaction	Effect on development of motor skills
Birth-1 Mo	
Reflexes	
Sucking and swallowing	Learns vertical orientation to world
Palmar grasp	Begins to strengthen postural muscles
Plantar grasp	Can lift head in prone position to clear airway
Asymmetrical tonic neck	
Tonic labyrinthine	
Galant	
Moro	
Startle	
Positive support	
Developmental reaction	
Head righting	
2-3 Mo	
Reflexes	
Traction response of arms in pull-to-sit action stronger	Can hold head up when held at shoulder
Sucking and swallowing reflexes weaker	Holds head to 90° briefly in prone position
Galant reflex inhibited	Bobs head upright in supported sitting position
Positive supporting reflex inhibited	Holds chest up in prone position with some
Stepping reflex inhibited	weight through forearms
Developmental reaction	
Optical and labyrinthine head righting developing	
4-5 Mo	
Reflexes	
ATNR integrated	Rolls from prone to supine position
Palmar grasp reflex integrated	Pivots in prone position
	Bears weight through extended arms in prone position
Developmental reactions	Begins forward propping in sitting position
Equilibrium reactions in prone position developing	Sits alone briefly
Protective extension forward in sitting position developing	Grasps and releases toys
Landau response becoming stronger	
6-7 Mo	
Reflexes	
STNR developing	Rolls from supine to prone position
Moro reflex inhibited	Holds weight on one hand to reach for toy
	Assumes sitting position without assistance
	Stands holding on

Modified from Ratliffe KT: *Clinical pediatric physical therapy,* St Louis, 1998, Mosby.
ATNR, Asymmetrical tonic neck reflex; *STNR,* symmetrical tonic neck reflex.

Continued

Table—cont'd

Developmental reaction	Effect on development of motor skills
6-7 Mo—cont'd	
Developmental reactions	
Protective extension sideward in sitting position developed	
Equilibrium reactions in supine position developed	
8-9 Mo	
Reflexes	
Plantar grasp inhibited	Assumes hands-and-knees position
STNR inhibited	Moves from sitting to prone position
	Sits without hand support
Developmental reaction	Creeps on hands and knees
Protective extension backward developing in sitting position	Cruises along furniture
10-11 Mo	
Developmental reaction	
Equilibrium responses emerging in quadruped position	Stands briefly without support
	Pulls to stand using half-kneel intermediate position
12-15 Mo	
Developmental reactions	
Equilibrium reactions emerging in standing position	Walks without support
Protective extension forward in standing position developed	Walks backward
	Walks sideways
16-24 Mo	
Developmental reaction	
Protective extension sideways and backward in standing position developed	Squats in play
	Kicks ball
	Propels ride-on toys

Modified from Ratliffe KT: *Clinical pediatric physical therapy,* St Louis, 1998, Mosby.

Ages at which Postural Reactions Acquired

Balance reactions	Age of acquisition
Righting Reactions	
Neck on body	
Immature	Birth
Mature	4-5
Body on body	
Immature	Birth
Mature	4-5
Body on head	
Prone	
Partial	1-2
Mature	4-5
Supine	5-6
Landau	
Immature	3
Mature	6-10
Flexion	
Partial (head in line)	3-4
Mature (head forward)	6-7
Vertical	
Partial (head in line)	2
Mature (head to vertical)	6
Protective Reactions	
Forward	6-7
Lateral	6-11
Backward	9-12
Equilibrium Reactions	
Prone	5-6
Supine	7-8
Sitting	7-10
Quadruped	9-12
Standing	12-21

Modified from Case-Smith J, Allen AS, Pratt PN, editors: *Occupational therapy for children*, ed 3, St Louis, 1996, Mosby.

Developmental Milestones

As children mature, they gain the abilities to perform certain skills at specific ages. These activities, known as *developmental milestones,* include gross motor skills, activities of daily living, speech and language skills, and psychosocial skills. Therapists who understand the normal sequences for the acquisition of these milestones can detect developmental delays promptly and establish realistic plans of care.

Pediatric Population

Developmental Checklist

Age level	Performance criteria
Neurological development to 5 yr	Tonic neck reflex
	TLR
	Response to touch
	Protective extension
	Body righting
1-3 mo	Lifts head
	Follows moving object with eyes
4-7 mo	Transfers toy hand to hand
	Approaches mirror
8-12 mo	Rises to sitting position
	Finger-feeds self
13-18 mo	Makes pencil marks
	Cooperates in dressing
19-24 mo	Squats in play
	Identifies pictures by pointing
	Feeds self with spoon
25-36 mo	Runs well
	Holds pencil with fingers
	Pulls on simple garment
37-48 mo	Alternates feet going upstairs or rides tricycle
	Copies circle
	Feeds self well (spoon and fork)
49-60 mo	Catches ball
	Copies crosses
	Distinguishes front and back of clothes or self
	Acts out fantasies in play
5-7 yr	Recites letters of alphabet
	Differentiates right from left
	Exhibits hand dominance
	Performs somersault
	Plays well with other children
7-10 yr	Performs well in competition sports with other children
	Verbalizes plans for adult life
	Reads and writes at grade level
	Can perform math at grade level
	Demonstrates independence in self-care
10-15 yr	Prefers peer group activities
	Enjoys one hobby
	Travels independently
	Attains grade-level academic performance (C− or better)
	Attains grade-level athletic performance (C− or better)
15-20 yr	Takes an active interest in community and world affairs
	Prepares for adult occupational role
	Attains grade-level academic performance
	Maintains satisfactory peer relationships

Modified from Pratt PN, Allen AS: *Occupational therapy for children,* ed 2, St Louis, 1989, Mosby.
TLR, Tonic labyrinthine reflex.

Developmental Gross and Fine Motor Skills

Gross motor skills	Fine motor skills

Newborn
Prone
Physiological flexion
Lifts head briefly
Head to side

Regards objects in direct line of vision
Follows moving object to midline
Forms fist with hand
Performs jerky arm movements
Performs purposeful or random movements

Supine
Performs physiological flexion
Rolls partly to side

Sitting
Demonstrates head lag in pull-to-sit motion

Standing
Performs reflex standing and walking

2-3 Mo
Prone
Lifts head 90 degrees briefly
Holds chest up in prone position with some
    weight through forearms
Rolls prone to supine

Can see further distances
Opens hands more
Visually follows through 180 degrees
Grasps reflexively
Uses palmar grasp

Supine
Demonstrates strong ATNR influence
Kicks legs reciprocally
Prefers head to side

Sitting
Exhibits variable head lag in pull-to-sit position
Needs full support to sit
Holds head upright but bobs

Standing
Bears weight poorly
Holds hips in flexion, behind shoulders

4-5 Mo
Prone
Bears weight on extended arms
Pivots in prone to reach toys

Grasps and releases toys
Uses ulnar-palmar grasp

Supine
Rolls from supine to side position
Plays with feet to mouth

Modified from Ratliffe KT: *Clinical pediatric physical therapy*, St Louis, 1998, Mosby.
ATNR, Asymmetrical tonic neck reflex.

Continued

Gross motor skills	Fine motor skills
4-5 Mo—cont'd	
Sitting	
Holds head steady in supported sitting position	
Turns head in sitting position	
Sits alone for brief periods	
Standing	
Bears all weight through legs in supported stand	
6-7 Mo	
Prone	
Rolls from supine to prone position	Approaches objects with one hand
Holds weight on one hand to reach for toy	Holds arm in neutral position when approaching toy
Supine	Performs radial-palmar grasp
Lifts head	"Rakes" with fingers to pick up small objects
	Exhibits voluntary release to transfer objects between hands
Sitting	
Lifts head and helps when pulled to sitting position	
Assumes sitting position without assistance	
Sits independently	
Standing	
Stands holding on to support surface when placed	
Bounces in standing	
Mobility	
May crawl backward	
8-9 Mo	
Prone	
Assumes hands-and-knees position	Develops active supination
	Develops radial-digital grasp
Supine	Uses inferior pincer grasp
Does not tolerate supine position	Extends wrist actively
	Points with index finger
Sitting	Pokes with index finger
Moves from sitting to prone position	Demonstrates more refined release of objects
Sits without hand support for longer periods	Takes objects out of containers
Pivots in sitting position	
Standing	
Stands with support of furniture	
Pulls to stand with support of furniture	
Lowers to sitting position from supported stand	
Mobility	
Crawls forward	
Walks along furniture (cruising)	

Modified from Ratliffe KT: *Clinical pediatric physical therapy,* St Louis, 1998, Mosby.

Gross motor skills	Fine motor skills
10-11 Mo	
Standing	
Stands without support briefly	Performs fine pincer grasp
Pulls to stand using half-kneel intermediate position	Puts objects into containers
Picks up objects from floor from supported standing position	Grasps crayons adaptively
Mobility	
Walks with both hands held	
Walks with one hand held	
Creeps on hands and feet (bear walk)	
12-15 Mo	
Mobility	
Walks without support	Marks paper with crayons
Walks fast	Builds tower using two cubes
Walks backward	Turns over small container to obtain contents
Walks sideways	
Bends over to look between legs	
Creeps or hitches upstairs	
Throws ball from sitting position	
16-24 Mo	
Squats in play	Folds paper
Walks upstairs and downstairs with one hand held and both feet on step	Strings beads
Propels ride-on toys	Stacks six cubes
Kicks ball	Imitates vertical and horizontal strokes with crayons on paper
Throws ball forward	Holds crayons with thumb and finger
Picks up toy from floor without falling	
2 Yr	
Rides tricycle	Turns knob
Walks backward	Opens and closes jar
Walks on tiptoe	Buttons large buttons
Runs on toes	Uses child-size scissors with help
Walks downstairs, alternating feet	Does 12- to 15-piece puzzles
Catches large ball	Folds paper or clothes
Hops on one foot	
Preschool Age (3-4 Yr)	
Throws ball 10 ft	Controls crayons more effectively
Walks on a line 10 ft	Copies a circle or cross
Hops 2-10 times on one foot	Matches colors
Jumps distances of up to 2 ft	Cuts with scissors
Jumps over obstacles up to 12 in	Draws recognizable human figure with head and two extremities
Throws and catches small ball	Draws squares
Runs fast and avoids obstacles	May demonstrate hand preference

Pediatric Population

Continued

Table—cont'd

Gross motor skills	Fine motor skills
Early School Age (5-8 Yr)	
Skips on alternate feet	Demonstrates obvious hand preference
Gallops	Prints well; starts to learn cursive writing
Can play hopscotch, balance on one foot, control hopping, and squat on one leg	Can button small buttons
Jumps with rhythm, control (jump rope)	
Bounces large ball	
Kicks ball with greater control	
Limbs growing faster than trunk allow greater speed, leverage	
Later School Age (9-12 Yr)	
Demonstrates mature patterns of movement in throwing, jumping, running	Develops greater control in hand use
Increases competitiveness, enjoys competitive games	Learns to draw
	Exhibits developed handwriting
Exhibits improved balance, coordination, endurance, attention span	
May develop preadolescent fat spurt (boys)	
May develop prepubescent and pubescent changes in body shape of hips, breasts (girls)	
Adolescence (13 Yr+)	
Demonstrates rapid growth in size and strength, boys more than girls	Develops greater dexterity in fingers for fine tasks (knitting, sewing, arts, crafts)
Develops changes in body proportions because of puberty (center of gravity rising toward shoulders for boys, lowering to hips for girls)	
May experience plateaus in balance skills, coordination, eye-hand coordination, endurance during growth spurt	

Modified from Ratliffe KT: *Clinical pediatric physical therapy,* St Louis, 1998, Mosby.

Ages at which Motor Milestones Acquired

Motor milestone	Age (months)
Head Control	
Prone	
Lifts head to 45°	2
Lifts head to 90°	4
Supine	
Maintains in midline	2
Lifts	6
Rolling	
Prone to supine	
Without rotation	4-6
With rotation	6-9
Supine to prone	
Without rotation	5-7
With rotation	6-9
Sitting	
Unsustained with arm support	4-5
Sustained with arm support	5-6
Unsustained without arm support	6-7
Sustained without arm support	7-9
Mobility	
Crawling	7-9
Creeping	9-11
Cruising	9-13
Walking	12-14

From Case-Smith J, Allen AS, Pratt PN, editors: *Occupational therapy for children,* ed 3, St Louis, 1996, Mosby.

Development of Stair Climbing and Jumping and Hopping Skills

Age	Skill
Stair Climbing	
15 mo	Creeps up stairs
18-24 mo	Walks up and down stairs while holding on
18-23 mo	Creeps backward down stairs
2-2½ + yr	Walks up and down stairs without support, marking time
2½-3½ yr	Walks up stairs, alternating feet
3-3½ yr	Walks down stairs, alternating feet
Jumping and Hopping	
2 yr	Jumps down from step
2½ + yr	Hops on one foot, few steps
3 yr	Jumps off floor with both feet
3-5 yr	Jumps over objects
3½-5 yr	Hops on one foot
3-4 yr	Gallops, leading with one foot and transferring weight smoothly and evenly
5 yr	Hops in straight line
5-6 yr	Skips on alternating feet, maintaining balance

Modified from Case-Smith J, Allen AS, Pratt PN, editors: *Occupational therapy for children*, ed 3, St. Louis, 1996, Mosby.

Typical Developmental Sequence of Toileting Skills

Approximate age	Toileting skill
10 mo	Indicates when wet or soiled
12 mo	Has regular bowel movements
15 mo	Sits on toilet when placed there and supervised (short time)
18-21 mo	Urinates regularly
20 mo	Demonstrates more toileting regulation
22 mo	Indicates need to go to the toilet
24 mo	Exhibits daytime control with occasional accidents
	Requires reminders to go to the bathroom
30 mo	Tells someone of need to go to the bathroom
	Seats self on toilet
34 mo	Goes to the bathroom independently
3-4 yr	May need help with clothing
4-5 yr	Demonstrates complete independence

Modified from Case-Smith J, Allen PS, Pratt PN, editors: *Occupational therapy for children*, ed 3, St Louis, 1996, Mosby.

Typical Developmental Sequence for Dressing

Age (yr)	Self-dressing skills
1	Cooperates with dressing (holds out arms and feet)
	Pulls off shoes, removes socks
	Pushes arms through sleeves and legs through pants
2	Removes unfastened coat
	Removes shoes if laces are untied
	Helps pull down pants
	Finds armholes in over-the-head shirt
2½	Removes pull-down pants with elastic waist
	Assists in pulling on socks
	Puts on front-button coat or shirt
	Unbuttons large buttons
3	Puts on over-the-head shirt with minimal assistance
	Puts on shoes without fasteners (may be on wrong foot)
	Puts on socks (may be with heel on top)
	Independently pulls down pants
	Zips and unzips jacket once on track
	Needs assistance to remove over-the-head shirt
	Buttons large front buttons
3½	Finds front of clothing
	Snaps or hooks front fastener
	Unzips from zipper on jacket, separating zipper
	Puts on mittens
	Buttons series of three or four buttons
	Unbuckles shoe or belt
	Dresses with supervision (needs help with front and back)
4	Removes pullover garment independently
	Buckles shoes or belt
	Zips jacket zipper
	Puts on socks correctly
	Puts on shoes with assistance to tie laces
	Laces shoes
	Consistently identifies front and back of garment
4½	Puts belt in loops
5	Ties and unties knots
	Dresses unsupervised
6	Closes back zipper
	Ties bow, buttons back buttons.
	Snaps back snaps

Modified from Klein MD: *Predressing skills*, San Antonio, 1984, Communication Skill Builders, The Psychological Corporation.

Pediatric Population

Developmental Sequence for Home Management Tasks

Age	Task
13 mo	Imitates housework
2 yr	Picks up and puts away toys with parental reminders
	Copies parents' domestic activities
3 yr	Carries things without dropping them
	Dusts with help
	Dries dishes with help
	Gardens with help
	Puts toys away with reminders
	Wipes spills
4 yr	Fixes dry cereal and snacks
	Helps sort laundry
5 yr	Puts toys away neatly
	Makes sandwiches
	Takes out trash
	Makes bed
	Puts dirty clothes away
	Answers telephone correctly
6 yr	Performs simple errands
	Performs household chores thoroughly (no need to redo)
	Cleans sink
	Washes dishes with help
	Crosses street safely
7-9 yr	Begins to cook simple meals
	Puts clean clothes away
	Hangs up clothes
	Manages small amounts of money
	Uses telephone correctly
10-12 yr	Cooks simple meals with supervision
	Completes simple repairs with appropriate tools
	Begins doing laundry
	Sets table
	Washes dishes
	Cares for pet with reminders
13-14 yr	Cleans laundry
	Cooks meals

Modified from Case-Smith J, Allan AS, Pratt PN, editors: *Occupational therapy for children,* ed 3, St Louis, 1996, Mosby.

Social, Language, Cognitive, and Adaptive Skills of Childhood

Age	Social skills	Language skills
Newborn	Maintains eye contact Molds body when held Relaxes when held Regards face	Cries to indicate needs Makes monotonous nasal cry Makes comfort sounds
2-3 mo	Watches speaker's eyes and mouth Responds with smile when socially approached Enjoys physical contact Vocalizes in response to conversation	Coos open-vowel sounds Cries in various pitches and volumes to indicate different needs Laughs Squeals
4-5 mo	Socializes with strangers Lifts arms to mother Enjoys social play Vocalizes pleasure and displeasure	Reacts to music Reacts to own name Babbles consonant chains ("bababa") Babbles to people
6-7 mo	Smiles at self in mirror Does not like to be separated from mother Recognizes mother visually Demonstrates anxiety toward strangers Yells to get attention Loves vigorous play	Babbles double consonants ("baba") Waves bye-bye Produces more consonant sounds when babbling
8-9 mo	Allows only mother to meet needs Explores environment enthusiastically Enjoys social games	Babbles single consonant ("ba") Mimics adult pattern of inflection in babbling Says "dada" or "mama" nonspecifically
10-11 mo	Tests parental reactions Extends toys to show, not give	Babbles monologue when alone Says "dada" or "mama" specifically Repeats sounds or gestures if they produce laughs Cannot talk while walking
12-15 mo	Displays tantrum behaviors Acts impulsively Enjoys imitating adult behaviors Says "no" and resists adult control Can be distracted	Uses exclamatory sentences ("uh-oh" "no-no") Uses words or word approximations to express self Has one- to three-word vocabulary Says "no" meaningfully May hit speech plateau as learns to walk
16-24 mo	Expresses affection Plays alone for short periods Gets frustrated easily Displays wide range of emotions, including jealousy of family members Exhibits parallel play Interacts with peers, using gestures and vocalizations	Imitates environmental sounds Uses two-word sentences Attempts to sing songs Exhibits expressive vocabulary up to 50 words Uses own name to refer to self Uses jargon mixed with intelligible words

Modified from Ratliffe KT: *Clinical pediatric physical therapy*, St Louis, 1998, Mosby.

Continued

Table—cont'd

Age	Social skills	Language skills
2 yr	Talks loudly Becomes bossy and demanding Obeys simple rules Demonstrates trouble with changes Separates easily from mother in familiar surroundings May have tantrums May demonstrate fears of unfamiliar things, such as animals or clowns	Gains language quickly, up to four words per day Uses three-word sentences Becomes frustrated when not understood Pronounces full name Recites simple nursery rhymes Sings phrases of songs
Preschool age (3-4 yr)	Enjoys making friends Plays cooperatively Needs praise and guidance from adults Enjoys helping with adult activities (shopping, setting table) Enjoys imitating adult behavior May exhibit continuation of fears	Talks to self at play and rest Uses rhythmic language Uses language actively Exhibits expressive vocabulary of up to 1000 words Learns entire songs and nursery rhymes Loves to talk

Age	Cognitive skills	Adaptive/self-help skills
Newborn	Stops crying when picked up Responds to voice Consoles self by sucking	Opens and closes mouth in response to food Begins to coordinate sucking, swallowing, and breathing
2-3 mo	Searches with eyes for sound Shows active interest in person or object for 1 min Inspects and plays with own hands	Brings hand to mouth Demonstrates better coordination of sucking, swallowing, and breathing Stays awake longer periods during day Sleeps for longer periods at night
4-5 mo	Looks for hidden voice Plays for 2-3 min with one toy Finds partially hidden objects Works to obtain objects out of reach	Holds bottle Eats pureed or strained foods Drinks from cup Naps 2-3 times per day Sleeps up to 12 hr at night
6-7 mo	Looks for family members when named Shakes toys to hear sound Plays peek-a-boo Plays with paper Imitates simple gestures	Mouths solid food Feeds self crackers Bites and chews toys Finger-feeds self
8-11 mo	Responds to simple verbal requests ("come here," "give to mommy") Throws and drops objects Looks at pictures when named Enjoys looking at pictures in books Stacks and unstacks rings Guides action toys manually Dances	Chews using munching pattern Sleeps up to 14 hr at night Holds spoon Extends arm or leg for dressing

Modified from Ratliffe KT: *Clinical pediatric physical therapy,* St Louis, 1998, Mosby.

Table—cont'd

Age	Cognitive skills	Adaptive/self-help skills
12-15 mo	Enjoys messy activities, such as finger-painting and feeding self Recognizes individuals outside family Helps turn pages	Brings spoon to mouth Holds cup and drinks with some spilling Indicates discomfort over dirty diapers Shows pattern of elimination behavior
16-24 mo	Can put things away Names six body parts Matches sounds to pictures of animals Sorts objects	Feeds self with spoon, with some spilling Uses rotary jaw movements to chew food Removes shoes Plays with food Helps wash hands Turns knob to open doors Begins toilet training
2 yr	Matches shapes Completes three- to four-piece puzzle Understands concept of one Understands concept of two Plays house Loves being read to Sorts colors, matches some colors	Undresses and dresses with help Uses spoon and fork Uses napkin Washes and dries hands Uses toilet consistently Hangs clothes on hooks Blows nose with help Insists on doing things without help
Preschool age (3-4 yr)	Identifies colors and shapes Can complete 30-piece puzzle or more Identifies paper money, coins Enjoys books Demonstrates vivid imagination May confuse fantasy with reality	Dresses and undresses independently (except back buttons) Uses toilet without help Uses utensils (forks, spoons) independently Brushes teeth with supervision May exhibit modesty while dressing, toileting, bathing

Age	Social skills	Language skills
Early school age (5-8 yr)	Prefers to play with peers rather than adults Refines social skills of giving, sharing, receiving Cares deeply what others think of self Likes to impress peers	Uses plurals, pronouns, tenses correctly Recites or sings rhymes, TV commercials, songs Demonstrates interest in new words Maintains vocabulary of 2000 to 4000 words
Late school age (9-12 yr)	Shows increased interest in group activities Demonstrates high spirit of adventure Displays interest in organized sports (athletes as heros) Shows interest in practicing skills to gain social approval and develop skills	Exhibits increasing vocabulary and maturity of language skills

Pediatric Population

Continued

Table—cont'd

Age	Social skills	Language skills
Adolescent (13-18 yr)	Demonstrates orientation toward peers Becomes self-conscious Develops interest in opposite sex Increases social maturity	Improves expressive writing skills

Age	Cognitive skills	Adaptive/self-help skills
Early school age (5-8 yr)	Learns to read Learns basic math skills of addition and subtraction Learns concept of conservation Learns to write (printing)	May suffer stomach aches related to school attendance Develops definite likes and dislikes with food Learns to use knife for spreading, cutting Learns to tie shoes
Late school age (9-12 yr)	Enjoys table games Able to think more abstractly Develops increased attention span Becomes intellectually curious Reads greater variety of materials, including nonfiction	Can bathe independently and wash hair with supervision Demonstrates independence in daily care activities Learns to cook Takes role in household tasks
Adolescent (13-18 yr)	Can develop hypotheses, theories Demonstrates increased attention span Expands interests beyond self to environment, those less fortunate, etc.	Takes on greater household roles (laundry, cooking, cleaning) Learns to drive

Modified from Ratliffe KT: *Clinical pediatric physical therapy*, St Louis, 1998, Mosby.

SPECIAL CONSIDERATIONS FOR PRETERM NEWBORNS AND INFANTS

Preterm newborns and infants comprise a unique population and require special considerations in several areas. The presence or absence of reflexes and responses depends on the length of the pregnancy. Some illnesses and problems affect preterm newborns and infants specifically, who display distinctive behaviors that signal they are under excessive stress. Effective care of preterm newborns and infants necessitates the complete understanding of such special considerations.

Preterm Neuromotor Development

Age	Development (Creger and Browne)

27-28 wk

Resting Posture
Generalized hypotonia

Response to Handling
Full range of motion without resistance demonstrated through heel-to-ear maneuver
No attempt to recoil arms into flexion when both arms extended parallel to body
No attempt to grasp with toes when pressure placed on ball of foot
Placing response absent
No attempt to align head and body when pulled to sitting position

Active Movement
Movements spasmodic and involve total extremity

29 wk

Resting Posture
Capability for increased variety in posture when compared with earlier hypotonia

Response to Handling
Continual demonstration of little resistance to passive movements, but manipulation of one extremity more likely to elicit response in opposite extremity
Incomplete but symmetric Moro response
Some attempt to pull body into flexion, using legs, in prone position
Some knee flexion in one leg in response to traction of other leg
Extreme head lag in pull-to-sit motion but attempts to right head anteriorly once in sitting position
Some active flexion at knee with attempt to elicit placing response
Minimal attempt to assume upright posture in supported standing, but evident stepping response

Active Movement
Movements remaining jerky
Movements continuing to be reflexive responses to handling
Movements predominant in legs

30 wk

Resting Posture
Some beginning flexion in lower extremities

Response to Handling
Arm recoil evident; grasp involving some arm flexion; grasp and traction beginning to lift infant's body from supporting surface
Head lag still extreme; once in sitting position, anterior and posterior head righting possible but position maintained only momentarily
No attempt to bear weight on legs in supported standing position; some resistance to supporting surface with feet; still little attempt to assume upright posture

Active Movement
Movement more purposeful and controlled (active movement still involving total extremity)

Pediatric Population

Creger PJ: *Developmental interventions for preterm and high-risk infants: self-study modules for professionals,* Tucson, 1989, Therapy Skill Builders.

Continued

Age	Development (Creger and Browne)
31 wk	**Resting Posture**
	Increased flexor tone in lower extremities when compared with more preterm infants
	Response to Handling
	More resistance to passive movements in legs than in arms (exhibited by the heel-to-ear maneuver)
	Recoil and traction more pronounced in lower extremities when compared with upper extremities
	Some attempt to maintain head in alignment with body while being pulled to sitting position; ability to right head anteriorly and posteriorly once in sitting position
	Still no attempt to bear weight on legs in supported standing; possible knee flexion and resistance to surface with feet; no attempt to align head with body
	Active Movement
	Flexion of arms and legs against gravity; movements not always smoothly coordinated (like tremors) and commonly observed in preterm infants
32 wk	**Resting Posture**
	Continual development of lower extremity flexion
	Response to Handling
	Decreased lower extremity range of passive movement
	Consistent and smooth head righting in pull-to-sit position
	More ability to maintain head aligned with body in supported sitting position compared with younger infants
	Supported stand; some weight on feet, beginning of head righting, some knee extension with some effort to extend trunk
	Moro: complete arm extension and abduction; no flexion and adduction component
	Active Movement
	More activity and smoother and more purposeful movements
	Brief periods of hand-to-mouth activity
33 wk	**Resting Posture**
	Increasingly stronger flexion of lower extremities
	Response to Handling
	Increasing resistance to passive knee extension through heel-to-ear maneuver
	Recoil and traction responses of upper and lower extremities stronger and more consistent
	Stronger attempts to align head with body in pull-to-sit; ability to right head anteriorly and posteriorly in supported sitting position; in ability to maintain head upright
	Some attempt to bear weight on legs and effort to extend trunk and align head with body when held in supported standing position
	Palmar and plantar grasps quick and easy
	Active Movement
	Spontaneous flexion and extension of arms and legs; movements smoother and more purposeful

Creger PJ: *Developmental interventions for preterm and high-risk infants: self-study modules for professionals,* Tucson, 1989, Therapy Skill Builders.

Age	Development (Creger and Browne)
34 wk	**Resting Posture** Development of hip flexion through assumption of froglike resting posture **Response to Handling** Ability to grasp and maintain traction with upper extremities Traction demonstrated in lower extremities; resistance to passive knee extension Hip and knee extension and head righting attempts when in supported sitting position Placing response demonstrated Ventral suspension; some flexion in elbows and knees; effort to lift head Moro: extension and abduction of arms; partial flexion and adduction **Active Movement** Vigorous kicks during more prolonged awake status; progressively more purposeful and reciprocal movements that involve flexion of trunk
35 wk	**Resting Posture** More consistent flexion in prone position **Response to Handling** Resistance to passive movements of knees and hips Purposeful head turns to either side when in prone position with head in midline Head righting and attempt to maintain head in alignment with body in pull-to-sit maneuver Supported stand: attempt to bear weight on legs and feet and to align head with upright body **Active Movement** Possibility of definite alert periods Movements of head and eyes less random and more purposeful
36 wk	**Resting Posture** Wide variety of resting postures Flexor tone domination in trunk and extremities **Response to Handling** Ability to elicit all newborn primary reflexes; Moro reflex complete; leg recoil brisk Resistance of knee extension and hip adduction Efforts to align head with body during pull-to-sit maneuver Pull into flexion with trunk and legs in prone position Stepping and placing responses **Active Movement** Wide variety; movements more smooth and purposeful
40 wk	**Resting Posture** All four extremities held in flexion; flexor tone never as good as that of full-term infant **Response to Handling** Resistance to full extension of knees, hips, and shoulders

Pediatric Population

Continued

Table—cont'd

Age	Development (Creger and Browne)
40 wk —cont'd	**Response to Handling—cont'd** Recoil of arms within 2-3 sec after release by examiner; flexion of arms at elbows at an angle of <100° Less shoulder muscle tone than full-term infant; possible inability to maintain head alignment with body when pulled to sitting position Usual weight bearing on legs but possible inability to reciprocally step like full-term infant **Active Movement** Active movement smooth and purposeful Primary reflexes consistent and complete Less flexor hypertonicity (result being general greater range of movement of preterm infant equivalent to full-term infant)

Creger PJ: *Developmental interventions for preterm and high-risk infants: self-study modules for professionals,* Tucson, 1989, Therapy Skill Builders.

Neurobehavioral Development of Preterm Newborns by Gestational Age

Neurobehavioral system	Developmental behaviors
≤30 Wk Gestation	
Autonomic	Breathing irregular and mainly abdominal
	Eyelids fluttering; limbs twitching and tremoring in jerky movements
Motor	Reflex smiling and startle response present
	Muscle tone flaccid; little head control or back support; movements jerky
	Inability to coordinate sucking, swallowing, and breathing
State	Little state differentiation; alert or drowsy states fleeting, not robust
	Sleep states predominating, with sleep frequently in restless undifferentiated state
	Rapid eye movement apparent, as is continuous tonguing and mouthing
	Waking periods occurring only in brief intervals
Attention and interaction	Visual acuity poor, with little accommodation
	Ability to fixate and follow face (not common)
	Apnea possible when visual stimuli present
	Hearing well developed; preference for mother's voice possible
Self-regulation	Easily stressed by environmental stimuli

Modified from Case-Smith J, Allen AS, Pratt PN, editors: *Occupational therapy for children,* ed 3, St Louis, 1996, Mosby.

Table—cont'd

Neurobehavioral system	Developmental behaviors
≤32 Wk Gestation	
Motor	Overall increase in motor tone with more flexion apparent
	Smooth motor movements evident
	Improved head control evident
State	Regular episodes of active and quiet sleep
	Active sleep decreasing as quiet sleep increasing
	Movements sporadic in active sleep
	Increase in alert awake time with decrease in drowsy state
34-36 Wk Gestation	
Autonomic	Color changes accompanying most stimulation
Motor	Beginning coordination of sucking, swallowing, and breathing apparent
	Head control incomplete
	Beginning of leg and trunk support noted when infant held upright
State	Quiet sleep distinguished by slow, regular respiration and limited body movement
	Overall, less random activity
	Active sleep and quiet sleep clearly defined and alternating regularly
	Awakening to stimulation, but awake state brief
	Crying states more frequent in response to discomfort, pain, or hunger
Attention and interaction	Ability to fixate up to 15 sec on visual stimulus
	Turning or widening of eyes as brief response to auditory stimulation
Self-regulation	Possibility of overarousal when stimulated
	Possible consolation through swaddling or stroking
	Hand-to-mouth maneuvers possible
37-40 Wk Gestation	
Motor	Possible self-support when placed upright
State	All states of consciousness evident
	Quiet sleep increasing with equal periods of active sleep
	Crying more closely approximating that of full-term newborn
Attention and interaction	Longer periods of alertness and evident alertness to sound possible
	Preferences for visual stimuli evident; tracking of objects

Pediatric Population

Reflex Development in Preterm Newborns

Gestational age (wk)	Palmar grasp	Galant	Rooting	Sucking	Gag and swallow
23-24	Slight, latent	Strong	Incomplete reflex	Arrythmic, brief reflex	Absent reflex
25-26	Improving	Strong	Slight reflex; yawn, upper lips and sides	Improving reflex	Absent reflex
27-28	Localized	Strong	Yawn, three phases, no lower lip	Chewing motions	Tongue protrusion
30	Less latent; vigorous in fingers and wrists	Strong	Incomplete fourth phase; poor head extension	Improved synchrony	Suck and swallow not coordinated with breathing
32	Stronger; traction beginning	Strong	Complete, intense, long lasting	Active, good reflex	Active, fair reflex
35	Firm, effective; head not following traction	Strong	Perfect; head extension still weak	Better reflex; expression of hunger	Better reflex
37	Vigorous, except for neck	Strong	Perfect; weak head extension	Reflex like that of full-term newborn	Reflex like that of full-term newborn

Modified from Case-Smith J, Allen AS, Pratt PN, editors: *Occupational therapy for children,* ed 3, St Louis, 1996, Mosby.

Moro	Plantar grasp	Automatic walking	Crossed extension	Doll's eye	Placing
Minimal (hand only)	Absent	Absent	Absent reflex	Absent	Absent
Better; slight upper-extremity extension	Constant	Trace	Questionable reflex	Absent	Absent
Present; upper-extremity extension, no abduction	Constant	Improving	Contralateral defense reaction	Absent	Absent
Vigorous, easily elicited	Constant	Improving	Improved reflex	Absent	Absent
Complete; abduction and extension of upper extremities	Constant	Present; tiptoes	Good flexion and extension; abduction beginning	Beginning	Absent
Complete, brisk	Constant	Present; not sustained	Reflex more like that of full-term newborn	Present	Weak
Perfect	Constant	Automatic; full plantar support	Complete reflex; toe fanning beginning	Present	Appearing

Characteristics of Preterm Newborns

Age	Muscle tone	Posture	Facial features	Hair and nails
Extremely preterm (25-30 wk)	Extreme hypotonicity	Lies with all extremities in full extension	Well defined, except cartilage unformed and ears able to be folded	Early hair (lanugo) forming over most of body; healthy scalp hair
Moderately preterm (31-36 wk)	Hypotonicity; some beginning flexor tone palpable and visible at rest	Lies with all extremities in moderate extension	Well defined; ear cartilage beginning to form	Fingernails and toenails present
Almost full term (37-38 wk)	Moderate flexor tone at rest	Lies with some flexion of extremities	Well defined	Lanugo and much of scalp hair possibly falling out, fingernails and toenails possibly ready for trimming
Full term (39-42 wk)	Strong physiological flexion	Lies with strong flexion of all extremities	Well defined	Lanugo and much of scalp hair possibly falling out; fingernails and toenails possibly ready for trimming

Modified from Ratliffe KT: *Clinical pediatric physical therapy*, St Louis, 1998, Mosby.

Age	Genitals	Skin	Head shape
Extremely preterm (25-30 wk)	Poorly developed Female: outer labia not covering inner labia and clitoris Males: scrotum small and smooth; testicles undescended	Thin, translucent with wrinkles; veins apparent; dusky-red color at birth	Skull bones thin and malleable; head often becoming elongated and flattened when exposed to gravity and uneven pressure
Moderately preterm (31-36 wk)	Undeveloped Females: outer labia not covering inner labia and clitoris Males: scrotum small and smooth; testicles undescended	Thin but more opaque; more fat under skin but still wrinkled	Skull bones thin and malleable; head often becoming elongated and flattened when exposed to gravity and uneven pressure
Almost full term (37-38 wk)	More fully developed Females: outer labia covering inner tissues Males: testicles possibly descending to fill scrotum	Opaque; healthy layer of fat under skin	Skull bones thicker in older preterm newborn; head shape not as typical of earlier preterm newborn
Full term (39-42 wk	Fully developed	Opaque; chubby appearance	Skull bones relatively round and shaped by more even pressure of uterus

Continued

Table—cont'd

Age	Movements	Behavior	Sleep
Extremely preterm (25-30 wk)	Jerky; unorganized	Poor state control; overwhelmed by sensory stimuli most of time	Sleep characterized by restlessness and occupies most of time
Moderately preterm (31-36 wk)	Jerky, unorganized but better controlled than in extremely preterm newborn	Poor state control; habituation to aversive or repetitive stimuli beginning	Sleep more quiet but still occupies most of time
Almost full term (37-38 wk)	More controlled; less excursion than in preterm preterm newborn	Emerging state control; ability to calm self newborn	Sleep mostly quiet; brief periods of wakefulness
Full term (39-42 wk)	Mostly smooth	Variable state control; possible ability to calm self	Sleep mostly quiet; brief periods of wakefulness

Modified from Ratliffe KT: *Clinical pediatric physical therapy,* St Louis, 1998, Mosby.

Common Medical Problems of Preterm Newborns and Infants

Problem	Description	Potential associated disorders of developmental significance
Respiratory		
Respiratory distress syndrome	Respiratory disorder that affects immature lungs and is characterized by grunting, retractions, nasal flaring, tachypnea, and cyanosis	May require prolonged mechanical ventilation that results in decreased movement, decreased stimulation or interaction, and decreased parent-infant interaction; associated with an increased incidence of neurodevelopmental deficits in infants who require prolonged ventilation resulting from respiratory complications; possible abnormal tone and movement patterns (for example, increased trunk and neck extension, shoulder retraction, decreased shoulder girdle stability); may be associated with secondary feeding problems
Atelectasis	Incomplete expansion of lungs at birth resulting from poor development of lung tissue and weak respiratory muscles	
Hyaline membrane disease	A respiratory disorder in which an inadequate amount of pulmonary surfactant lines the terminal respiratory units of the mature fetal lung; results in subsequent inadequate fetal lung development	

Modified from Pratt PN Allen AS: *Occupational therapy for children,* ed 2, St Louis, 1989, Mosby.

Table—cont'd

Problem	Description	Potential associated disorders of developmental significance
Respiratory— cont'd		
Bronchopulmonary dysplasia	A chronic lung disease characterized by abnormal development of the lung and bronchi that occurs in many survivors of respiratory therapy for hyaline membrane disease	Increased incidence of hospitalization secondary to lower-respiratory infections; increased incidence of asthma and asthmalike conditions
Meconium aspiration	Inspiration of meconium, a fetal fecal substance passed during delivery when hypoxia occurs; may result in obstruction of the airway, interference with gas exchange, and respiratory distress	
Apnea	The transient cessation of breathing	
Cardiovascular		
Patent ductus arteriosus	Failure of the fetal heart openings to close; most common cause of congestive heart failure in newborns	Inadequate nutrition resulting from fluid restriction; risk of chronic pulmonary abnormalities with prolonged ventilation
Hemorrhage	Bleeding resulting from deficiency of several clotting factors in the blood, combined with the fragility of the capillary walls (especially in small vessels as in the brain), and leading to intraventricular or intracranial bleed	Neurological insults and subsequent neurodevelopmental deficits
Metabolic		
Hyperbilirubinemia	An excess of bilirubin (a red bile pigment) in the blood, which creates the appearance of jaundice	Neurological deficits in severe cases
Metabolic acidosis	A pathological condition resulting from accumulation of acid or loss of base in the body; characterized by decreased pH	Jitteriness, neurological deficits in severe cases
Hypocalcemia	Reduction of the blood calcium below normal	Jitteriness, convulsions
Hypoglycemia	An abnormally diminished content of glucose in the blood	Hyperirritability, jitteriness, apnea, cyanosis, irregular respiration, convulsions

Pediatric Population

Continued

Table—cont'd

Problem	Description	Potential associated disorders of developmental significance
Nutritional and Gastrointestinal		
Necrotizing enterocolitis	An acute superficial necrosis of the mucosa of the small intestine and colon characterized by profound shock and dehydration	Long-term feeding problems and behavioral complications
Temperature Regulation		
Subnormal body temperature	Results from poor heat production or increased heat loss; cold exposure possibly causing an increased metabolic rate and oxygen consumption with subsequent acidosis, apnea, hypoglycemia, and pulmonary hemorrhage	Possible neurological deficits in severe cases
Immunity		
Pneumonia	Inflammation of the lungs	Respiratory distress, temperature instability, acidosis, poor feeding, lethargy, seizures, potential hearing loss secondary to ototoxic antibiotic medication
Septicemia	Presence in the blood of bacterial toxins	
Meningitis	Inflammation of meninges of the brain	
Urinary tract infection	Infection of the urinary tract	
Ophthalmological		
Retrolental fibroplasia	Characterized by the presence of opaque tissue behind the lens, leading to retinal detachment and arrest of eye growth; generally attributed to use of high concentrations of oxygen in the care of the preterm newborn	Myopia, strabismus, poor central acuity, retinal detachment, blindness, problems with depth perception

Modified from Pratt PN Allen AS: *Occupational therapy for children*, ed 2, St Louis, 1989, Mosby.

Additional Common Medical Problems of Preterm Newborns and Infants

Problem	Description	Potential associated disorders of developmental significance
Neurological		
Asphyxia	Anoxia and increased carbon dioxide tension in blood and tissues	Abnormal tone, poor interactive skills, irritability, feeding problems, decreased spontaneous movement, cerebral palsy, mental retardation, developmental disabilities, and related problems
Intraventricular hemorrhage	Bleeding into the ventricles of the brain	
Seizure	Abnormal electrical activity in the brain	
Congenital Anomalies		
Trisomy	Presence of an additional chromosome of one type in an otherwise diploid cell, as in Down syndrome	Abnormal muscle tone, mental retardation
Limb deficiency	Absence at birth of a portion of one or more extremity	Temporary movement and functional disorders
Cleft lip or palate	Longitudinal opening or fissure (occurring in the embryo) in the lip or palate	Feeding problems, speech difficulties
Tracheal-esophageal fistula	Abnormal passage or communication between trachea and esophagus	Feeding problems
Birth Weight		
Small for gestational age	Weight for age falling in the 0 to 10th percentile range	Impaired attachment process; jittery, irritable
Large for gestational age	Weight for age falling in the 90th to 100th percentile range	Frequently poor tone
Birth Trauma		
Head injury	Damage to the cranium or underlying structures	Neurological sequelae, depending on nature of injury
Nerve injury	Damage to neural tissues	Temporarily impaired movement
Fracture	A break or crack in bone	
Other		
Substance abuse (maternal)	Use of narcotics or other illegal drugs or the overuse of prescription medications by the mother	Jitteriness, irritability, impaired attachment
Failure to thrive	Inability of infant to gain weight and sustain life	Feeding or behavioral problems, abnormal muscle tone and head growth, developmental delay

Pediatric Population

Modified from Pratt PN, Allen AS: *Occupational therapy for children*, ed 2, St Louis, 1989, Mosby.

Stress Versus Stability

Signs of stress	Signs of stability
Thrashing or grimacing in sleep	Well-defined sleep states
Abrupt state changes	Gradual state changes
Periods of extremely increased or decreased alertness	Alertness
Fussiness	Self-quieting behavior
Color changes from pink to mottled to gray	Pink color
Irregular breathing	Regular breathing
Whimpering or weak cries	Strong cries
Seizure activity	Absence of seizure activity
Hiccuping, gagging, or spitting up	Absence of hiccuping, gagging, or spitting up
Blank stares	Focused gazes
Panicked expressions	Cooing and smiling
Finger splays, trunk arching, and fisting	Controlled posture
Fluctuating tone	Consistent tone
Uncontrolled movements	Controlled movements

FREQUENTLY ENCOUNTERED PEDIATRIC PROBLEMS

Many disabilities and impairments that develop later in the life cycle originate during infancy and childhood. Effective management of these disabilities and impairments requires early recognition and intervention. By detecting these problems as early as possible and providing appropriate interventions, therapists minimize functional limitations.

Asthma

Asthma is a condition in which the airways become hypersensitive to irritants, resulting in contraction of the muscles that control airway diameter, inflammation of the mucous membranes, and increased production of mucous. All of these problems lead to breathing difficulties and bouts of wheezing that vary in severity. A variety of environmental factors and genetic predispositions are known to cause asthma. The condition is treated through medication, avoidance of trigger factors, and a healthy lifestyle that includes monitored exercise.

Triggers or Irritants of Childhood Asthma

Trigger or irritant	Examples
Exercise	Running, team sports; swimming being the least asthma-provoking form of exercise
Infections	Respiratory infections (bacterial and viral), colds, sinus infections
Allergies	Outdoor allergens (pollens, molds), indoor allergies (house dust, feathers, molds, pets), foods (milk, soy, eggs)
Irritants	Cigarette smoke, air pollution, strong odors, aerosol sprays, paint fumes
Weather	Cold air, weather that allows proliferation of molds or pollens
Emotions	Emotional responses that triggers deep breathing such as laughing, crying, yelling, anger, frustration, anxiety

Modified from Ratliffe KT: *Clinical pediatric physical therapy,* St Louis, 1998, Mosby.

Clinical Estimation of Severity for Children with Asthma Attacks

	Respiratory rate	Level of alertness	Ability to speak	Accessory muscle use	Psychological state	Skin color
Mild	Normal to 30% higher than normal*	Alert	Speaking clearly in full sentences	Mild use of inter-costal muscles	Normal to mildly anxious	Normal
Moderate	30% to 50% higher than normal	Alert	Speaking in phrases or short sentences	Moderate use of intercostal muscles, chest hyperinflation, use of sternocleido-mastoid and neck muscles	Moderately anxious	Normal to pale
Severe	More than 50% higher than normal	Possibly decreased	Speaking in single words or short phrases	Clear retractions, use of all accessory muscles, nasal flaring, chest hyperinflation	Severely anxious	Pale; may exhibit some blueness (cyanosis) around mouth and nail beds

Modified from Ratliffe KT: *Clinical pediatric physical therapy*, St Louis, 1998, Mosby.
*Normal respiratory rates vary for children, with younger children having higher rates. A rule of thumb in breaths per minute is as follows:
Newborns and infants up to 1 yr: 30-35
Toddlers 1-4 yr: 23-29
School-age children 5-11 yr: 19-22
Adolescents 12 yr+: 16-18

Pediatric Population

Burns

Although burns may result from contact with thermal, electrical, chemical, or radioactive agents, thermal burns are most common in children. Small children generally encounter hot water or hot beverage scalds, whereas older children more commonly come in contact with flames. Prognostic indicators for children with burns include the percentage of body area involved (Figure 2-6) and the classification of the burn. Debridement, exercise programs, positioning, and splinting are important interventions therapists may use with children who have sustained burns.

Classifications of Burns

| | Partial thickness | | | Full thickness | Full thickness plus Underlying tissue |
| | Superficial | | Deep | | Char |
	1st degree	2nd degree		3rd degree	4th degree
Depth of Burn	Superficial skin only	Epidermis and small part of dermis	Epidermis and deeper portion of dermis	All of epidermis and dermis	Epidermis, dermis and under-lying structures of fat, muscle, and bone
Appearance	Red, dry; blanches with pressure	Red blisters, moist; blanches with pressure	Marbled white, red, mottled; blisters	White, brown-black, dry, tough; no blanches with pressure	White, brown-black, dry, tough; no blanches with pressure
Sensation	Pain	Extreme pain	Extreme pain	No pain or temperature sensation	No pain or temperature sensation
Type of Burn	Sunburn, brief scald	Scald, flash flame	Scald, flash flame	Flame, contact with hot object	Flame, contact with hot object

Modified from Ratliffe KT: *Clinical pediatric physical therapy*, St Louis, 1998, Mosby.

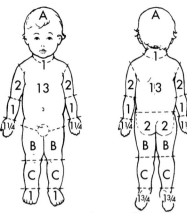

Relative percentages of areas affected by growth

AREA	BIRTH	AGE 1 YR	AGE 5 YR
A = ½ of head	9½	8½	6½
B = ½ of one thigh	2¾	3¼	4
C = ½ of one leg	2½	2½	2¾

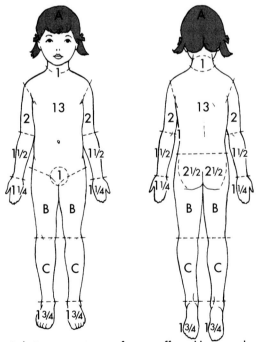

Relative percentages of areas affected by growth

AREA	AGE 10 YR	AGE 15 YR	ADULT
A = ½ of head	5½	4½	3½
B = ½ of one thigh	4½	4½	4¾
C = ½ of one leg	3	3¼	3½

FIGURE 2-6 Estimation of total body surface area in children. (From Wong DL: *Whaley and Wong's nursing care of infants and children,* ed 5, St Louis, 1995, Mosby.)

Common Splints for Burns Crossing Joints

Joint or body area	Optimal position	Potential contracture	Splint or position
Anterior neck	Neutral flexion and extension	Cervical flexion	Neck conformer—maintains chin-to-chest distance No pillow in bed
Posterior neck	Neutral flexion and extension	Cervical extension	Neck conformer—maintains length in posterior neck Pillow in supine position Pillow under chest in prone position
Anterior chest	Shoulder retraction	Shoulder protraction	Body jacket with neck conformer No pillow in supine position, shoulder abduction and external rotation
Axilla	Shoulder abduction	Shoulder adduction	Airplane splint—maintains shoulder in abduction
Anterior elbow	Extension	Elbow flexion	Posterior splint
Anterior wrist and hand	Neutral wrist flexion and extension, extension and abduction of fingers	Wrist and hand and finger flexion	15° wrist extension splint, finger troughs for finger abduction
Posterior wrist	Neutral flexion and extension of wrist	Wrist extension	15° wrist flexion splint
Anterior hip	Extension	Hip flexion	Prone positioning Supine position with hip and knee extended, externally rotated, and abducted; pillow under hips for increased extension
Posterior knee	Extension	Knee flexion	Posterior knee splint No pillow under knees in supine position
Posterior or anterior ankle	Neutral flexion and extension	Ankle plantar flexion or dorsiflexion	Ankle foot orthosis at 90° Anterior ankle conformer

Modified from Ratliffe KT: *Clinical pediatric physical therapy,* St Louis, 1998, Mosby.

Cancers

Cancers, characterized by uncontrolled proliferations of cells, are responsible for more children's death than any other cause except injuries. Although cancer strikes all age groups, childhood cancers are more active than adulthood cancers; at the time of diagnosis 80% of children have cancers that have spread to other sites, compared with 20% of adults. In addition, the types of cancers common to childhood differ from those adults more often experience. Cancers of the lungs, colon, breast, prostate, and pancreas are more common in adults, whereas cancers of the blood, brain, bones, muscles, and nervous system more frequently affect children. Medical interventions include radiation therapy, chemotherapy, surgery, and bone marrow transplants.

Types of Pediatric Cancers

Type	Total pediatric cancers (%)
Leukemia	39
Brain and nervous system	22
Lymphomas (cancers of the lymph system)	10
Kidney	6
Bone	6
Soft tissue (muscle)	5
Other	12
TOTAL	100

Modified from Ratliffe KT: *Clinical pediatric physical therapy*, St Louis, 1998, Mosby.

Pediatric Population

Types of Nervous System Tumors in Children

Type of tumor	Symptoms	Prognosis	Treatment
Astrocytoma Affects almost half of children with brain tumors; two major types			
Cerebellar: Comprise about 10%–20% of childhood CNS tumors	Ataxia, clumsiness, awkward gait, vomiting, headache, irritability, personality changes, fatigue, anorexia	70%–90% cure rate	Surgery
Supratentorial: Comprise about 35% of childhood CNS tumors	Visual disturbances, seizures, headaches, vomiting, irritability, personality changes, fatigue, anorexia	75%–85% cure rate for low grade, lower for high grade	Surgery, radiation, chemotherapy
Medulloblastoma Affects about 15% of children with CNS tumors; usually occurs in the cerebellum	Ataxia, headache, vomiting, irritability, personality changes, fatigue, anorexia	50% cure rate; highest for low grade, lower for high grade	Surgery, irradiation
Brain Stem Glioma Affects about 15% of children with CNS tumors	Cranial nerve dysfunction, gait disturbances	Poor prognosis	Irradiation
Ependymoma Affects 5%–10% of children with CNS tumors	Seizures, ataxia, clumsiness, hemiparesis, hydrocephalus in infants, headache, vomiting, irritability, personality changes, fatigue, anorexia	50% cure rate	Surgery, irradiation
Craniopharyngioma Affects 6%–9% of children with CNS tumors	Visual disturbances, headaches, vomiting, endocrine disturbances	Benign tumor	Surgery, irradiation (if necessary)
Neuroblastoma Arises in the sympathetic nervous system, with common sites being adrenal glands or paraspinal ganglions; affects young children	Pain, abdominal mass, persistent diarrhea, bone pain, pallor, weakness, irritability, anorexia, weight loss	75% for children younger than 1 year, 50% for children older than 1 year; may spontaneously regress	Surgery, chemotherapy, irradiation (if necessary)

Cancer Interventions and Residual Effects

Treatment	Types of cancer	Side effects, residual effects
Surgery	Brain and nervous system tumors Lymphomas (Hodgkin's disease, non-Hodgkin's lymphoma) Kidney Bone (osteosarcoma) Soft tissue tumors	Amputation, limb deficiency Poor wound healing Infection Poor body image
Irradiation	Leukemia (some CNS prophylaxis) Brain and nervous system tumors Lymphomas (Hodgkin's disease, non-Hodgkin's lymphoma) Kidney Bone (Ewing's sarcoma) Soft tissue tumors	Impairment of intellectual function Impairment of motor function Delayed or deficient growth Hormonal dysfunction Decreased fertility or sterility Skeletal deformities, including scoliosis, leg length discrepancy, skull and facial disfigurement Osteoporosis Pathological fractures Dental caries Postirradiation somnolence 5-8 wk after CNS irradiation and for 4-15 days (fever, nausea, vomiting, anorexia)
Chemotherapy	Leukemia Brain and nervous system tumors Lymphomas (Hodgkin's disease, non-Hodgkin's lymphoma) Kidney Bone Soft tissue tumors	Infection Bleeding Anemia Nausea, vomiting Anorexia Mucosal ulceration Severe constipation Foot drop, weakness, numbing of extremities Jaw pain Alopecia (hair loss) Hemorrhagic cystitis
Immunotherapy	Leukemia	Similar to chemotherapy
Bone marrow transplantation	Leukemia	Infection Skin breakdown Delayed wound healing Death

Modified from Ratliffe KT: *Clinical pediatric physical therapy,* St Louis, 1998, Mosby.
CNS, Central nervous system.

Pediatric Population

Cerebral Palsy

Cerebral palsy refers to a group of conditions that produce neurological and motor deficits in developing children as a result of brain damage. Although cerebral palsy occurs in a variety of patterns, motor involvements, and severities, the impaired ability to maintain normal posture is characteristic of all those with the condition. Medical management includes medications that address spasticity and seizures, orthopedic surgeries that help correct deformities and improve comfort and function, and dorsal rhizotomies that help decrease spasticity. Bracing and splinting of the lower and upper extremities are vital to the reduction of deformities and the optimization of functions.

Cerebral palsy is classified according to the evaluator's preference. Some individuals classify the condition based on quality of muscle tone, whereas others use the pattern of motor expression or area of brain involvement. Other evaluators prefer to use the less complicated, more subjective classification that is based on severity. The following table presents the four major cerebral palsy classification systems and their possible categories.

Classifications of Cerebral Palsy

Quality of muscle tone	Pattern of motor expression	Area of brain involvement	Severity
Hypotonic	Whole-body involvement	Generalized	Mild or Moderate or Severe
Rigid			
Ataxic		Extrapyramidal Cerebellar	
Fluctuating tone, athetoid, dystonic		Extrapyramidal Basal ganglia	
Spastic, hypertonic	Monoplegia	Pyramidal Motor tracts	
	Diplegia, paraplegia		
	Hemiplegia		
	Triplegia		
	Quadriplegia		
Mixed		Multiple areas	

Modified from Ratliffe KT: *Clinical pediatric physical therapy,* St Louis, 1998, Mosby.

Comparison of Clinical Signs for Hypotonic, Hypertonic (Spastic), and Athetoid Cerebral Palsy

	Characteristics	Distribution	Range of motion	Risk for contractures and deformities
Hypo-tonicity	Low, floppy, "rag doll"	Generalized, symmetrical	Excessive range, too much joint movement; stiffness caused by lack of movement in older children	Risk for dislocation (jaw, hip, atlantoaxial joint), risk for contractures caused by lack of movement in older children
Hyper-tonicity	High—spastic, stiff, rigid	Generalized, often asymmetrical	Limited range; contractures developing with age	Risk for contractures (flexor), dislocation (hip), deformities (scoliosis, kyphosis)
Athetosis	Fluctuating, writhing, constantly moving	Generalized, possibly asymmetrical	Full range of motion resulting from constant movement through range	Risk for deformities (scoliosis, lordosis), risk for joint contractures if spasticity and athetosis both present

Modified from Ratliffe KT: *Clinical pediatric physical therapy,* St Louis, 1998, Mosby.

Continued

Pediatric Population

Table—cont'd

	Deep tendon reflexes	Integration of primitive reflexes	Achievement of motor milestones	Influence of body position
Hypo-tonicity	Weak	Weak display of reflexes, sometimes delayed integration	Delayed (amount of delay corresponding to severity of hypotonicity)	Tone remaining same
Hyper-tonicity	Abnormally strong	Often delayed integration, possible obligatory reflexes	Delayed (amount of delay corresponding to severity of hypertonicity)	Tone fluctuating with change in body position
Athetosis	Abnormally strong	Often delayed integration, possible obligatory reflexes	Delayed (amount of delay corresponding to severity of tone deviations)	Tone fluctuating with change in body position

Modified from Ratliffe KT: *Clinical pediatric physical therapy,* St Louis, 1998, Mosby.

Consistency of muscles	Respiratory problems	Speech problems	Feeding problems
Soft, doughy	Shallow breathing, choking because of weakness in pharyngeal muscles	Shallow breathing, difficulty sustaining voice sounds	Weak gag reflex, open mouth, protruding tongue, poor coordination of swallowing and breathing
Hard, rocklike	Decreased thoracic mobility, limited inspiration and expiration	Dysarthria secondary to hypertonicity in oral muscles	Abnormally strong gag reflex, tongue thrust, bite reflex, rooting reflex
String, elastic	Decreased thoracic mobility and shallow breathing related to poor control of respiratory muscles	Dysarthria secondary to poor motor control in oral muscles	Abnormally strong gag reflex, tongue thrust, poor coordination of oral muscles for chewing and swallowing

Pediatric Population

Overview of Lower-Extremity Orthotics and Splints

Splints	Materials	Indications	Benefits	Precautions
Orthotics				
Dynamic ankle-foot orthotics	Polypropylene	Neuromuscular disorder	Produce even pressure distribution through contours Varying degrees of ankle support Holds forefoot and hindfoot in alignment	Monitor splint fit as child grows to prevent skin breakdown.
Dynamic ankle-foot orthotics with free plantar flexion	Polypropylene	Mild or severely abnormal lower-extremity tone	Allows dorsiflexion and plantar flexion Allows maximal lower leg contact during crawling Does not interfere with balance reactions	Monitor splint fit as child grows to prevent skin breakdown.
Solid-backed dynamic ankle-foot orthotics	Polypropylene	Inability to place voluntary foot flat during stance	May eliminate hyperextension of knee Keeps heel down in splint May prevent shortening of calf muscles	Observe for redness and poor skin tolerance.
Floor reaction brace	Polypropylene	Crouch gait caused by weakness (myelodysplasia)	Blocks ankle dorsiflexion Permits easy donning and doffing Encourages hip and knee extension	Child experiences poor intrinsic foot control. Brace does not work well for children with crouch gait because of high tone (spastic diplegia).
Splints				
Resting splints	Low temperature Thermoplastics Polypropylene	Plantar flexion contracture not managed by daytime splinting	Provide prolonged stretch on soft tissues Can be worn at night Promote static standing	Splint is not designed for ambulation.
Foot orthotics	Polyethylene foam Polypropylene	Hypotonicity Hypermobility of feet with good control of muscle activity	Support weight-bearing surface of foot Help with balance Improve mild discrepancies in alignment	Device does not control spastic foot or help with foot that fixes into a poorly aligned position.

Splints	Materials	Indications	Benefits	Precautions
Static				
Dorsal resting hand splint Volar resting hand splint	Low-temperature thermoplastics	Cerebral palsy Head injury Arthrogryposis Limb deficiency Juvenile rheumatoid arthritis Burns Trauma	Costs little Features lightweight design Provides durability Features attractive design Helps maintain comfort Provides broad contact area (decreased pressure) Can be easily remolded	Monitor splint fit as child grows to prevent skin breakdown. Prolonged use may produce joint stiffness.
Static thumb index webspace splint	Low-temperature thermoplastics	Cerebral palsy Head injury Spasticity Fisted thumb	Inhibits spastic muscles Maintains range for thumb opposition Places thumb in functional position	Monitor splint edges around thumb because this can be area of increased pressure.
Semidynamic				
Sof-Splint Joe Cool thumb splint Good Samaritan splint Neoprene webspace splint Benik Corporation thumb abduction splint	Neoprene Neoplush	Marked thumb adduction Cerebral palsy Webspace tightness Increased tone in hand Limited active use of thumb Excessive thumb joint mobility	Allows controlled arc of motion Provides stable and functional thumb position Can be fabricated quickly and easily Costs little Allows sensory exposure of hand Prevents too much pressure because of elasticity	Do not use with fixed deformity, bony changes, or strong flexion pattern at wrist. With Neoprene webspace splint, skin must be monitored closely because it has poor ventilation.
Dynamic				
Orthokinetic wrist splint MacKinnon splint	Low-temperature thermoplastics Dowel Straps Latex tubing	Spastic cerebral palsy Hemiplegia with fixed posture of upper extremity	Inhibits spastic flexor muscles Facilitates extensor muscles Encourages bilateral hand use	Device should not be used for children with fisted hands, cortical thumb, or severe radial or ulnar deviation.

Pediatric Population

Modified from Ratliffe KT: *Clinical pediatric physical therapy*, St Louis, 1998, Mosby.

Cystic Fibrosis

Cystic fibrosis is an inherited disorder characterized by an impermeability of the body's epithelial cells to chloride, which causes the exocrine glands to produce thick secretions that ultimately block the lungs, digestive tract, and pancreatic ducts. The blockage leads to serious pulmonary disease, infection, pneumothorax, and right ventricular hypertrophy. Children with cystic fibrosis exhibit persistent coughing, respiratory retractions (Figure 2-7), clubbing of the fingers and toes, and barrel-shaped chests. Medical management includes antibiotics for multiple infections, expulsion of secretions (Figures 2-8 and 2-9), and lung transplants.

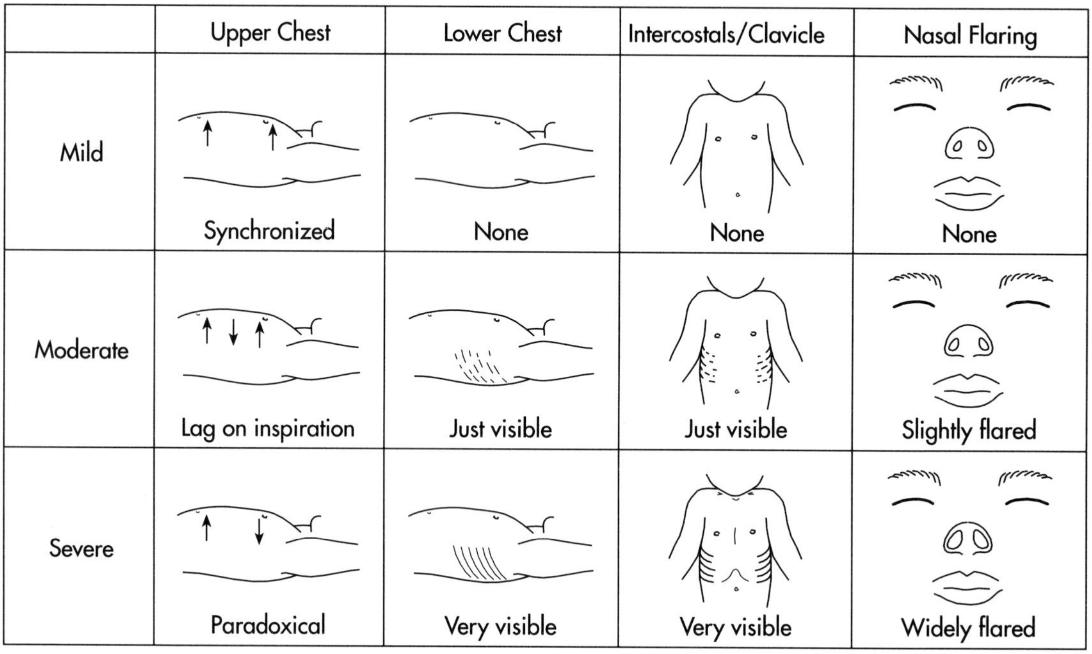

	Upper Chest	Lower Chest	Intercostals/Clavicle	Nasal Flaring
Mild	Synchronized	None	None	None
Moderate	Lag on inspiration	Just visible	Just visible	Slightly flared
Severe	Paradoxical	Very visible	Very visible	Widely flared

FIGURE 2-7 Respiratory retractions. (From Ratliffe KT: *Clinical pediatric physical therapy,* St Louis, 1998, Mosby.)

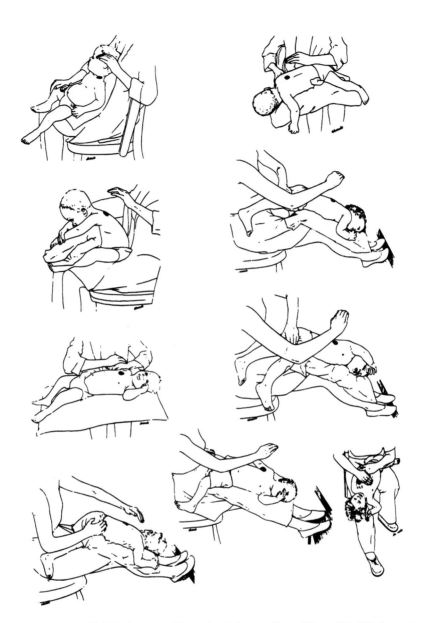

FIGURE 2-8 Bronchial drainage positions for infants. (From Wong DL: *Whaley and Wong's nursing care of infants and children,* ed 5, St Louis, 1995, Mosby.)

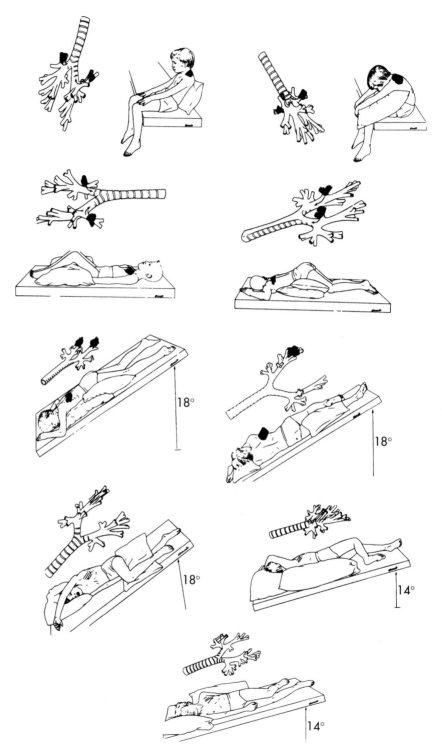

FIGURE 2-9 Bronchial drainage positions for children. (From Chernick V, editor: *Kendig's disorders of the respiratory tracts of children*, ed 5, Philadelphia, 1990, WB Saunders.)

Fractures

Fractures occur commonly in children as a result of injuries or pathological conditions. Because children's bones are more flexible and thinner than adults' bones, the fracture patterns also differ (Figure 2-10). Fractures involving epiphyseal plates are especially worrisome because these plates are the growth centers of bones; injuries in such spots can lead to permanent growth disturbances (Figure 2-11). Symptoms of fractures include inflammation, erythema, pain, deformity, and muscle guarding. Immediate intervention and correction of bone alignment is imperative in the prevention of permanent deformities resulting from serious fractures (Figure 2-12).

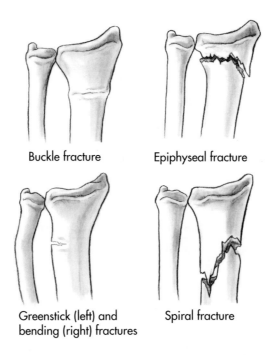

Buckle fracture   Epiphyseal fracture

Greenstick (left) and Spiral fracture
bending (right) fractures

FIGURE 2-10 Common fracture patterns in children. (From Ratliffe KT: *Clinical pediatric physical therapy,* St Louis, 1998, Mosby.)

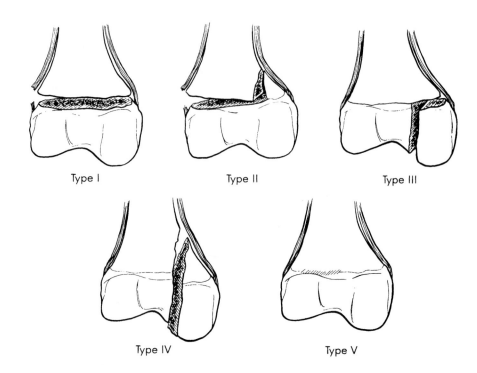

Salter-Harris Classifications of Epiphyseal Plate Injuries

Type	Injury and growth effects	Mechanism
I	Complete separation of epiphysis along plate; growing cells remain with plate	Shearing force
II	Complete separation of epiphysis with fracture into metaphysis; growth cells remain with plate	Bending and shearing forces
III	Incomplete separation along epiphyseal plate, fracture through epiphysis; growth cells not damaged	Intraarticular
IV	Fracture through epiphysis, through plate, and into metaphysis	Intraarticular
V	No separation or fracture, but epiphysis and plate have received severe blow sufficient to interrupt growth	Crushing force through epiphysis

FIGURE 2-11 Salter-Harris classifications of epiphyseal plate injuries. (Modified from Case-Smith J et al: *Occupational therapy for children*, ed 3, St Louis, 1996, Mosby.)

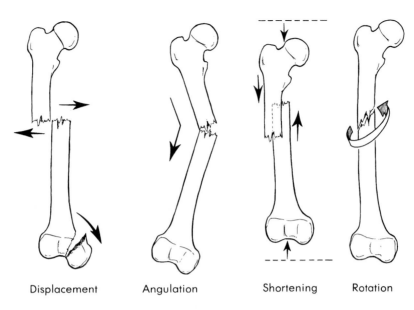

| Displacement | Angulation | Shortening | Rotation |

FIGURE 2-12 Deformities caused by fractures. (From Case-Smith J et al: *Occupational therapy for children,* ed 3, St Louis, 1996, Mosby.)

Genetic Disorders

Genetic disorders occur when genes mutate or duplicate incorrectly during cell division. The results of such disorders include genetic defects, which are expressed as chromosome abnormalities, or defects in specific genes. Chromosome abnormalities result in incorrect numbers of chromosomes (for example, Down Syndrome), sex chromosome deviations (for example, Klinefelter syndrome), or partial deletions (for example, cri du chat syndrome). Specific gene defects are autosomal dominant defects (for example, osteogenesis imperfecta), autosomal recessive defects (for example, sickle cell anemia) (Figure 2-13), and sex-linked defects (for example, fragile X syndrome). The effects of and interventions for genetic disorders vary depending on the type of disorder.

Pediatric Population

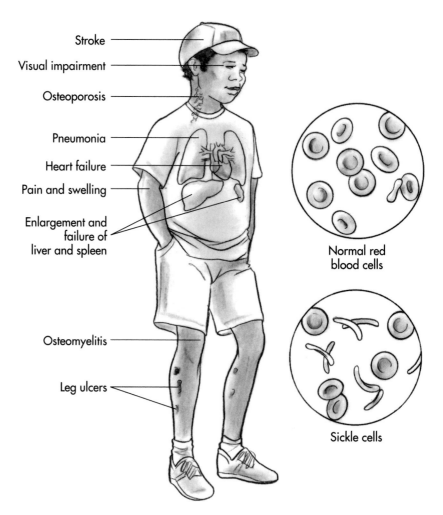

FIGURE 2-13 Differences between normal and sickled blood cells. (From Ratliffe KT: *Clinical pediatric physical therapy,* St Louis, 1998, Mosby.)

Typical Clinical Symptoms of Genetic Disorders

Type of disorder	Name of disorder	Clinical features
Chromosome Abnormalities		
Deviation in number of chromosomes	Down syndrome (trisomy 21)	Characteristic facial features, including flat occiput, flat face, upward slanting eyes; hypotonicity; broad, short feet and hands; protruding abdomen; mental retardation; possible cardiac anomalies
	Edwards syndrome (trisomy 18)	Small stature, long and narrow skull, low-set ears, hypotonicity, rocker-bottom feet, scoliosis, profound mental retardation
	Patau syndrome (trisomy 13)	Microcephaly, cleft lip and palate, polydactyly of hands and feet, severe to profound mental retardation
Deviation in sex chromosomes	Turner syndrome (XO syndrome)	Congenitally webbed neck, growth retardation, ptosis of upper eyelids, lack of sexual development, congenital heart and kidney disease, scoliosis, low normal intelligence
	Klinefelter syndrome (XXY)	Long limbs; tall and slender build until adulthood, when obesity becomes problem (if no testosterone replacement therapy); small penis and testes; low average to mild mental retardation; tremors; behavior problems
Partial deletion syndrome	Cri du chat syndrome (5p-)	High-pitched, catlike cry in infancy; microcephaly; low-set ears; hypotonicity; severe mental retardation; scoliosis; clubfeet; dislocated hips
	Prader-Willi syndrome (15q-)	Low tone with feeding disorder in infancy; insatiable appetite in toddlerhood; moderate mental retardation; hyperflexibility; obesity; characteristic facial features, including almond-shaped eyes; small stature; small hands and feet; small penis
	Williams syndrome (deletion near elastin gene on chromosome 7)	Characteristic facial abnormalities, including prominent lips, medial eyebrow flare, and open mouth; mild microcephaly; mild growth retardation; short nails; mild to moderate mental retardation; cardiovascular anomalies

Continued

Modified from Ratliffe KT: *Clinical pediatric physical therapy,* St Louis, 1998, Mosby.

Pediatric Population

Table—cont'd

Specific Gene Defects

Type of disorder	Name of disorder	Clinical features
Autosomal dominant	Neurofibromatosis	Areas of hyperpigmentation or hypopigmentation of skin, including "café au lait" spots or axillary "freckling;" tumors along nerves and in connective tissue, eyes, or meninges; macrocephaly; short stature; possible skeletal abnormalities, including scoliosis, bowing of long bones, and dislocations
	Tuberous sclerosis	Brain lesions causing seizures and mental retardation, skin lesions on cheeks and around nose, "café au lait" spots; cystlike areas in bones of fingers, kidney and teeth abnormalities
	Osteogenesis imperfecta	Type I: Small stature, thin bones, bowing of bones, fractures of long bones, hyperextensible joints, kyphoscoliosis, flat feet, thin skin, deafness in adult life, blue sclerae of eyes, blue or yellow teeth. Type II: Prenatal growth deficiency, short limbs, multiple fractures, hypotonia, hydrocephalus, frequent early death. Type III: Short stature, bowing and angulation of long bones, multiple fractures, kyphoscoliosis. Type IV: Osteoporosis leading to fractures, variable mild deformity of long bones, normal sclerae of eyes, possibility of poor teeth
Autosomal recessive	Spinal muscular atrophy	Progressive muscle atrophy and weakness; normal intelligence; normal sensation; weakness beginning before birth, in early childhood, or in late childhood
	Sickle cell disease	Group of diseases characterized by blood disorders related to hemoglobin defects; mostly seen in people of African or infrequently of Mediterranean descent; sickle-shaped red blood cells causing anemia and crises of blockages in veins, causing a variety of conditions, including leg ulcers, arthritis, acute pain, and problems in major organ systems (spleen, liver, kidney, bones, heart, and central nervous system); children possibly exhibiting weakness, pain or fever, or growth retardation
	Hurler syndrome	Normal or rapid growth during first year, with deterioration during second year; coarse facial features characterized by full lips, flared nostrils, thick eyebrows, low nasal bridge, and prominent forehead; stiff joints; small stature; small teeth, enlarged tongue; kyphosis, short neck; clawhand, hip dislocation and other joint deformities; mental retardation

Phenylketonuria	Inability to metabolize phenylalanine; causes mental retardation, growth retardation, hypertonicity, seizures, pigment deficiency of hair and skin if left untreated; successful treatment through limitation on amount of phenylalanine in diet

Sex-Linked Disorders (Boys Only)

Fragile X syndrome	One of most common causes of mental retardation in boys; characteristic facial features including elongated face, large ears, and prominent jaw; enlarged testicles in adulthood; prolapse of the mitral valve in the heart; mental retardation usually severe, sometimes with aggressive behavior; some boys exhibiting poor coordination and hypotonia
Duchenne muscular dystrophy	Progressive weakness beginning between 2 to 5 years; characteristic gait disturbances, including toe walking, abducted gait, lordosis, waddling gait; progressive weakness leading to wheelchair use, decreased independence in all areas, and eventual death from respiratory or cardiac failure
Lowe syndrome	Progressive mental deterioration, leading to moderate to severe mental retardation; renal dysfunction; cortical cataracts, with or without glaucoma, leading to blindness later in life; hypotonicity; joint hyperextensibility; growth retardation; large low-set ears; pale skin; and blond hair
Lesch-Nyhan syndrome	Moderate to severe mental retardation; hypertonicity, leading to dislocated hips; club foot; growth retardation; movement disorders, including chorea, ballistic movements, and tremor; characterized by self-mutilating behaviors, including lip-biting and fingertip-biting

Pediatric Population

Modified from Ratliffe KT: *Clinical pediatric physical therapy*, St Louis, 1998, Mosby.

Effect of Onset of Osteogenesis Imperfecta

Type	Severity	Effect
Fetal	Most severe	Fractures occur in utero and during birth. Mortality is high.
Infantile	Moderately severe	Many fractures occur in early childhood. Severe limb deformities and growth disturbances also develop.
Juvenile	Least severe	Fractures begin in late childhood. By puberty, bones often begin to harden and fewer fractures occur. Dental problems may be present.

Modified from Case-Smith J, Allen AS, Pratt PN, editors: *Occupational therapy for children,* ed 3, St Louis, 1996, Mosby.

Hearing Loss

Hearing loss affects many children to some degree. Early detection can help minimize future problems. Therapists who work closely with children must recognize signs of hearing loss and their functional consequences. Using devices that help enhance hearing (for example, aids and amplifiers), following guidelines that help improve communication, and learning the manual alphabet (Figure 2-14) or some basic sign language (Figure 2-15) together allow the therapist to work effectively with hearing-impaired children.

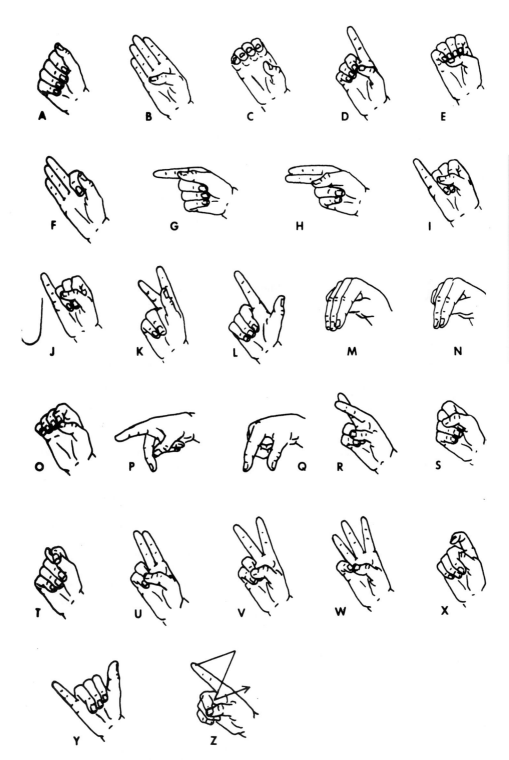

FIGURE 2-14 American one-hand manual alphabet. (From Case-Smith J et al: *Occupational therapy for children,* ed 3, St Louis, 1996, Mosby.)

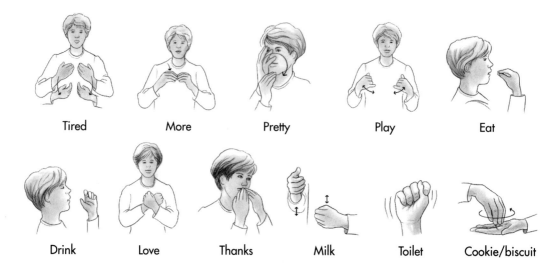

FIGURE 2-15 Basic sign language for children. (From Ratliffe KT: *Clinical pediatric physical therapy,* St Louis, 1998, Mosby.)

Signs That Indicate Possible Hearing Loss

Possible hearing impairment must be considered in the following instances:

- A newborn does not exhibit a startle (Moro) reflex in response to a sharp clap 3 to 6 feet away.
- A 3-month-old child has not developed auditory-orienting responses as indicated by not becoming alert to toys that make noise.
- An 8- to 12-month-old child does not turn to a whispered voice.
- An 8- to 12-month-old child does not turn to sounds, such as a rattle 3 feet to the rear.
- A 1-year-old child does not understand a variety of words, such as "bye-bye" and "doggie."

- A 2-year-old child does not use words.
- A 2-year-old child cannot identify an object with a verbal clue alone, such as "Show me the ball."
- A 3-year-old child has largely unintelligible speech.
- A 3-year-old child omits beginning consonants.
- A 3-year-old child does not use two- and three-word sentences.
- A 3-year-old child uses mostly vowel sounds.
- A child of any age speaks in a voice that is too loud, too soft, of poor quality, or of a quality that does not fit the child's age and sex.
- A child always sounds as if suffering a cold.

Modified from Case-Smith J, Allen AS, Pratt PN, editors: *Occupational therapy for children,* ed 3, St Louis, 1996, Mosby.

Effects of Hearing Loss on Function

Hearing level (decibel)	Degree of loss	Type	Missed sounds	Effect	Intervention
16-25	Slight	Conductive, sensorineural	10% speech sounds	Misses fast-paced peer interactions, experiences fatigue in listening	Hearing aid or FM system, seating in front, antibiotics, myringotomy
26-40	Mild	Conductive, sensorineural	25%–40% speech sounds, distant sounds, unvoiced consonants, plurals, and tenses	Misses 50% of class discussion, has problems suppressing background noise	Seating in front, hearing aid or FM system, language therapy, antibiotics, myringotomy
41-55	Moderate	Conductive, sensorineural	50%-80% speech sounds	Exhibits articulation deficits, limited vocabulary, learning dysfunction	Hearing aid or FM system, resource help, speech-language therapy, speech reading
56-70	Moderate-severe	Sensorineural or mixed	100% speech information	Demonstrates delayed language, syntax, atonal voice, reduced speech intelligibility	Full-time amplification, special education class, speech-language therapy
71-90	Severe	Sensorineural or mixed	All speech sounds; can hear loud environmental noises	Exhibits undeveloped or deteriorated speech, learning deficits	Full-time program for deaf, signing or total communication, amplification
>90	Profound	Sensorineural or mixed	All speech and other sounds; feels vibration	Demonstrates same as above	Same as above, cochlear implant

Modified from Anderson KI, Matkin ND: Hearing conservation in the public schools revisited, *Semin Hearing* p. 12, 1991.

Suggestions for the Use of Total Communication

1. Face the child squarely at eye level.
2. Position yourself so that the child can see your face and hands at the same time without strain.
3. Make sure you have the child's attention.
4. Avoid light behind you. If the child has to look into the light, your lips may not be clearly visible.
5. Use a normal tone of voice. Do not exaggerate mouth movements; this practice may confuse the lipreader.
6. Speak the word and give the sign at the same time, not in sequence.
7. Use appropriate pauses between words, especially when using finger spelling.
8. Sit close to the child, rather than across the room, to obtain better results.
9. Keep instructions simple and to the point.
10. Be consistent, especially with the young child.
11. Above all, talk to the child, who needs the same amount of input as a hearing child, although the method may be altered.

Modified from Case-Smith J, Allen AS, Pratt PN, editors: *Occupational Therapy for Children,* ed 3, St Louis, 1996, Mosby.

Hip Dysplasias

A hip dysplasia is a condition that occurs in the developing hip when abnormal growth of the acetabulum or proximal femur occurs as a result of hip joint malalignment. Signs of hip dysplasias include asymmetrical groin or buttock folds or movements of the femur in and out of the acetabulum with manual traction or femoral shortening (Figure 2-16). Ortolani's sign is one screening test therapists can use to detect hip dysplasias. A positive result on this test may indicate some type of hip dysplasia. Bracing or splinting, traction, casting, or surgical interventions often are necessary in the effective management of such conditions.

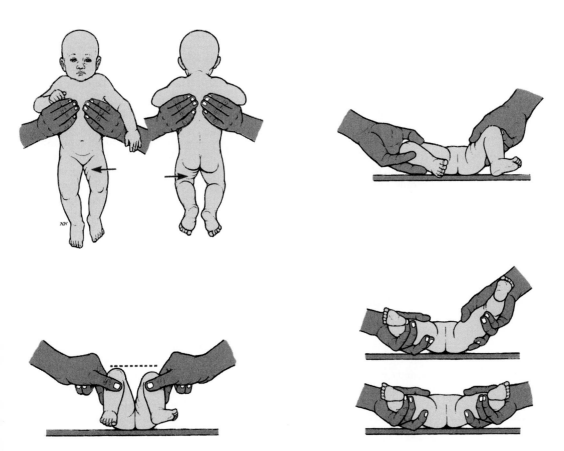

FIGURE 2-16 Signs of developmental hip dysplasia. (From Wong D: *Wong and Whaley's clinical essentials of pediatric nursing*, ed 5, St Louis, 1997, Mosby.)

Types of Developmental Dysplasia of the Hip in Infancy

Type	Definition	Treatment considerations
Complete	The acetabulum may be shallow or small, with poor lateral borders. Acetabular dysplasia may occur alone or with any level of femoral deformity or displacement.	The hip must be kept abducted and flexed with the femoral head centered in the acetabulum. In this position the acetabulum continues to deepen, maintaining a correct shape, and the ligaments and joint capsule tighten to provide extra joint stability.
Subluxatable	The femoral head can be partially displaced to the rim of the acetabulum. It slides laterally, but not all the way out of the socket.	
Dislocatable	The femoral head is in the socket, but it can be displaced completely outside the acetabulum with manual pressure.	
Dislocated	The femoral head lies completely outside the hip socket but can be reduced with manual pressure.	
Teratologic	The femoral head lies completely outside the hip socket and cannot be reduced with manual pressure. Deformity of the joint surfaces is significant and usually related to another severe developmental anomaly, such as arthrogryposis or myelomeningocele.	Surgery is needed to reconstruct the joint. Pain may accompany some hip movements, and the child likely may suffer significant limitation in some ranges of motion (most likely abduction and extension).

Modified from Ratliffe KT: *Clinical pediatric physical therapy*, St Louis, 1998, Mosby.

Handling Strategies for Children in Spica Casts

Turning

1. Use proper body mechanics, getting up on the bed if necessary, to turn the child.
2. Seek help. Usually two people are needed to safely turn a child who weighs more than 50 pounds (with the cast) in a spica cast.
3. Make sure that the child knows what will happen and is ready. Initially the child may be in significant pain. Think about premedicating the child 30 minutes before turning.
4. The child should be turned as one unit, in a "log roll." Do not twist the child's trunk during the turn.
5. Do not use the cast as a lever when turning the child. The cast should be grasped firmly, with attention paid to prevention of excessive pressure through the legs when turning the child.
6. The child should be positioned (if in supine position) with pillows under the head and shoulders and possibly under the legs until the child is comfortable after being turned. If the child is in the prone position, pillows should be placed under the abdomen and chest. Make sure the edges of the cast are not digging into the child. Make sure any diapers are positioned appropriately to avoid accidents.

Lifting

1. Use proper body mechanics to lift the child.
2. Obtain the help of another individual or a mechanical lift if the child weighs more than 50 pounds (with the cast).
3. Always plan the lift thoroughly before actually lifting the child. Know how to lift, where the hand holds will be, where the child is going, and the reason for the lift.
4. Always get the child to help, even if the child is only counting in preparation for the lift.
5. For a two-person lift, the individual at the head is always in charge. This individual ensures the environment is safe and the other(s) are ready and initiates the count.

Positioning

Supine. The head and shoulders should be supported with pillows. If the child is in a bed, a trapeze should be set up to allow the child independent weight shifts and assist with transfers.

Positioning—cont'd

The legs may need to be elevated slightly with pillows.
Prone. Pillows should be placed under the child's chest and abdomen, with a small pillow under the head. The head of the bed may be elevated or the child may be placed on a wedge to allow the child to see the environment more easily.
Side-lying. Full side-lying position is not possible in a spica cast; however, in either the prone or supine position, the child may and should be placed in a partial side-lying position. Pillows should be placed under one side of the child and cast to prop the child in a partial side-lying position. Make sure that the child and the cast are aligned and not twisted.

Mobility

Small child. An adult reclining wheelchair, with the legrests removed and possibly the armrests too, works well. Make sure antitippers are in place to prevent the chair from falling over backward because of the posterior shift in the center of gravity.

A wagon, lawn cart, or automobile scooterboard may be adapted to position and transport a child in a spica cast. A dolly (for carrying heavy boxes) or tilt table are also acceptable mobility devices. Beware of the width of the cast and the narrowness of doorways.

A gurney or special cart may be used to transport a child in a spica cast. This type of device takes a lot of room and is almost impossible to transport in a car.
Larger child. A hospital bed provides the most stable positioning and greatest potential mobility in the house for a larger child in a spica cast. An older child always should have a trapeze attachment on the bed frame to assist with transfers, bed mobility, and turning. The trapeze also helps maintain upper-extremity strength and range of motion.

Another option is an adult wheelchair with elevating legrests and a wide board across the leg rests to support the width of the cast. The cast may need to be tied loosely to the frame of the wheelchair to prevent it from falling.

Because transferring is so difficult with a large child, floor-level mobility devices, such as scooterboards, are not recommended.

Modified from Ratliffe KT: *Clinical pediatric physical therapy,* St Louis, 1998, Mosby.

Pediatric Population

Common Surgical Hip Procedures for Children

Type of surgery	Disorder	Explanation
Myotomy	Cerebral palsy	Soft tissue releases, usually of the adductor muscles, can reduce abnormal pressures that cause subluxation and potential dislocation of the femoral head.
Fixation in situ	Slipped capital femoral epiphysis	A pin is driven through the femoral neck into the femoral head to stabilize the head on the neck.
Proximal femoral derotation osteotomy	Cerebral palsy	The femoral head is rotated to decrease the angle of anteversion. This procedure usually is done with a varus osteotomy.
Proximal femoral varus osteotomy	Developmental dysplasia of the hip Legg-Calvé-Perthes disease Cerebral palsy	A wedge is cut out of the femoral neck so that the neck-to-shaft angle is reduced (the neck sticking out more from the shaft). The femur has increased stability because it can be seated more directly in the acetabulum with less tendency to slide out.
Innominate pelvic osteotomy	Developmental dysplasia of the hip Legg-Calvé-Perthes disease Cerebral palsy	If the acetabulum faces more anteriorly and laterally than normal, the hip is not stable in a normal weight-bearing position. This procedure rotates the acetabulum so that it faces more downward and provides more stability for the femoral head during weight bearing.
Pemberton pelvic osteotomy	Developmental dysplasia of the hip Legg-Calvé-Perthes disease Cerebral palsy	The acetabulum is deepened and rotated downward to provide more stability to the femoral head. This procedure is used for the younger child with a shallow, dish-shaped acetabulum.

Modified from Ratliffe KT: *Clinical pediatric physical therapy*, St Louis, 1998, Mosby.

Muscular Dystrophies

Muscular dystrophies describe conditions that change the biochemistries and structures of muscle cells, resulting in muscle weakness and deformities. Muscular dystrophies occur in three major patterns: limb-girdle, facioscapulohumeral, and pseudohypertrophic (Figure 2-17). Pseudohypertrophic, or Duchenne's Muscular Dystrophy, is the most common form of this condition in children and predominately affects boys. Early signals include tripping, falling, fatigue, and Gowers' sign (Figure 2-18). Medical interventions include surgical procedures, bracing, medications, and therapy.

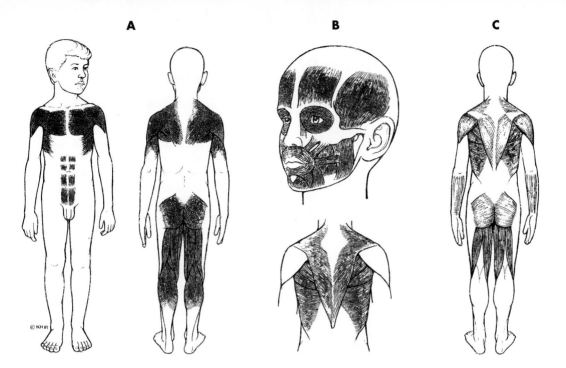

FIGURE 2-17 Initial muscle groups involved in muscular dystrophies. A, Pseudohypertrophic. **B,** Facioscapulohumeral. **C,** Limb-girdle. (From Wong DL: *Whaley and Wong's essentials of pediatric nursing,* 4th ed, St Louis, 1993, Mosby.)

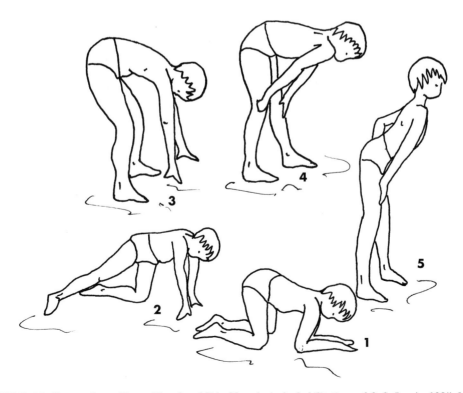

FIGURE 2-18 Gower sign. (From Umphred DA: *Neurological rehabilitation,* ed 3, St Louis, 1995, Mosby.)

Common Types of Muscular Dystrophy in Childhood

Type	Age of onset and mechanism of inheritance	Typical clinical progression
Congenital myotonic	Birth (autosomal dominant)	Hypotonia, severe mental retardation, speech disturbances, spinal deformities, muscle weakness and other problems associated with myotonic dystrophy, frequent early death, born to mothers with myotonic dystrophy
Duchenne's (pseudohypertrophic)	1-5 yr (X-linked)	Progressive weakness from proximal to distal muscles, loss of walking skills by preteen years, progressive loss of other self-care skills, death by late teens or twenties from respiratory or cardiac causes
Becker	5-10 yr (X-linked)	Similar to Duchenne's but much slower progression, walking until late teens, death in adult life from respiratory compromise
Facioscapulohumeral	Variable from infancy to adulthood (autosomal dominant)	Characterized by facial weakness and shoulder girdle weakness, possible hearing or visual problems, wide clinical spectrum
Limb-girdle	Adolescence to adulthood (autosomal recessive)	Progressive weakness of proximal muscles of shoulder and hip girdle, variable age of onset and progression, lower-extremity disability preceding upper-extremity disability
Myotonic	Adolescence (autosomal dominant)	Muscle weakness, delay in relaxation time of muscle, stiffness, distal weakness often occurring before proximal weakness, cardiac problems, cataracts, and endocrine problems

Modified from Ratliffe KT: *Clinical pediatric physical therapy,* St Louis, 1998, Mosby.

Physical Therapy Interventions by Age of Child

Age	Clinical features	Physical therapy interventions
Birth to 2 yr	Possibly learning to walk late	Monitor developmental and functional skills, strength, and range of motion
3-5 yr	Falling; toe walking; clumsiness; reluctance to run; hypertrophy in calves and deltoids; weakness of neck flexors, abdominals, and shoulder and hip extensor muscles; Gower's sign	Teach family range of motion; of gastrocsoleus and tensor fascia lata groups, positioning, and a general exercise program, such as swimming; monitor strength and range of motion
6-8 yr	Toe walking, lordosis, lack of reciprocal arm swing, inability to climb stairs without support, fatigue, limited ambulation distance, walk exhibiting wide-based gait, trendelenberg, inability to rise from floor without help	Implement a general exercise program, such as swimming; monitor strength and range of motion; consult with family and school on how to modify activities to avoid fatigue; develop standing and walking program; teach breathing exercises; consult with physical education instructor for range-of-motion program in school; prescribe night splints for ankles; monitor spinal alignment
9-11 yr	Walking with braces, possible tenotomy surgeries to prolong ambulation or surgery to stabilize scoliosis, respiratory insufficiency, beginning scoliosis, possible loss of ambulation skills without surgery or braces	Fit and prescribe knee-ankle-foot orthoses; prescribe and teach to use Rollator walker or parapodium or reciprocating gait orthosis; develop program to integrate walking into school activities; use intervention before and after surgery for strengthening and gait training; develop breathing exercises; use manual wheelchair for longer distances with appropriate seating and positioning supports; consider motorized scooter for independent seated mobility; provide range of motion and positioning, monitor scoliosis and limb contractures
12-14 yr	Loss of ambulation skills; increasing respiratory difficulty; obesity; increasing contractures at hips, knees, ankles and elbows; progression of scoliosis; osteoporosis; dependent transfers, increasing need for assistance in activities of daily living	Continue with standing program as long as possible; manage obesity and contractures; use power wheelchair for independent mobility; instruct family and school on use of mechanical lifting device (Hoyer or other); recommend commode chair, shower chair, other equipment, as needed; work with teacher and other team members to develop positioning in classroom and access to computer to facilitate academic work

Modified from Ratliffe KT: *Clinical pediatric physical therapy*, St Louis, 1998, Mosby.

Pediatric Population

Table—cont'd

Age	Clinical features	Physical therapy interventions
15-17 yr	Dependence in many activities of daily living, possible need for assisted ventilation, increased respiratory compromise	Use adapted equipment to assist with activities of daily living, including a ball-bearing feeder; develop regular schedule and method for pressure relief and monitor skin; adapt power or manual chair for mechanical ventilation, if indicated; teach family-assisted coughing, breathing exercises, and postural drainage; monitor respiratory function and consider mechanical or power-control bed; use comfort mattress, such as air flow or alternating pressure pad; work with child, family and team to assist in planning vocational goals for child
18+ yr	Need for assisted ventilation, dependence in all activities of daily living, death after period of declining respiratory function	Adapt controls of power chair to sip and puff or other control that is accessible to individual with Duchenne's muscular dystrophy; perform skin care, manage contractures, positioning, and consultation regarding access to higher-educational or vocational activities; provide support to individual and family; provide family information about accessible transportation for family and child

Modified from Ratliffe KT: *Clinical pediatric physical therapy*, St Louis, 1998, Mosby.

Seizures

Seizures occur when the brain's electrical system malfunctions, resulting in periods of inappropriate behavior, unusual motor or sensory activity, or lapses in consciousness. Pathological conditions, fever, and unknown sources can cause seizures, which vary significantly depending on the type. Seizures can have long-lasting effects, especially in developing children. Medical interventions include medications and the prevention of serious injuries during seizure activity.

Classification of Seizures

International classification	Older terms	Manifestations
Generalized Seizure	Generalized seizure	Seizure generalized to the entire body; always involves the loss of consciousness
Tonicoclonic seizure	Grand mal seizure	Beginning with tonic contraction (stiffening) of the body, then changing to clonic movements (jerking)
Tonic seizure		Stiffening of the entire body
Clonic seizure	Minor motor seizure	Myoclonic jerks starting and stopping abruptly
Atonic seizure	Drop attack	Sudden lack of muscle tone
Absence seizure	Petit mal seizure	Nonconvulsive seizure with a loss of consciousness; blinking, staring, or minor movements lasting a few seconds
Akinetic seizure		Lack of movement, "freezing" in place
Partial Seizure	Focal seizure	Seizure not generalized to the entire body; variety of sensory and motor symptoms accompanying this seizure
Simple partial seizure	Jacksonian seizure	No loss of consciousness or awareness
With motor symptoms		Jerking beginning in one small part of the body and spreading to other parts; usually limited to one half of the body
With sensory symptoms		Sensory aura preceding motor seizure
Complex partial seizure	Psychomotor seizure	Loss of consciousness occurring during seizure, either at beginning or end of
	Temporal lobe seizure	episode; may develop from a simple partial seizure or into a generalized seizure; possible automatisms, such as lip smacking, staring, or laughing
Unclassified Seizure		Seizures that do not fit into the above categories, including some neonatal and febrile seizures

Modified from Ratliffe KT: *Clinical pediatric physical therapy,* St Louis, 1998, Mosby.

Pediatric Population

Spina Bifida

Spina bifida, also referred to as *myelomeningocele, neural tube defect, myelodysplasia,* or *congenital spinal cord defect,* occurs when the laminae of one or more vertebrae do not completely close during prenatal development. This incomplete closure can occur at any level along the spinal cord, but it most frequently affects the lumbosacral region of the spine (Figure 2-19). The degree of spinal cord involvement varies from an open spine with no cord involvement to protrusion of the meninges through the opening to herniation of the meninges and spinal cord (Figure 2-20). The level of impairment depends on the level and degree of spinal cord involvement. Medical management includes surgery to repair the herniations, reduce the risk of infection, and preserve the spinal nerves; medications to control seizures or infections; and therapy to facilitate development, prevent deformities, and optimize function. Surgical intervention also may be necessary to manage other complications of spina bifida, such as cleft palate, scoliosis, hip dysplasia, and hydrocephalus.

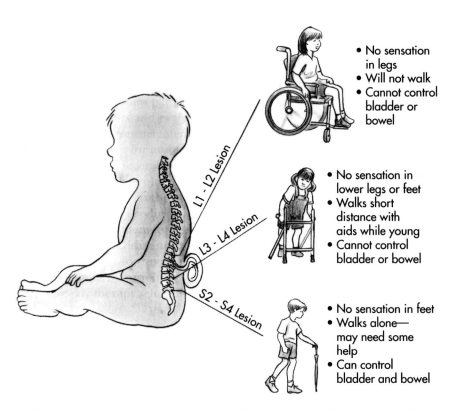

L1 - L2 Lesion
- No sensation in legs
- Will not walk
- Cannot control bladder or bowel

L3 - L4 Lesion
- No sensation in lower legs or feet
- Walks short distance with aids while young
- Cannot control bladder or bowel

S2 - S4 Lesion
- No sensation in feet
- Walks alone— may need some help
- Can control bladder and bowel

FIGURE 2-19 Levels of spinal cord defects. (Modified from Ratliffe KT: *Clinical pediatric physical therapy,* St Louis, 1998, Mosby.)

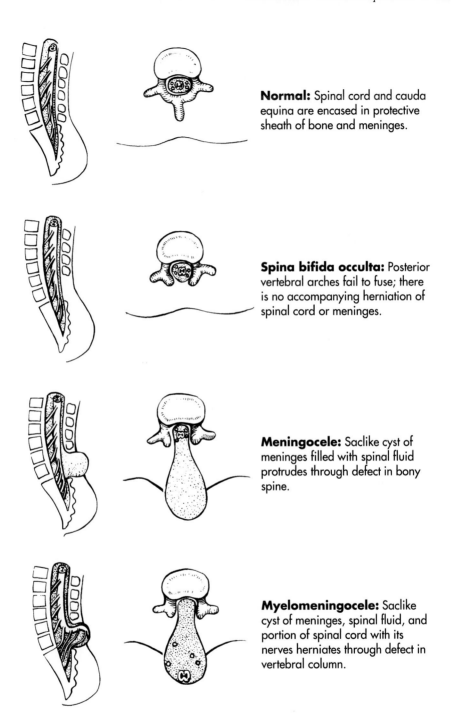

Normal: Spinal cord and cauda equina are encased in protective sheath of bone and meninges.

Spina bifida occulta: Posterior vertebral arches fail to fuse; there is no accompanying herniation of spinal cord or meninges.

Meningocele: Saclike cyst of meninges filled with spinal fluid protrudes through defect in bony spine.

Myelomeningocele: Saclike cyst of meninges, spinal fluid, and portion of spinal cord with its nerves herniates through defect in vertebral column.

Pediatric Population

FIGURE 2-20 Normal spine and three forms of spina bifida. (Modified from Whaley L, Wong D: *Nursing care of infants and children,* ed 2, St Louis, 1983, Mosby.)

Classification of Spina Bifida

Spinal defect	Neurological classification	Level of disability	Functional prognosis
Occulta (not visible)	No tissue protrusion from nonfused spinous processes	None	Usually no neurological or orthopedic problems (excellent)
Acculta (visible)	Meningocele—tissue protrusion in sac, but neurological tissue rarely involved	None	Usually no neurological or orthopedic problems (excellent)
	Myelomeningocele—abnormal neural elements part of protruding sac	Dependent on level of involvement	Innervation of neck, upper limb, shoulder girdle, and trunk musculature
		Thoracic level	No volitional lower limb movements present; for lesions below T10, possible weakness in lower trunk muscles; wheelchair for necessary mobility; development of hydrocephalus likely
		L1-2	Weak hip movements; possible dislocated hips; with assistive devices, such as a knee-ankle-foot orthosis, (crutches, walker), ambulation possible short distances, especially in young children, but wheelchair necessary for longer distances; no bowel and bladder control; development of hydrocephalus likely
		L3	Strong hip flexion and adduction; some knee extension, knee-ankle-foot orthosis and crutches necessary for household and short-distance community ambulation and wheelchair for longer distances, no bowel and bladder control, development of hydrocephalus likely

L4	Possibly active knee flexion and ankle dorsiflexion with stronger knee extension, community ambulation with ankle-foot orthosis, and crutches, development of foot deformities possible; wheelchair possibly necessary for long community distances; no bowel and bladder control; development of hydrocephalus less likely
L5	Weak hip extension and abduction, good knee flexion against gravity, weak plantar flexion with eversion, and strong dorsiflexion with inversion possibly leading to foot deformities; walking possible with no orthoses but crutches necessary for long distances because of fatigue; bicycle use possible; no bowel and bladder control, development of hydrocephalus less likely
S1	Improved hip stability leading to independent walking without support, weakness in hip abductors and plantar flexors leading to gait deviations, no bowel and bladder control
	Good ambulation with weak push-off and decreased stride length with rapid movement, possible impaired bladder and bowel control, foot orthoses possibly necessary for support

Modified from Ratliffe KT: *Clinical pediatric physical therapy*, St Louis, 1998, Mosby.

Pediatric Population

Spinal Curvatures

The normal spine displays slight cervical and lumbar lordosis and slight thoracic kyphosis. However, muscle imbalances, bone deformities, pathological conditions, and unknown causes produce excessive curves (Figure 2-21). Scoliosis, the lateral curvature of the spine, is one of the most common excessive spinal curves in children, especially girls. Appropriate screening (Figure 2-22) and early recognition are vital parts of successful management. Treatments include bracing, electrical stimulation, biofeedback, strengthening, and surgery.

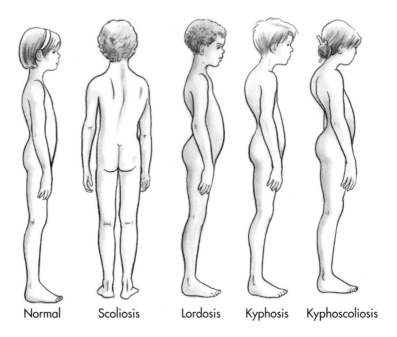

| Normal | Scoliosis | Lordosis | Kyphosis | Kyphoscoliosis |

FIGURE 2-21 Spinal curves. (From Ratliffe KT: *Clinical pediatric physical therapy*, St Louis, 1998, Mosby.)

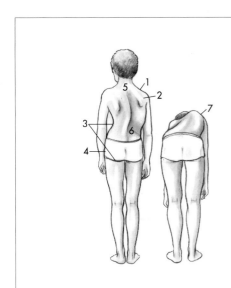

Standing

The child stands and faces away from examiner.

1. Assess symmetry of the shoulders. (Shoulder may be elevated on the convex side.)
2. Assess symmetry of scapulae and posterior rib cage. (Scapula may be high and rib cage may be prominent on the convex side of the curve.)
3. Assess symmetry of the waist and gluteal folds. (The waist may appear fuller on the convex side of the curve. Gluteal folds may be asymmetrical.)
4. Assess symmetry of the hips. (One hip may protrude.)
5. Drop plumb line from occiput to assess trunk alignment. (Plumb line may fall lateral to gluteal crease. If it falls over gluteal crease, check for a compensatory curve.)
6. Assess symmetry of spinous processes.

Bending Forward

The child bends forward from the waist as if to touch the ground. The arms should swing freely.

7. As the child bends forward, assess symmetry of the ribcage. (Rib hump may appear posteriorly on the convex side.)

FIGURE 2-22 Screening for scoliosis. (From Ratliffe KT: *Clinical pediatric physical therapy,* St Louis, 1998, Mosby.)

Pediatric Population

Categorization of Scoliosis

A. Age of Onset
Congenital: Birth to 3 years
Juvenile: 3 years to puberty
Adolescent: During or after puberty

B. Magnitude of Curve
Mild: 0-20 degrees
Moderate: 20-40 degrees
Severe: More than 40 degrees

C. Specifics of Curves
Direction: Right or left apex
Location: Cervical, cervicothoracic, thoracic, thoracolumbar, or lumber curves
Size: Minor or major curve
Number: Single or double curve

D. Type and Etiology of Curve

Type of curve	Etiology
Functional (also called postural, nonstructural) No structural changes Bending or postural correction *Structural* Changes in vertebrae and supporting tissues Decreased flexibility Rotation of vertebrae usually present Related changes to rib cage, pelvis, hips	Possible relation to poor posture Possible relation to musculoskeletal anomalies **Congenital** Malformation of vertebrae at 3 to 5 weeks of gestation *Neuromuscular (paralytic)* Association with neuromuscular diseases, such as cerebral palsy, muscular dystrophy, or myelomeningocele; diseases with orthopedic manifestations, such as arthrogryposis and osteogenesis imperfecta, also being included *Idiopathic* Cause unknown Possible familial tendency for scoliosis Prognosis varying with age of onset (variable) Most common form of scoliosis *Traumatic onset* Association with spinal fractures, irradiation, tumors, or metabolic disorders (rickets)

Modified from Ratliffe KT: *Clinical pediatric physical therapy,* St Louis, 1998, Mosby.

Common Surgical Procedures for Spinal Stabilization

Type of procedure	Description	Indication	Rehabilitation needs
Dwyer anterior fusion	Resection of a rib and cutting through of diaphragm to expose vertebrae; screws applied to each vertebra with wires between them to stabilize spine	Procedure only for low curves in thoracolumbar or lumbar areas	All procedures use bony fusion of spine with instrumentation to stabilize fusion. Most require postsurgical orthosis. Newer procedures allow children to get up within first few days of surgery and increase their activities gradually over first year. Physical therapy input includes: • Teaching child and family to use postsurgical orthosis • Teaching child and family body mechanics and functional skills, including getting in and out of bed, transfers, dressing, and ambulation • Teaching child and family general range-of-motion and strengthening exercises • Emphasizing importance of early ambulation • Monitoring fit and use of orthosis • Monitoring neurological signs and skin for stability of instrumentation
Zielke anterior fusion	Same description as Dwyer but newer procedure with better screws used with rods to stabilize segments	Procedure only for low curves in thoracolumbar or lumbar areas	
Harrington rod posterior instrumentation	Older procedure not often used; two rods attached by hooks to posterior spinal segments—distraction rod on concave side of curve and compression rod on convex side; no control of sagittal plane correction; postsurgical spine immobilization always required	Formerly standard procedure for spinal stabilization; currently infrequently used because of long rehabilitation time and poor correction in sagittal plane	
Cotrel-Dubousset posterior instrumentation	Two rods with compression and distraction hooks attached to pedicles or lamina of vertebrae; normal spinal curves in sagittal plane obtainable through contouring of rods; spinal orthosis after surgery possibly unnecessary in children who have idiopathic scoliosis with good correction	Commonly used for idiopathic scoliosis and neuromuscular scoliosis	
Luque procedure (posterior)	Two L-shaped rods attached to each level with wiring; good stabilization and allowance for lumbar lordosis and pelvic stability	Good procedure for children with poor bone, skin, or muscle quality; associated with higher risk for neurological damage	

Modified from Ratliffe KT: *Clinical pediatric physical therapy,* St Louis, 1998, Mosby.

Traumatic Brain Injuries

Traumatic brain injuries include injuries to the scalp, skull meninges, or brain and present major medical problems for children in the United States. These injuries are classified either as closed (injury causing no open or penetrating wound) or open (penetration or laceration occurring). Initial damage to the central nervous system is the result of impact or penetration, but secondary damage often also results from increased intracranial pressure, hematoma, inflammation of the brain, and embolus, to name a few, and such an injury often results in a coma. The degree of neurological development and prognosis for the return of function depends on the structures involved. Because children's brains still are developing, younger children have poorer prognoses than older children. Regardless of age, traumatic brain injuries often result in permanent cognitive and motor function impairments.

Pediatric Coma Scale

Category of assessment	Score	>1 yr	<1 yr	
Opening of eyes	4	Spontaneous response	Spontaneous response	
	3	Response to verbal command	Response to shout	
	2		Response to pain	
	1	Response to pain	No response	
		No response		
		>1 yr	**<1 yr**	
Best motor response	6	Obedience		
	5	Localization of pain	Localization of pain	
	4	Flexion withdrawal	Flexion withdrawal	
	3	Flexion—abnormal (decorticate rigidity)	Flexion—abnormal (decorticate rigidity)	
	2	Extension (decerebrate rigidity)	Extension (decerebrate rigidity)	
	1	No response	No response	
		>5 yr	**2-5 yr**	**0-23 mo**
Best verbal response	5	Orientation and conversation	Appropriate words and phrases	Appropriate smiles, coos, cries
	4	Disorientation and conversation	Inappropriate words	Cries
	3	Inappropriate words	Cries or screams	Inappropriate crying or screaming
	2			
	1	Incomprehensible sounds	Grunts	Grunts
		No response	No response	No response
TOTAL	3-15			

Modified from Wong DL and others: *Clinical manual of pediatric nursing,* St Louis, 1990, Mosby.

Pediatric Population

Brain Structures and Implications of Injury

Brain structure	Functions	Results after injury
Frontal lobes of cerebrum	Abstract thinking, recognition of cause-and-effect relationships, expressive language, basis for social interaction; posterior portion containing cells that control motor activity throughout body	Personality changes, altered intellectual functioning, memory deficits, language deficits, impaired motor skills
Parietal lobes of cerebrum	Appreciation of sensation, somatic (sensory) interpretation and integration	Language dysfunction, aphasia (inability to formulate and use symbols such as words), apraxia (inability to carry out on request complex or skilled movements); motor and sensory loss in lower extremities; atopognosia (inability to localize tactile stimuli)
Occipital lobe of cerebrum	Visual cortex, spatial orientation, visual recognition	Impaired vision, functional blindness
Temporal lobes of cerebrum	Reception and interpretation of stimuli for taste, vision, sound, smell; conversion of crude visual impressions into recognizable images, interpretation of images; primary speech, hearing, receptive language	Inability to interpret sensory stimuli, difficulty in understanding higher levels of meaning of body sensory experiences, aphasia (ability to formulate and use symbols such as words), hearing dysfunction
Cerebellum	Refinement and coordination of all muscle movements, including walking, talking, control of muscle tone, and balance	Dysmetria, ataxia, dysarthria (inability to form words), hypotonia, nystagmus, dystonia, tremors at rest
Basal ganglia	Unconscious or automatic control of lower motor centers; excitation causing inhibition of muscle tone throughout body	Movement disorders, including chorea, athetosis, dystonia, tremors at rest
Diencephalon (thalamus and hypothalamus)	Major relay station for sensory impulses to cerebral cortex, activation of cerebral cortex Vital control centers for involuntary functions (for example, blood pressure, satiety, hunger, rage, feeding, water conservation, temperature, sleep regulation, libido), secretion of tropic hormones	Impaired consciousness Alterations in vegetative functions, somnolence, coma, anorexia, loss of weight, fever, diabetes insipidus, loss of libido, endocrine disorders
Brain stem (mesencephalon, pons, and medulla)	All cranial nerves except I, eye movement, vital centers for respiration and vasomotor control	Impaired eye movement; deep, rapid, or periodic breathing; impaired function of facial muscles; flaccid muscle tone; absent deep tendon reflexes; no response to stimuli; impaired vital functions (for example, respiration, vasomotor control)

Modified from Ratliffe KT: *Clinical pediatric physical therapy,* St Louis, 1998, Mosby.

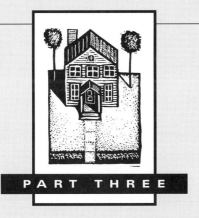

PART THREE

Adult Population

ADULT ENVIRONMENTAL EVALUATION

ADULT AFFECTIVE EVALUATION

ADULT ACTIVITIES OF DAILY LIVING SKILLS EVALUATION

ADULT MOBILITY EVALUATION

ADULT FINE MOTOR EVALUATION

ADULT NEUROLOGICAL EVALUATION

ADULT INTEGUMENTARY EVALUATION

ADULT CARDIOPULMONARY EVALUATION

ADULT ENVIRONMENTAL EVALUATION

Home situations set the tone for patient care. Some patients have ready access to reliable caregivers with excellent coping skills, active social support systems, and ideal home layouts. Other patients reside alone with minimal social support in homes requiring numerous adaptations to facilitate the rehabilitation process. Environmental evaluations provide valuable information about the home situations of patients, including caregivers' abilities and dynamics, informal caregiving availability, and physical environment safety and accessibility. Home care therapists use this information to distinguish the realistic abilities of informal caregivers more objectively and to determine the physical environmental adaptations required to assist the rehabilitation in the home. Associated caregiver guidelines offer referral suggestions for caregivers seeking varying levels of assistance to care for their loved ones. Associated environmental guidelines provide specifications for making homes accessible and suggestions for ameliorating common home safety hazards.

Caregiver Assessments
Caregiver Strain Index

The Caregiver Strain Index (CSI) is a screening tool that assesses the degree of caregiver strain. It examines the presence of potential stressors experienced by caregivers, such as confinement, inconvenience, and overwhelment. The CSI is a self- or therapist-administered tool. The total score ranges from 1 to 13. Higher scores denote a greater potential risk for and/or presence of caregiver strain.

Adult Population

CSI Form

	Yes = 1	No = 0
My sleep is disturbed because _____ is in and out of bed or wanders around at night.	_____	_____
It (caregiving) is inconvenient (e.g., because helping takes so much time or it's a long drive over to help).	_____	_____
It (caregiving) is a physical strain (e.g., because lifting in and out of a chair, effort, or concentration is required).	_____	_____
It (caregiving) is confining (e.g., helping restricts free time or cannot go visiting).	_____	_____
There have been family adjustments (e.g., because helping has disrupted routines or there is no privacy).	_____	_____
There have been changes in personal plans (e.g., had to turn down a job, could not go on vacation).	_____	_____
There have been other demands on my time (e.g., from other family members).	_____	_____
There have been emotional adjustments.	_____	_____
Some behavior is upsetting (incontinence or not being able to remember; care receiver accuses people of taking things).	_____	_____
It is upsetting to find that _____ has changed so much from his or her former self (e.g., is a different person than he or she used to be).	_____	_____
There have been work adjustments (e.g., because of having to take time off).	_____	_____
It (caregiving) is a financial strain.	_____	_____
(I am) feeling completely overwhelmed (e.g., because of worry about _____, concerns about how you will manage).	_____	_____
TOTAL SCORE (count yes responses)	_____	

Modified from Robinson B: Validation of a caregiver strain index, *J Gerontol* 38:345, 1983.

Cost of Care Index

The Cost of Care Index (CCI) is a case management tool that identifies actual or potential problem areas of families caring for older adults. It examines five areas of caregiving related to the "costs" of providing care to dependent older adults. These five areas include personal and social restrictions experienced by caregivers, physical and emotional health of caregivers, value that caregivers place in providing care, provocation by patients that may precipitate mistreatment by caregivers, and economic burden of care provision. The CCI is a self- or therapist-administered tool. The total score ranges from 20 to 80. Higher scores denote greater caregiver perception of personal costs.

CCI Form

	Strongly disagree	Disagree	Agree	Strongly agree
1. I feel that meeting the psychological needs of my elderly relative for feeling wanted and important is not worth the effort.	1	2	3	4
2. I feel that my elderly relative is an overly demanding individual to care for.	1	2	3	4
3. I feel that caring for my elderly relative has negatively affected my family or my physical health.	1	2	3	4
4. I feel that as a result of caring for my elderly relative I do not have enough time for myself.	1	2	3	4
5. I feel that caring for my elderly relative is causing me to dip into savings meant for other things.	1	2	3	4
6. I feel that meeting the health needs of my elderly relative is not worth the effort.	1	2	3	4
7. I feel that my elderly relative tries to manipulate me.	1	2	3	4
8. I feel that caring for my elderly relative has negatively affected my appetite.	1	2	3	4
9. I feel that caring for my elderly relative has put a strain on family relationships.	1	2	3	4
10. I feel that my family and I must give up necessities because of the expenses to care for my elderly relative.	1	2	3	4
11. I feel that caring for my elderly relative disrupts my routine in my home.	1	2	3	4
12. I feel that caring for my elderly relative has caused my family and me much aggravation.	1	2	3	4
13. I feel that meeting the daily needs of my elderly relative is not worth the effort.	1	2	3	4
14. I feel that caring for my elderly relative has caused me to be physically fatigued.	1	2	3	4
15. I feel that my family and I cannot afford those little extras because of the expenses to care for my elderly relative.	1	2	3	4
16. I feel that my elderly relative makes unnecessary requests of me for care.	1	2	3	4
17. I feel that meeting the social needs of my elderly relative for companionship is not worth the effort.	1	2	3	4
18. I feel that caring for my elderly relative has caused me to become anxious.	1	2	3	4
19. I feel that caring for my elderly relative interferes with my friends or friends of my family coming to my home.	1	2	3	4
20. I feel that caring for my elderly relative is too expensive.	1	2	3	4

Adult Population

Modified from Kosberg JI, Cairl RE: The cost of care index: a case management tool for screening informal care providers, *The Gerontologist* 26(3):273-278, 1986.

Stress Assessment Score of the Caregiver

The Stress Assessment Score of the Caregiver (SASC) evaluates the level of stress and strain experienced by caregivers. It examines potential caregiver stressors such as finances, personal medical and social history, and available support systems. The SASC is a therapist-administered tool. The total score ranges from 0 to 26. Higher scores denote greater presence of or risk for caregiver stress.

SASC Form

A. Personal Data Section (Caregiver)

Data	2 points	1 point	0 points	Score
Age	70 and over	45-69	Under 45	
Physical health	Poor	Good	Excellent	
Mental health	Poor	Good	Excellent	
Income	Under $7,000	$7,000-$14,000	$14,000 or more	
Dependents (not older adults)	2 or more	1	None	
SUBTOTAL: (A. Personal Data [sum of above, range 0 to 10])				

B. Stress Factors Section (Caregiver)

Scoring: 1 point for a "yes"; 0 points for a "no" or "don't know"	Score
Alcoholism or substance abuse?	
Mental retardation?	
History or observation of family violence?	
Change in lifestyle to assume care of older adult?	
Financial help from the older adult?	
Limited time for own personal activities?	
Personal stressors (i.e., marital problems, empty nest)?	
Staying at home, mostly or always (inability to leave older adult)?	
Absence of support system (family, friends, community)?	
Frustrations, resentment in care of older adult?	
Treatment of older adult as a child?	
Limited knowledge of the aging process?	
Belief that any care at home is better than nursing home?	
Minimization or denial of dependency toward the older adult?	
Show of dependency toward the older adult?	
Authoritative manner with the older adult?	
SUBTOTAL: (B. Stress Factors [sum of above, range 0 to 16])	
SASC (sum of subtotals A and B, range 0 to 26)	

Modified from Hamilton GP: Prevent elder abuse using a family system approach, *J Gerontol Nurs* 15(3):21-26, 1989.

Social Support Assessments
Abbreviated 23-Item Duke Social Support Index

The Abbreviated 23-Item Duke Social Support Index measures the type and quality of social support available to patients. It examines three subscales of social support, including social interaction, subjective support, and instrumental support. The Abbreviated 23-Item Duke Social Support Index is a self- or therapist-administered tool.

Abbreviated 23-Item Duke Social Support Index Form

Social Interaction Subscale

1. Number of family members within 1 hour that you can depend on or feel close to
2. Number of times in the past week you spent time with someone not living with you
3. Number of times in the past week you talked with friends or relatives on the phone
4. Number of times in the past week you attended meetings of clubs, religious groups, or other groups that you belong to (other than work)

Subjective Support Subscale

5. Do family and friends understand you?	Yes	No
6. Do you feel useful to family and friends?	Yes	No
7. Do you know what is happening with family and friends?	Yes	No
8. Do you feel family and friends listen to you?	Yes	No
9. Do you feel you have a definite role in your family or among your friends?	Yes	No
10. Can you talk about your deepest problems?	Yes	No
11. How satisfied are you with relationships with family and friends?	Yes	No

Instrumental Support Subscale

Do family members or friends ever help you in any of the following ways?

12. Help out when you are sick?	Yes	No
13. Shop or run errands for you?	Yes	No
14. Give you gifts (presents)?	Yes	No
15. Help you out with money?	Yes	No
16. Fix things around your house?	Yes	No
17. Keep house for you or do household chores?	Yes	No
18. Give you advice on business or financial matters?	Yes	No
19. Provide companionship to you?	Yes	No
20. Listen to your problems?	Yes	No
21. Give you advice on dealing with life's problems?	Yes	No
22. Provide transportation for you?	Yes	No
23. Prepare or provide meals for you?	Yes	No

Modified from Koenig HG and others: Abbreviating the Duke Social Support Index for use in chronically ill elderly individuals, *Psychosomatics* 34(1):61-69, 1993.

Adult Population

Older American Resource and Services Social Resources Scale

The Older American Resource and Services (OARS) Social Resources Scale identifies social resources available to patients. It examines the extent and perceived adequacy of existing social contacts with friends and families, the presence of confidants, and the availability of help from friends in times of need. Items 1 to 9 are self-administered or therapist administered, whereas item 10 is therapist administered. The total score ranges from 1 to 6. Higher scores denote greater social impairment.

OARS Social Resources Scale Form

Now I'd like to ask you some questions about your family and friends.

1. Are you single, married, widowed, divorced, or separated?
   1   Single
   2   Married
   3   Widowed
   4   Divorced
   5   Separated
   —   Not answered

2. Who lives with you?
   (Check "yes" or "no" for each of the following.)
   Yes   No
   _____ _____ No one
   _____ _____ Husband or wife
   _____ _____ Children
   _____ _____ Grandchildren
   _____ _____ Brothers and sisters
   _____ _____ Other relatives (does not include in-laws covered in the above categories)
   _____ _____ Friends
   _____ _____ Nonrelated paid help (includes free room)
   _____ _____ Others (specify) _____

3. How many individuals do you know well enough to visit in their homes?
   3   Five or more
   2   Three to four
   1   One to two
   0   None
   —   Not answered

4. About how many times did you talk to someone—friends, relatives, or others—on the telephone in the past week (either you called them or they called you)? (If the patient has no phone, the question still applies.)
   3   Once a day or more
   2   Two to six times
   1   Once
   0   Not at all
   —   Not answered

5. How many times during the past week did you spend some time with someone who does not live with you; that is, you went to see them, or they came to see you, or you went out to do things together? (This applies to relationships at work, relationships outside of work, and visits with agency personnel.)
   3   Once a day or more
   2   Two to six times
   1   Once
   0   Not at all
   —   Not answered

Modified from Fillenbaum GG: *Multidimensional functional assessment of older adults: the Duke Older American Resource and Services Procedure,* Hillsdale, NJ, 1988, Lawrence Erlbaum Associates.

Box—cont'd

6. Do you have someone in whom you can trust and confide?
   1 Yes
   0 No
   — Not answered

7. Do you find yourself feeling lonely quite often, sometimes, or almost never?
   0 Quite often
   1 Sometimes
   2 Almost never
   — Not answered

8. Do you see your relatives and friends as often as you want?
   1 As often as wants to
   0 Not as often as wants to
   — Not answered

9. Is there someone who would give you help if you were sick or disabled (e.g., your husband or wife, a member of your family, or a friend)?
   1 Yes
   0 No one willing and able to help
   — Not answered

   If "yes" ask *a* and *b*.

   a. Is there someone who would take care of you as long as needed, or only for a short time, or only someone who would help you now and then (e.g., taking you to the physician, fixing lunch occasionally)?
      3 Someone who would take care of the patient indefinitely (as long as needed)
      2 Someone who would take care of the patient for a short time (a few weeks to 6 months)
      1 Someone who would help the patient now and then (taking him or her to the physician or fixing lunch, etc.)
      — Not answered

   b. Who is this individual?
      Name _____
      Relationship _____

Rate the current social resources of the individual being evaluated along the 6-point scale presented below. Circle the *one* number that best describes the individual's present circumstances.

1. *Excellent social resources:* Social relationships are very satisfying and extensive; at least one individual would take care of him or her indefinitely.

2. *Good social resources:* Social relationships are fairly satisfying and adequate, and at least one individual would take care of him or her indefinitely; *or* social relationships are very satisfying and extensive, and only short-term help is available.

3. *Mildly socially impaired individual:* Social relationships are unsatisfactory, of poor quality, and few, but at least one person would take care of him or her indefinitely; *or* social relationships are fairly satisfactory and adequate, and only short-term help is available.

4. *Moderately socially impaired individual:* Social relationships are unsatisfactory, of poor quality, and few, and only short-term care is available; *or* social relationships are at least adequate or satisfactory, but help would only be available now and then.

5. *Severely socially impaired individual:* Social relationships are unsatisfactory, of poor quality, and few, and help would only be available now and then; *or* social relationships are at least satisfactory or adequate, but help is not even available now and then.

6. *Totally socially impaired individual:* Social relationships are unsatisfactory, of poor quality, and few, and help is not even available now and then.

Adult Population

Elder Abuse Assessments
The HALF Assessment of Elder Abuse in the Family

The HALF Assessment of Elder Abuse in the Family assesses for the presence of potentially contributing factors to abuse of older adults. These contributing factors are the health status of patients, caregiver and patient attitudes toward the aging process, current living arrangements, and finances. The HALF Assessment of Elder Assessment in the Family is a therapist-administered tool. The number of checks and the columns in which they fall indicate the presence or absence of abuse (or its risk), the severity of abuse, and/or the need for intervention.

The HALF Assessment Form

	Almost always	Some of the time	Never
Health			
1. Older adult risk dynamics			
1.1 Is in poor health	___	___	___
1.2 Is an overly dependent adult child	___	___	___
1.3 Was extremely dependent on spouse who is now deceased	___	___	___
1.4 Persists in advising, admonishing, and directing the adult child, on whom he or she is dependent	___	___	___
2. Older adult abuse dynamics			
2.1 Has an unexplained or repeated injury	___	___	___
2.2 Shows evidence of dehydration and/or malnutrition without obvious cause	___	___	___
2.3 Has been given inappropriate food, drink, and/or drugs	___	___	___
2.4 Shows evidence of overall poor care	___	___	___
2.5 Is notably passive and withdrawn	___	___	___
2.6 Has muscle contracture due to being restricted	___	___	___
3. Adult child and caregiver risk dynamics			
3.1 Abused or battered child	___	___	___
3.2 Poor self-image	___	___	___
3.3 Limited capacity to express own needs	___	___	___
3.4 Alcohol or drug abuser	___	___	___
3.5 Psychologically unprepared to meet dependency needs of parent	___	___	___
3.6 Denial of parent's illness	___	___	___

Modified from Ferguson D, Beck C: H.A.L.F.—a tool to assess elder abuse within the family, *Ger Nurs* September/October: 301-304, 1983.

Box—cont'd

		Almost always	Some of the time	Never

Health—cont'd

4. Adult child and caregiver abuse dynamics

4.1	Shows evidence of loss of control or fear of losing control	___	___	___
4.2	Presents contradictory history	___	___	___
4.3	Projects cause of injury onto third party	___	___	___
4.4	Has delayed unduly in bringing the older adult in for care; shows detachment	___	___	___
4.5	Overreacts or underreacts to the seriousness of the situation	___	___	___
4.6	Complains continuously about irrelevant problems unrelated to injury	___	___	___
4.7	Refuses consent for further diagnostic studies	___	___	___

Attitudes toward Aging

5.1	Older adult views self negatively due to aging process	___	___	___
5.2	Adult child views older adult negatively due to aging process	___	___	___
5.3	Has a negative attitude toward aging	___	___	___
5.4	Adult child has unrealistic expectations of self or older adult	___	___	___

Living Arrangements

6.1	Older adult insists on maintaining old patterns of independent functioning that interfere with child's needs or endanger older adult	___	___	___
6.2	Older adult is intrusive; allows adult child no privacy	___	___	___
6.3	Adult child is socially isolated	___	___	___
6.4	Adult child has no one to provide relief when "uptight" with older adult	___	___	___
6.5	Older adult is socially isolated	___	___	___
6.6	Older adult has no one to provide relief when "uptight" with adult child	___	___	___

Finances

7.1	Older adult uses gift of money to control others, particularly adult children	___	___	___
7.2	Older adult refuses to apply for financial aid	___	___	___
7.3	Older adult has no savings	___	___	___
7.4	Adult child financially unprepared to meet dependency needs of older adult	___	___	___

High Risk Placement Worksheet

The High Risk Placement Worksheet (HRPW) assesses the quantitative and qualitative characteristics of high risk older patients, caregivers, and family systems. It screens for elder abuse risk factors such as patient gender and dependence, caregiver inexperience and economic dependence, and family system traits such as overcrowding or intrafamily problems. The HRPW is a therapist-administered tool. Higher frequencies of risk factors denote greater potential for abuse of older adults.

HRPW Form

Name of Client _____

A. Characteristics of Older Adult	Existence of risk
1. Female	_____
2. Advanced in age	_____
3. Dependent	_____
4. Problem drinker	_____
5. Intergenerationally conflicted	_____
6. Internalizer	_____
7. Excessively loyal	_____
8. Previously abused	_____
9. Stoic	_____
10. Isolated	_____
11. Impaired	_____
12. Provocative behavior	_____

B. Characteristics of Caregiver	Existence of risk
1. Problem drinker	_____
2. Medication or drug abuser	_____
3. Has senile dementia or confusion	_____
4. Mentally or emotionally ill	_____
5. Inexperienced	_____
6. Economically troubled	_____
7. Abused as a child	_____
8. Stressed	_____
9. Unengaged outside the home	_____
10. Blamer	_____
11. Unsympathetic	_____
12. Not understanding	_____

Modified from Kosberg JI: Preventing elder abuse: identification of high risk factors to prior placement decisions, *The Gerontologist* 28(1):43-50, 1988.

Box—cont'd

B. Characteristics of Caregiver—cont'd	Existence of risk
13. Has unrealistic expectations	_____
14. Economically dependent (on care receiver)	_____
15. Hypercritical	_____

C. Characteristics of Family System	Existence of risk
1. Lack of family support	_____
2. Reluctant caregiver	_____
3. Overcrowded	_____
4. Isolated	_____
5. Has marital conflict	_____
6. Has economic pressures	_____
7. Has intrafamily problems	_____
8. Has a desire for institutionalization of older adult	_____
9. Is in disharmony in shared responsibility	

D. Congruity of Perceptions between Older Adult and (Potential) Caregiver   Existence of risk

1. Quality of past relationships   _____
   a. Perception of older adult

   _____

   b. Perception of caregiver

   _____

2. Quality of present relationship   _____
   a. Perception of older adult

   _____

   b. Perception of caregiver

   _____

3. Preferred placement location   _____
   a. Perception of older adult

   _____

   b. Perception of caregiver

   _____

4. Ideal placement location   _____
   a. Perception of older adult

   _____

   b. Perception of caregiver

   _____

Risk of Elder Abuse in the Home

The Risk of Elder Abuse in the Home (REAH) is a two-part assessment consisting of the SASC and the Vulnerability Assessment Score of the Aged Person (VASAP). The SASC component evaluates the level of caregiver stress, and the VASAP component examines the degree of patient dependence on caregivers. The REAH is a therapist-administered tool. The total score, the sum of SASC and VASAP scores, ranges from 0 to 41. Higher scores denote greater strains and the potential for abuse of older adults.

REAH Form

A. Personal Data Section (Older Adult)

Data	2 points	1 point	0 points	Score
Age	85 or older	75-84	74 or younger	
Gender		Female	Male	
Health	Frail	Average	Robust	
SUBTOTAL: (A. Personal Data [sum of above, range 0 to 5])				

B. Dependency Needs Section (Older Adult)

Scoring: 1 point for a "yes"; 0 points for a "no" or "don't know"	Score
Has intellectual or severe mental impairment?	
Lives in home with caregiver?	
Needs help bathing?	
Needs help dressing?	
Needs help toileting (or is incontinent or has catheter)?	
Needs help eating?	
Depends on caregiver for all social interaction?	
Allows caregiver to assume parental role?	
Is demanding and authoritative to caregiver?	
Is financially dependent on caregiver?	
SUBTOTAL: (B. Dependency Needs [sum of above, range 0 to 10])	
VASAP (sum of subtotals A and B, range 0 to 15)	

Modified from Hamilton GP: Prevent elder abuse using a family system approach, *J Gerontol Nurs* 15(3):21-26, 1989.

Home Assessments
Functional Environmental Assessment

The Functional Environmental Assessment objectively assesses the safety of patient homes. It evaluates the degrees of home hazard risks and the frequency patients encounter home hazards. The Functional Environmental Assessment is a therapist-administered tool. For each living area evaluated, interviewers multiply the hazard score by the frequency (HS*F) then sum all the (HS*F) scores to obtain a total score. Higher scores denote greater numbers of potential home hazards.

Functional Environmental Assessment Form

The hazard identification and score is based on the patient's ability to maneuver around in his or her environment. Following are guidelines for assessing potential hazards. Any hazardous items not listed should be identified and scored as "other." The hazard score should reflect "potential" risk and is based on the patient's mobility performance and the condition of his or her environment.

1. Into House

Ask the patient to show how he or she gets into his or her house:

Access

Check the condition of the stairs, railing, and porch as the patient goes into the house. Absence of railing in the presence of stairs should be given a hazard score of at least 1 for all patients.

Doorway

Have the patient open the door and assess (e.g., the way he or she handles door knobs, opens and closes doors).

Threshold

Cross over into the home and note structural items such as obstacles, steps, or raised thresholds that are potentially hazardous.

2. Living Room

Assess the following:

Lighting

Ask the patient to turn on the lights. Assess the accessibility and illumination.

Flooring

Assess the carpeting (including throw rugs), cracks, or uneven surfaces.

Furniture

Have the patient sit and rise from favorite seating. Have the patient perform one or two habitual activities (e.g., turn on television or stereo/radio, get book off shelf).

2. Living Room—cont'd

Storage

Assess cabinets and shelves that the patient typically uses.

Other

Assess cords and clutter (other furniture may be considered clutter).

3. Kitchen

Assess the following:

Lighting

Ask the patient to turn on the lights. Assess the accessibility and illumination.

Flooring

Assess thresholds, uneven surfaces, and carpeting (including throw rugs).

Furniture

Assess the accessibility and difficulty of maneuvering around the stove, kitchen table, chairs, and refrigerator.

Storage

Ask the patient to open and close two or three of the most commonly used cabinets, preferably one high and one low. Check to see whether the patient can reach the items most commonly used. If a stepping stool is needed, ask the patient to demonstrate.

Other

Assess clutter or cords.

Modified from Chandler JR and others: Reliability of a new instrument: the functional environmental assessment, *Phys Ther* 71 (suppl 6):S86, 1991.

Continued

Adult Population

4. Bedroom

Assess the following:

Lighting

Ask the patient to turn on the lights. Assess the accessibility and illumination.

Flooring

Assess the carpets (including throw rugs), uneven surfaces, and cracks.

Furniture

Have the patient lie in the bed. Assess the patient's performance getting up and down from the bed, turning the light on or off (if he or she usually does), and going to the bathroom as if it were night time.

Storage

Ask the patient to go to his or her closet and demonstrate the way he or she reaches for items. Check the lighting. Ask the patient to go to the dresser, then open and close commonly used drawers.

Other

Assess clutter or cords.

5. Bathroom

Assess the following:

Lighting

Ask the patient to turn on the lights. Assess the accessibility and illumination.

5. Bathroom—cont'd

Flooring

Assess nonskid surface mats outside the tub or shower, cracks, and carpeting (throw rugs).

Storage

Assess the accessibility of medicine cabinets.

Furniture

Assess the accessibility into the shower, on and off the commode (toilet paper), to the sink (towel racks nearby). The absence of a nonskid surface in the bath or shower should be given a hazard score of at least 1 for all patients.

Other

Assess clutter or cords.

6. Other Relevant Pathways

Assess the following:

Lighting

Ask the patient to turn on the lights. Assess the accessibility and illumination.

Flooring

Assess the carpets (including throw rugs), uneven surfaces, and cracks.

7. Other Outside Access

Same as #1

Scoring system

Hazard Score

0 = No risk

1 = Low to mild risk—The patient may demonstrate some difficulty maneuvering around this item 10%-40% of the time the item is encountered.

2 = Moderate to high risk—The patient has difficulty maneuvering around the item, or it appears that he or she would have difficulty frequently (50%-100% of the time the hazard is encountered).

Frequency

Assign a frequency rating to each hazard that is encountered.

Frequency rating scale

0 = Never

1 = Less than once per month

2 = Less than once per week

3 = 2 to 3 times per week

4 = 1 to 2 times per day

5 = More than 2 times per day

Modified from Chandler JM and others: Reliability of a new instrument: the functional environmental assessment, *Phys Ther* 71 (suppl 6):S86, 1991.

Box—cont'd

HS * F (Hazard Score * Frequency)

Multiply the frequency by the hazard score. Then total the column (cumulative score of all the hazards for that pathway) to obtain the total score for that pathway.

Total Score (for Each Pathway)

S = Total score (sum of HS * F)

Total Score for FEA

TS = Total score (sum of all S's)

	Hazards	Hazard score	Frequency	HS*F
Into House				
Access				
railing	_____	_____	_____	_____
steps	_____	_____	_____	_____
Door	_____	_____	_____	_____
Threshold	_____	_____	_____	_____
Other	_____	_____	_____	_____
			S =	_____
Living Room				
Lighting				
access	_____	_____	_____	_____
illumination	_____	_____	_____	_____
Floor				
threshold(s)	_____	_____	_____	_____
carpet	_____	_____	_____	_____
surface	_____	_____	_____	_____
Furniture				
chair	_____	_____	_____	_____
television	_____	_____	_____	_____
Storage				
cabinets	_____	_____	_____	_____
closets	_____	_____	_____	_____
Other	_____	_____	_____	_____
	_____	_____	_____	_____
			S =	_____
Kitchen				
Lighting				
access	_____	_____	_____	_____
illumination	_____	_____	_____	_____
Floor				
threshold(s)	_____	_____	_____	_____
carpet	_____	_____	_____	_____
surface	_____	_____	_____	_____
Storage				
cabinets	_____	_____	_____	_____

Adult Population

Continued

Box—cont'd

	Hazards	Hazard score	Frequency	HS*F
Kitchen—cont'd				
Furniture				
kitchen table				
chair				
Appliances				
refrigerator				
sink				
stove				
Other				
				S = _____
Bedroom				
Lighting				
access				
illumination				
Floor				
threshold(s)				
carpet				
surface				
Storage				
closets				
dressers				
Furniture				
bed				
night stand				
Other				
				S = _____
Bathroom				
Lighting				
access				
illumination				

Modified from Chandler JM and others: Reliability of a new instrument: the functional environmental assessment, *Phys Ther* 71 (suppl 6):S86, 1991.

Box—cont'd

	Hazards	Hazard score	Frequency	HS*F
Bathroom—cont'd				
Floor				
threshold	_____	_____	_____	_____
carpet	_____	_____	_____	_____
surface	_____	_____	_____	_____
Furniture				
commode	_____	_____	_____	_____
sink	_____	_____	_____	_____
tub or shower	_____	_____	_____	_____
Storage				
medicine cabinet	_____	_____	_____	_____
Other	_____	_____	_____	_____
			S =	_____
Other Relevant Pathways				
Lighting				
access	_____	_____	_____	_____
illumination	_____	_____	_____	_____
Floor				
threshold(s)	_____	_____	_____	_____
carpet	_____	_____	_____	_____
surface	_____	_____	_____	_____
Other	_____	_____	_____	_____
	_____	_____	_____	_____
			S =	_____
Other Outside Access				
Access				
railings	_____	_____	_____	_____
steps	_____	_____	_____	_____
Door	_____	_____	_____	_____
Threshold	_____	_____	_____	_____
Other	_____	_____	_____	_____
			S =	_____
TOTAL FEA SCORE			TS =	_____

Home Safety Checklist

The Home Safety Checklist is a narrative tool examining the safety of home environments. It is a therapist-administered tool. Therapists perform home safety checks and record safety problems observed in patient homes.

Home Safety Checklist Form

Type of Home
House: Apartment: Single-level dwelling: Multilevel dwelling (elevator):
Multilevel dwelling (no elevator):
Urban dwelling: Suburban dwelling: Rural dwelling:

Outside the Home
Pathway to patient's primary entrance (describe key elements):
Outside steps: Hand rail (yes/no; side going up/down):
Entrance porch (yes/no):   Entrance (describe in relation to the patient's needs):
Door(s) (describe lock, type and weight of door, presence of screen or storm door, height of door
    sill in relation to the patient's needs):
Other (describe other critical items that may affect patient independence):

Inside the Home
Lighting
    Adequacy of overall lighting (describe):
    Light switches that are easily accessible near all room entrances (list exceptions):
    Night lights in bedroom: Night lights in bathroom: Night lights in hallway:
Pathways
    Width of hallways: Width of bathroom door: Width of bedroom door:
    Special problems (describe width of hazards or specific needs):
Living areas
    Accessibility of chair or sofa (describe):
    Accessibility of telephone: Accessiblity of television: Accessibility of radio:
        Accessibility of side table:
    Special problems (describe hazards or specific needs):
Dining area
    Space for the patient to get to and from table: Seating arrangements:

Modified from May BJ: *Home health and rehabilitation: concepts of care,* Philadelphia, 1993, FA Davis.

Box—cont'd

Inside the Home—cont'd

Kitchen
  Accessibility and useability (comment):
  Stove: Refrigerator:
  Sink: Cupboards:
  Countertop: Table:
  Floor covering (describe):
  Special problems (describe hazards or specific needs):
Laundry
  Laundry facilities in home (yes/no):   Accessibility:
Bathroom
  Accessibility and useability (comment):
  Bathtub:
  Shower:
  Toilet:
  Sink:
  Floor covering (describe):
  Presence or absence of grab bars:
  Special equipment:
Bedroom
  Accessibility and useability (comment):
  Bed: Night table: Dresser:
  Closet:
  Special problems (describe hazards or specific needs):

General Considerations

Describe the floor covering in the various rooms, noting problems and hazards (deep pile, scatter rugs, etc.):
Describe safety hazards in the home (frayed electrical cords, rough flooring, sharp furniture edges, crowded conditions):
Determine whether the telephone is accessible to the patient for emergencies.
Determine whether the patient can leave the home in an emergency.
Other

Recommendations

Please list any specific recommendations or suggestions discussed with the patient and caregivers:

Securing a Functional Environment with the Anemaet-Trotter Home Observation and Modification Evaluation

The Securing a Functional Environment with the Anemaet-Trotter Home Observation and Modification Evaluation (SAFE AT HOME) is a comprehensive tool evaluating the presence of risks, safety problems, and architectural barriers in patient homes. It is a therapist-administered tool. Therapists assess the home and document all deficiencies. They use ordinal scales to rate the required assistance level, difficulty level, equipment use, and degree of safety. Higher scores denote greater numbers of safety problems in the home.

SAFE AT HOME Form

Objective SAFE AT HOME	Assistance	Difficulty	Equipment	Safety	Comments
Environmental Areas					
Driveway ☐ Yes ☐ No Paved surface _____ ☐ Yes ☐ No Level surface ☐ Yes ☐ No Adequate walking space _____ Feet to home entrance					
Access to Mailbox ☐ Yes ☐ No Paved surface _____ ☐ Yes ☐ No Level surface ☐ Yes ☐ No Box that patient opens easily ☐ Yes ☐ No Steps: number _____ _____ Feet from home entrance					
Primary Path to Home Entrance ☐ Yes ☐ No Paved surface _____ ☐ Yes ☐ No Level surface ☐ Yes ☐ No Adequate lighting ☐ Yes ☐ No Adequate walking space ☐ Yes ☐ No Steps: number _____ ☐ Yes ☐ No Rails: number _____ ☐ Yes ☐ No Secure rails ☐ Yes ☐ No Door mat ☐ Yes ☐ No Nonskid mat backing					
Home Entrance Doorway ☐ Yes ☐ No Door that opens into home ☐ Yes ☐ No Enough room to open door ☐ Yes ☐ No Threshold ☐ Yes ☐ No Self-closing door ☐ Yes ☐ No Door that closes securely					
Electrical Areas					
Light Switches ☐ Yes ☐ No Accessible locations ☐ Yes ☐ No Switches in working order					
Outlets ☐ Yes ☐ No Accessible locations ☐ Yes ☐ No Outlets in working order ☐ Yes ☐ No Electrical hazards ☐ Yes ☐ No Visible bare wires					

Modified from Anemaet WK, Moffa-Trotter ME: *The user friendly home care handbook*, Washington, DC, 1997, LEARN Publications.

Objective SAFE AT HOME—cont'd

	Assistance	Difficulty	Equipment	Safety	Comments
Electrical Areas—cont'd					
Smoke Detectors ☐ Yes ☐ No Appropriate locations ☐ Yes ☐ No Detectors in working order _____ Type: Battery/electrical/none _____ Number of detectors					
Electrical Cords ☐ Yes ☐ No Obstructive cords ☐ Yes ☐ No Appropriate use of cords ☐ Yes ☐ No Cords that are secured with tape					
Phone ☐ Yes ☐ No Accessible phone locations ☐ Yes ☐ No Emergency number (posted nearby)					
Garage					
Negotiation ☐ Yes ☐ No Scatter rugs ☐ Yes ☐ No Nonskid rug backing ☐ Yes ☐ No Adequate lighting ☐ Yes ☐ No Obstructed path ☐ Yes ☐ No Automatic door opener ☐ Yes ☐ No Steps: number _____ _____ Flooring type					
Kitchen					
Negotiation ☐ Yes ☐ No Scatter rugs ☐ Yes ☐ No Nonskid rug backing ☐ Yes ☐ No Adequate lighting ☐ Yes ☐ No Obstructed path _____ Flooring type					
Stove ☐ Yes ☐ No In working order ☐ Yes ☐ No Door that opens easily ☐ Yes ☐ No Adequate height ☐ Yes ☐ No Flammable items out of range					

Adult Population

Continued

Objective SAFE AT HOME—cont'd

	Assistance	Difficulty	Equipment	Safety	Comments
Kitchen—cont'd					
Refrigerator					
☐ Yes ☐ No In working order					
☐ Yes ☐ No Door that opens easily					
☐ Yes ☐ No Accessible necessary items					
_____ Door handle (on left or right)					
_____ Type (side-by-side, top freezer, etc.)					
Cupboards and Drawers					
☐ Yes ☐ No Appropriate height					
☐ Yes ☐ No Doors that open easily					
☐ Yes ☐ No Accessible necessary items					
Sink					
☐ Yes ☐ No Appropriate height					
☐ Yes ☐ No Appropriate depth					
☐ Yes ☐ No Water temperature < 120°F					
☐ Yes ☐ No Faucet in working order					
Dishwasher					
☐ Yes ☐ No In working order					
☐ Yes ☐ No Appropriate height					
☐ Yes ☐ No Door that opens easily					
Microwave					
☐ Yes ☐ No In working order					
☐ Yes ☐ No Appropriate height					
☐ Yes ☐ No Appropriate location					
☐ Yes ☐ No Door that opens easily					
Counters					
☐ Yes ☐ No Appropriate height					
☐ Yes ☐ No Rough or sharp edges					
☐ Yes ☐ No Overly cluttered counters					
Eating Area					
Negotiation					
☐ Yes ☐ No Scatter rugs					
☐ Yes ☐ No Nonskid rug backing					
☐ Yes ☐ No Adequate lighting					
☐ Yes ☐ No Obstructed path					
_____ Flooring type					

Modified from Anemaet WK, Moffa-Trotter ME: *The user friendly home care handbook,* Washington, DC, 1997, LEARN Publications.

Objective SAFE AT HOME—cont'd

	Assistance	Difficulty	Equipment	Safety	Comments
Eating Area—cont'd					
Table					
☐ Yes ☐ No Appropriate location					
☐ Yes ☐ No Adequate height					
☐ Yes ☐ No Adequate leg clearance					
☐ Yes ☐ No Stable table					
Chair					
☐ Yes ☐ No Adequate height					
☐ Yes ☐ No Arm rests					
☐ Yes ☐ No Stable chair					
_____ Swivels/gliders/rollers					
Living Room					
Negotiation					
☐ Yes ☐ No Scatter rugs					
☐ Yes ☐ No Nonskid rug backing					
☐ Yes ☐ No Adequate lighting					
☐ Yes ☐ No Obstructed path					
_____ Flooring type					
Patient's Preferred Seating					
☐ Yes ☐ No Adequate seat height					
☐ Yes ☐ No Arm rests					
☐ Yes ☐ No Arm rests with proper height					
☐ Yes ☐ No Proper seat depth					
☐ Yes ☐ No Stable seating					
☐ Yes ☐ No Swivels/rocks/wheels					
_____ Type of furniture					
Halls					
Negotiation					
☐ Yes ☐ No Scatter rugs					
☐ Yes ☐ No Nonskid rug backing					
☐ Yes ☐ No Adequate lighting					
☐ Yes ☐ No Obstructed path					
_____ Flooring type					

Adult Population

Continued

Objective SAFE AT HOME—cont'd

	Assistance	Difficulty	Equipment	Safety	Comments
Bedroom					
Negotiation					
☐ Yes ☐ No Scatter rugs					
☐ Yes ☐ No Nonskid rug backing					
☐ Yes ☐ No Adequate lighting					
☐ Yes ☐ No Obstructed path					
_____ Flooring type					
Bed					
☐ Yes ☐ No Adequate height					
☐ Yes ☐ No Firm mattress					
☐ Yes ☐ No Appropriate location					
☐ Yes ☐ No Bed rails					
☐ Yes ☐ No Electric blanket (in use)					
_____ Bed size					
Dresser					
☐ Yes ☐ No Opens with ease					
☐ Yes ☐ No Appropriate height					
☐ Yes ☐ No Accessible necessary items					
_____ Necessity of one or two hands to open drawers					
Closet					
☐ Yes ☐ No Opens with ease					
☐ Yes ☐ No Accessible necessary items					
☐ Yes ☐ No Appropriate rod/shelf height					
_____ Necessity of one or two hands to open doors					
_____ Size					
Laundry					
Negotiation					
☐ Yes ☐ No Scatter rugs					
☐ Yes ☐ No Nonskid rug backing					
☐ Yes ☐ No Adequate lighting					
☐ Yes ☐ No Obstructed path					
_____ Flooring type					
Washer/Dryer					
☐ Yes ☐ No Accessible controls					
☐ Yes ☐ No Accessible necessary items					
_____ Washer/dryer type: front load/top load					

Modified from Anemaet WK, Moffa-Trotter ME: *The user friendly home care handbook*, Washington, DC, 1997, LEARN Publications.

Objective SAFE AT HOME—cont'd

	Assistance	Difficulty	Equipment	Safety	Comments
Bathroom					
Negotiation					
☐ Yes ☐ No Scatter rugs					
☐ Yes ☐ No Nonskid rug backing					
☐ Yes ☐ No Adequate lighting					
☐ Yes ☐ No Obstructed path					
_____ Flooring type					
Toilet					
☐ Yes ☐ No Adequate height					
☐ Yes ☐ No Accessible location					
☐ Yes ☐ No Accessible toilet paper					
☐ Yes ☐ No Grab bars					
_____ Adaptive equipment type					
Shower/Tub					
☐ Yes ☐ No Shower seat					
☐ Yes ☐ No Hand-held shower head					
☐ Yes ☐ No Grab bars					
☐ Yes ☐ No Water temperature <120°F					
☐ Yes ☐ No Accessible toiletries					
☐ Yes ☐ No Accessible faucets					
☐ Yes ☐ No Accessible towel bars					
☐ Yes ☐ No Nonskid surface					
_____ Type: tub/walk-in shower					
_____ LxWxH of step/tub wall					
Sink					
☐ Yes ☐ No Appropriate height					
☐ Yes ☐ No Water temperature <120°F					
☐ Yes ☐ No Accessible faucets					
☐ Yes ☐ No Accessible toiletries					
☐ Yes ☐ No Accessible towel bars					

Other

☐ Yes ☐ No Windows that open easily
☐ Yes ☐ No Stairs in residence: number _____ location(s) _____ Stair surface type _____
☐ Yes ☐ No Stair railings: number _____
_____ Number of floors
Residence type:
_____ house _____ mobile home _____ condominium _____ apartment _____ assisted living facility

Continued

Objective SAFE AT HOME—cont'd

Other safety concerns:

Equipment needs and recommendations:

Scoring

Home area	Assistance score	Difficulty score	Equipment score	Safety score	Total score
Environmental areas					
Electrical areas					
Garage					
Kitchen					
Eating area					
Living room					
Halls					
Bedroom					
Laundry					
Bathroom					
TOTAL					

Scoring Key

Assistance score	Difficulty score	Equipment score	Safety score
1 = Unable 2 = Maximum assistance (75%-100%) 3 = Moderate assistance (25%-50%) 4 = Minimal assistance (up to 25%) 5 = Contact guard assistance 6 = Supervised assistance 7 = No assistance needed independent	1 = Unable 2 = Moderate difficulty (requires rest period after activity) 3 = Minimal difficulty (increased effort to perform) 4 = No difficulty	1 = Assistive device and/or adaptive equipment required 2 = No equipment required	1 = Unsafe 2 = Safe

Modified from Anemaet WK, Moffa-Trotter ME: *The user friendly home care handbook,* Washington, DC, 1997, LEARN Publications.

Caregiver Support Guidelines
Checklist of Concerns and Resources for Caregivers

My relative . . .	Services needed	Resources
. . . really needs to get out and do something.	**Socialization and Volunteering** Programs designed to provide opportunities for socialization with peers and to offer services without compensation	• Area churches and synagogues • City recreation departments • Day care centers • Friendly visitors • Local hospice volunteer program • Nutrition sites • Senior centers • YMCA/YWCA
. . . can do light housecleaning, but needs assistance with heavy tasks.	**Chore Services** Window washing, lawn care, roof repairs, minor housing repairs	• Area churches or synagogues • Fraternal orders • Neighborhood clubs • Social service agencies • Youth groups
. . . has some legal matters that need attention.	**Legal** Assistance with matters pertaining to law	• Adult protective services • Banking institutions • Legal counsels for older adults • Local bar associations
. . . is grieving over the death of a loved one.	**Bereavement** Dealing with the normal grieving process	• Area churches or synagogues • Local hospice • Support groups
. . . cannot drive or use public transportation, and taxicabs are too expensive.	**Transportation** Special transportation for older adults	• Area churches or synagogues • City transportation services for older adults • Transportation for individuals with disabilities • Private transportation • Social service agencies
. . . is unable to remain in his or her current housing.	**Housing** Special residential options available to older adults	• Assisted living facilities • Group homes • House sharing • Public housing • Retirement communities • Skilled nursing facilities • Nursing homes
. . . needs help with food preparation, housekeeping, or laundry.	**Homemaker Services** Nonmedical assistance to help older adults remain in their homes	• Home health agencies • Private homemakers • Social service agencies

Adult Population

Modified from American Association of Retired Persons: *Miles away and still caring,* , Washington, DC, 1987, The Association.

Continued

Table—cont'd

My relative . . .	Services needed	Resources
	Home Health or Personal Care Services	
. . . needs assistance with personal care (bathing, dressing, grooming, toileting).	Personal and basic health care provided by specialists	• Home health agencies • Private nurses • Public health nurses • Social service agencies
	Nutrition	
. . . does not eat properly.	Nutritious meals provided at homes or in group settings	• Home-delivered meals • Meals on Wheels • Nutrition sites • Weekend meals program
	Companionship	
. . . cannot be left alone during the day.	Volunteers who visit older adults or a facility that provides constant supervision	• Adult day care • Foster homes • Home health agencies • Live-in attendants • Social service agencies
	Services for Individuals with Disabilities	
. . . needs special services for physical limitations and impairments.	Services to help older adults accommodate to physical limitations and impairments	• Disease-specific organizations • Local office of physical disabilities
	Health Care Cost Containment	
. . . has extraordinary health care costs.	Reduction in costs of quality health care	Local insurance companies: • Medicare and Social Security office • Medicaid Department of Human Services
	Mental Health	
. . . is depressed, is suspicious, is frequently angry, or just sits all day.	Evaluation of psychological stability	• Area churches and synagogues • City mental health department • Crisis intervention units • Psychiatric nursing • Psychiatric hospitals • Social service agencies
	Geriatric Evaluation	
. . . is acting strange; could he or she be senile?	Complete medical, psychological, and social testing of older adults	• Alzheimer's Association • Mental health workers • Neurologist • Physician • Psychiatrist

Modified from American Association of Retired Persons: *Miles away and still caring*, Washington, DC, 1987, The Association.

Table—cont'd

I sometimes feel . . .	Services needed	Resources
	Private Nurses or Nursing Homes	
. . . really needs 24-hour supervision even though he or she fights it.	Privately paid nursing care in the home or homes for older adults, offering 24-hour medical supervision	• Homes for older adults • Home health agencies • Local ombudsman • Private nursing associations • Social service agencies
	Hospice	
. . . has a terminal illness and wants to return home instead of dying in a hospital.	Medical and social services designed for terminally ill patients	• Area churches or synagogues • Cancer Society • National Hospice Organization • Social service agencies
	Information and Referral	
. . . overwhelmed; I have so many unanswered questions about aging and services for older adults.	Method of providing knowledge of particular services and recommendations of places providing those services	• Area agency on aging • City information and referral • Local office on aging • Social service agencies
	Counseling and Support	
. . . I honestly need to share my feelings with someone who understands.	One-on-one consultation or meetings with other caregivers who share problems and coping skills	• City family services • Pastoral counseling • Social service agencies • Support group for caregivers of older adults
	Family Counseling	
. . . other family members are not helping enough.	Meeting of relatives to discuss responsibilities for care of older adults	• Family service agencies • Family therapists • Private therapists • Social service agencies
	Physical Examination, Stress Management, and Complete Medical Examination	
. . . my caregiving responsibilities are negatively affecting my work, personal life, and health.	Techniques designed to alleviate stress and/or increase coping skills	• Caregivers in the work place • Employee personnel or employer counselors • Employee medical physicians or nurses • Private therapists • Stress clinics

Home Accessibility Guidelines
Specifications for the Accommodation of Individuals with Disabilities

Size of Adult Wheelchair

Seat height	19 in (48.5 cm)
Armrest height	30 in (76 cm)
Push-handle height	36 in (91.5 cm)
Toe height	8 in (20.5 cm)
Lap height	27 in (68.5 cm)
Eye level	43-51 in (109-129.5 cm)
Chair width	26 in (66 cm)
Chair width plus hands	30 in (76 cm)
Chair length	42 in (106.5 cm)
Chair length plus feet	48 in (122 cm)
Footrest width	18 in (45.5 cm)

Space Required for Turns

U turn between walls	60 in (152.5 cm) minimum
U turn completion length	78 in (196.5 cm)
Turning space (180 to 360 degrees)	60 in (152.5 cm) diameter minimum
Aisle width (T shape)	36 in (91.5 cm) minimum each

Passageway Widths

Doorways (clear space)	32 in (81.5 cm) minimum
Aisle (one wheelchair)	36 in (91.5 cm) minimum
Aisle (one wheelchair plus one walking person)	48 in (122 cm) minimum
Aisle (two wheelchairs)	60 in (152.5 cm) minimum

Ramps

Slope 1:12 rise	30 in (76 cm) maximum
Slope 1:12 run	30 ft (9 m) maximum

Ramps—cont'd

Slope 1:16 rise	30 in (76 cm) maximum
Slope 1:16 run	40 ft (12 m) maximum
Slope 1:20 rise	30 in (76 cm) maximum
Slope 1:20 run	50 ft (15 m) maximum
Curb spacing	36 in (91.5 cm) minimum
Curb height	2 in (5 cm) minimum (width to suit)
Clearance between two handrails	36 in (91.5 cm) minimum
Clearance between handrail and ramp edge	12 in (30.5 cm) minimum (no curb); 1.5 in (3.8 cm) minimum (with curb or wall)
Handrail size (diameter)	1.9 in (4.8 cm) maximum
Curb ramps:	
Slope	1:12
Width	48 in (122 cm) minimum

Elevator Floor Space

Width (center opening)	80 in (203 cm) minimum
Width (side opening)	68 in (173 cm) minimum
Back to door space	54 in (137 cm) minimum
Back to wall space	51 in (129.1 cm) minimum
Door opening	32 in (81.5 cm) minimum

Modified from Rothstein JM, Roy SH, Wolf SL: *The rehabilitation specialist's handbook,* Philadelphia, 1991, FA Davis.

Box—cont'd

Reach Heights

Controls (side reach)	54 in (137 cm) maximum (ANSI); 48 in (122 cm) maximum (federal regulations)
Gross (side reach)	9 in (23 cm) minimum
Over counter (side reach)	46 in (117 cm) maximum
Controls (front reach)	48 in (122 cm) maximum
Over 20 in (51 cm) counter (front reach)	48 in (122 cm) maximum
Over 24 in (61 cm) counter (front reach)	44 in (112 cm) maximum
Clothes rods	54 in (137 cm) maximum

Drinking Fountains

Spout height	36 in (91.5 cm)
Knee clearance	27 in (68.5 cm) minimum
Projection from wall	17-19 in (43-48.5 cm)

Kitchens

Aisle width	40 in (101.5 cm) minimum
Aisle where U turn is required	60 in (152.5 cm) minimum
Work shelf width	30 in (76 cm) minimum
Work shelf height:	36 in (91.5 cm)
Alternate	32 in (81.5 cm) adjustable
Alternate	28 in (71 cm) adjustable
Work shelf thickness	2 in (5 cm) maximum
Wall cabinets (bottom height)	48 in (122 cm) maximum

Kitchens—cont'd

Leg space (width)	30 in (76 cm) minimum
Leg space (height)	27 in (68.5 cm) minimum
Leg space (depth)	19 in (48.5 cm) minimum

Bathroom Lavatory

Lavatory projection	17 in (43 cm) minimum
Knee clearance (height)	29 in (73.5 cm) minimum
Knee clearance (depth)	8 in (20.5 cm) minimum
Toe clearance (height)	9 in (23 cm) minimum
Toe clearance (depth)	6 in (15 cm) maximum
Mirror height (bottom)	40 in (101.5 cm) maximum
Floor space (width)	30 in (76 cm) minimum
Floor space (depth)	48 in (122 cm) minimum

Bathroom Toilet

Seat height	17-19 in (43-48.5 cm)
Seat center to sidewall	18 in (45.5 cm) minimum
Seat center to lavatory	18 in (45.5 cm) minimum
Toilet paper dispenser height	19 in (48.5 cm) minimum
Toilet paper dispenser from back wall	36 in (91.5 cm) maximum
Standard stall width	60 in (152.5 cm)
Standard stall depth wall mounting	56 in (142 cm) minimum
Standard stall area (depth floor mounting)	59 in (150 cm) minimum

Adult Population

Home Safety Guidelines
Home Safety Checklist

In all areas of the home, check all of the following:
- Electrical and telephone cords
- Rugs, runners, and mats
- Smoke detectors
- Electrical outlets and switches
- Light bulbs
- Space heaters
- Woodburning stoves
- Emergency exit plan

Cords stretched across walkways may cause people to trip.

Are lamp, extension, and telephone cords out of the flow of traffic?	• Arrange furniture so that outlets are available for lamps and appliances without the use of extension cords. • If extension cords are necessary, place them on the floor against the wall so individuals will not trip over them. • Move phones so that the cords will not lie where individuals walk.

Furniture resting on cords can damage them, creating fire and shock hazards. Electrical cords running under rugs may cause fires.

Are cords out from beneath furniture, rugs, and carpeting?	• Remove cords from under furniture and carpeting. • Replace damaged or frayed cords.

Nails or staples can damage cords, presenting fire and shock hazards.

Are cords attached to walls, baseboards, and other areas with nails or staples?	• Remove nails or staples from cords. • Check wiring for damage. • Use electrical tape to attach cords to walls or floors.

Damaged cords may cause shocks or fires.

Are electrical cords in good condition (not frayed or cracked)?	• Replace frayed or cracked cords.

Overloaded extension cords may cause fires. Standard 18-gauge extension cords can carry 1250 volts.

Do extension cords carry more than their proper load, as indicated by the ratings labeled on the cords and appliances?	• Use extension cords with sufficient wattage or amperage ratings. • Change the cords to higher rated ones, or unplug some appliances. • Decrease loads carried on cords by unplugging some appliances.

Modified from United States Product Safety Commission, *Safety for older consumer home safety checklist,* Publication #4701, Washington, DC, 1986.

Box—cont'd

Tripping over rugs, runners, and mats is a frequent cause of falls.	
Are all small rugs, runners, and mats slip resistant?	• Remove rugs, runners, and mats that slide. • Apply double-faced adhesive carpet tape or rubber matting to the backs of rugs, runners, and mats. • Purchase rugs with slip-resistant backing. • Check rugs, runners, and mats periodically to determine whether backing needs to be replaced. • Place rubber matting under rugs.
In case of emergency, telephone numbers for police, fire, and poison control, along with a neighbor's number, should be readily available.	
Are emergency numbers posted on or near telephones?	• Write the numbers in large print, and tape them to the telephones or place them where they are easily seen.
Is there access to telephones if someone falls or experiences some other emergency that prevents him or her from standing and reaching wall telephones?	• Have at least one telephone located where it would be accessible in the event of an accident that leaves someone unable to stand.
Many home fire injuries and deaths are caused by smoke and toxic gases, rather than fires themselves. Smoke detectors provide an early warning and can wake individuals in the event of fires.	
Are smoke detectors present and properly working?	• Purchase smoke detectors if there are not any. • Check and replace batteries and bulbs according to manufacturer instructions. • Vacuum the grillwork of smoke detectors. • Replace smoke detectors that cannot be repaired.
At least one smoke detector should be placed on every floor of the home.	
Are smoke detectors properly located?	• Read the instructions that come with smoke detectors for advice on the best place to install them. • Make sure smoke detectors are placed near bedrooms, either on the ceiling or 6 to 12 inches below the ceiling on the wall. • Locate smoke detectors away from air vents.
Unusually warm or hot outlets or switches may indicate that an unsafe wiring condition exists.	
Are any outlets and switches unusually warm or hot to touch?	• Unplug cords from outlets, and do not use switches. • Have an electrician check the wiring as soon as possible.

Adult Population

Continued

Box—cont'd

Exposed wiring presents shock hazards.	
Do all outlets and switches have cover plates so that no wiring is exposed?	• Add coverplates.
Bulbs of too high wattage or wrong types may lead to fires through overheating. Ceiling fixtures, recessed lights, and "hooded" lamps trap heat.	
Are light bulbs the appropriate size and type for the lamps and fixtures?	• Replace with bulbs of the correct types and wattage. • If the wattage is unknown, replace with bulbs no larger than 60 watts.
The grounding features of space heaters provided by three-hole receptacles or adapters for two-hole receptacles are safety features designed to lessen the risk of shock.	
Are space heaters that come with three-prong plugs being used in three-hole outlets or with properly attached adapters?	• Never defeat grounding features. • If there are not any three-hole outlets, use adapters to connect three-prong plugs. • Make sure adapter ground wires or tabs are attached to outlets.
Heaters can cause fires or serious burns if they cause people to trip or if they are knocked over.	
Are small stoves and heaters placed where they cannot be knocked over, and away from furnishings and flammable materials such as curtains and rugs?	• Relocate heaters away from passageways. • Relocate heaters away from flammable materials.
Unvented heaters should be used with room doors open or windows slightly open to provide ventilation. The correct fuel, as recommended by manufacturers, should always be used. Vented heaters should have proper venting, and the venting system should be checked frequently. Improper venting is the most frequent cause of carbon monoxide poisoning.	
Are the installation and operation instructions for kerosene heaters, gas heaters, or propane gas heaters used in the home understandable?	• Review installation and operation instructions. • Call the local fire department with additional questions.
Qualified individuals should install woodburning stoves according to local building codes.	
Is woodburning equipment installed properly?	• Local building code officials or fire marshals can provide requirements and recommendations for installation.
After fires start, they spread rapidly. Because there may be a lot of confusion and little time to get out, it is important that everyone knows what to do.	
Is there an emergency exit plan and an alternative exit plan in case of fire?	• Develop an emergency exit plan. • Choose a meeting place outside of the home to be sure everyone is safe. • Practice the plan periodically. • Make sure everyone is capable of following the emergency plan.

Modified from United States Product Safety Commission, *Safety for older consumer home safety checklist,* Publication #4701, Washington, DC, 1986.

Box—cont'd

After fires start, they spread rapidly. Because there may be a lot of confusion and little time to get out, it is important that everyone knows what to do.—cont'd	
In the kitchen, check the following:	• Range area • Electrical cords • Lighting • Step stool • Throw rugs and mats • Telephone area
Placing or storing noncooking equipment such as potholders, dish towels, or plastic utensils on or near ranges may result in fires or burns.	
Are towels, curtains, and other flammable items located away from the range?	• Store flammable and combustible items away from ranges and ovens. • Remove towels hanging on oven handles. • Remove towels that hang close to burners. • Shorten or remove curtains that can brush against heat sources.
Long sleeves are more likely to catch fire than short sleeves. Long sleeves are also more apt to catch on pot handles, overturning pots and pans, resulting in scalds.	
Does the clothing worn during cooking have short or close-fitting sleeves?	• Wear short sleeves or close-fitting sleeves while cooking. • Roll back long sleeves while cooking.
Indoor air pollutants may accumulate to unhealthful levels in kitchens where gas or kerosene-fire appliances are in use.	
Are kitchen ventilation systems or range exhausts functioning properly, and are they in use during cooking?	• Use ventilation systems or open windows to clear the air of vapors and smoke. • Hire a qualified individual to repair broken ventilation systems.
Electrical appliances and power cords can cause shocks or electrocution if they come in contact with water. Excess heat can also damage cords.	
Are all extension cords and appliance cords located away from sinks or range areas?	• Move cords and appliances away from sink areas and hot surfaces. • Move appliances closer to wall outlets or to different outlets so extension cords are not needed. • If extension cords must be used, install wiring guides so that cords do not hang near sink, range, or working areas. • Consider adding new outlets for convenience and safety.

Adult Population

Continued

Box—cont'd

Low lighting and glare can contribute to burns or cuts.	
Does good, even lighting exist over stoves, sinks, and work areas, especially where food is cut or sliced?	• Open curtains or blinds unless this causes too much glare. • Use the maximum wattage bulbs allowed by fixtures. • Reduce glare by using frosted bulbs, indirect lighting, and shades or globes on light fixtures, as well as by partially closing curtains or blinds. • Install additional light fixtures (e.g., under cabinet or over countertop lighting).
Standing on chairs, boxes, or other makeshift items to reach high shelves can result in falls.	
Is there a step stool that is stable and in good repair?	• Buy step stools with handrails. • Before climbing on any step stool, make sure it is fully open and stable. • Tighten screws and braces on step stools. • Discard step stools with broken parts.
In the living room or family room, check the following:	• Rugs and runners • Electrical and telephone cords • Lighting • Fireplace and chimney • Telephone areas • Passageways
Clogged chimneys can cause poorly burning fires to result in poisonous fumes and gases coming back into the home.	
Are chimneys clear from accumulations of leaves and other clogging debris?	• Have registered or licensed professionals check chimneys. • Do not use chimneys until blockages are removed.
Burning wood can cause build-up of tarry substances (creosote) inside chimneys. These materials can ignite and result in serious chimney fires.	
Has the chimney been cleaned in the past year?	• Have registered or licensed professionals check the chimney.
Shadowed or dark areas can hide tripping hazards.	
Are hallways and passageways between rooms and other heavy traffic areas well lit?	• Use the maximum wattage bulbs allowed by fixtures. • Install night lights. • Reduce glare by using frosted bulbs, indirect lighting, and shades or globes on light fixtures, as well as by partially closing blinds or curtains. • Consider using additional lamps or light fixtures.

Modified from United States Product Safety Commission, *Safety for older consumer home safety checklist,* Publication #4701, Washington, DC, 1986.

Box—cont'd

Furniture, boxes, and/or other items can be obstructions or tripping hazards, especially in the event of emergencies such as fires.

Are exits and passageways kept clear?

In the bathroom, check the following:

- Rearrange furniture to open passageways and walkways.
- Remove boxes and clutter.
- Bathtub and shower areas
- Water temperature
- Rugs and mats
- Lighting
- Small electrical appliances
- Storage areas for medications

Wet, soapy tiles or porcelain surfaces are especially slippery and may contribute to falls.

Are bathtubs and showers equipped with nonskid mats, abrasive strips, or surfaces that are not slippery?

- Apply textured strips or appliqués on the floors of tubs and showers.
- Use nonskid mats in tubs, showers, and bathroom floors.

Grab bars can help getting into and out of tubs or showers and can help prevent falls.

Do bathtubs and showers have at least one (preferably two) grab bars?

- Check existing grab bars for strength and stability, and repair if necessary.
- Attach grab bars through tiles to structural supports in walls, or install bars specifically designed to attach to the sides of bathtubs.
- If unsure of the way to install grab bars, get someone qualified for assistance.

Water temperatures above 120°F can cause tap water scalds.

Is the water temperature 120°F or lower?

- Lower the setting on hot water heaters to "low" or 120°F.
- If unfamiliar with hot water heater controls, have someone qualified provide help.
- If hot water heaters are controlled by landlords, ask them to lower the setting.
- If hot water heaters do not have temperature settings, use thermometers.
- Always check the water temperature by hand before entering the bath or shower.
- Taking baths, rather than showers, reduces the risk of a scald from suddenly changing water temperatures.

A light switch near the door prevents individuals from walking through dark areas.

Is a light switch located near the bathroom entrance?

- Install a light switch outside the bathroom entrance.
- Install night lights.
- Consider replacing existing switches with "glow switches" that can be seen in the dark.

Adult Population

Continued

Box—cont'd

Even appliances that are not turned on can be potentially hazardous if left plugged in. If it falls into water while plugged in, it could cause lethal shock.

Are small electrical appliances such as hairdryers, shavers, and curling irons unplugged when not in use?

- Unplug all small appliances when not in use.
- Never reach into water to retrieve appliances that have fallen in without being sure they are unplugged.
- Install ground fault circuit interrupters (GFCIs) in the bathroom outlets to protect against electrical shocks.

Medications that are not clearly marked and accurately labeled can be easily mixed up. Taking the wrong medications or missing dosages of necessary medicine can be dangerous.

Are all medicines stored in the containers in which they came, and are they clearly marked?

- Be sure all containers are clearly marked with the contents, physician's instructions, expiration dates, and patient's name.
- Dispose of outdated medications properly.
- Request nonchild-resistant closures from pharmacists only when unable to use child-resistant closures.

In bedrooms, check the following:

- Rugs, mats, and runners
- Electrical and telephone cords
- Areas around beds

Lamps or switches located close to each bed enable individuals getting up at night to see where they are going.

Are lamps or light switches within reach of each bed?

- Rearrange furniture closer to switches, or move lamps closer to beds.
- Install night lights.

Burns are a leading cause of accidental death. Smoking in bed is a major contributor to this problem.

Are ash trays, smoking materials, or other fire sources(heaters, hot plates, tea pots, etc.) located away from beds or bedding?

- Remove sources of heat or flame from areas around beds.
- Do not smoke in bed.

"Tucking in" electrical blankets or placing additional covers on top of them can cause excessive heat build-up, which can start fires.

Is anything covering the electric blanket when in use?

- Use electrical blankets according to manufacturer instructions.
- Do not allow anything on top of the blanket while it is in use (e.g., other blankets, pets).
- Do not set electrical blankets so high that they can burn someone who falls asleep while they are on.

Never go to sleep with heating pads if they are turned on because they can cause serious burns even at relatively low settings.

Are heating pads turned on while individuals sleep?

- Turn heating pads off before going to sleep.

Modified from United States Product Safety Commission, *Safety for older consumer home safety checklist,* Publication #4701, Washington, DC, 1986.

Box—cont'd

In case of emergencies, it is important to be able to reach the telephone without getting out of bed.	
Is there a telephone close to the bed?	• Keep a telephone near the bed.
In the basement, garage, workshop, and storage areas, check the following:	• Lighting
	• Fuse boxes or circuit breakers
	• Appliances and power tools
	• Electrical cords
	• Flammable liquids

Good lighting reduces the chances of injuries when working with power tools.	
Are work areas, especially areas where power tools are used, well lit?	• Install additional lighting.
	• Avoid working with power tools in areas with poor lighting.

Basements, garages, workshops, and storage areas can contain many tripping hazards and sharp or pointed tools that make falls even more hazardous.	
Can individuals turn on the lights without first having to walk through dark areas?	• Keep an operating flashlight handy.
	• Have an electrician install switches at each entrance to dark areas.

Replacing correct size fuses with larger size fuses can present serious fire hazards. If the fuses in the box are rated higher than those intended for the circuit, excessive current will be allowed to flow and possibly overload the outlet and house wiring to the point that fires can begin.	
If fuses are used, are they the correct size for the circuit?	• Be certain that correct size fuses are used.
	• If unsure of what size fuses should be used, hire an electrician to identify and label the sizes to be used.

Power tool safety features reduce the risk of electrical shock.	
Are power tools equipped with three-prong plugs or marked to show that they are double insulated?	• Use properly connected three-prong adapters for connecting three-prong plugs to two-hole receptacles.
	• Consider replacing old tools that have neither three-prong plugs nor double insulation.

Power tools used with guards removed pose a serious risk of injury from sharp edges or moving parts.	
Are power tool guards in place?	• Replace guards that have been removed from power tools.

Improperly grounded appliances can lead to electrical shock.	
Have the grounding features on any three-prong plugs been defeated by removal of the grounding pin or by improper use of adapters?	• Check with a service individual or an electrician if in doubt of the grounding status.
	• Do not use appliances that have had grounding pins removed.

If containers are not tightly closed, vapors from volatile liquids may escape that may be toxic when inhaled.	
Are containers of volatile liquids tightly capped?	• Check containers periodically to make sure they are tightly closed.

Adult Population

Continued

Box—cont'd

Gasoline, kerosene, and other flammable liquids should be stored out of living areas in properly labeled, nonglass safety containers.

Are gasoline, kerosene, paints, solvents, or other products that give off vapors or fumes stored away from ignition sources?

For all stairways, check the following:

- Remove these products from the areas near heat or flame, such as heaters, furnaces, water heaters, ranges, and other gas appliances.
- Lighting
- Handrails
- Condition of steps and coverings

Stairs should be lighted so that each step, particularly the step edges, can be clearly seen while individuals are going up and down stairs. The lighting should not produce glare or shadows along the stairway.

Are stairs well lit?

- Use the maximum wattage bulbs allowed by light fixtures.
- Reduce glare by using frosted bulbs, indirect lighting, and shades or globes on light fixtures, as well as partially closing blinds and curtains.
- Have a qualified individual add additional lighting fixtures.

Even for those familiar with the stairs, lighting is an important factor in preventing falls. Individuals should be able to turn on the lights before using the stairway from either end.

Are light switches located at both the top and bottom of the stairs?

- If no other light source is available, keep an operating flashlight in a convenient location at the top and bottom of the stairs.
- Install night lights at nearby outlets.
- Consider installing switches at the top and bottom of the stairs.

Worn treads or worn or loose carpeting can lead to insecure footing, resulting in slips or falls.

Do the steps allow secure footing?

- Try to avoid wearing only socks or smooth-soled shoes or slippers when using stairs.
- Make certain the carpet is firmly attached to the steps all along the stairs.
- Consider refinishing or replacing worn treads or replacing worn carpeting.
- Paint outside steps with paint that has rough textures, or use abrasive strips.

Modified from United States Product Safety Commission, *Safety for older consumer home safety checklist,* Publication #4701, Washington, DC, 1986.

Box—cont'd

Even small differences in step surfaces or riser heights can lead to falls.	
Are steps even and of the same size and height?	• Mark any steps that are especially narrow, or have risers that are higher or lower than the others.

Worn or torn coverings or nails sticking out from coverings could snag feet or cause individuals to trip.	
Are the coverings on the steps in good condition?	• Repair coverings. • Remove coverings. • Replace coverings.

Falls may occur if the edges of the steps are blurred or hard to see.	
Can individuals clearly see the edges of the steps?	• Paint edges of outdoor steps white to see them better at night. • Add extra lighting. • If planning to carpet stairs, avoid deep pile carpeting or patterned or dark colored carpeting that can make it difficult to see the edges of the steps clearly.

Individuals can trip over objects left on stairs, particularly in the event of emergencies or fires.	
Is anything stored on the stairway, even temporarily?	• Remove all objects from stairways.

ADULT AFFECTIVE EVALUATION

Therapists often overlook the role patient affective components play in rehabilitation. For example, clinical depression can easily be mistaken for poor motivation for rehabilitation, resulting in improper clinical decision making that seriously jeopardizes achievement of patient potential. Adult affective evaluations include tools to assess cognition, the presence of depressive symptoms and delirium, the degree of patient stress, morale, and the type of pain patients experience. The results of these assessments allow therapists to set therapy goals more accurately, anticipate the amount of caregiver assistance required to fulfill the plan of care, and determine the need for referral to other team members such as medical social workers, occupational therapists, speech-language pathologists, or psychiatric nurses. Associated standards provide information about distinguishing dementia, depression, and delirium. Associated guidelines offer suggestions for overcoming motivational barriers in the home.

Adult Population

Cognitive Assessments
Mini Mental State Examination

The Mini Mental State Examination (MMSE) assesses the cognitive aspects of mental functions. It evaluates intellectual capacities such as orientation, memory, and language. The MMSE is a therapist-administered tool. The total score ranges from 0 to 30. In older adults, scores of 15 or less indicate severe cognitive impairment, scores of 16 to 20 indicate moderate cognitive impairment, scores of 21 to 24 indicate mild cognitive impairment, and scores greater than 24 indicate normal cognitive functioning.

MMSE Form

	Maximum score	Score	Instructions
Orientation			
What is the (year) (season) (date) (day) (month)?	5	_____	Ask for the date. Then proceed to ask other parts of the question. Score 1 point for each correct segment of the question.
Where are we: (street number) (street) (city) (country) (state)?	5	_____	Ask for the street address, then proceed to ask other parts of the question. Score 1 point for each correct segment of the question.
Registration			
Name three objects (bed, apple, shoe). Ask the patient to repeat them.	3	_____	Name the objects slowly, 1 second for each. Ask the patient to repeat. Score by the number of objects repeated. Take time here for the patient to learn the series of objects, up to six trials, to use later for the memory test.
Attention/Calculation			
Count backwards by sevens. Start with 100. Stop after five calculations. *Alternate Question:* Spell the word "world" backwards.	5	_____	Score the total number correct (93, 86, 79, 72, 65). Score the number of letters in correct order (dlrow = 5, dlorw = 3).

Modified from Folstein MF, Folstein SE, McHugh PR: Mini-mental state: a practical method for grading the cognitive state of patients for the clinician, *J Psych Res* 12:189-198, 1975.

Box—cont'd

	Maximum score	Score	Instructions
Recall			
Ask the patient to repeat the three objects mentioned earlier (bed, apple, shoe).	3	_____	Score 1 point for each correct answer (bed, apple, shoe).
Language			
Naming: Name this object: (watch, pencil).	2	_____	Hold the object. Ask the patient to name it. Score 1 point for each correct answer.
Repeating: Repeat the following: "No *if*s, *and*s, or *but*s."	1	_____	Allow one trial only. Score 1 point for the correct answer.
Following a three-stage command: "Take the paper in your right hand, fold it in half, and put it on the floor."	3	_____	Use a blank sheet of paper. Score 1 point for each part correctly executed.
Writing: Write a sentence.	1	_____	Provide paper and a pencil. Allow the patient to write any sentence. It must contain a noun and a verb, and it must be sensible.
Reading: Read and obey the following: Close your eyes.	1	_____	The instruction should be printed on paper. Allow the patient to read it. Score 1 point for a correct response.
Copying: Copy this design	1	_____	All 10 angles must be present. Figures must intersect. Ignore tremor and rotation.

Level of Consciousness

Circle one of the following: Alert   Drowsy   In a stupor   In a coma

MINI MENTAL STATE TOTAL SCORE   **(MAX 30)** _____

Short Portable Mental Status Questionnaire

The Short Portable Mental Status Questionnaire (SPMSQ) assesses the presence and degree of intellectual impairment in older adults. It evaluates five aspects of cognitive functioning, including short-term memory, long-term memory, orientation to surroundings, information about current events, and the capacity to perform serial mathematical tasks. The SPMSQ is a therapist-administered tool. Patients receive 1 point for each correct response. The total score ranges from 0 to 10. Scores of 0 to 2 indicate severe intellectual impairment, scores of 3 to 5 indicate moderate intellectual impairment, scores of 6 to 7 indicate mild intellectual impairment, and scores of 8 to 10 indicate intact intellectual functioning.

SPMSQ Form

1. What is the date today (month/day/year)? _____
2. What day of the week is it? _____
3. What is the name of this place? _____
4. What is your telephone number? (If no phone, what is the street address?) _____
5. How old are you? _____
6. When were you born (month/day/year)? _____
7. Who is the current president of the United States? _____
8. Who was the president just before him? _____
9. What was your mother's maiden name? _____
10. Subtract 3 from 20 and keep subtracting each new number until you get all the way down. _____

TOTAL SCORE _____

Modified from Pfeiffer E: A short portable mental status questionnaire for the assessment of organic brain deficit in elderly patients, *J Am Ger Soc* 23(10):433-441, 1975.

Delirium Assessments

Reversible Cognitive Dysfunction Scale

The Reversible Cognitive Dysfunction Scale (RCDS) predicts cognitive improvement in older patients. It assesses the presence of clinical signs such as incoherent speech, reduced psychomotor activity, and conscious level. The RCDS is a therapist-administered tool, and a baseline MMSE score is required for scoring. The total score ranges from 0 to 54. Scores less than 15/16 are associated with subsequent improvement in cognitive function.

RCDS Form

Clinical sign	Score
Incoherence of Speech 0 = Absent 1 = Possibly present 2 = Mild 3 = Moderate 4 = Severe	
Contact with Patient 0 = Absent 1 = Possibly present 2 = Mild 3 = Moderate 4 = Severe	
Reduced Psychomotor Activity 0 = Absent 1 = Possibly present 2 = Mild 3 = Moderate 4 = Severe	
Fluctuating Attention at Interview 0 = Absent 1 = Possibly present 2 = Mild 3 = Moderate 4 = Severe	
Awareness of Surroundings 0 = Fully aware of surroundings 1 = Occasionally unaware of distant surroundings 2 = Frequently unaware of distant surroundings 3 = Continually unaware of distant surroundings	
Consciousness Level 0 = Alert 1 = Slightly drowsy 2 = Significantly drowsy 3 = Asleep; easily rousable 4 = Asleep; briefly rousable 5 = Unrousable Subscore Mini Mental State Examination (MMSE) score at baseline Subtotal (MMSE − subscore) TOTAL SCORE (Add 30 points to subtotal.)	

Modified from Treloar AJ, Macdonald AJD: Outcome of delirium diagnosed by DSM-III-R, ICD-10 and CAMDEX and derivation of the reversible cognitive dysfunction scale among acute geriatric inpatients, *Int J Ger Psychiatry* 12:609-613, 1997.

Adult Population

Shortened Confusion Assessment Method

The Shortened Confusion Assessment Method (CAM) identifies delirium in older adults. It assesses four features of delirium, including acute onset and fluctuating course, inattention, disorganized thinking, and altered level of consciousness. The CAM is a therapist-administered tool. A diagnosis of delirium is likely if features 1 and 2, as well as 3 or 4, are present.

Shortened CAM Form

Feature	Diagnostic algorithm	Yes	No
1. Acute onset	a. Is there evidence of an acute change in mental status from the patient's baseline? b. Did the (abnormal) behavior fluctuate during the day (i.e., tend to come and go, or increase and decrease in severity)?		
2. Inattention	a. Did the patient have difficulty focusing attention (e.g., being easily distractible, or having difficulty keeping track of what was being said)? (1) Not present at any time during the interview (2) Present at some time during the interview, but in mild form (3) Present at some time during the interview, in marked form (4) Uncertain b. If present or abnormal: Did this behavior fluctuate during the interview (i.e., tend to come and go or increase and decrease in severity)? (1) Yes (2) No (3) Uncertain (4) Not applicable		
3. Disorganized thinking	Was the patient's thinking disorganized or incoherent, resulting in conversation that was rambling or irrelevant, consisted of an unclear or illogical flow of ideas, or contained unpredictable switching from subject to subject?		
4. Altered level of consciousness	a. Overall, how would you rate the patient's level of consciousness? (1) Alert (normal) (2) Vigilant (hyperalert, overly sensitive to environmental stimuli, startled easily) (3) Lethargic (drowsy, easily aroused) (4) In a stupor (difficult to arouse) (5) In a coma (unarousable) (6) Uncertain		

Modified from Inoye SK and others: Clarifying confusion: the confusion assessment method, *Ann Int Med* 113(12):941-949, 1990.

Depression Assessments
Geriatric Depression Screening Scale

The Geriatric Depression Screening Scale (GDS) screens for the presence of depressive symptoms in older adults. It assesses patient agreement with feelings relevant to depression experienced over the past week, such as self-image, agitation, and somatic complaints. The GDS is a self- or therapist-administered tool. The examiner should score 1 point if patients answer "no" to statements 1, 5, 7, 9, 15, 19, 21, 27, 29, and 30. The examiner should score 1 point if patients respond "yes" to items 2, 3, 4, 6, 8, 10, 11, 12, 13, 14, 16, 17, 18, 19, 20, 22, 23, 24, 25, 26, and 28. The total score ranges from 0 to 30. A total score of 0 to 10 is normal, a score of 11 to 19 indicates mild depression, and a score of 20 to 30 indicates severe depression.

GDS Form

1.	Are you basically satisfied with your life?	Yes	No
2.	Have you dropped many of your activities and interests?	Yes	No
3.	Do you feel that your life is empty?	Yes	No
4.	Do you often get bored?	Yes	No
5.	Are you hopeful about the future?	Yes	No
6.	Are you bothered by thoughts you can't get out of your head?	Yes	No
7.	Are you in good spirits most of the time?	Yes	No
8.	Are you afraid that something bad is going to happen to you?	Yes	No
9.	Do you feel happy most of the time?	Yes	No
10.	Do you often feel helpless?	Yes	No
11.	Do you often get restless and fidgety?	Yes	No
12.	Do you prefer staying at home rather than going out and doing new things?	Yes	No
13.	Do you frequently worry about the future?	Yes	No
14.	Do you feel that you have more problems with memory than most?	Yes	No
15.	Do you think it is wonderful to be alive now?	Yes	No
16.	Do you often feel downhearted and blue?	Yes	No
17.	Do you feel pretty worthless the way you are now?	Yes	No
18.	Do you worry a lot about the past?	Yes	No
19.	Do you find life very exciting?	Yes	No
20.	Is it hard for you to get started on new projects?	Yes	No
21.	Do you feel full of energy?	Yes	No
22.	Do you feel that your situation is hopeless?	Yes	No
23.	Do you think that most individuals are better off than you are?	Yes	No
24.	Do you frequently get upset over little things?	Yes	No
25.	Do you frequently feel like crying?	Yes	No
26.	Do you have trouble concentrating?	Yes	No
27.	Do you enjoy getting up in the morning?	Yes	No
28.	Do you prefer to avoid social gatherings?	Yes	No
29.	Is it easy for you to make decisions?	Yes	No
30.	Is your mind as clear as it used to be?	Yes	No

Adult Population

Modified from Yesavage JA and others: Development and validation of a geriatric depression screening scale: a preliminary report, *J Psych Res* 17(1): 37-49, 1983.

Revised Brief Depression Scale

The Revised Brief Depression Scale screens for major depression among medically ill older adults. It assesses patient agreement with statements associated with depression, such as tension, contentedness, hopelessness, sadness, cognition, life fulfillment, and activity. The Revised Brief Depression Scale is a self- or therapist-administered tool. The therapist should score 1 point if patients answer "no" to statements 3, 5, and 8. The therapist should score 1 point if patients respond "yes" to all other items. The total score ranges from 0 to 11. A total score greater than 2 indicates depressive symptoms.

Revised Brief Depression Scale Form

During the past week . . .		
1. I often became bored.	Yes	No
2. I often became restless and fidgety.	Yes	No
3. I felt in good spirits.	Yes	No
4. I felt I had more problems with memory than most other people.	Yes	No
5. I could concentrate easily when reading the papers.	Yes	No
6. I preferred to avoid social gatherings.	Yes	No
7. I felt downhearted and blue.	Yes	No
8. I felt happy most of the time.	Yes	No
9. I often felt helpless.	Yes	No
10. I felt worthless and ashamed about myself.	Yes	No
11. I often wished I was dead.	Yes	No

Modified from Koenig HG, Blumenthal J, Moore K: New version of brief depression scale, *J Am Ger Soc* 43(12) : 1447, 1995.

Life Stress and Morale Assessments

Recent Life Changes Questionnaire

The Recent Life Changes Questionnaire (RLCQ) evaluates levels of life stress that adults experience. It is a self- or therapist-administered tool, with patients and/or caregivers circling the events that have occurred in the past year. The total score ranges from 0 to 3545. Scores greater than 500 denote high recent life stress.

RLCQ Form

For the past year, circle the events that have occurred.

Health

An injury or illness that resulted in the following:

Kept you in bed a week or more, or sent you to the hospital	74
Was less serious than above	44
Major dental work	26
Major change in eating habits	27
Major change in sleeping habits	26
Major change in your usual type and/or amount of recreation	28

Work

Change to a new type of work	51
Change in your work hours or conditions	35

Change in your responsibilities at work:

More responsibilities	29
Fewer responsibilities	21
Promotion	31
Demotion	42
Transfer	32

Troubles at work:

With your boss	29
With coworkers	35
With individuals under your supervision	35
Other work troubles	28
Major business adjustment	60
Retirement	52

Loss of job:

Laid off from work	68
Fired from work	79
Correspondence course to help you in your work	18

Home and Family

Major change in living conditions	42

Change in residence:

Move within the same town or city	25
Move to a different town, city, or state	47
Change in family get-togethers	25

Modified from Miller MA, Rahe RH: Life changes scaling for the 1990s, *J Psych Som Res* 43(3):279-292, 1997.

Adult Population

Continued

Box—cont'd

Major change in health or behavior of family member	55
Marriage	50
Pregnancy	67
Miscarriage or abortion	65
Gain of a new family member:	
Birth of a child	66
Adoption of a child	65
A relative moving in with you	59
Spouse beginning or ending work	46
Child leaving home:	
To attend college	41
Due to marriage	41
For other reasons	45
Change in arguments with spouse	50
In-law problems	38
Change in the marital status of your parents:	
Divorce	59
Remarriage	50
Separation from spouse:	
Due to work	53
Due to marital problems	76
Divorce	96
Birth of a grandchild	43
Death of spouse	119
Death of other family member:	
Child	123
Brother or sister	102
Parent	100

Personal and Social Changes

Change in personal habits	26
Beginning or ending of school or college	38
Change of school or college	35
Change in political beliefs	24
Change in religious beliefs	29
Change in social activities	27
Vacation	24
New, close, personal relationship	37

Modified from Miller MA, Rahe RH: Life changes scaling for the 1990s, *J Psych Som Res* 43(3):279-292, 1997.

Box—cont'd

Personal and Social Changes—cont'd

Engagement to marry	45
Girlfriend or boyfriend problems	39
Sexual difficulties	44
"Falling out" of a close personal relationship	47
An accident	48
Minor violation of the law	20
Imprisonment	75
Death of a close friend	70
Major decision regarding your immediate future	51
Major personal achievement	36

Financial Changes

Major change in finances:

Increased income	38
Decreased income	60
Investment and/or credit difficulties	56
Moderate purchase	30
Major purchase	37
Foreclosure on a mortgage or loan	58

Revised Philadelphia Geriatric Center Morale Scale

The Revised Philadelphia Geriatric Center (PGC) Morale Scale assesses the inner state of older adults. It determines patient agreement with statements concerning three factors of morale: agitation, attitude toward own aging, and lonely dissatisfaction. The PGC Morale Scale is a self- or therapist-administered tool. The therapist should score 1 point if patients answer "no" to statements 1 to 7, 9, 14, 15, and 17. The therapist should score 1 point if patients respond "yes" to items 8, 11, and 13. The therapist should score 1 point if patients answer "better" to statement 10. The therapist should score 1 point if patients answer "not much" to statement 12. The therapist should score 1 point if patients answer "satisfied" to statement 16. The total score ranges from 0 to 23. Higher scores denote greater presence of high morale.

Revised PGC Morale Scale Form

1. Little things bother me more this year.	Yes	No
2. I sometimes worry so much that I cannot sleep.	Yes	No
3. I am afraid of a lot of things.	Yes	No
4. I get mad more than I used to.	Yes	No
5. I take things hard.	Yes	No
6. I get upset easily.	Yes	No
7. Things keep getting worse as I get older.	Yes	No
8. I have as much pep as I had last year.	Yes	No
9. As I get older I am less useful.	Yes	No
10. As I get older, things are better/worse than I thought they would be.	Better	Worse
11. I am as happy now as when I was younger.	Yes	No
12. I feel lonely not much/a lot.	Not much	A lot
13. I see enough of my friends and relatives.	Yes	No
14. I sometimes feel that life is not worth living.	Yes	No
15. Life is hard for me much of the time.	Yes	No
16. I am satisfied/unsatisfied with my life today.	Satisfied	Unsatisfied
17. I have a lot to be sad about.	Yes	No

Modified from Lawton MP: The Philadelphia Geriatric Center Morale Scale: a revision, *J Gerontol* 30(1):85-89, 1975.

Pain Assessments

Functional Interference Estimate

The Functional Interference Estimate (FIE) assesses pain-related impairment of function. It measures the degree to which chronic pain interferes with five significant motor and psychosocial functions. The FIE is a self- or therapist-administered tool. The total score ranges from 0 to 25. Higher scores denote greater interference of pain with daily functioning.

FIE Form

For each question below, please circle the appropriate number according to the following scale:

0	1	2	3	4	5
Pain usually or severely interferes			Pain occasionally interferes		Pain rarely interferes

1. Rate your ability to stand or sit.	0	1	2	3	4	5
2. Rate your ability to engage in social activities (clubs, visiting relatives).	0	1	2	3	4	5
3. Rate your ability to walk.	0	1	2	3	4	5
4. Rate your ability to participate in recreational activities (dancing, etc.).	0	1	2	3	4	5
5. Rate your ability to perform work.	0	1	2	3	4	5

Modified from Toomey TC and others: Psychometric characteristics of a brief measure of pain-related functional impairment, *Arch Phys Med Rehabil* 74:1305-1308, 1993.

Pain and Impairment Relationship Scale

The Pain and Impairment Relationship Scale (PAIRS) examines the extent to which individuals with chronic pain endorse the belief that pain necessarily impedes them from normal function. It examines a range of cognitive factors potentially related to level of impairment and patient response to treatment such as disability perceptions and self-imposed limitations to pain. The PAIRS is a self-administered tool. The therapist should score items 1, 6, and 14 such that patients accrue 7 points for "completely disagree," scaling down to 1 point for "completely agree." Therapists score all other items in the opposite manner, with 7 points assigned for "completely agree" and 1 point for "completely disagree." The total score ranges from 15 to 75. Higher scores denote greater degrees to which patients link pain with impairment and experience, resulting in decreased physical functioning.

PAIRS Form

1. I can still be expected to fulfill my work and family responsibilities despite my pain.

| Completely disagree | Disagree | Disagree somewhat | Neutral | Agree somewhat | Agree | Completely agree |

2. An increase in pain is an indication that I should stop what I am doing until the pain decreases.

| Completely disagree | Disagree | Disagree somewhat | Neutral | Agree somewhat | Agree | Completely agree |

3. I cannot go about my normal life activities when I am in pain.

| Completely disagree | Disagree | Disagree somewhat | Neutral | Agree somewhat | Agree | Completely agree |

4. If my pain would go away, I could be every bit as active as I used to be.

| Completely disagree | Disagree | Disagree somewhat | Neutral | Agree somewhat | Agree | Completely agree |

5. I should have the same benefits as individuals with disabilities because of my chronic pain problems.

| Completely disagree | Disagree | Disagree somewhat | Neutral | Agree somewhat | Agree | Completely agree |

6. I owe it to myself and those around me to perform my usual activities even when my pain is bad.

| Completely disagree | Disagree | Disagree somewhat | Neutral | Agree somewhat | Agree | Completely agree |

7. Most people expect too much of me, considering that I have chronic pain.

| Completely disagree | Disagree | Disagree somewhat | Neutral | Agree somewhat | Agree | Completely agree |

8. I have to be careful not to do anything that might make my pain worse.

| Completely disagree | Disagree | Disagree somewhat | Neutral | Agree somewhat | Agree | Completely agree |

Modified from Riley JF, Ahern DK, Follick MJ: Chronic pain and functional impairment: assessing beliefs about their relationship, *Arch Phys Med Rehabil* 69:579-582, 1988. *Continued*

Adult Population

Box—cont'd

9. As long as I am in pain, I'll never be able to live as well as I did before.

Completely disagree	Disagree	Disagree somewhat	Neutral	Agree somewhat	Agree	Completely agree

10. When my pain gets worse, I find it very hard to concentrate on anything else.

Completely disagree	Disagree	Disagree somewhat	Neutral	Agree somewhat	Agree	Completely agree

11. I have come to accept that I am a disabled individual because of my chronic pain.

Completely disagree	Disagree	Disagree somewhat	Neutral	Agree somewhat	Agree	Completely agree

12. There is no way that I can return to doing the things that I used to do unless I first find a cure for my pain.

Completely disagree	Disagree	Disagree somewhat	Neutral	Agree somewhat	Agree	Completely agree

13. I find myself frequently thinking about my pain and what it has done to my life.

Completely disagree	Disagree	Disagree somewhat	Neutral	Agree somewhat	Agree	Completely agree

14. Although my pain is always present, I often do not notice it at all when I'm keeping myself busy.

Completely disagree	Disagree	Disagree somewhat	Neutral	Agree somewhat	Agree	Completely agree

15. All my problems would be solved if my pain would go away.

Completely disagree	Disagree	Disagree somewhat	Neutral	Agree somewhat	Agree	Completely agree

Modified from Riley JF, Ahern DK, Follick MJ: Chronic pain and functional impairment: assessing beliefs about their relationship, *Arch Phys Med Rehabil* 69:579-582, 1988.

Pain Disability Index

The Pain Disability Index (PDI) measures general and more specific indexes of disability related to chronic pain. Patients rate their overall level of disability in seven activities, including family and home responsibilities, recreation, social activity, occupation, sexual behavior, self-care, and life-support activity. The PDI is a self- or therapist-administered tool. The total score ranges from 0 to 70. Higher scores denote greater levels of pain-related disability.

PDI Form

1. *Family/Home Responsibilities.* This category refers to activities related to the home or family. It includes chores and duties performed around the house (e.g., yard work) and errands or favors for other family members (e.g., driving the children to school).

0	1	2	3	4	5	6	7	8	9	10

No disability   Total disability

2. *Recreation.* This category include hobbies, sports, and other similar leisure time activities.

0	1	2	3	4	5	6	7	8	9	10

No disability   Total disability

3. *Social Activity.* This category refers to activities which involve participation with friends and acquaintances other than family members. It includes parties, theater, concerts, dining out, and other social functions.

0	1	2	3	4	5	6	7	8	9	10

No disability   Total disability

4. *Occupation.* This category refers to activities that are a part of or directly related to one's job. This includes nonpaying jobs as well, such as that of a housewife or volunteer worker.

0	1	2	3	4	5	6	7	8	9	10

No disability   Total disability

5. *Sexual Behavior.* This category refers to the frequency of sexual encounters and quality of sex life.

0	1	2	3	4	5	6	7	8	9	10

No disability   Total disability

6. *Self Care.* This category includes activities that involve personal maintenance and independent daily living (e.g., taking a shower, driving, getting dressed).

0	1	2	3	4	5	6	7	8	9	10

No disability   Total disability

7. *Life-Support Activity.* This category refers to basic life-supporting behaviors such as eating, sleeping, and breathing.

0	1	2	3	4	5	6	7	8	9	10

No disability   Total disability

From Tait RC and others: The pain disability index: psychometric and validity data, *Arch Phys Med Rehabil* 68:438-441, 1987.

Adult Population

Short Form McGill Pain Questionnaire

The Short Form McGill Pain Questionnaire measures the qualitative and quantitative aspects of pain. It is a combination of three pain-assessment tools. The shortened version of the McGill Pain Questionnaire provides valuable information about the sensory, affective, and evaluative dimensions of pain. The Present Pain Intensity (PPI) Scale and the Visual Analog Scale (VAS) provide data on pain intensity. The Short Form McGill Pain Questionnaire is a self-administered tool. To obtain the VAS score, the therapist should measure to the nearest millimeter the pain intensity marked by patients. The therapist should then sum the Short McGill, VAS, and PPI scores to obtain the total score. The total score ranges from 0 to 75. Higher scores denote greater levels of pain perceived by patients.

Short Form McGill Pain Questionnaire Form

Type of pain	None	Mild	Moderate	Severe
Throbbing	1) _____	2) _____	3) _____	4) _____
Shooting	1) _____	2) _____	3) _____	4) _____
Stabbing	1) _____	2) _____	3) _____	4) _____
Sharp	1) _____	2) _____	3) _____	4) _____
Cramping	1) _____	2) _____	3) _____	4) _____
Gnawing	1) _____	2) _____	3) _____	4) _____
Hot or burning	1) _____	2) _____	3) _____	4) _____
Aching	1) _____	2) _____	3) _____	4) _____
Heavy	1) _____	2) _____	3) _____	4) _____
Tender	1) _____	2) _____	3) _____	4) _____
Splitting	1) _____	2) _____	3) _____	4) _____
Tiring or exhausting	1) _____	2) _____	3) _____	4) _____
Sickening	1) _____	2) _____	3) _____	4) _____
Fearful	1) _____	2) _____	3) _____	4) _____
Punishing or cruel	1) _____	2) _____	3) _____	4) _____

Present Pain Intensity

0 = None   _____
1 = Mild   _____
2 = Discomforting _____
3 = Distressing   _____
4 = Horrible   _____
5 = Excruciating _____

Visual Analog Scale

No pain ├─────────────────────────────────┤ Worst possible pain

Modified from Melzack R: The Short-Form McGill Pain Questionnaire, *Pain* 30:191-197, 1987.

Dementia, Depression, and Delirium Standards
Diagnostic Criteria for Delirium with Multiple Etiologies

A. Disturbance of consciousness (i.e., reduced clarity of awareness of the environment) with reduced ability to focus, sustain, or shift attention
B. Change in cognition (e.g., memory deficit, disorientation, language disturbance) or the development of a perceptual disturbance that is not better accounted for by a preexisting, established, or evolving dementia
C. Disturbance developing over a short period (usually hours to days) and tending to fluctuate during the course of the day
D. Evidence from the history, physical examination, or laboratory findings that the delirium has more than one etiology (e.g., more than one etiological general medical condition, a general medical condition plus substance intoxication or medication side effect

Modified from American Psychiatric Association: *Diagnostic and statistical manual of mental disorders,* ed 4, Washington, DC, 1994, The Association.

Diagnostic Criteria for Dementia of the Alzheimer's Type

A. The development of multiple cognitive deficits are manifested by both of the following:
  1. Memory impairment (impaired ability to learn new information or to recall previously learned information)
  2. One (or more) of the following cognitive disturbances:
     • aphasia (language disturbance)
     • apraxia (impaired ability to carry out motor activities despite intact motor function)
     • agnosia (failure to recognize or identify objects despite intact sensory function)
     • disturbance in executive functioning (i.e., planning, organizing, sequencing, abstracting)
B. The cognitive deficits in criteria *A1* and *A2* cause significant impairment in social or occupational functioning and represent a significant decline from a previous level of functioning.
C. The course is characterized by gradual onset and continuing cognitive decline.
D. The cognitive deficits in criteria *A1* and *A2* are not due to any of the following:
  1. Other central nervous system conditions that cause progressive deficits in memory and cognition (e.g., cerebrovascular disease, Parkinson's disease, Huntington's disease, subdural hematoma, normal-pressure hydrocephalus, brain tumor)
  2. Systemic conditions that are known to cause dementia (e.g., hypothyroidism, vitamin B_{12} or folic acid deficiency, niacin deficiency, hypercalcemia, neurosyphilis, HIV infection)
  3. Substance-induced conditions
E. The deficits do not occur exclusively during the course of a delirium.
F. The disturbance is not better accounted for by another Axis I disorder (e.g., major depressive disorder, schizophrenia).

Modified from American Psychiatric Association: *Diagnostic and statistical manual of mental disorders,* ed 4, Washington, DC, 1994, The Association.
HIV, Human immunodeficiency virus.

Adult Population

Diagnostic Criteria for Major Depressive Episode

A. Five (or more) of the following symptoms have been present during the same 2-week period and represent a change from previous functioning; at least one of the symptoms is (1) a depressed mood or (2) loss of interest or pleasure.
   NOTE: Do not include symptoms that are clearly due to a general medical condition, or mood-incongruent delusions or hallucinations.
   1. Depressed mood most of the day, nearly every day, as indicated by a subjective report (e.g., feels sad or empty) or observation made by others (e.g., appears tearful); NOTE: in children and adolescents, can be irritable mood
   2. Markedly diminished interest or pleasure in all, or almost all, activities most of the day, nearly every day (as indicated by a subjective account or observation made by others)
   3. Significant weight loss when not dieting or weight gain (e.g., a change of more than 5% of body weight in a month), or decrease or increase in appetite nearly every day; NOTE: in children, consider failure to make expected weight gains
   4. Insomnia or hypersomnia nearly every day
   5. Psychomotor agitation or retardation nearly every day (observable by others, not merely subjective feelings of restlessness or being slowed down)
   6. Fatigue or loss of energy nearly every day
   7. Feelings of worthlessness or excessive or inappropriate guilt (which may be delusional) nearly every day (not merely self-reproach or guilt about being sick)
   8. Diminished ability to think or concentrate, or indecisiveness, nearly every day (by a subjective account or as observed by others)
   9. Recurrent thoughts of death (not just fear of dying), recurrent suicidal ideation without a specific plan, or a suicide attempt or a specific plan for committing suicide
B. The symptoms do not meet criteria for a mixed episode.
C. The symptoms cause clinically significant distress or impairment in social, occupational, or other important areas of functioning.
D. The symptoms are not due to the direct physiological effects of a substance (e.g., a drug of abuse, a medication) or a general medical condition (e.g., hypothyroidism).
E. The symptoms are not better accounted for by bereavement (i.e., after the loss of a loved one, the symptoms persist for longer than 2 months or are characterized by marked functional impairment, morbid preoccupation with worthlessness, suicidal ideation, psychotic symptoms, or psychomotor retardation).

Modified from American Psychiatric Association: *Diagnostic and statistical manual of mental disorders,* ed 4, Washington, DC, 1994, The Association.

Comparison of Delirium, Depression, and Dementia

	Delirium	Depression	Dementia
Onset	Is rapid (hours to days)	Is rapid (weeks to months)	Is gradual (years)
Course	Shows wide fluctuations; may continue for weeks if cause not found	May be self-limited or may become chronic without treatment	Is chronic; slow but continuous decline
Level of consciousness	Fluctuates from hyperalert to difficult to arouse	Is normal	Is normal
Orientation	Is disoriented, confused	May seem disoriented	Is disoriented, confused
Affect	Fluctuates	Is sad, depressed, worried, guilty	Is labile; displays apathy in later stages
Attention	Is always impaired	Has difficulty concentrating; may check and recheck all actions	May be intact; may focus on one thing for long periods
Sleep	Is always disturbed	Is disturbed; experiences excess sleeping or insomnia, especially early-morning waking	Is usually normal
Behavior	Is agitated, restless	May be fatigued, apathetic; may occasionally be agitated	May be agitated or apathetic; may wander
Speech	Is sparse or rapid; may be incoherent	Is flat, sparse; may have outbursts; is understandable	Is sparse or rapid; is repetitive; may be incoherent
Memory	Is impaired, especially for recent events	Varies day to day; has slow recall; often has short-term deficit	Is impaired, especially for recent events
Cognition	Shows disordered reasoning	May seem impaired	Shows disordered reasoning and calculation
Thought content	Is incoherent, confused, delusional, stereotyped	Is negative; is hypochondriacal; has thoughts of death; is paranoid	Is disorganized; displays rich content; is delusional; is paranoid
Perception	Experiences misinterpretations, illusions, hallucinations	Is distorted; may have auditory hallucinations; has negative interpretation of people and events	Shows no change
Judgment	Is poor	Is poor	Is poor; displays socially inappropriate behavior
Insight	May be present in lucid moments	May be impaired	Is absent
Performance on mental status examination	Is poor but variable; improves during lucid moments and with recovery	Is memory impaired; does not usually have impairments with calculation, drawing, following directions; gives frequent "I don't know" answers	Is consistently poor; progressively worsens; attempts to answer all questions

Adult Population

Modified from Holt J: How to help confused patients, *Am J Nurs* pp 32-36, 1993.

Motivation Guidelines*
Principle 1: Be an Effective Teacher

Often noncompliance occurs simply because patients do not understand the purpose of tasks or directions to complete them correctly. Patients may be too embarrassed to ask therapists for assistance, so they continue to do tasks incorrectly or not at all. In these instances, therapists must maximize their teaching skills to encourage full patient participation from the first visit.

1. **Be clear and concise**—When providing verbal or written instructions, therapists should use simple words and terminology to facilitate understanding.

2. **Provide written instructions**—Patients often have several home health services, each independently asking them to learn new information such as nutrition education, home programs, and medication information. Because all this new information is important, therapists must provide patients with written information to enhance their recall. After providing written instructions, therapists should ask patients to read the instructions back and ask pertinent questions about the instructions to ensure patients are able to read them correctly and understand the content.

3. **Tailor the teaching**—Patients, like therapists, have specific learning styles that work best for them. For example, some patients respond best to written explanations, whereas others learn more quickly from demonstrations. Therapists should tailor their teaching styles to meet the needs of patients and promote more expedient learning. Therapists should ask patients about their best learning styles and incorporate them into each treatment for quicker and more accurate communication and learning.

4. **Explain the purpose and goal**—Sometimes patients elect not to do activities or tasks as requested because they simply do not understand the reason they are being asked to do them. Therefore therapists must always explain the reasons for a task and relate its purpose to functional activities in a way patients can readily understand. For example, if working on unilateral stance with patients with hip fractures, the therapist should explain how hip abductor strengthening improves not only balance but also the "limp" they have when walking by improving hip abductor strength. Because patients usually desire "normal" gait patterns, they are much more interested in complying with the task when aware of the functional purpose.

5. **Observe patient performance**—Just because therapists have taught patients tasks, provided written instructions, and answered questions, therapists should never assume patients understand completely what was just taught. Regardless of the simplicity of the instructions, therapists should always have patients demonstrate the task. This allows therapists to assess safe and effective carryover more accurately than simply relying on patient statements that they understand "what to do."

6. **Provide positive feedback**—Everyone follows through with instructions when given encouragement and positive feedback. Feedback tells patients that therapists are watching and interested in their rehabilitation. Patients are more

---

*This section is modified from Anemaet WK, Moffa-Trotter ME: *The user friendly home care handbook,* Washington, DC, 1997, LEARN Publications.

likely to comply with therapy programs when they realize someone is taking a sincere interest in them.

Principle 2: Be a Supportive Partner

Gone are the days when therapists "get patients better." Today, therapists serve as partners to patients, showing them the things they need to do to get better. Sometimes, therapists do not provide proper direction or support for patients, allowing patients to take on passive roles in their rehabilitation and fostering relationships in which patients depend on therapists. This makes eventual attainment of independence slower and more difficult.

1. **Set realistic and patient-oriented goals**—Sometimes therapists set goals that are too easy for patients or incongruent with what patients hope to obtain after rehabilitation. At other times, therapists set goals that are too aggressive, and work toward functional goals in which patients do not have a vested interest, such as working toward ambulating without a cane when the patient feels insecure without it but confident and independent with it. To avoid mismatched goals, therapists ask patients about their personal goals for rehabilitation and set goals accordingly. Any modifications suggested are discussed so that both parties work with, rather than against, each other toward the same goals.

2. **Give patients choices**—At times, patients fall into passive roles after extended hospitalizations and nursing home stays, in part because decisions about what to eat, when to sleep, and what to do have been made by others. Taking away decision making disempowers patients and does not inspire high compliance or motivation with therapy. To assist patients in regaining some control over their daily routines and promote active participation in therapy, therapists offer patients choices during treatment. For example, therapists allow patients to decide what to do first or last in treatment sessions or which goal to focus on for the coming week.

3. **Give patients purposeful active roles**—Therapists prevent patients from being passive participants in their rehabilitation by instructing them on the evaluation of their responsibilities, such as compliance with home programs. In this way, patients learn in the early stages of treatment that the task of getting well again truly rests on their own shoulders.

4. **Encourage caregiver involvement**—Caregiver involvement benefits patients, caregivers, and therapists for several reasons. First, caregivers assist therapists by monitoring patient compliance with therapy instructions. Second, active caregivers take on more involved roles, perhaps assisting patients with home programs or even performing the exercises with patients. Third, involving caregivers in therapy programs and education gives therapists witnesses—another pair of eyes and ears—that can support them when patients claim they were never told to do a certain task. Finally, caregiver participation in therapy allows patients to foster a working relationship with their caregivers, which eases the transition after therapy discharge. Of course, there are instances in which caregiver involvement may be detrimental (e.g., when the caregiver has too many responsibilities, when a poor marital relationship is a factor). Therefore therapists must screen caregiver-patient dynamics carefully before involving the caregiver.

Adult Population

5. **Update patients**—Therapists act as supportive partners when encouraging patients in meaningful ways. Perhaps the most effective method for motivating patients is to update them weekly about the progress made with therapy. Everyone likes to feel that things are improving, yet many patients lack the ability to objectively view their progress. If patients feel their functional status has not changed, they are less likely to participate in therapy or comply with home programs.

Principle 3: Be a Positive Role Model

Patients look to therapists for advice, direction, encouragement and guidance. Therapists with upbeat attitudes and good teaching skills foster much better patient relationships compared with therapists who take little time with their patients or seem detached. Therapists must be role models for patients and encourage them to be motivated and to participate.

1. **Address ageist thoughts and excuses**—Sometimes patients limit their own abilities and participate less in therapy because of erroneous beliefs or stereotypes about the aging process. For example, patients with arthritis may not do an exercise program because they believe that exercise increases pain. Other patients may not comply with strengthening programs because they feel too old to get stronger. Therapists can use the numerous clinical studies published to address these counterproductive beliefs and prevent patients from relying on excuses not to comply with therapy.

2. **Use individualized therapy**—When therapists realize that they are using the same treatment interventions each day with all or most of their patients and changing little or nothing in their patients' programs or status they are using "canned" therapy. Patients often notice this and may view therapists as unenthusiastic and uninterested in their therapy programs. This turns therapists into poor role models, and subsequently patient participation and motivation may suffer.

3. **Join the crowd**—Being a good role model involves setting good examples for patients. Patients, especially those with little experience exercising or being active, are more inclined to comply when therapists perform the exercises or tasks with them.

4. **Make it fun**—Like most people, patients are more enthusiastic and participate more in therapy if the activities are fun. As role models, therapists must creatively develop home programs and therapy interventions and make tasks enjoyable. For example, instead of having a patient perform repetitive weight shifts, the therapist can make the activity more exciting and purposeful by using balls or cones. Therapists should incorporate patients' hobbies, such as crafts, golf, or tennis, into therapy sessions to maintain patient interest in specific tasks.

ADULT ACTIVITIES OF DAILY LIVING SKILLS EVALUATION

Activities of daily living (ADL) are tasks such as feeding, grooming, bathing, dressing, toileting, and maintaining continence. Conversely, instrumental activities of daily living (IADL) more complex tasks such as taking medications, obtaining transportation, preparing meals, managing finances, doing laundry, and housekeeping. Together, ADL and IADL comprise critical tasks that must be performed if patients are to function in their home environments with minimal assistance. One of the main benefits of the home health setting is the immediate applicability of therapy intervention to the restoration of ADL and IADL performance or compensation for problems performing ADL and IADL. ADL and IADL assessment tools provide therapists with standardized methods to objectively evaluate deficits, target treatment interventions, and after a reevaluation, demonstrate material progress to claims reviewers. Specific glossaries define ADL and incontinence terminology. Associated guidelines address recommendations and tips for daily living skills deficits.

Basic Activities of Daily Living Assessments
Barthel Index

The Barthel Index scores the ability of patients to care for themselves. It examines nine tasks, including feeding, transferring, toileting, toilet transferring, bathing, ambulation or propelling a wheelchair, stair climbing, dressing, and maintaining continence. The Barthel Index is a self- or therapist-administered tool. The total score ranges from 0 to 100. Higher scores denote greater independence in performing ADL.

Barthel Index Form

The following presents the items or tasks scored in the Barthel Index with the corresponding values for independent performance of the tasks:

	Can do by myself	Can do with help of someone else	Cannot do at all
Self-Care Index			
1. Drinking from a cup	4	0	0
2. Eating	6	0	0
3. Dressing upper body	5	4	0
4. Dressing lower body	7	4	0
5. Putting on brace or artificial limb	0	2	0 (Not applicable)
6. Grooming	5	0	0
7. Washing or bathing	6	0	0
8. Controlling urination	10	5 (Accidents)	0 (Incontinence)
9. Controlling bowel movements	10	5 (Accidents)	0 (Incontinence)

Modified from Mahoney FI, Barthel DW: Functional evaluation: the Barthel Index, *Maryland St Med J* 14(2):61-65, 1965.

Continued

Table—cont'd

	Can do by myself	Can do with help of someone else	Cannot do at all
Mobility Index			
10. Getting in and out of chair	15	7	0
11. Getting on and off toilet	6	3	0
12. Getting in and out of tub or shower	1	0	0
13. Walking 50 yards on the level	15	10	0
14. Walking up and down one flight of stairs	10	5	0
15. If not walking, propelling or pushing wheelchair	5	0	0 (Not applicable)

BARTHEL TOTAL: Best score is 100; worst score is 0.

   NOTE: Tasks 1-9, the Self-Care Index (which includes control of bladder and bowel sphincters), have a total possible score of 53. Tasks 10-15, the Mobility Index, have a total possible score of 47. The two groups of tasks combined make up the total Barthel Index, with a total possible score of 100.

Modified from Mahoney FI, Barthel DW: Functional evaluation: The Barthel Index, *Maryland St Med J* 14(2):61-65, 1965.

Basic Activities of Daily Living Disability Continuum Scale

The Basic Activities of Daily Living (BADL) Disability Continuum Scale assesses the level of difficulty and dependence in ADL function in older adults. It evaluates six tasks, including bathing, dressing, bed-to-chair transferring, feeding, toileting, and grooming. The BADL Disability Continuum Scale is a self- or therapist-administered tool. Patients are considered "independent without difficulty" if they do not require assistance or report difficulty with any ADL. Patients are considered "independent with difficulty" if they do not require assistance but report difficulty with at least one activity; patients are considered "dependent" if they require assistance with at least one ADL.

BADL Disability Continuum Scale Form

Basic Activities of Daily Living	Do you need help?		How much difficulty on average do you have?		
Bathing	Yes	No	None	Some	A lot
Dressing	Yes	No	None	Some	A lot
Bed-to-chair transferring	Yes	No	None	Some	A lot
Eating	Yes	No	None	Some	A lot
Toileting	Yes	No	None	Some	A lot
Grooming	Yes	No	None	Some	A lot

Modified from Gill TM, Robinson JT, Tinetti ME: Difficulty and dependence: two components of the disability continuum among community-living older persons, *Ann Int Med* 128:96-101, 1998.

Index of Activities of Daily Living

The Index of Activities of Daily Living evaluates overall performance in ADL. It examines the ability of patients to independently perform six functional tasks, including bathing, dressing, toileting, transferring, feeding, and maintaining continence. The Index of Activities of Daily Living is a therapist-administered tool. The total score ranges from grade A to G, with grade A indicating independence in performing ADL and grade G indicating dependence in performing ADL.

Index of Activities of Daily Living Form

For each area of functioning listed below, check the description that applies. (The word *assistance* means supervision, direction, or personal assistance.)

Bathing—taking either sponge bath, tub bath, or shower

☐
Receives no assistance (gets in and out of tub by self if tub is usual means of bathing)

☐
Receives assistance in bathing only one part of the body (such as back or a leg)

☐
Receives assistance in bathing more than one part of the body (or has not bathed)

Dressing—getting clothes from closets and drawers, including underclothes, outer garments, and fasteners (including braces if worn)

☐
Gets clothes and gets completely dressed without assistance

☐
Gets clothes and gets dressed without assistance (except receives assistance in tying shoes)

☐
Receives assistance in getting clothes or in getting dressed, or stays partly or completely undressed

Toileting—going to the toilet room for bowel and urine elimination, cleaning self after elimination, and arranging clothes

☐
Goes to toilet room, cleans self, and arranges clothes without assistance (may use object such as cane, walker, or wheelchair for support; may use night bedpan or commode and empty it in morning)

☐
Receives assistance in going to toilet room in cleansing self, in arranging clothes after elimination, or in using night bedpan or commode

☐
Does not go to appropriate room for the elimination process

Transferring

☐
Moves in and out of bed and chair without assistance (may use object such as cane or walker for support)

☐
Moves in and out of bed or chair with assistance

☐
Does not get out of bed

Maintaining Continence

☐
Controls urination and bowel movement completely by self

☐
Has occasional "accidents"

☐
Needs supervision to help control urination or bowel movements; uses catheter or is incontinent

Modified from Katz S and others: Studies of illness in the aged, *J Am Med Assoc* 185(12):914-919, 1963.

Adult Population

Continued

Feeding

☐

Feeds self without assistance

☐

Feeds self independently but gets assistance in cutting meat or buttering bread

☐

Receives assistance feeding or is fed partly or completely by using tubes or intravenous fluids

The Index of Independence in Activities of Daily Living is based on an evaluation of the functional independence or dependence of patients in bathing, dressing, going to the toilet, transferring, continence, and eating. Specific definitions of functional independence and dependence appear after the index.

A—Independent in feeding, continence, transferring, going to the toilet, dressing, and bathing
B—Independent in all but one of these functions
C—Independent in all but bathing and one additional function
D—Independent in all but bathing, dressing, and one additional function
E—Independent in all but bathing, dressing, going to the toilet, and one additional function
F—Independent in all but bathing, dressing, going to the toilet, transferring, and one additional function
G—Dependent in all six functions
Other—Dependent in at least two functions, but not classifiable as C, D, E, or F

Independent means without supervision, direction, or active personal assistance, except as specifically noted below. This is based on actual status and not on ability. A patient who refuses to perform a function is considered as not performing the function, even though he is deemed able.

Bathing (Sponge, Shower, or Tub)
Independent: receives assistance only in bathing a single part (such as back or disabled extremity) or bathes self completely
Dependent: receives assistance in bathing more than one part of body; receives assistance in getting in or out of tub or does not bathe self

Dressing
Independent: gets clothes from closets and drawers; puts on clothes, outer garments, braces; manages fasteners (act of tying shoes is excluded)
Dependent: does not dress self or remains partly undressed

Toileting
Independent: gets to the toilet; gets on and off the toilet; arranges clothes; cleans self (may manage own bedpan used at night only and may be using mechanical supports)
Dependent: uses bedpan or commode or receives assistance in getting to and using the toilet

Transferring
Independent: moves in and out of bed independently and moves in and out of chair independently (may be using mechanical supports)
Dependent: receives assistance in moving in or out of bed and/or chair; does not perform one or more transfers

Maintaining Continence
Independent: controls urination and defecation entirely independently
Dependent: experiences partial or total incontinence in urination or defecation; experiences partial or total control by enemas, catheters, or regulated use of urinals or bedpans

Feeding
Independent: gets food from plate or its equivalent into mouth (precutting meat and preparing food, such as buttering bread, not included in evaluation)
Dependent: receives assistance in feeding (see above); does not eat at all or receives parenteral feeding

Modified from Katz S and others: Studies of illness in the aged, *J Am Med Assoc* 185(12):914-919, 1963.

Physical Self-Maintenance Scale

The Physical Self-Maintenance Scale (PSMS) measures the ability of patients to independently perform ADL. It evaluates the level of independence in performing toileting, eating, dressing, grooming, locomotion, and bathing tasks. The PSMS is a self- or therapist-administered tool. The total score ranges from 0 to 6. Higher scores denote greater independence in performing ADL.

PSMS Form

Task	Score
Toileting	
1 = Cares for self at the toilet completely, experiences no incontinence	
0 = Needs to be reminded or needs help in cleaning self, or has rare (weekly at most) accidents	
0 = Soils or wets while asleep more than once a week	
0 = Soils or wets while awake more than once a week	
0 = Has no control of bowels or bladder	
Feeding	
1 = Feeds self without assistance	
0 = Feeds self with minor assistance at meal times and/or with special preparation of food, or help in cleaning up after meals	
0 = Feeds self with moderate assistance and is untidy	
0 = Requires extensive assistance for all meals	
0 = Does not feed self at all and resists efforts of others to help	
Dressing	
1 = Dresses, undresses, and selects clothes from own wardrobe	
0 = Dresses and undresses with minor assistance	
0 = Needs moderate assistance in dressing or selecting clothes	
0 = Needs major assistance in dressing or selecting clothes	
0 = Is completely unable to dress self and resists efforts of others to help	
Grooming (Neatness, Hair, Nails, Hands, Face, Clothing)	
1 = Grooms self without assistance and is always neatly dressed and well-groomed	
0 = Grooms self adequately and receives occasional minor assistance (e.g., with shaving)	
0 = Needs moderate and regular assistance or supervision in grooming	
0 = Needs total grooming care, but can remain well-groomed after help from others	
0 = Actively resists all efforts of others to assist with grooming	

Modified from Lawton MP, Brody EM: Assessment of older people: self-maintaining and instrumental activities of daily living, *Gerontologist* 9:179-186, 1969.

Continued

Table—cont'd

Task	Score
Physical Ambulation 1 = Goes about grounds or city 0 = Ambulates within residence or about 1-block distance 0 = Ambulates with assistance of the following (check one): ( ) Another person ( ) Railing ( ) Cane ( ) Walker ( ) Wheelchair _____ gets in and out without help _____ needs help getting in and out 0 = Sits unsupported in chair or wheelchair, but cannot propel self without help 0 = Is bedridden more than half the time **Bathing** 1 = Bathes self (e.g., in tub, in shower, by sponge bath) 0 = Bathes self with help in getting in and out of tub 0 = Washes face and hands only, but cannot bathe rest of body 0 = Does not wash self but is cooperative with those who assist 0 = Does not try to wash self and resists efforts to assist	

Modified from Lawton MP, Brody EM: Assessment of older people: self-maintaining and instrumental activities of daily living, *Gerontologist* 9:179-186, 1969.

Instrumental Activities of Daily Living Assessments
Five-Item IADL Questionnaire

The Five-Item IADL Questionnaire evaluates the capacity of adults to live independently in the community. It measures the ability of patients to independently perform transportation, shopping, meal preparation, housework, and money management tasks. The Five-Item IADL Questionnaire is a self- or therapist-administered tool. The total score ranges from 0 to 5. Higher scores denote greater independence with IADL.

Five-Item IADL Questionnaire Form

Can you get to places out of walking distance . . .
1   without help (alone on buses or taxis, or by driving your own car)?
0   with some help (i.e., someone to help you or go with you when traveling), or are you unable to travel unless emergency arrangements are made for a specialized vehicle such as an ambulance?
—   Not answered

Can you go shopping for groceries or clothes (assuming you have transportation) . . .
1   without help (taking care of all shopping needs yourself, assuming you had transportation)?
0   with some help (need someone to go with you on all shopping trips) or are you completely unable to do any shopping?
—   Not answered

Can you prepare your own meals . . .
1   without help (plan and cook full meals yourself)?
0   with some help (can prepare some things but unable to cook full meals yourself), or are you completely unable to prepare any meals?
—   Not answered

Can you do your housework . . .
1   without help (can scrub floors, etc.)?
0   with some help (can do light housework but need help with heavy work), or are you completely unable to do any housework?
—   Not answered

Can you handle your own money . . .
1   without help (write checks, pay bills, etc.)?
0   with some help (manage day-to-day buying but need help with managing your checkbook and paying your bills), or are you completely unable to handle money?
—   Not answered

Modified from Fillenbaum GG: Screening the elderly: a brief instrumental activities of daily living measure, *J Am Ger Soc* 33:698, 1985.

Adult Population

IADL Scale

The IADL Scale measures independence in performing IADL. It evaluates the ability of patients to independently perform eight tasks, including using the telephone, housekeeping, and taking medication. The IADL Scale is a self- or therapist-administered tool. The total score ranges from 0 to 8. Higher scores denote greater independence with IADL.

IADL Scale Form

Task	Score

Ability to Use Telephone
1 = operates telephone on own initiative (looks up and dials numbers, etc.)
1 = dials a few well-known numbers
1 = answers telephone but does not dial
0 = does not use telephone at all

Shopping
1 = takes care of all shopping needs independently
0 = shops independently for small purchases
0 = needs to be accompanied on any shopping trip
0 = is completely unable to shop

Food Preparation
1 = plans, prepares, and serves adequate meals independently
0 = prepares adequate meals if supplied with ingredients
0 = heats and serves prepared meals, or prepares meals but does not maintain
      adequate diet
0 = needs to have meals prepared and served

Housekeeping
1 = maintains house alone or with occasional assistance (e.g., "heavy work-domestic help")
1 = performs light daily tasks such as dishwashing and bedmaking
1 = performs light daily tasks but cannot maintain acceptable level of cleanliness
1 = needs help with all home maintenance tasks
0 = does not participate only in housekeeping tasks

Laundry
1 = does personal laundry completely
1 = launders small items (rinses socks, stockings, etc.)
0 = requires all laundry to be done by others

Mode of Transportation
1 = travels independently on public transportation or drives own car
1 = arranges own travel via taxi, but does not otherwise use public transportation
1 = travels on public transportation when assisted or accompanied by another
1 = travels only in taxi or automobile with assistance of another (*score 0 if patient is male*)
0 = does not travel at all

Responsibility for Own Medications
1 = is responsible for taking medication in correct dosages at correct time
0 = takes responsibility if medication is prepared in advance in separate dosages
0 = is not capable of dispensing own medication

Ability to Handle Finances
1 = manages financial matters independently (budgets, writes checks, pays rent, pays
      bills, goes to bank), collects and keeps track of income
1 = manages day-to-day purchases, but needs help with banking, major purchases, etc.
0 = is incapable of handling money

Modified from Lawton MP, Brody EM: Assessment of older people: self-maintaining and instrumental activities of daily living, *Gerontologist* 9:179-186, 1969.

Basic and Instrumental Activities of Daily Living Assessments
Activities of Daily Living-Instrumental Activities of Daily Living Scale

The ADL-IADL Scale measures functional problems with ADL and IADL in older adults. It evaluates dependence and difficulty with 18 ADL and IADL tasks. The ADL-IADL Scale is a self- or therapist-administered tool. The total score ranges from 18 to 54. Higher scores denote greater dependence with ADL and IADL tasks.

ADL-IADL Scale Form

Task	Independently and easily	Independently but with some difficulty	Dependently or with supervision
Eating and drinking (ADL)	1	2	3
Washing face and hands (ADL)	1	2	3
Using the toilet (ADL)	1	2	3
Arising from chair (ADL)	1	2	3
Getting in and out of bed (ADL)	1	2	3
Moving inside house (ADL)	1	2	3
Dressing (ADL)	1	2	3
Performing "light" house-cleaning activities (IADL)	1	2	3
Washing oneself completely (ADL)	1	2	3
Moving outdoors on flat ground (ADL)	1	2	3
Preparing dinner (IADL)	1	2	3
Preparing breakfast and lunch (IADL)	1	2	3
Going up and down stairs (ADL)	1	2	3
Making bed (IADL)	1	2	3
Caring for feet and nails (ADL)	1	2	3
Washing and ironing clothes (IADL)	1	2	3
Shopping (IADL)	1	2	3
Performing "heavy" house-cleaning activities (IADL)	1	2	3

Modified from Kempken GIJM, Suurmeijer TPBM: The development of a hierarchial polychotomous ADL-IADL Scale for noninstitutionalized elders, *Gerontologist* 30(4):497-502, 1990.

Older American Resource and Services Activities of Daily Living Questionnaire

The OARS ADL Questionnaire measures the extent or capacity of adults to perform select tasks needed for continued independent living in the community. It assesses ADL tasks, including feeding and dressing, and IADL tasks, including telephone use and meal preparation. The OARS ADL Questionnaire is a self- or therapist-administered tool. Therapists complete the performance rating scale for ADL. The total score of the performance rating scale for ADL ranges from 1 to 6. Higher scores denote greater impairment in ADL-IADL capacity. The total score for the ADL Questionnaire ranges from 0 to 29. Higher scores denote greater independence with ADL.

Adult Population

OARS ADL Questionnaire Form

Task	Score

Instrumental Activities of Daily Living

Can you use the telephone . . .
2 = without help, including looking up numbers and dialing?
1 = with some help (can answer phone or dial operator in an emergency, but need a special phone or help in getting the number or dialing)?
0 = not at all? (completely unable to use the phone)
— not answered

Can you get to places out of walking distance . . .
2 = without help (drive your own car or travel alone on buses, taxis)?
1 = with some help (need someone to help you or go with you when traveling)?
0 = not at all, unless emergency arrangements are made for a specialized vehicle such as an ambulance?
— not answered

Can you go shopping for groceries or clothes (assuming you have transportation) . . .
2 = without help (taking care of all shopping needs yourself, assuming you had transportation)?
1 = with some help (need someone to go with you on all shopping trips)?
0 = not at all? (completely unable to do any shopping)
— not answered

Can you prepare your own meals . . .
2 = without help (plan and cook full meals yourself)?
1 = with some help (can prepare some things but unable to cook full meals yourself)?
0 = not at all? (completely unable to prepare any meals)
— not answered

Can you do your housework . . .
2 = without help (can clean floors, etc.)?
1 = with some help (can do light housework but need help with heavy work)?
0 = not at all? (completely unable to do housework)
— not answered

Can you take your own medicine . . .
2 = without help (in the right dose at the right time)?
1 = with some help (able to take medicine if someone prepares it for you and/or reminds you to take it)?
0 = not at all? (completely unable to take your own medicine)
— not answered

Can you handle your own money . . .
2 = without help (write checks, pay bills, etc.)?
1 = with some help (manage day-to-day buying but need help with managing your checkbook and paying your bills)?
0 = not at all? (completely unable to handle money)
— not answered

Modified from Fillenbaum GG: *Multidimensional functional assessment of older adults: the Duke older American resource and services procedure.* Hillsdale, NJ, 1988, Lawrence Erlbaum Associates.

Task	Score
Physical Activities of Daily Living	

Physical Activities of Daily Living

Can you eat . . .
2 = without help (able to feed yourself completely)?
1 = with some help (need help with cutting, etc.)?
0 = not without help? (completely unable to feed yourself)
— not answered

Can you dress and undress yourself . . .
2 = without help (able to pick out clothes, dress and undress yourself)?
1 = with some help?
0 = not at all? (completely unable to dress and undress yourself)
— not answered

Can you take care of your own appearance (e.g., combing your hair and [for men] shaving) . . .
2 = without help?
1 = with some help?
0 = not at all? (completely unable to maintain your appearance yourself)
— not answered

Can you walk . . .
2 = without help (except from a cane)?
1 = with some help (from an individual or with the use of a walker, crutches, etc.)?
0 = not at all? (completely unable to walk)
— not answered

Can you get in and out of bed . . .
2 = without help?
1 = with some help (from an individual or with the aid of some device)?
0 = not without someone else to lift you? (i.e., totally dependent)
— not answered

Can you take a bath or shower . . .
2 = without help?
1 = with some help (need help getting in and out of the tub, or need special attachments on the tub)?
0 = not by yourself?
— not answered

Do you ever have trouble getting to the bathroom on time?
2 = no
0 = yes
1 = have catheter or colostomy
— not answered
(if "yes," ask *a*)
a. How often do you wet or soil yourself (either day or night)?
   1 = once or twice a week
   0 = three times a week or more
   — not answered

Adult Population

Continued

Table—cont'd

Task	Score
Is there someone who helps you with tasks such as shopping, housework, bathing, dressing, and getting around? 1 = yes 0 = no — not answered (if "yes," ask *a* and *b*) a. Who is your major helper? _____ relationship _____ b. Who else helps you? _____ relationship _____	

Performance Rating Scale for Activities of Daily Living

Excellent ADL capacity
Can perform all activities of daily living without assistance and with ease

Good ADL capacity
Can perform all activities of daily living without assistance

Mildly impaired ADL capacity
Can perform all but one to three of the activities of daily living; requires some help with one to three, but not necessarily every day; can get through any single day without help; is able to prepare his or her meals

Moderately impaired ADL capacity
Regularly requires assistance with at least four activities of daily living but is able to get through any single day without help; or regularly requires help with meal preparation

Severely impaired ADL capacity
Needs help each day but not necessarily throughout the day or night with many of the activities of daily living

Completely impaired ADL capacity
Needs help throughout the day and/or night to carry out the activities of daily living

Modified from Fillenbaum GG: *Multidimensional functional assessment of older adults: the Duke older American resource and services procedure.* Hillsdale, NJ, 1988, Lawrence Erlbaum Associates.

Incontinence Assessments
Clinical Score of Fecal Incontinence

The Clinical Score of Fecal Incontinence assesses the characteristics of fecal incontinence that adults experience. It specifically measures the frequency, type, quantity, and timing of incontinent episodes, as well as feces-retention ability. The Clinical Score of Fecal Incontinence is a self- or therapist-administered tool. The total score ranges from 0 to 17. Higher scores denote greater problems with fecal incontinence.

Clinical Score of Fecal Incontinence Form

Aspect of incontinence	Score
Frequency of Soiling Per 7 Days 0 = 0 times 1 = 1-3 times 2 = 4-7 times 3 = >7 times	
Incontinent to . . . 1 = flatus only 2 = feces too	
If Soiling with Feces, are Feces . . . 1 = watery? 2 = loose? 3 = solid?	
Quantity of Soiling 1 = minor (causing minor soiling of underclothes or pads) 2 = major (causing clothing change immediately)	
Time of Soiling 1 = night only 2 = day also	
Ability to Retain Feces 1 = more than 15 minutes 2 = 10-14 minutes 3 = 5-9 minutes 4 = 2-4 minutes 5 = less than 2 minutes	

Modified from Guillemot F and others: Biofeedback for the treatment of fecal incontinence, *Dis Colon Rectum* 38(4):393-397, 1994.

Adult Population

Incontinence Scoring System

The Incontinence Scoring System assesses the characteristics of fecal incontinence that adults experience. It specifically examines the frequency and type of fecal incontinence. The Incontinence Scoring System is a self- or therapist-administered tool. The total score ranges from 0 to 20. Higher scores denote greater degrees of fecal incontinence.

Incontinence Scoring System Form

Type of incontinence	Never (0)	Rarely (<1/month)	Sometimes (<1/week; ≥1/month)	Usually (<1/day; ≥1/week)	Always (≥1/day)
Solid	0	1	2	3	4
Liquid	0	1	2	3	4
Gas	0	1	2	3	4
Wears pad	0	1	2	3	4
Alters lifestyle	0	1	2	3	4

Modified from Jorge JMN, Wexner SD: Etiology and management of fecal incontinence, *Dis Colon Rectum* 36(3):77-97, 1993.

Incontinence Questionnaire

The Incontinence Questionnaire assesses the characteristics of urinary incontinence that adults experience. It examines aspects such as frequency, duration, type, and timing. The Incontinence Questionnaire is a self- or therapist-administered tool.

Incontinence Questionnaire Form

1. When did the incontinence begin? _____

2. How often do you experience incontinence? _____

3. How much urine do you leak? _____

4. What have you tried to manage the incontinence? _____

5. What events, if any, produce incontinence (e.g., coughing, sneezing, laughing, exercise, lifting, straining, urgency, sexual intercourse)? _____

6. Do you notice more problems with incontinence in colder weather? _____

7. Does the sound of running water precipitate incontinence? _____

8. Does the incontinence occur as you reach the bathroom or prepare to urinate? _____

9. Does incontinence occur after you have urinated and risen from the toilet? _____

10. Do you have pain with urination? _____

11. Do you urinate frequently? _____

12. Do you have blood in your urine? _____

13. Do you empty your bladder fully? _____

14. Do you have fecal incontinence? _____

15. Do you urinate at night? How often? _____

16. Are you using pads or other protective devices? _____

Modified from McIntosh LJ, Richardson DA: 30-minute evaluation of incontinence in the older woman, *Geriatrics* 49(2):35-44, 1994.

Indexes of Incontinence

The Index of Incontinence evaluates urinary incontinence in adults. It assesses urinary characteristics such as frequency, amount, urgency, and bothersomeness related to incontinence. The Index of Incontinence is a self- or therapist-administered tool. The total score ranges from 0 to 12. Higher scores denote greater degrees of urinary incontinence.

Indexes of Incontinence

Aspect of incontinence	Score
Frequency of Incontinent Episodes	
0 = none	
1 = 1 to 3 times per week	
2 = 4 to 6 times per week	
3 = 1 or more times per day	
Leakage Amount	
0 = none	
1 = slight leakage	
2 = 1 to 2 pads a day	
3 = 3 or more pads a day	
Urgency	
0 = none	
1 = little	
2 = moderate	
3 = strong	
Bothersomeness Related to Incontinence	
0 = none	
1 = little	
2 = moderate	
3 = strong	
TOTAL SCORE	

Modified from Kondo A and others: Bladder neck support prosthesis: a nonoperative treatment for stress or mixed urinary incontinence, *J Urol* 157:824-827, 1997.

Adult Population

Severity Index

The Severity Index assesses the degree of urinary incontinence. It specifically measures frequency and quantity of leakage. The Severity Index is a self- or therapist-administered tool. The results of the questions should be multiplied to obtain the total score. The total score ranges from 0 to 8. Scores of 1 to 2 indicate slight incontinence, scores of 3 to 4 indicate moderate incontinence, and scores of 6 to 8 indicate severe incontinence.

Severity Index Form

Aspect of incontinence	Score
How Often Do You Experience Urinary Leakage? 0 = never 1 = less than once a month 2 = one or several times a month 3 = one or several times a week 4 = every day and/or night	
How Much Urine Do You Lose Each Time? 1 = drops or little 2 = more	
TOTAL SCORE	

From Sandvik H and others: Validation of a severity index in female urinary incontinence and its implementation in an epidemiological survey, *J Epidemiol Comm Health* 47:497-499, 1993.

Activities of Daily Living Glossary

Activities of daily living (ADL)	Instrumental activities of daily living (IADL)
Mobility Bed mobility Wheelchair mobility Transfers Ambulation	**Home Management** Shopping Planning meals Preparing meals Cleaning Doing laundry Caring for children Recycling
Self-Care Dressing Self-feeding Toileting Bathing Grooming	**Community Living Skills** Managing money and finances Using public transportation Driving Shopping Having access to recreation activities
Communication Writing Typing or using computer Telephoning Using special communication devices	**Health Management** Handling medication Knowing health risks Making medical appointments
Environmental Hardware Keys Faucets Light switches Windows and doors .	**Safety Management** Fire safety awareness Ability to call 911 Response to smoke detector Identification of dangerous situations
	Environmental Hardware Vacuum cleaner Can opener Stove and oven Refrigerator Microwave oven

Modified from Pedretti LW, ed: *Occupational therapy practice skills for physical dysfunction,* ed 4, St Louis, 1996, Mosby.

Incontinence Glossary

Absorbent products. Pads and garments, either disposable or reusable, worn to contain incontinence or uncontrolled leakage. Absorbent products include shields, guards, undergarment pads, combination pad-pant systems, diaperlike garments, and bed pads.

Behavioral techniques. Specific interventions designed to alter the relationship between the patient's symptoms and his or her behavior and/or environment for the treatment of maladaptive voiding problems.

Adult Population

a. *Biofeedback.* A behavioral technique by which information about a normally unconscious physiological process is presented to the patient and the clinician as a visual, auditory, or tactile signal. The signal is derived from a measurable physiological parameter, which is subsequently used in an educational process to accomplish a specific therapeutic result. The signal is displayed in a quantitative way, and the patient is taught how to alter it and thus control the physiological process.

b. *Bowel/bladder training.* A behavioral technique that requires the patient to resist or inhibit the sensation of urgency (the strong desire to urinate or defecate), to postpone voiding, and to void according to a timetable rather than to urge to void.

c. *Habit training.* A behavioral technique that calls for scheduling toileting at regular intervals. Unlike bowel or bladder training, there is no systemic effort to motivate the patient to delay voiding and resist urge.

d. *Pelvic muscle exercises.* A behavioral technique that requires repetitive active exercise of the pubococcygeus muscle to improve urethral resistance and urinary control by strengthening the periurethral and pelvic muscles.

e. *Prompted voiding.* A behavioral technique for use primarily with dependent individuals or individuals with cognitive impairments. Prompted voiding is used to teach individuals with incontinence awareness of their incontinence status and to request toileting assistance, either independently or after being prompted by a caregiver.

f. *Voiding record.* Also called an *incontinence chart.* A record maintained by the patient or caregiver that is used to record the frequency, timing, amount of voiding, and other factors associated with incontinence.

Fecal incontinence. Involuntary loss of solid, liquid, or gaseous contents.

a. *Major incontinence.* Deficient control of stool of normal consistency.

b. *Minor incontinence.* Partial soiling or incontinence of flatus or liquid stool.

Urinary incontinence. Involuntary loss of urine sufficient to be a problem.

a. *Mixed urinary incontinence.* The combination of urge and stress urinary incontinence.

b. *Overflow incontinence.* The involuntary loss of urine associated with overdistension of the bladder. Overflow incontinence results from urinary retention that causes the capacity of the bladder to be overwhelmed. Continuous or intermittent leakage of small amounts of urine results.

c. *Stress urinary incontinence.* A form of urinary incontinence characterized by the involuntary loss of urine from the urethra during physical exertion (e.g., during coughing). The stress incontinence symptom or complaint may be confirmed by observing urine loss coincident with an increase in abdominal pressure in the absence of detrusor contraction or an overdistended bladder.

d. *Urge incontinence.* The involuntary loss of urine associated with an abrupt and strong desire to void. Urge incontinence is usually associated with the urodynamic findings of involuntary detrusor (smooth muscle in the wall of the bladder that contracts the bladder and expels urine) contractions or detrusor overactivity.

Activities of Daily Living Guidelines
ADL Techniques for Limited Range of Motion and Strength

Limited Range of Motion and Strength

The major problem for individuals with limited joint range of motion (ROM) is compensation for the lack of reach and joint excursion through means such as environmental adaptation and assistive devices. Individuals who lack muscle strength may require some of the same devices or techniques to compensate and conserve energy. Some adaptations and devices are outlined here.

Dressing activities

The following are general suggestions for facilitating dressing:

1. Use front-opening garments, one size larger than needed and made of fabrics that have some stretch.
2. Use dressing sticks with a garter on one end and a neoprene-covered coat hook on the other (Figure 3-1) for pushing and pulling garments off and on feet and legs and to push a shirt or blouse over the head. Use a pair of dowels with a cup hook on the end of each to pull socks on if a loop tape is sewn to the tops of the socks.
3. Use larger buttons or zippers with a loop on the pull tab.
4. Replace buttons, snaps, hooks, and eyes with Velcro or zippers (for patients who cannot manage traditional fastenings).
5. Eliminate the need to bend to tie shoelaces or use finger joints in this fine activity by using elastic shoelaces or other adapted shoe fasteners.

Dressing activities—cont'd

6. Facilitate donning stockings without bending to the feet by using stocking aids made of garters attached to long webbing straps or by buying those that are commercially available (Figure 3-2).
7. Use one of several types of commercially available button-hooks (Figure 3-3) if finger ROM is limited.
8. Use reachers (Figure 3-4) for picking up socks and shoes, arranging clothes, removing clothes from hangers, picking up objects on the floor, and donning pants.

Feeding activities

The following are assistive devices that can facilitate feeding:

1. Built-up handles on eating utensils can accommodate limited grasp or prehension (Figure 3-5).
2. Elongated or specially curved handles on spoons and forks may be needed to reach the mouth. A swivel spoon or spoon-fork combination can compensate for limited supination (Figure 3-6).
3. Long plastic straws and straw clips on glasses or cups can be used if neck, elbow, or shoulder ROM limits hand-to-mouth motion or if grasp is inadequate to hold the cup or glass.

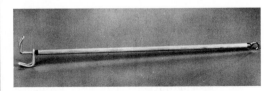

FIGURE 3-1 Dressing stick, or reacher.
(Sammons Preston, an Ability One Company, Bolingbrook, Ill.)

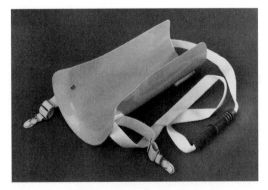

FIGURE 3-2 Sock aid. (Sammons Preston, an Ability One Company, Bolingbrook, Ill.)

Adult Population

Modified from Pedretti LW, ed: *Occupational therapy practice skills for physical dysfunction,* ed 4, St. Louis, 1996, Mosby.

Continued

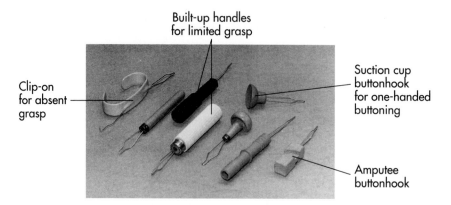

FIGURE 3-3 Buttonhooks to accommodate individuals with amputations or limited or special types of grasp.

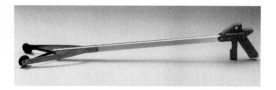

FIGURE 3-4 Extended handled reacher.

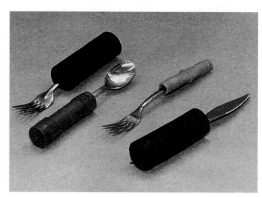

FIGURE 3-5 Eating utensils with built-up handles.

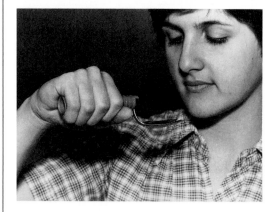

FIGURE 3-6 Swivel spoon compensates for incoordination or limited supination.

Feeding activities—cont'd

4. Universal cuffs or utensil holders can be used if grasp is very limited and built-up handles do not work (Figure 3-7).
5. Plate guards or scoop dishes may be useful to prevent food from slipping off the plate.

Hygiene and grooming

Environmental adaptations that can facilitate bathing and grooming are as follows:

1. A handheld shower head on flexible hose for bathing and shampooing hair can eliminate the need to stand in the shower and offers the user control of the direction of the spray. The handle can be built up or adapted for limited grasp.
2. A long-handled bath brush or sponge with a soap holder (Figure 3-8) or long cloth scrubber can allow the user to reach legs, feet, and back. A wash mitt (Figure 3-9) and soap on a rope can aid limited grasp.

Modified from Pedretti LW, ed: *Occupational therapy practice skills for physical dysfunction*, ed 4, St Louis, 1996, Mosby.

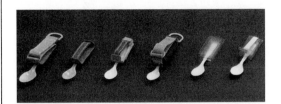

FIGURE 3-7 Utensil holders, universal cuffs. (Sammons Preston, an Ability One Company, Bolingbrook, Ill.)

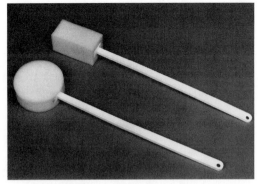

FIGURE 3-8 Long-handled bath sponges. (Sammons Preston, an Ability One Company, Bolingbrook, Ill.)

Hygiene and grooming—cont'd

3. A position-adjustable hair dryer described by Feldmeier and Poole may be helpful for those who prefer a hair style more elaborate than one that can be air-dried. This device is useful for patients with limited ROM, upper extremity weakness, incoordination, or use of only one upper extremity. The dryer is adapted from a desk lamp with spring-balanced arms and a tension-control knob at each joint. The lamp is removed, and the hair dryer is fastened to the spring-balanced arms. The device is mounted on a table or countertop and can be adjusted for various heights and direction of air flow. It frees the patient's hands to manage brushes or combs used to style the hair. The reader is referred to the original source for specifications for constructing this device.

4. Long handles on a comb, brush, toothbrush, lipstick, mascara brush, and safety or electric razor may be useful for limited hand-to-head or hand-to-face movements. Extensions may be constructed from inexpensive wooden dowels or pieces of PVC pipe found in local hardware stores.

5. Spray deodorant, hair spray, and spray powder or perfume can extend the reach by the distance the material sprays. Some individuals may require special adaptations to operate the spray mechanism (Figure 3-10).

6. An electric toothbrush and a Water-Pik may be easier to manage than a standard toothbrush.

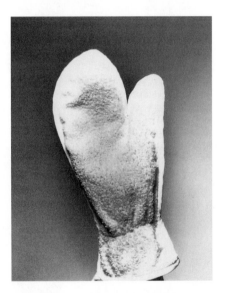

FIGURE 3-9 Terry cloth bath mitt. (Sammons Preston, an Ability One Company, Bolingbrook, Ill.)

Hygiene and grooming—cont'd

7. A short reacher can extend reach for using toilet paper. Several types of toilet aids are available in catalogues that sell assistive devices.

8. Dressing sticks can be used to pull garments up after using the toilet. An alternative is the use of a long piece of elastic or webbing with garters on each end that can be hung around the neck and fastened to pants or panties, preventing them from slipping to the floor during use of the toilet.

Adult Population

Continued

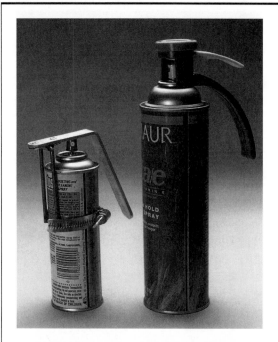

FIGURE 3-10 Spray can adapters. (Sammons Preston, an Ability One Company, Bolingbrook, Ill.)

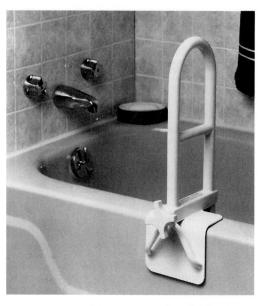

FIGURE 3-11 Bathtub safety rail. (Sammons Preston, an Ability One Company, Bolingbrook, Ill.)

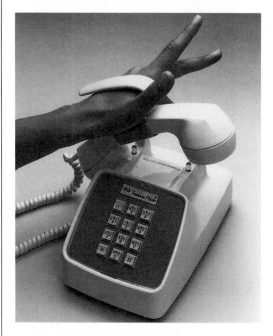

FIGURE 3-12 Telephone clip holder. (Sammons Preston, an Ability One Company, Bolingbrook, Ill.)

Hygiene and grooming—cont'd

9. Safety rails (Figure 3-11) can be used for bathtub transfers, and safety mats or strips can be placed in the bathtub bottom to prevent slipping.
10. A transfer tub bench, shower stool, or regular chair set in the bathtub or shower stall can eliminate the need to sit on the bathtub bottom or stand to shower, thus increasing safety.
11. Grab bars can be installed to prevent falls and ease transfers.

Communication and environmental hardware adaptations

The following are examples of environmental adaptations that can facilitate communication and hardware management:

1. Extended or built-up handles on faucets can accommodate limited grasp.
2. Telephones should be placed within easy reach. A clip-type receiver holder (Figure 3-12), extended receiver holder, speaker phone, or voice-activated phone (Figure 3-13) may be necessary. Dialing sticks and push-button phones are other adaptations.

Modified from Pedretti LW, ed: *Occupational therapy practice skills for physical dysfunction,* ed 4, St Louis, 1996, Mosby.

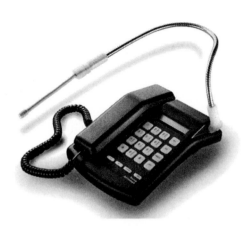

FIGURE 3-13 Voice activated speaker phone.

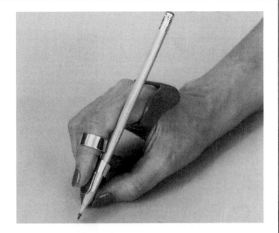

FIGURE 3-14 Wanchik writing aid.
(Sammons Preston, an Ability One Company, Bolingbrook, Ill.)

Communication and environmental hardware adaptations—cont'd

3. Built-up pens and pencils to accommodate limited grasp and prehension can be used. A Wanchik writer and several other commercially available or custom fabricated writing aids are possible (Figure 3-14).
4. Electric typewriters or personal computers and book holders can facilitate communication for patients with limited or painful joints.
5. Lever-type doorknob extensions (Figure 3-15), car door openers, and adapted key holders can compensate for hand limitations.

Mobility and transfer skills

The individual who has limited ROM without significant muscle weakness may benefit from the following assistive devices:

1. A glider chair that is operated by the feet can facilitate transportation if hip, hand, and arm motion is limited.
2. Platform crutches can prevent stress on hand or finger joints and accommodate limited grasp.
3. Enlarged grips on crutches, canes, and walkers can accommodate limited grasp.
4. A raised toilet seat can be used if hip and knee motion is limited.
5. A walker with padded grips and forearm troughs can be used if marked hand, forearm, or elbow joint limitations are present.
6. A walker or crutch bag or basket can facilitate the carrying of objects.

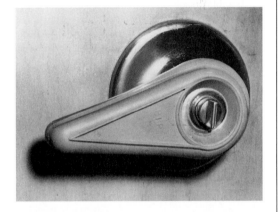

FIGURE 3-15 Rubber doorknob extension.
(Sammons Preston, an Ability One Company, Bolingbrook, Ill.)

Home management activities

Home management activities can be facilitated by a wide variety of environmental adaptations, assistive devices, energy conservation methods, and work simplification techniques. The principles of joint protection are essential for patients with rheumatoid arthritis. The following are suggestions to facilitate home management for individuals with limited ROM:

1. Store frequently used items on the first shelves of cabinets just above and below counters or on counters where possible.

Continued

Box—cont'd

Home management activities—cont'd

2. Use a high stool to work comfortably at counter height , or attach a drop-leaf table to the wall for planning and a meal preparation area if a wheelchair is used.
3. Use a utility cart of comfortable height to transport several items at once.
4. Use reachers to get lightweight items (e.g., cereal box) from high shelves.
5. Stabilize mixing bowls and dishes with non-slip mats.
6. Use lightweight utensils, such as plastic or aluminum bowls and aluminum pots.
7. Use electric can openers and electric mixers.
8. Use electric scissors or adapted loop scissors to open packages (Figure 3-16).
9. Eliminate bending by using extended and flexible plastic handles on dust mops, brooms, and dustpans.
10. Use adapted knives for cutting (Figure 3-17).
11. Use pull-out shelves to organize cupboards and eliminate bending.

Home management activities—cont'd

12. Eliminate bending by using wall ovens, countertop broilers, and microwave ovens.
13. Eliminate leaning and bending by using a top-loading automatic washer and elevated dryer. Wheelchair users can benefit from front-loading appliances.
14. Use an adjustable ironing board to make it possible to sit while ironing.
15. Elevate the playpen and diaper table, and use a bathinette or a plastic tub on the kitchen counter for bathing to reduce the amount of bending and reaching for the ambulatory mother during child care. The crib mattress can be in a raised position until the child is 3 or 4 months of age.
16. Use larger and looser fitting garments with Velcro fastenings on children.
17. Use a reacher to pick up clothing and children's toys.

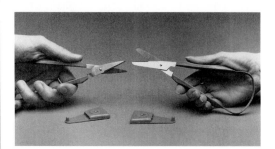

FIGURE 3-16 Loop scissors. (Sammons Preston, an Ability One Company, Bolingbrook, Ill.)

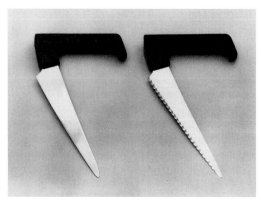

FIGURE 3-17 Right-angle knife. (Sammons Preston, an Ability One Company, Bolingbrook, Ill.)

Modified from Pedretti LW, ed: *Occupational therapy practice skills for physical dysfunction,* ed 4, St Louis, 1996, Mosby.

Problems of Incoordination

Incoordination in the form of tremors, ataxia, athetoid, or choreiform movements can result from a variety of central nervous system (CNS) disorders, such as Parkinson disease, multiple sclerosis, cerebral palsy, and head injuries. The major problems encountered in activities of daily living (ADL) performance are safety and adequate stability of gait, body parts, and objects to complete the tasks.

Fatigue, emotional factors, and fears may influence the degree of incoordinated movement. The patient must be taught appropriate energy conservation and work simplification techniques, along with appropriate work pacing and safety methods to avoid the fatigue and apprehension that can increase incoordination and affect performance.

When muscle weakness is not a major deficit for the individual with incoordination, the use of weighted devices can help with stabilization of objects. A Velcro-fastened weight can be attached to the patient's arm to decrease ataxia, or the device being used can be weighted, such as eating utensils, pens, and cups. Another technique that can be used throughout all ADL tasks is stabilizing the involved upper extremity. This technique is accomplished by propping the elbow on a counter or table top, pivoting from the elbow and only moving the forearm, wrist, and hand in the activity. Stabilizing the arm reduces some of the incoordination and may allow the individual to accomplish gross and fine motor movements without assistive devices.

Dressing activities

Potential dressing difficulties can be reduced by using the following adaptations:

1. Front-opening garments that fit loosely can facilitate donning and removing garments.
2. Large buttons, Velcro, or zippers with loops on the tab can facilitate opening and closing fasteners. A buttonhook with a large, weighted handle may be helpful.
3. Elastic shoelaces. Velcro closures, other adapted shoe closures, and slip-on shoes eliminate the need for bow tying.
4. Trousers with elastic tops for women or Velcro closures for men are easier to manage than those with hooks, buttons, and zippers.

Dressing activities—cont'd

5. Brassieres with front openings or Velcro replacements for the usual hook and eye may facilitate donning and removing this garment. A slipover elastic-type brassiere or bra-slip combination also may eliminate the need to manage brassiere fastenings. Regular brassieres may be fastened in front at waist level, then slipped around to the back and the arms put into the straps, which are then worked up over the shoulders.
6. Men can use clip-on ties.
7. Dressing should be performed while sitting on or in bed or in a wheelchair or chair with arms to avoid balance problems.

Feeding activities

For patients with problems of incoordination, eating can be a challenge. Lack of control during feeding is not only frustrating, but can cause embarrassment and social rejection. Therefore it is important to make eating safe, pleasurable, and as neat as possible. The following are some suggestions for achieving this goal:

1. Use plate stabilizers, such as nonskid mats, suction bases, or even damp dishtowels.
2. Use a plate guard or scoop dish to prevent pushing food off the plate. The plate guard can be carried away from home and clipped to any ordinary dinner plate (Figure 3-18).
3. Prevent spills during the plate-to-mouth excursion by using weighted or swivel utensils to offer stability. Weighted cuffs may be placed on the forearm to decrease involuntary movement (Figure 3-19).

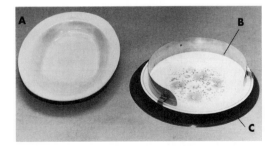

FIGURE 3-18 Eating aids. A, Scoop dish. **B,** Plate with plate guard. **C,** Nonskid mat.

Adult Population

Modified from Pedretti LW, ed: *Occupational therapy practice skills for physical dysfunction*, ed 4, St Louis, 1996, Mosby.

Continued

Box—cont'd

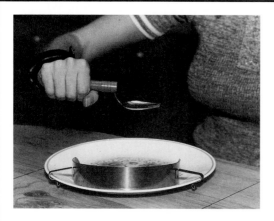

FIGURE 3-19 Weighted wrist cuff and swivel utensil. This device can sometimes compensate for incoordination or involuntary motion and limited supination.

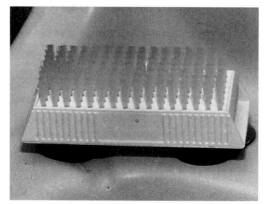

FIGURE 3-20 Suction brush. Attaches to bathroom sink for dentures or fingernails. Can also be used in kitchen to wash vegetables and fruit.

Feeding activities—cont'd
4. Use long plastic straws with a straw clip on a glass or cup with a weighted bottom to eliminate the need to carry the glass or cup to the mouth, thus avoiding spills. Plastic cups with covers and spouts may be used for the same purpose.
5. Use a resistance or friction-type arm brace similar to a mobile arm support, which was shown to help control patterns of involuntary movement during feeding activities of adults with cerebral palsy and athetosis. Such a brace may help many patients with severe incoordination achieve some degree of independence in feeding.

Hygiene and grooming
Stabilization and handling of toilet articles may be achieved by the following suggestions:
1. Articles such as a razor, lipstick, and a toothbrush can be attached to a cord if frequent dropping is a problem. An electric toothbrush may be more easily managed than a regular one.
2. Weighted wrist cuffs may be helpful during the finer hygiene activities, such as applying make-up, shaving, and hair care.

Hygiene and grooming—cont'd
3. The position-adjustable hair dryer described earlier for patients with limited ROM can be useful for patients with incoordination as well.
4. An electric razor rather than a blade razor offers stability and safety. A strap around the razor and hand can prevent dropping.
5. A suction brush attached to the sink or counter can be used for nail or denture care (Figure 3-20).
6. Soap should be on a rope and can be worn around the neck or hung over a bathtub or shower fixture during a bath or shower to keep it in easy reach. A leg from a pair of pantyhose with a bar of soap in the toe may be tied over a faucet to keep soap within reach and will stretch for use.
7. An emery board or small piece of wood with fine sandpaper glued to it can be fastened to the table top for filing nails. A nail clipper can also be stabilized in the same manner.
8. Large roll-on deodorants are preferable to sprays or creams.
9. Sanitary pads that stick to undergarments may be easier to manage than tampons.

Modified from Pedretti LW, ed: *Occupational therapy practice skills for physical dysfunction*, ed 4, St Louis, 1996, Mosby.

Box—cont'd

Hygiene and grooming—cont'd

10. A bath mitt with a pocket to hold the soap can be used for washing and eliminates the need for frequent soaping and rinsing and wringing a washcloth.
11. Nonskid mats should be used inside and outside the bathtub during bathing. Their suction bases should be fastened securely to the floor and bathtub before use. Safety grab bars should be installed on the wall next to the bathtub or fastened to the edge of the bathtub. A bathtub seat or shower chair provides more safety than standing while showering or transferring to a bathtub bottom. Many uncoordinated clients require supervisory assistance during this hazardous activity. Sponge bathing while seated at a bathroom sink may substitute for bathing or showering several times a week.

Communication and environmental hardware adaptations

The following adaptations can facilitate communication for patients who have incoordination:

1. Doorknobs may be managed more easily if adapted with lever-type handles or covered with rubber or friction tape (Figure 3-15).
2. A holder for a telephone receiver, large button phones, or speaker phones may be helpful.
3. Writing may be managed by using a weighted, enlarged pencil or pen. An electric typewriter or computer with a keyboard guard is an extremely helpful aid to communication. A computer mouse may frequently be substituted for the keyboard.
4. Keys may be managed by placing them on an adapted key holder that is rigid and offers more leverage for turning the key. Inserting the key in the keyhole may be very difficult, however, unless the incoordination is relatively mild.
5. Extended lever-type faucets are easier to manage than knobs that turn and push-pull spigots. Cold water should be turned on first and hot water added gradually to prevent burns during bathing and kitchen activities.
6. Lamps that require a wall switch only, a light touch to turn on, or a signal-type device can eliminate turning a small switch.

Mobility and transfers

Patients with problems of incoordination may use a variety of ambulation aids, depending on the type and severity of incoordination. In degenerative diseases, it is sometimes necessary to help the client recognize the need for and to accept ambulation aids. This problem may mean graduation from a cane to crutches to a walker and finally to a wheelchair for some individuals. Patients with incoordination can improve stability and mobility by the following suggestions:

1. Instead of lifting objects, slide them on floors or counters.
2. Use suitable ambulation aids.
3. Use a utility cart, preferably a custom-made cart that is heavy and has some friction on the wheels.
4. Remove doorsills, throw rugs, and thick carpeting.
5. Install banisters on indoor and outdoor staircases.
6. Substitute ramps for stairs wherever possible.

Home management activities

The therapist must make a careful assessment of homemaking activities performance to determine (1) which activities can be done safely, (2) which activities can be done safely if modified or adapted, and (3) which activities cannot be done adequately or safely and should be assigned to someone else. The major problems are stabilization of foods and equipment to prevent spilling and accidents, as well as the safe handling of appliances, pots, pans, and household tools to prevent cuts, burns, bruises, electric shock, and falls. The following are suggestions for the facilitation of home management tasks:

1. Use a wheelchair and wheelchair lapboard, even if ambulation is possible with devices. The wheelchair saves energy and increases stability if balance and gait are unsteady.
2. If possible, use convenience and prepared foods to eliminate as many processes as possible (e.g., peeling, chopping, slicing, and mixing).
3. Use easy-open containers or store foods in plastic containers once opened. A jar opener is also useful.

Continued

Home management activities—cont'd

4. Use heavy utensils, mixing bowls, and pots and pans to increase stability.
5. Use nonskid mats on work surfaces.
6. Use electrical appliances such as crock pots, electric fry pans, toaster-ovens, and microwave or convection ovens because they are safer than using the range.
7. Use a blender and countertop mixer, because they are safer than handheld mixers and easier than mixing with a spoon or whisk.
8. If possible, adjust work heights of the counters, sink, and range to minimize leaning, bending, reaching, and lifting, whether the patient is standing or using a wheelchair.
9. Use long oven mitts, which are safer than potholders.
10. Use pots, pans, casserole dishes, and appliances with bilateral handles, because they may be easier to manage than those with one handle.
11. Use a cutting board with stainless steel nails (Figure 3-21) to stabilize meats and vegetables while cutting. When not in use the nails should be covered with a large cork. The bottom of the board should have suction cups or should be covered with stair tread, or the board should be placed on a nonskid mat to prevent slippage when in use.
12. Use heavy dinnerware, which may be easier to handle, because it offers stability and control to the distal part of the upper extremity. On the other hand, unbreakable dinnerware may be more practical if dropping and breakage are problems.
13. Cover the sink, utility cart, and countertops with protective rubber mats or mesh matting to stabilize items.
14. Use a serrated knife for cutting and chopping because it is easier to control.
15. Use a steamer basket or deep-fry basket for preparing boiled foods to eliminate the need to carry and drain pots with hot liquids in them.
16. Use tongs to turn foods during cooking and to serve foods because they may offer more control and stability than a fork, spatula, or serving spoon.
17. Use blunt-ended loop scissors to open packages.
18. Vacuum with a heavy upright cleaner, which may be easier for the ambulatory patient. The wheelchair user may be able to manage a lightweight tank type vacuum cleaner or electric broom.

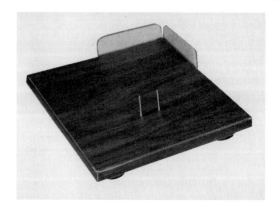

FIGURE 3-21 Cutting board with stainless steel nails, suction cup feet, and a corner for stabilizing bread. Useful for patients who are uncoordinated or can only use one hand. (Sammons Preston, an Ability One Company, Bolingbrook, Ill.)

Home management activities—cont'd

19. Use dust mitts for dusting.
20. Eliminate fragile knickknacks, unstable lamps, and dainty doilies.
21. Eliminate ironing by using no-iron fabrics or a timed dryer or by assigning this task to other members of the household.
22. Use front-loading washers, a laundry cart on wheels, and premeasured detergents, bleaches, and fabric softeners.
23. Sit while working with an infant and use foam-rubber bath aids, an infant bath seat, and a wide, padded dressing table with safety straps with Velcro fastening to offer enough stability for bathing, dressing, and diapering an infant. (Child care may not be possible unless the incoordination is mild.)
24. Use disposable diapers with tape fasteners because they are easier to manage than cloth diapers and pins.
25. Do not feed the infant with a spoon or fork unless the incoordination is very mild or does not affect the upper extremities. This task may need to be performed by another household member.
26. Provide clothing for the child that is large, loose, with Velcro fastenings, and made of nonslippery stretch fabrics.

Modified from Pedretti LW, ed: *Occupational therapy practice skills for physical dysfunction*, ed 4, St Louis, 1996, Mosby.

REFERENCES FOR BOXES ON DAILY LIVING GUIDELINES

Activities of daily living for patients with incoordination, limited range of motion, paraplegia, quadriplegia, and hemiplegia, Cleveland, 1968, Rev 1989, Metro Health Center for Rehabilitation, Metro Health Medical Center, Unpublished.

Klinger JL: *Mealtime manual for people with disabilities and the aging,* Camden, NJ, 1978, Campbell Soup.

Malick MH, Almasy BS: Activities of daily living and homemaking. In Hopkins HL, Smith HD, eds, *Willard and Spackyman's occupational therapy,* ed 7, Philadelphia, JB Lippincott.

Melvin JL: *Rheumatic disease: occupational therapy and rehabilitation,* ed 2, Philadelphia, 1982, FA Davis.

The Professional Manual Subcommittee of the Educational Committee, Allied Health Professional Section of the Arthritis Foundation: *Arthritis manual for allied health professionals,* New York, 1973, The Arthritis Foundation.

Trombly CA: Activities of daily living. In Trombly CA, ed: *Occupational therapy for physical dysfunction,* ed 2, Baltimore, 1983, Williams & Wilkins.

Incontinence Guidelines
Fecal Incontinence
Bowel training program

Interventions for Bowel Elimination

1. Assess bowel patterns for usual habits, stool characteristics, and frequency of incontinence.
2. Establish a time for daily defecation, preferably 30 minutes to 1 hour after a meal.
3. Inform the patient to drink 2 to 3 L of fluids per day if permitted.
4. Encourage bowel movement at regular times by offering warm fluids, abdominal massage, and digital stimulation of anal area. Allow 1 hour for defecation.
5. Administer an enema at regular times to empty the bowel until the next scheduled defecation. Suppositories may also be used.
6. Tell the patient to avoid foods that produce gas and foods that may produce diarrhea and stool incontinence.
7. Encourage a routine time each day for bowel elimination. Provide bathroom facilities, a bedpan, or a commode at that time.
8. Revise the training program if it is not successful. Report any failure to achieve goals.

Modified from Jaffe M, Skidmore-Roth L: *Home health nursing care plans,* ed 2, St Louis, 1995, Mosby.

Urinary Incontinence
Bladder training program

Contraction of the bladder causes passing of water. Normally, the bladder does not contract until it is convenient to pass water. In other words, the bladder contractions are under the control of the brain. In some individuals this ability of the brain to control the bladder is lost. The bladder is then liable to contract at any time, even if its owner does not want it to. These uncontrolled bladder contractions are not dangerous but are a common cause of frequency, urgency, and leakage of urine.

The aim of bladder training is to re-establish the brain's control over the bladder. Provided the exercises are performed with real determination, the results are excellent and urgency and leakage are cured. Your own attitude is one of the most important aspects of this treatment.

You will be given a chart and a measuring jug. Every time you experience a desire to pass water you should write down the time in the first column. You must then try hard to regain control of your bladder by relaxing it and holding on to your water. If you succeed, the desire to void will soon pass and you should put a cross in the "no leak" column. If leakage occurs before the desire to void passes, you should put a cross in the "leakage" column. If you are unable to hold on and have to pass your water, you must measure the volume passed and write it down in the fourth column.

You must aim to do the following:

(*a*) abolish leakage

(*b*) hold your water for 4 hours

(*c*) pass a volume of 400 ml

At first, you will probably find you have to pass water fairly frequently and in small amounts, but if you persevere, you will soon see a great improvement. You will have to continue the exercises for about 3 months, by which time you should have regained control of your bladder, and the improvement will be permanent.

Modified from Pengelly AW, Booth CM: A prospective trial of bladder training as treatment for detrusor instability, *Br J Urol* 52:463-466, 1980.

Voiding diary

Time	Amount urinated in toilet	Small accident	Large accident	Reason for accident	Fluid intake
___	___	___	___	___	___
___	___	___	___	___	___
___	___	___	___	___	___
___	___	___	___	___	___
___	___	___	___	___	___

Type of pads used _____

Number of pads used today _____

Comments _____

_____

_____

_____

From Colling J: Noninvasive techniques to manage urinary incontinence among care-dependent persons, *J Wound Ost Care Nurs* 23(6):302-308, 1996.

ADULT MOBILITY EVALUATION

Purpose of Mobility Evaluations

Mobility encompasses the performance of bed mobility, transfers, wheelchair negotiation, and gait. These subset activities of daily living are intimately associated with the ability of patients to regain their prior levels of function and reduce reliance on caregivers for everyday tasks such as accessing bathrooms or retrieving mail. Mobility assessment tools for bed mobility, transfers, balance, and gait offer methods to objectify observed levels of dependence, compensatory techniques, and abnormal body mechanics. Therapists use this information to establish baseline deficits, target treatment interventions, and after reevaluations, demonstrate material progress to claims reviewers. Associated standards inform therapists of normative mobility data for older adults, posture and gait characteristics with age, and segmental descriptions of proper transfer techniques. Associated guidelines address assistive device fit, hierarchy of balance reaction facilitation, and training guidelines containing research-based suggestions for improving key mobility aspects.

Bed Mobility and Transfer Assessments
Bed Mobility and Transfer Assessment Form

Levels of assistance			
Abbreviation	**Description**	**Abbreviation**	**Description**
I	Independent	MIN A	<25% physical assistance required
S	Supervision	MOD A	25%-50% physical assistance required
SBA	Standby assistance	MAX A	>50% physical assistance required
VC	Verbal cueing	D	Dependent—unable to provide any assistance
CGA	Contact guard assistance	U	Unable—unable to perform task

Mobility tasks		
Bed Mobility	**Assistance level**	**Comments (e.g., quality, time to complete task)**
Moving in bed		
Bridging		
Scooting toward head of bed		
Scooting toward foot of bed		
Scooting to the left side		
Scooting to the right side		
Rolling to the left		
Rolling to the right		
Seated, scooting along edge of bed		

Mobility tasks		
Transfers	**Assistance level**	**Comments (e.g., quality, time to complete task)**
Supine to sit		
Sit to supine		
Side to sit		
Sit to side		
Sit to stand		
Stand to sit		
Stand pivot to left		
Stand pivot to right		
Sliding board		
Toilet transfer		
Bath/shower transfer		
Floor to stand		
Stand to floor		
Vehicle transfer		

Modified Bed Rise Difficulty Scale

The Modified Bed Rise Difficulty (MBRD) Scale assesses the movements that occur during rising from bed in older patients. It evaluates the completion time and three specific mobility aspects, including the use of upper extremities, the relationship of the trunk and lower extremities, and lower extremities. The total score ranges from 0 to 7. Higher scores denote greater difficulty rising from bed.

MBRD Scale Form

Aspect of bed rise task	Absent	Present
Use of Upper Extremities to Push Off on Bed Surface		
Long duration pushes (score both extremities together)	0	1
Repeated pushes	0	1
Push indicating substantial force or effort used	0	1
Relationship of Trunk and Lower Extremities		
Discontinuity of trunk elevation and leg motion off the bed surface	0	1
Multiple adjustments of the shoulder and pelvic girdle	0	1
Use of Lower Extremities		
Multiple motion adjustments of the legs	0	1
Poor vertical clearance of heels off the surface of the bed	0	1
Rise time(s)		
TOTAL BRD SCORE (0-7)		

Modified from Boffelli S and others: Assessment of functional ability with the bed rise difficulty scale in a group of elderly patients, *Gerontology* 42:294-300, 1996.

Wheelchair Mobility and Negotiation Assessments
Wheelchair Mobility and Negotiation Assessment Form

		Levels of assistance	
Abbreviation	**Description**	**Abbreviation**	**Description**
I	Independent	MIN A	<25% physical assistance required
S	Supervision	MOD A	25%-50% physical assistance required
SBA	Standby assistance	MAX A	>50% physical assistance required
VC	Verbal cueing	D	Dependent—unable to provide any assistance
CGA	Contact guard assistance	U	Unable—unable to perform task

Continued

Adult Population

Table—cont'd

Mobility tasks	Assistance level	Comments (e.g., quality, time to complete task)
Wheelchair to bed		
Toilet to wheelchair		
Wheelchair to toilet		
Bath/shower to wheelchair		
Wheelchair to bath/shower		
Stand pivot to left		
Stand pivot to right		
Sit to stand		
Stand to sit		
Wheelchair to floor		
Floor to wheelchair		
Chair/couch to wheelchair		
Wheelchair to couch/chair		
Vehicle to wheelchair		
Wheelchair to vehicle		

Wheelchair negotiation	Assistance level	Comments (e.g., quality, time to complete task)
Forward propulsion		
Backward propulsion		
Left turn		
Right turn		
180-degree turn		
360-degree turn		
Opening of door		
Closing of door		
Ramp ascension		
Ramp descension		
Curb/step ascension		
Curb/step descension		
Level surfaces		
Uneven surfaces		

Balance and Gait Assessments
Balance Scale

The Balance Scale rates the ability of patients to maintain balance while performing 14 movements required in everyday living. These 14 tasks include transfers, forward reaching, 360-degree turns, and unilateral stance. The total score ranges from 0 to 56 points. Higher scores denote greater balance.

Balance Scale Form

Item description	Score (0-4)
1. Sitting to standing	_____
2. Standing unsupported	_____
3. Sitting unsupported	_____
4. Standing to sitting	_____
5. Transferring	_____
6. Standing with eyes closed	_____
7. Standing with feet together	_____
8. Reaching forward with outstretched arm	_____
9. Retrieving object from floor	_____
10. Turning to look behind	_____
11. Turning 360 degrees	_____
12. Placing alternate foot on stool	_____
13. Standing with one foot in front	_____
14. Standing on one foot	_____
TOTAL	_____

General Instructions

Please demonstrate each task and/or give instructions as written. When scoring, please record the lowest response category that applies for each item.

In most items, the patient is asked to maintain a position for a specific time. Progressively, more points are deducted if the time or distance requirements are not met, if the patient's performance warrants supervision, or if the patient touches an external support or receives assistance from the therapist. Patients should understand that they must maintain their balance while attempting the tasks. The choices of which leg to stand on or how far to reach are left to the patient. Poor judgment adversely influences the performance and the scoring.

Equipment required for testing are a stopwatch or watch with a second hand, as well as a ruler or other indicator of 2, 5, and 10 inches (5, 12, and 25 cm). Chairs used during testing should be of reasonable height. A step or a stool (of average step height) may be used for item #12.

1. Sitting to standing
   Instructions: Please stand up. Try not to use your hands for support.
   ( )4 able to stand without using hands and stabilize independently
   ( )3 able to stand independently using hands
   ( )2 able to stand using hands after several tries
   ( )1 needs minimal aid to stand or to stabilize
   ( )0 needs moderate or maximal assistance to stand

2. Standing unsupported
   Instructions: Please stand for 2 minutes without holding.
   ( )4 able to stand safely 2 minutes
   ( )3 able to stand 2 minutes with supervision
   ( )2 able to stand 30 seconds unsupported
   ( )1 needs several tries to stand 30 seconds unsupported
   ( )0 unable to stand 30 seconds unassisted

Modified from Berg KO and others: Measuring balance in the elderly: validation of an instrument, *Can J Pub Health* 83 (suppl 2):S7-11, 1992.

Continued

Adult Population

Box—cont'd

If a patient is able to stand 2 minutes unsupported, score full points for sitting unsupported. Proceed to item #4.

3. Sitting with back unsupported but feet supported on floor or on a stool
   Instructions: Please sit with arms folded for 2 minutes.
   ( )4 able to sit safely and securely 2 minutes
   ( )3 able to sit 2 minutes under supervision
   ( )2 able to sit 30 seconds
   ( )1 able to sit 10 seconds
   ( )0 unable to sit without support 10 seconds

4. Standing to sitting
   Instructions: Please sit down.
   ( )4 sits safely with minimal use of hands
   ( )3 controls descent by using hands
   ( )2 uses back of legs against chair to control descent
   ( )1 sits independently but has uncontrolled descent
   ( )0 needs assistance to sit

5. Transferring
   Instructions: Arrange chair(s) for a pivot transfer. Ask the patient to transfer one way toward a seat with armrests and one way toward a seat without armrests. You may use two chairs (one with and one without armrests) or a bed and a chair.
   ( )4 able to transfer safely with minor use of hands
   ( )3 able to transfer safely; definitely needs hands
   ( )2 able to transfer with verbal cueing and/or supervision
   ( )1 needs one individual to assist
   ( )0 needs two individuals to assist or supervise to be safe

6. Standing unsupported with eyes closed
   Instructions: Please close your eyes and stand still for 10 seconds.

( )4 able to stand 10 seconds safely
( )3 able to stand 10 seconds with supervision
( )2 able to stand 3 seconds
( )1 unable to keep eyes closed 3 seconds but stays steady
( )0 needs help to keep from falling

7. Standing unsupported with feet together
   Instructions: Place your feet together and stand without holding.
   ( )4 able to place feet together independently and stand 1 minute safely
   ( )3 able to place feet together independently and stand for 1 minute with supervision
   ( )2 able to place feet together independently but unable to hold for 30 seconds
   ( )1 needs help to attain position but able to stand 15 seconds with feet together
   ( )0 needs help to attain position and unable to hold for 15 seconds

8. Reaching forward with outstretched arm while standing
   Instructions: Lift arm to 90 degrees. Stretch out your fingers and reach forward as far as you can. (The therapist places a ruler at the end of the fingertips when the arm is at 90 degrees. The fingers should not touch the ruler while the patient reaches forward. The recorded measure is the distance forward that the fingers reach while the patient is in the most forward lean position. When possible, ask the patient to use both arms when reaching to avoid rotation of the trunk.)
   ( )4 can reach forward confidently >25 cm (10 inches)
   ( )3 can reach forward >12 cm safely (5 inches)
   ( )2 can reach forward >5 cm safely (2 inches)
   ( )1 reaches forward but needs supervision
   ( )0 loses balance while trying; requires external support

Modified from Berg KO and others: Measuring balance in the elderly: validation of an instrument, *Can J Pub Health* 83 (suppl 2):S7-11, 1992.

Box—cont'd

9. Picking up object from the floor from a standing position
Instructions: Pick up the shoe or slipper, which is placed in front of your feet.
- ( )4 able to pick up slipper safely and easily
- ( )3 able to pick up slipper but needs supervision
- ( )2 unable to pick up slipper but reaches 2-5 cm (1-2 inches) from slipper and keeps balance independently
- ( )1 unable to pick up slipper and needs supervision while trying
- ( )0 unable to try; needs assistance to keep from losing balance or falling

10. Turning to look behind, over left and right shoulders while standing
Instructions: Turn to look **directly** behind you, over toward your left shoulder. Repeat to the right. The therapist may pick an object to look at directly behind the patient to encourage a better twist turn.
- ( )4 looks behind from both sides and shifts weight well
- ( )3 looks behind one side only other side shows less weight shift
- ( )2 turns sideways only but maintains balance
- ( )1 needs supervision when turning
- ( )0 needs assistance to keep from losing balance or falling

11. Turning 360 degrees
Instructions: Turn completely around in a full circle. Pause. Then turn a full circle in the other direction.
- ( )4 able to turn 360 degrees safely in 4 seconds or less
- ( )3 able to turn 360 degrees safely one side only in 4 seconds or less
- ( )2 able to turn 360 degrees safely but slowly
- ( )1 needs close supervision or verbal cueing
- ( )0 needs assistance while turning

12. Placing alternate foot on step or stool while standing unsupported
Instructions: Place each foot alternately on the step or stool. Continue until each foot has touched the step or stool four times.
- ( )4 able to stand independently and safely and complete eight steps in 20 seconds
- ( )3 able to stand independently and complete eight steps in >20 seconds
- ( )2 able to complete four steps without aid with supervision
- ( )1 able to complete >2 steps; needs minimal assistance
- ( )0 needs assistance to keep from falling; unable to try

13. Standing unsupported with one foot in front
Instructions: (Demonstrate to patient) Place one foot directly in front of the other. If you feel that you cannot place your foot directly in front, try to step far enough ahead that the heel of your forward foot is ahead of the toes of the other foot. (To score 3 points, the length of the step should exceed the length of the other foot and the width of the stance should approximate the patient's normal stride width.)
- ( )4 able to place foot tandem independently and hold 30 seconds
- ( )3 able to place foot ahead of other independently and hold 30 seconds
- ( )2 able to take small step independently and hold 30 seconds
- ( )1 needs help to step but can hold 15 seconds
- ( )0 loses balance while stepping or standing

14. Standing on one leg
Instructions: Stand on one leg as long as you can without holding.
- ( )4 able to lift leg independently and hold >10 seconds
- ( )3 able to lift leg independently and hold 5-10 seconds
- ( )2 able to lift leg independently and hold = or >3 seconds
- ( )1 tries to lift leg; unable to hold 3 seconds but remains standing independently
- ( )0 unable to try or needs assistance to prevent fall

- ( ) TOTAL SCORE (Maximum = 56)

Functional Reach Test

The Functional Reach Test (FRT) is a balance measure that represents the maximum distance patients can reach forward beyond arm's length while maintaining a fixed base of support in standing. Patients stand with their dominant arm extended and their fisted hand at the edge of a ruler taped to a wall at the level of the acromion. Therapists instruct patients to "reach as far forward as you can without taking a step" (Figure 3-22). The further patients reach forward, the lower their risk for falls. Distances of 0 to 1 inches indicate patients are 28 times more likely to fall. Distances of 1 to 6 inches indicate patients are 4 times more likely to fall. Distances of 6 to 10 inches indicate patients are 2 times as likely to fall. Distances greater than 10 inches indicate patients are unlikely to fall.

FRT Form

Distance reached (inches)	
Score (check one)	**Risk for falling**
>10 inches	Unlikely to fall
6-10 inches	2 times more likely to fall
1-6 inches	4 times more likely to fall
Unwilling to reach	28 times more likely to fall

Modified from Duncan PW and others: Functional reach: a new clinical measure of balance, *J Gerontol* 45(6):M192-197, 1990.

Modified Get-Up and Go Test

The Modified Get-Up and Go Test assesses balance and risk for falls. It evaluates patient performance during the tasks of rising from a chair, walking 3 meters, turning around, and attempting to sit. Therapists rate the balance of patients during these tasks and not concurrent factors such as gait deviations, unless they put patients at risk for falling during the test. The total score ranges from 1 to 5. Scores higher than 2 indicate patients are at risk for falling.

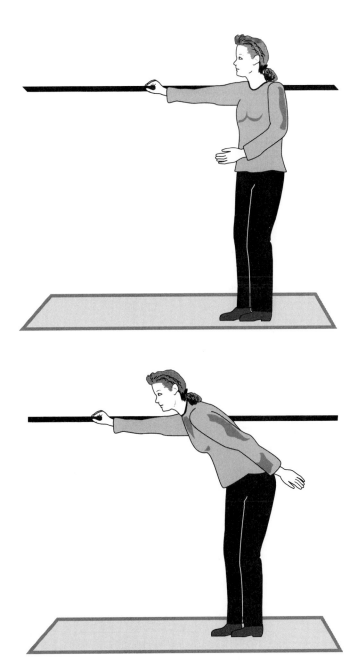

FIGURE 3-22 Functional reach test. (From Umphred DA: *Neurological rehabilitation,* ed 3, St Louis, 1995, Mosby.)

Modified Get-Up and Go Test Form

Key

Normal—patient gives no evidence of being at risk of falling during the test or at any other time

Intermediate—presence of undue slowness, hesitancy, abnormal movements of the trunk or upper limbs, staggering, or stumbling, indicating the possibility of falling in less favorable circumstances

Severely abnormal—patient appears at risk of falling during the test

Task	Score
Rising from Chair 1 = normal 2 = slightly abnormal 3 = mildly abnormal 4 = moderately abnormal 5 = severely abnormal	
Walking 10 Feet 1 = normal 2 = slightly abnormal 3 = mildly abnormal 4 = moderately abnormal 5 = severely abnormal	
Turning Around 1 = normal 2 = slightly abnormal 3 = mildly abnormal 4 = moderately abnormal 5 = severely abnormal	
Sitting Down in Chair 1 = normal 2 = slightly abnormal 3 = mildly abnormal 4 = moderately abnormal 5 = severely abnormal	
SUMMED SCORE	
TOTAL SCORE (summed score divided by four)	

Modified from Mathias S, Nayak USL, Isaacs B: Balance in elderly patients: the "get-up and go" test, *Arch Phys Med Rehabil* 67:387-389, 1986.

Modified Falls Efficacy Scale

The Modified Falls Efficacy Scale (MFES) measures self-perceived fear of falling during performance of 14 common activities. The 14 activities include simple meal preparation, transfers, light housekeeping, and crossing roads. The MFES is a self- or therapist-administered tool. The total score ranges from 0 to 140. Higher scores denote greater perceived self-confidence with daily activities.

MFES Form

Task	Not confident at all				Fairly confident				Completely confident		
Get dressed and undressed	0	1	2	3	4	5	6	7	8	9	10
Prepare a simple meal	0	1	2	3	4	5	6	7	8	9	10
Take a bath or shower	0	1	2	3	4	5	6	7	8	9	10
Get in and out of a chair	0	1	2	3	4	5	6	7	8	9	10
Get in and out of a bed	0	1	2	3	4	5	6	7	8	9	10
Answer the door or telephone	0	1	2	3	4	5	6	7	8	9	10
Walk around the inside of your house	0	1	2	3	4	5	6	7	8	9	10
Reach into cabinets or closet	0	1	2	3	4	5	6	7	8	9	10
Perform light housekeeping	0	1	2	3	4	5	6	7	8	9	10
Perform simple shopping	0	1	2	3	4	5	6	7	8	9	10
Use public transportation	0	1	2	3	4	5	6	7	8	9	10
Cross roads	0	1	2	3	4	5	6	7	8	9	10
Perform light gardening or hang out the washing*	0	1	2	3	4	5	6	7	8	9	10
Use front or rear steps at home	0	1	2	3	4	5	6	7	8	9	10
TOTAL SCORE											

Modified from Hill KD and others: Fear of falling revisited, *Arch Phys Med Rehabil* 77:1025-1029, 1996.
*Rate most commonly performed of these activities.

Modified Gait Abnormality Rating Scale

The Modified Gait Abnormality Rating Scale (MGARS) is a gait rating system that describes the qualitative abnormalities of gait and predicts risk for falls. It examines seven aspects of gait associated with an increased risk for falling. The seven aspects include variability, guardedness, staggering, foot contact, hip range of motion, shoulder extension, and arm-heel strike synchrony. The total score ranges from 0 to 21. Scores greater than 9 indicate an increased risk for falls in community dwelling older adults.

MGARS Form

Aspects of gait	Score

Staggering
Sudden, unexpected, laterally-directed loss of balance
0 = no loss of balance to the side
1 = a single lurch to the side
2 = two lurches to the side
3 = three or more lurches to the side

Arm-Leg Synchrony
Contralateral arm and leg movement
0 = good contralateral arm and leg motion
1 = arm and leg control out of phase 25% of time
2 = arm and leg moderately out of phase 25%-50% of time
3 = little or no synchrony present

Variability
Stepping-arm movement consistency and rhythm
0 = fluid and predictably paced limb movements
1 = occasional interruptions (changed velocity) <25% of time
2 = unpredictability of rhythm <25%-75% of time
3 = random timing of limb movements

Foot Contact
Heel strike
0 = very obvious angle of impact of heel
1 = barely visible impact of heel
2 = entire foot striking the ground
3 = anterior foot striking ground before the heel

Hip Range of Motion
The degree of hip range of motion during gait
0 = obvious hip extension (10 degrees) at double stance
1 = just barely visible hip extension
2 = no hip extension
3 = thigh flexion during double stance

Shoulder Extension
Arm swing
0 = 15 degrees of flexion, 20 degrees of extension
1 = shoulder flexion slightly anterior only
2 = shoulder coming to 0 degrees only with flexion
3 = shoulder staying in extension through the arm swing

Guardedness
Propulsion rate and arm swing and step commitment
0 = good forward momentum and no apprehension
1 = center of gravity of HAT (head, arms, trunk) projecting only slightly forward in front of pushoff, but still good arm-leg coordination
2 = HAT held over anterior aspect of foot, moderate loss of smooth reciprocation
3 = HAT held over rear aspect of stance foot and great tenativity in stepping
TOTAL SCORE

Modified from Wolfson L and others: Gait assessment in the elderly: a gait abnormality rating scale and its relation to falls, *J Gerontol* 45(1):M12-19, 1990.

Short Physical Performance Battery

The Short Physical Performance Battery assesses gait, balance, and lower extremity strength and endurance. It specifically measures standing balance, walking speed, and chair stand ability. The total score ranges from 0 to 12. Higher scores denote greater lower extremity function and less self-reported disability.

Short Physical Performance Battery Form

Standing balance	Score
0 = <10 seconds on side-by-side stand (feet right next to each other in Romberg position) and <10 seconds on semi-tandem (heel of one foot placed to the side of the first toe of the other foot) stand 1 = 10 seconds on side-by-side stand and <10 seconds on semi-tandem stand 2 = 10 seconds on semi-tandem stand and <3 seconds on full tandem (heel of one foot directly in front of the toes of other foot in Sharpened Romberg position) stand 3 = 10 seconds on semi-tandem stand and <10 seconds on full-tandem stand 4 = 10 seconds on semi-tandem stand and 10 seconds on full-tandem stand **Walking Speed** Over an 8-foot course at usual speed 0 = unable to complete task 1 = ≥5.7 seconds 2 = 4.1 to 5.6 seconds 3 = 3.2 to 4.0 seconds 4 = ≤3.1 seconds **Chair Stand Ability** Five chair stands with arms across chest 0 = inability to complete task 1 = ≥16.7 seconds 2 = 13.7 to 16.6 seconds 3 = 11.2 to 13.6 seconds 4 = ≤11.1 seconds SUMMARY PERFORMANCE SCALE SCORE	

Data from Guralnick JM and others: A short performance battery assessing lower extremity function: association with self-reported disability and prediction of mortality and nursing home admission, *J Gerontol* 49(2):M85-94, 1994.

Tinetti Assessment Tool

The Tinetti Assessment Tool evaluates balance and gait characteristics and predicts risk for falls. It evaluates nine facets of balance, including sitting balance and turning 360 degrees. It also evaluates seven facets of gait, including step symmetry and walking stance. The total score ranges from 0 to 28. Scores less than 19 indicate a high risk for falls, scores of 19 to 23 indicate a moderate risk for falls, and scores greater than 23 indicate a low risk for falls.

Tinetti Assessment Tool Form

Balance test—patient sits in hard, armless chair	Score

Sitting Balance
0 = leans or slides in chair
1 = is steady and safe

Arising
0 = is unable without help
1 = is able, uses arms to help
2 = is able without using arms

Attempt to Rise
0 = is unable without help
1 = is able, requires >1 attempt
2 = is able to arise on first attempt

Immediate Standing Balance (First 5 Seconds)
0 = is unsteady (swaggers, moves feet, sways trunk)
1 = is steady but uses assistive device or support
2 = is steady without assistance

Standing Balance
0 = is unsteady
1 = is steady but has wide stance and uses assistive device or support
2 = has narrow stance without support

Sternal Nudge
With feet as close together as possible, patient is given three sternal nudges
0 = begins to fall
1 = staggers, grabs, catches self
2 = is steady

Eyes Closed
Same position as in sternal nudge
0 = is unsteady
1 = is steady

360-Degree Turn
0 = Uses discontinuous steps
1 = Uses continuous steps
0 = is unsteady (grabs, staggers)
1 = is steady

Sitting Down
0 = is unsafe (misjudges distance, falls into chair)
1 = uses arms or not a smooth motion
2 = is safe, uses smooth motion

BALANCE SCORE

Modified from Tinetti ME, Williams TW, Mayewski R: Fall risk index for elderly patients based on number of chronic disabilities, *Am J Med* 80: 429-434, 1986.

Box—cont'd

Gait test—patient stands and walks down hallway or across room at "usual" pace using usual assistive devices	Score

Gait Initiation (Immediately after Told to "Go")
0 = shows hesitancy or multiple attempts to start
1 = shows no hesitancy

Step Length
0 = right swing foot does not pass left stance foot
1 = right swing foot passes left stance foot
0 = left swing foot does not pass right stance foot
1 = left swing foot passes right stance foot

Step Height
0 = right foot does not clear floor completely with step
1 = right foot clears floor completely
0 = left foot does not clear floor completely with step
1 = left foot clears floor completely

Step Symmetry
0 = right and left step length not equal
1 = right and left step length appear equal

Step Continuity
0 = stopping or discontinuity between steps
1 = steps appear continuous

Path
In relation to floor tiles, observe excursion of 12 inches over 10 feet of the course
0 = shows marked deviation
1 = shows mild or moderate deviation or uses assistive device
2 = completes straight path without assistive device

Trunk
0 = shows marked sway or uses assistive device
1 = shows no sway but flexion of knees or back, or spreads arms out while walking
2 = shows no sway, no flexion, and no use of arms, and uses no assistive device

Walking Stance
0 = has heels apart
1 = has heels almost touching while walking

GAIT SCORE

TOTAL SCORE (balance and gait score)

Normative Data for Mobility
Range of Motion
Normative data for range of motion—shoulder abduction

	Shoulder abduction AROM (degrees)		
Age	Female	Male	
65-74	123	128	
75+	112	120	

n: 378 females and 379 males; no screening for disease or disability
Method: measured in sitting, left shoulder only

Data from Bassey EJ and others: Normal values of shoulder abduction in men and women aged over 65 years, *Ann Human Biol* 6(3):249-257, 1989.
AROM, Active range of motion.

Normative data for range of motion—elbow

	Elbow AROM (degrees)			
	Female		Male	
Age	Flexion	Extension	Flexion	Extension
55-84	150	0	146	1

n: 30 females and 30 males; healthy adults with no musculoskeletal problems affecting the elbow
Method: measured with a 360-degree goniometer in supine position; obtained no differences in left and right elbows

Data from Smith JR, Walker JM: Knee and elbow range of motion in healthy older individuals, *Phys Occup Ther Ger* 2(4):31-38, 1983.
AROM, Active range of motion.

Normative data for range of motion—wrist

Wrist AROM (degrees)

Age	Female				Male			
	Flexion	Extension	Abduction	Adduction	Flexion	Extension	Abduction	Adduction
0-19	85.5	55.9	37.3	24.6	85.0	53.9	36.8	27.1
20-29	77.3	52.3	30.3	20.5	74.3	45.9	30.6	21.3
30-39	87.4	51.6	36.4	25.3	82.9	51.1	30.5	23.1
40-49	80.2	42.0	24.4	24.6	82.3	48.4	28.7	20.5
50-80	81.2	46.5	27.7	21.2	81.2	41.4	30.2	25.8

n: 39 females and 38 males; healthy Caucasians
Method: measured sitting at a table; left wrist only

Data from Bird HA, Stowe J: The wrist, *Clin Rheum Dis* 8(3): 550-568, 1982.
AROM, Active range of motion.

Normative data for range of motion—hip

Hip AROM (degrees)

Age	Female						Male					
	Flexion	Extension	Medial rotation	Lateral rotation	Abduction	Adduction	Flexion	Extension	Medial rotation	Lateral rotation	Abduction	Adduction
12-20	106.0	24.7	41.7	53.6	57.2	45.5	110.0	24.5	43.1	64.5	60.6	41.8
20-30	117.5	21.5	31.8	43.0	54.5	37.0	113.7	27.5	34.2	41.3	45.0	45.2
30-40	116.7	20.0	41.0	48.3	54.0	42.3	117.7	21.3	35.5	43.2	43.0	33.2
40-50	102.2	15.3	38.7	51.0	45.5	39.4	118.3	14.3	42.7	78.7	49.7	50.3
50-60	96.0	10.0	26.7	49.3	41.7	32.3	87.5	11.3	25.8	44.0	30.0	30.0
60-70	96.4	17.7	38.6	48.6	44.3	42.9	93.0	6.6	22.6	53.0	29.6	36.0
70-80	72.1	7.1	35.9	44.6	32.3	35.9	89.1	10.1	33.6	51.9	32.9	38.3
80+	75.0	2.5	37.5	50.0	30.0	40.0	86.6	2.3	27.7	56.7	26.7	30.0

n: 80 females and 60 males
Method: measured with a 360-degree goniometer

Data from Ellis MI, Stowe J: The hip, *Clin Rheum Dis* 8(3):655-675, 1982.
AROM, Active range of motion.

Adult Population

Normative data for range of motion—knee

	Knee AROM (degrees)			
	Female		Male	
Age	Flexion	Extension	Flexion	Extension
55-64	143	0	141	1
65-74	144	0	141	1
75-84	140	0	141	1

n: 30 females and 30 males; healthy adults with no musculoskeletal problems

Data from Smith JR, Walker JM: Knee and elbow range of motion in healthy older individuals, *Phys Occup Ther Ger* 2(4):31-38, 1983.
AROM, Active range of motion.

Normative data for range of motion—ankle

	Ankle AROM (degrees)							
	Female				Male			
Age	Plantar-flexion	Dorsi-flexion	Inversion	Eversion	Plantar-flexion	Dorsi-flexion	Inversion	Eversion
11-20	52.0	29.0	36.8	24.1	52.0	29.0	36.8	34.1
21-30	56.6	25.7	35.3	25.1	40.8	25.7	35.3	25.1
31-40	54.2	27.3	33.5	24.2	43.0	27.3	33.5	24.2
41-50	52.6	24.3	33.4	23.6	40.8	30.7	38.2	23.6
51-60	54.4	18.0	29.7	22.5	35.7	26.6	35.4	22.5
61-70	45.4	26.7	30.7	16.0	31.0	29.5	30.7	16.0
71-80	38.4	25.0	32.0	19.9	38.4	25.0	32.0	19.9

n: 140 normal males and females
Method: measured with a 360-degree goniometer with the ankle stabilized in an apparatus to prevent substitution

Data from Alexander RE and others: The ankle and subtalar joints, *Clinics in Rheumatic Diseases* 8(3):703-711, 1982.
AROM, Active range of motion.

Balance

Normative data for balance—unilateral stance

| Age | Unilateral stance (seconds) | |
	Eyes open	Eyes closed
20-29	30.0	28.8
30-39	30.0	27.8
40-49	29.7	24.2
50-59	29.4	21.0
60-69	22.5	10.2
70-79	14.2	4.3

n: 184 males and females without vertigo, neurological, or orthopedic dysfunction of trunk or lower extremities
Method: shoes on, 30-second maximum, best of five trials

Data from Bohannon RW and others: Decrease in timed balance test scores with aging, *Phys Ther* 64(7):1067, 1984.

Normative data for balance—female unilateral stance

| Age | Female unilateral stance (seconds) | | | |
| | Dominant leg | | Nondominant leg | |
	Eyes open	Eyes closed	Eyes open	Eyes closed
60-64	38.48	5.74	34.13	8.33
65-69	24.31	4.27	23.88	4.49
70-74	18.46	3.68	19.60	2.82
75-79	10.81	2.34	11.97	3.21
80-86	10.65	2.80	10.17	2.74

n: 71 females who ambulate independently without an assistive device and are independent with activities of daily living; no serious musculoskeletal or neurological disorders
Method: shoes on, 45-second maximum, best of three trials

Data from Briggs RC and others: Balance performance among noninstitutionalized elderly women, *Phys Ther* 69(9):748-756, 1989.

Normative data for balance—female sharpened Romberg

Age	Female sharpened Romberg (seconds)	
	Eyes open	Eyes closed
60-64	56.37	24.58
65-69	55.93	31.58
70-74	48.61	24.19
75-79	39.65	14.13
80-86	45.49	21.71

n: 71 females who ambulate independently without an assistive device and are independent with activities of daily living; no serious musculoskeletal or neurological disorders

Method: shoes on, 60-second maximum, dominant foot lead, best of three trials

Data from Briggs RC and others: Balance performance among noninstitutionalized elderly women, *Phys Ther* 69(9):748-756, 1989.

Normative data for balance—male sharpened Romberg

Age	Male sharpened Romberg (seconds)	
	Eyes open	Eyes closed
60-90	54.70	24.62

n: 54 males independent with activities of daily living; ambulation without an assistive device; no heart disease, neurological problems, or joint replacement

Method: shoes on, 60-second maximum, dominant foot lead, best of three trials

Data from Iverson BD and others: Balance performance, force production, and activity levels in noninstitutionalized men 60-90 years of age, *Phys Ther* 70(6):348-355, 1990.

Gait

Normative data for gait—gait characteristics

	Gait characteristics							
	Female				Male			
Age	Velocity (m/min)	Steps/min	Stride length (m)	Heart rate (bpm)	Velocity (m/min)	Steps/min	Stride length (m)	Heart rate (bpm)
6-12	68.29	119.19	1.148	118.33	70.72	120.35	1.178	111.32
13-19	73.16	107.21	1.364	102.75	73.41	99.84	1.465	90.12
20-59	77.67	117.59	1.319	103.21	81.58	108.15	1.511	96.10
60-80	71.83	112.85	1.272	105.85	76.64	105.85	1.450	97.15

n: 126 females and 124 males; subjects without orthopedic or neurological disease and no assistive
   device with gait
Method: tested on a level outdoor track at customary gait speed

Data from Waters RL and others: Energy-speed relationship of walking: standard tables, *J Ortho Res* 6(2):215-222, 1988.

Normative data for gait—male gait characteristics

	Male gait characteristics			
Age	Velocity (cm/s)	Stride length (cm)	Stride width (cm)	Cycle duration (s)
20-25	150	154	8	1.05
30-35	143	151	9	1.09
40-45	159	151	9	0.98
50-55	157	160	9	1.04
60-65	145	151	8	1.07
67-73	118	136	9	1.18
74-80	123	141	10	1.15
81-87	118	126	10	1.10

n: 64 males, all with WNL range of motion and strength; no neurological deficits

Data from Murray MP, Kory RC, Clarkson BH: Walking patterns in healthy old men, *J Gerontol* 24:169-178, 1969.
WNL, Within normal limits.

Posture Characteristics

Posture Characteristics in Older Adults

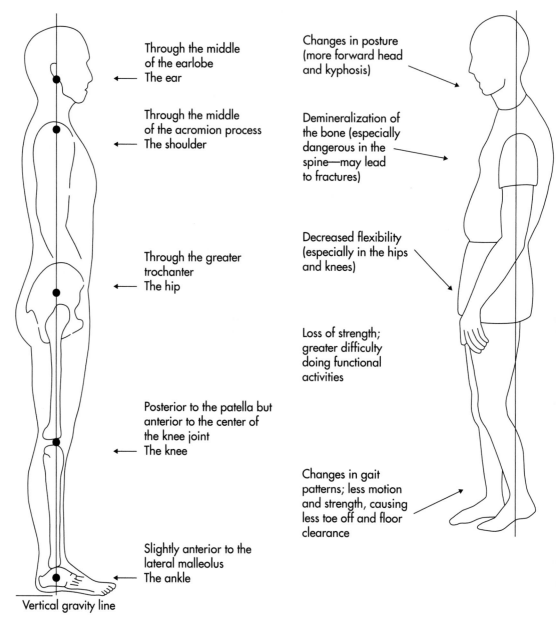

Through the middle of the earlobe
← The ear

Through the middle of the acromion process
← The shoulder

Through the greater trochanter
← The hip

Posterior to the patella but anterior to the center of the knee joint
← The knee

Slightly anterior to the lateral malleolus
← The ankle

Vertical gravity line

Changes in posture (more forward head and kyphosis)

Demineralization of the bone (especially dangerous in the spine—may lead to fractures)

Decreased flexibility (especially in the hips and knees)

Loss of strength; greater difficulty doing functional activities

Changes in gait patterns; less motion and strength, causing less toe off and floor clearance

FIGURE 3-23 Posture characteristics of older adults. (Modified from Lewis CB, editor: *Aging: the health care challenge*, ed 3, Philadelphia, 1996, FA Davis.)

Gait Characteristics
Gait Characteristics in Older Adults

Gait aspect	Healthy older men	Healthy older women
Gait velocity	Decreased	Decreased
Stride length	Decreased	Decreased
Step length	Not assessed	Decreased
Stride width	Increased*	Increased*
Stance phase duration	Increased	Not assessed
Swing phase duration	Decreased	Not assessed
Vertical excursion of the head	Decreased	Decreased*
Lateral excursion of the head	Increased*	Increased*
Shoulder extension ROM	Increased	Not assessed
Shoulder flexion ROM	Decreased	Not assessed
Elbow extension	Decreased	Not assessed
Pelvic rotation	Decreased*	Unchanged
Pelvic obliquity	Not assessed	Decreased
Hip flexion ROM	Decreased*	Not assessed
Knee flexion ROM	Decreased*	Not assessed
Ankle ROM	Decreased	Decreased
Toe-to-foot clearance	Increased	Not assessed

Modified from Murray MP, Kory RC, Clarkson BH: Walking patterns in healthy old men, *J Gerontol* 24:169-178, 1969; Hageman PA, Blanke DJ: Comparison of gait of young women and elderly women, *Phys Ther* 66(9):1382-1387, 1986.
ROM, Range of motion.
*Statistical significance attained.

Gait Characteristics in Older Men

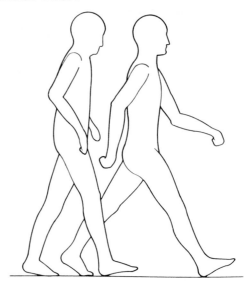

FIGURE 3-24 Differences between sagittal body positions of older *(left)* **and younger** *(right)* **individuals at the instant of heel strike.** Older individuals have a shorter step length, decreased excursions of hip flexion-extension, decreased angle extension and decreased heel elevation in rear limb, a decreased heel-floor angle and decreased toe elevation in forward limb, decreased shoulder flexion on forward arc of arm swing, and decreased elbow extension on backward arc of arm swing. (Modified from Murray MP, Draught AB, Kory RC: Walking patterns of normal men, *J Bone Joint Surg Am* 46(2):335-360, 1964.)

Transfer Standards
Supine-to-Sit Transfer Standards

Components of Supine-to-Sit Transfers

Pivot component	Pelvis motion as indicated by thigh abduction
Early pivot phase	First 30 degrees of thigh abduction
Middle pivot phase	30 to 60 degrees of thigh abduction
Late pivot phase	Greater than 60 degrees of thigh abduction until both thighs attain 90 degrees of flexion with legs dangling off the surface

Trunk elevation component	The angle made between the trunk and the horizontal surface in the sagittal/vertical plane
Early elevation phase	First 30 degrees of trunk elevation
Middle elevation phase	30 to 60 degrees of trunk elevation
Late elevation phase	Greater than 60 degrees of trunk elevation until the head and trunk are aligned and flexing toward the pelvis and lower extremities

NOTE: 9% of young and 18% of older subjects used an alternate rise technique consisting of rolling to the ipsilateral side before trunk elevation.

Strategies Used by Older Adults Compared with Younger Individuals

- Supine-to-sit transfers initiated with upper extremities only
- Greater use of lateral trunk flexion and rotation, especially in the late pivot phase to decrease sagittal plane trunk elevation
- Greater and earlier weightbearing on hip and gluteal areas
- Greater use of elbow contact on the surface to broaden the pivot base during the middle trunk elevation phase

Average Time to Complete Supine-to-Sit Transfers

	Including individuals using rolling technique		Excluding individuals using rolling technique	
	Young (mean age 23.5 years)	Old (mean age 73.8 years)	Young (mean age 23.5 years)	Old (mean age 73.8 years)
Time (seconds)	2.3 ± 0.5	3.3 ± 1.8	2.2 ± 0.4	2.9 ± 0.6

Modified from Alexander NB and others: Healthy young and old women differ in their trunk elevation and hip pivot motions when rising from supine to sitting, *J Am Ger Soc* 43:338-343, 1995.

Adult Population

Sit-to-Stand Transfer Standards

Components of Sit-to-Stand Transfers
Phase One: anterior weight shift
Phase Two: liftoff from seating surface

Requirements for Successful Sit-to-Stand Transfers
Phase One: total body mass center must move horizontally to within the area of foot support
Phase Two: enough joint torque strength must be generated for individual to rise from the seating surface

Strategies Used by Older Individuals Compared with Younger Individuals
Older adults able to rise without use of hands
• Greater percentage of time in Phase One when not using hands to rise
• Greater thigh and trunk flexion when not using hands to rise
• Greater thigh flexion when using hands to rise
Older adults unable to rise without use of hands
• Greater total time to rise
• Less thigh extension
• Greater trunk flexion
• Greater use of armrests compared with older individuals able to rise without use of hands

Average Time to Complete Sit-to-Stand Transfers

Phase	Subject group	With hands (seconds)	Without hands (seconds)
Phase One	Young (mean age 23.2)	0.59 ± 0.15	0.63 ± 0.15
	Old, able without hands (mean age 72.1)	0.65 ± 0.17	0.84 ± 0.41
	Old, unable without hands (mean age 84.4)	1.21 ± 0.57	Unable
Phase Two	Young (mean age 23.2)	0.98 ± 0.15	0.93 ± 0.23
	Old, able without hands (mean age 72.1)	0.91 ± 0.31	0.99 ± 0.34
	Old, unable without hands (mean age 84.4)	1.95 ± 1.1	Unable

Modified from Alexander NB, Schultz AB, Warwick DN: Rising from a chair: effects of age and functional ability on performance biomechanics, *J Gerontol* 46(3):M91-98, 1991.

Gait Standards

	Lower extremity range of motion during customary gait	
Gait aspect	Young adults (in degrees)	Older adults (in degrees)
Hip extension	10 ± 9	8 ± 6
Hip flexion	26 ± 8	29 ± 8
Knee extension	−3 ± 4	−7 ± 4
Knee flexion	66 ± 4	69 ± 5
Ankle dorsiflexion	12 ± 5	14 ± 3
Ankle plantarflexion	28 ± 8	24 ± 6

Data from Ostrosky KM and others: A comparison of gait characteristics in young and old subjects, *Phys Ther* 74(7):637-644, 1994.

Gait Phases and Definitions

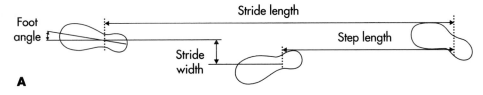

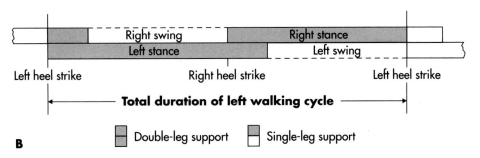

B

Double-leg support   Single-leg support

FIGURE 3-25 Stride length and left walking cycle. A, Schematic representation of stride dimensions: step and stride length, stride width, and foot angle. **B,** Schematic representation of left walking cycle showing temporal relationship of swing, double-limb support, and single-limb support. (Modified from Murray MP, Draught AB, Kory RC: Walking patterns of normal men, *J Bone Joint Surg Am* 46(2):335-360, 1964.)

Assistive Device Guidelines
Types of Assistive Devices

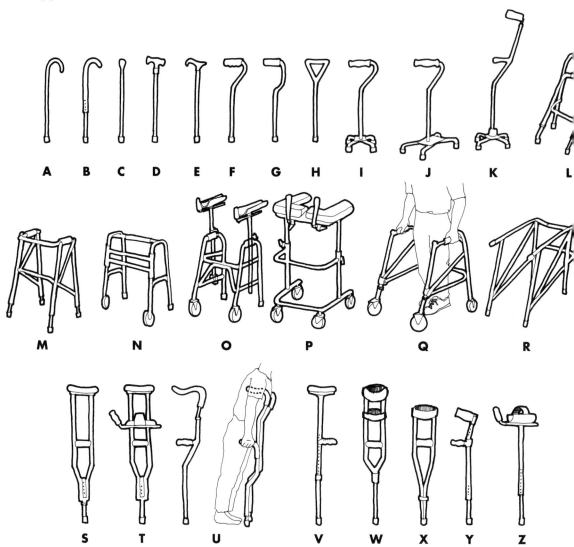

FIGURE 3-26 Gait aids. A, C-handle (J-handle or crook-top) wooden straight cane. **B,** C-handle adjustable aluminum straight cane. **C,** Ball-top straight cane. **D,** Functional grip cane. **E,** Slant-handled straight cane. **F,** Curved-top straight cane. **G,** Adjustable offset cane (e.g.,Ortho-cane). **H,** Shovel-handle (stirruplike) straight cane. **I,** Narrow-based quadruped ("quad") cane. **J,** Wide-based quadruped ("quad") cane. **K,** Forearm quadruped ("quad") cane. **L,** Walk-cane, or hemi-walker, or side-stepper cane. **M,** Nonfolding standard walker. (Folding type not shown.) **N,** Rolling, or gliding, walker. **O,** Bilateral platform walker. **P,** Rolling triceps walker. **Q,** Reverse rollator, or posture-control, walker. **R,** Stair-climbing walker. **S,** Adjustable axillary crutch (aluminum or wooden). **T,** Axillary crutch with platform. **U,** Ortho-crutch. **V,** Telescoping underarm (axillary) aluminum crutch. **W,** Triceps crutch (e.g., Canadian elbow extensor crutches). **X,** Forearm crutch with closed cuff (e.g., Kenny stick). **Y,** Adjustable forearm crutch (Lofstrand crutch). **Z,** Platform, or forearm support, crutch. (From Tan JC: *Practical manual of physical medicine and rehabilitation,* St Louis, 1998, Mosby.)

Critical Measurements for Assistive Device Prescription*
Canes

With the patient standing with the hands relaxed and at the sides, the cane handle should be level with the wrist. When holding the cane, the patient should have the elbow slightly flexed.

Axillary crutches

With the patient standing with the hands relaxed and at the sides, the crutches should rest under the arms with room for two to three fingers to fit between the crutch pads and the axilla. The crutch handles should be level with the patient's wrists.

Lofstrand crutches

With the patient standing with the hands relaxed and at the sides, the arm cuffs should be just below the elbows and the hand grips at the level of the wrists.

Walker

With the patient standing with the hands relaxed and at the sides, the walker handles should be level with the wrists. When holding the walker, the patient should have the elbows slightly flexed.

*This section modified from Anemaet WK, Moffa-Trotter ME: The user friendly home care handbook, Washington, DC, 1997, LEARN.

Adult Population

Wheelchair Guidelines
Types of Manual Wheelchairs

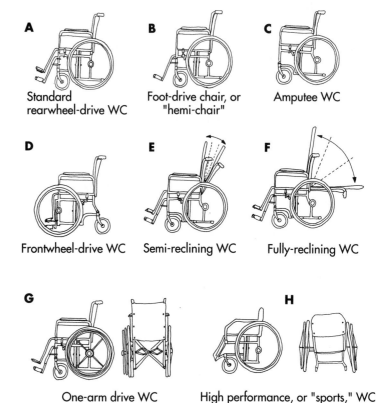

FIGURE 3-27 Types of manual wheelchairs (WCs). A, Standard WC. **B,** Seat of foot-drive or hemi-chair is about 2 inches lower than a standard and has only one front rigging. **C,** Amputee WC has rear wheels moved about 1.25 to 2 inches (3 to 5 cm) toward rear to compensate for posterior shift of center of gravity of individuals who have bilateral amputations. **D,** Frontwheel drive WC is typically used indoors. **E,** Semi-reclining WC has back upholstery that is 5 inches (13 cm) higher than that of a standard WC, and wheel is set back 1.25 inch (3 cm) toward rear. **F,** Fully reclining WC has back upholstery that is 7 inches (17 cm) higher than that of a standard WC, and wheel is set back 5 inches (12 cm) toward rear. **G,** One-arm drive WC (left-hand drive shown here) has driving wheels interconnected so that either or both can be controlled from one side through a dual set of handrims. **H,** High performance, or "sports," WC is very light and has wider camber (i.e., lower part of wheel tilted outward). (From Tan JC: *Practical manual of physical medicine and rehabilitation,* St Louis, 1998, Mosby.)

Parts of Manual Wheelchairs

FIGURE 3-28 Parts of a manual wheelchair. *1* through *4,* Types of tires. *1,* Solid hard rubber tire; *2,* pneumatic inner tube: *3,* semipneumatic tire with coil-reinforced zero pressure tire (ZPT inner tube); *4,* semipneumatic tire with solid foam ZPT inner tube. (From Tan JC: *Practical manual of physical medicine and rehabilitation,* St. Louis, 1998, Mosby.)

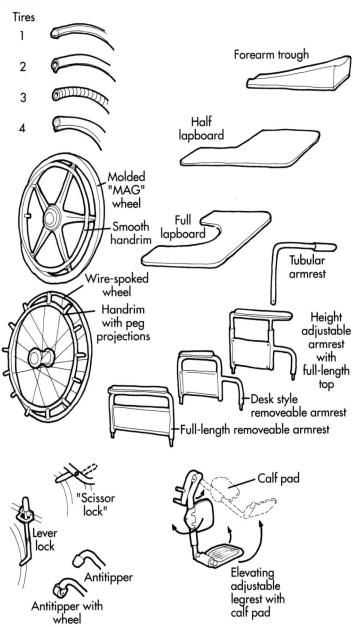

Continued

FIGURE 3-28 Parts of a manual wheelchair—cont'd. *a* through *d*, Types of casters. *a*, Standard 8-inch diameter with solid rubber tire; *b*, 8-inch diameter with semipneumatic tire; *c*, 8-inch diameter with pneumatic tire; *d*, 5-inch diameter with solid rubber tire. *A* through *F*, Types of pressure-relief seat cushions. *A*, Contoured foam (Veterans Administration spinal injury orthosis [VASIO]); *B*, contoured foam base with gel-filled pad (Jay cushion); *C*, viscoelastic foam with casing; *D*, polyurethane foam; *E*, gel enclosed in a nonbreathing plastic casing; *F*, air-filled villous ROHO cushion; *G*, water-filled seat cushion. (From Tan JC: *Practical manual of physical medicine and rehabilitation*, St. Louis, 1998, Mosby.)

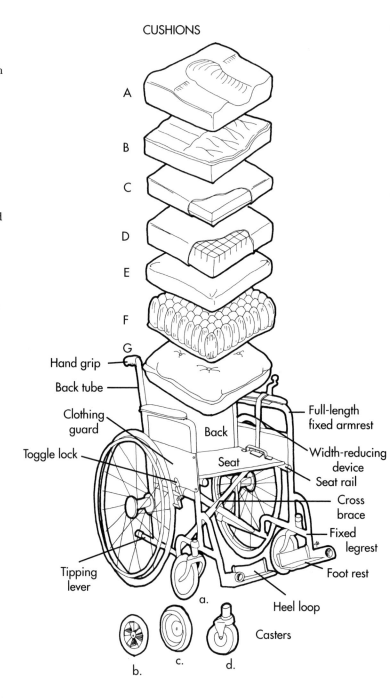

CUSHIONS

A
B
C
D
E
F
G

Hand grip
Back tube
Clothing guard
Back
Full-length fixed armrest
Toggle lock
Seat
Width-reducing device
Seat rail
Cross brace
Fixed legrest
Tipping lever
Foot rest
a.
Heel loop
b.
c.
d.
Casters

Critical Measurements for Wheelchair Prescription

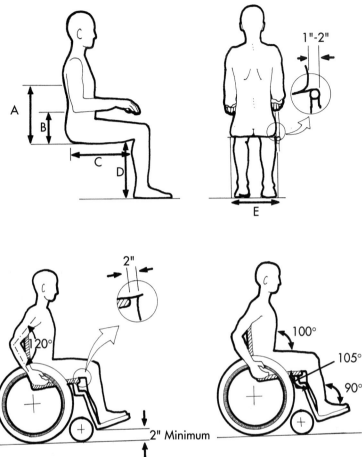

FIGURE 3-29 **Critical measurements for wheelchair prescription.** *A,* Back height (from seat): distance from bottom of buttocks to level of scapulae; *B,* arm height: distance from bottom of buttocks to olecranon with elbow fixed to 90°; *C,* seat depth: distance between popliteal and back of buttocks. (Add 1 to 2 inches so that popliteal fold is clear from anterior edge of seat, or adjust the back cushion or footrest until the fold is cleared.); *D,* seat height (from floor): length of leg from bottom of heel to popliteal fold. (Add 2 inches to provide clearance of footrest is to adjust seat cushion or footrest.); *E,* seat width (between uprights): widest distance across hips. (Add 1 to 2 inches for patient's clothing or braces.) The bottom figures show proper elbow, hip, knee, and ankle angles as well as proper footrest and popliteal clearances. (From Tan JC: *Practical manual of physical medicine and rehabilitation,* St Louis, 1998, Mosby; Wilson A: *Wheelchairs: a prescription guide,* New York, 1992, Demos.)

Balance Guidelines
Six Steps to Better Balance

Step	Purpose	Components
Step One: **Shake, Rattle,** **and Roll**	To promote trunk stability and initiate weight shifting in the sitting position	• Static sitting • Looking around • Reaching • Elevating UE • Shifting weight side to side • Shifting weight forward and back • Doing trunk clocks • Pushing therapy ball • Passing kickball • Catching kickball • Throwing kickball
Step Two: **Have a Ball**	To promote trunk stability and facilitate weight shifting in the sitting position, with a moveable base of support	• Static sitting • Looking around • Shifting weight • Doing trunk clocks • Reaching • Elevating UE • Bouncing • Marching • Using long arc quads • Using single limb support • Performing around the world
Step Three: **Stand Firm**	To promote static stability and facilitate weight shifting in the standing position	• Static standing • Shifting weight side to side • Shifting weight forward and back • Using body clocks • Using tandem weight shifts • Shifting weight in sharpened Romberg position

Modified from Anemaet WK, Moffa-Trotter ME: Six steps to better balance, *ADVANCE for Physical Therapists* 7(6):7,66, 1996.
UE, Upper extremity.

Table—cont'd

Step	Purpose	Components
Step Four: **Do Not be** **Swayed**	To enhance static stability and promote early dynamic standing balance	• Bouncing the ball to self • Bouncing the ball to therapist • Catching and tossing ball • Performing heel raises • Marching • Performing partial squats • Sidestepping • Maintaining single limb stance
Step Five: **The Minister of** **Funny Walks**	To facilitate weight shifting during dynamic gait skills	• Toe walking • Using backwards gait • Using crossovers • Braiding • Performing tandem gait • Heel walking
Step Six: **The Final** **Frontier**	To promote balance, coordination, and weight acceptance during unilateral stance	• Performing unilateral heel raises • Performing unilateral partial squats • Performing step ups • Performing lateral step ups • Performing step overs • Walking and tossing a ball • Walking and bouncing a ball • Static kicking of a ball • One step kicking of a ball • Ball traveling

Adult Population

Training Guidelines
Exercises to Improve Dynamic Postural Stability

Exercise Frequency
Two times a week for four 10- to 12-week sessions

Exercise Duration
60 minutes

Exercise Program
Warm-up period
5 minutes
- Moderately paced walking
- Arm movements added after 2-3 minutes to increase heart rate

Conditioning period
35 minutes
Aerobic exercises:

Lower extremity movements:
- sidestepping
- fast walking
- forward stepping
- backward stepping
- leg lifts
- knee bends
- forward lunges
- side lunges
- placing foot to the front
- placing foot to the side
- placing foot to the back

Trunk movements:
- upper body twists
- body bends
- cervical flexion
- cervical rotation
- knee lifts
- opposite elbow to raised knee
- pelvic rocking
- pelvic floor contractions
- belly dancing techniques

Upper extremity movements:
- arm circles
- bench presses
- upright rows
- short- and long-arm shoulder levers
- mock boxing
- shoulder rolls
- shoulder shrugs

Balance exercises:
- Unilateral stance
- Rope skills:
  - running under a skipping rope
- Ball skills:
  - static one-hand ball catch
  - dynamic one-hand ball catch
  - ball throw to moving target
  - ball kick
  - team ball games

Strengthening exercises:
- Modified push-ups
- Isometrics

Stretching period
15 minutes
- 20-second stretch in sitting of all major muscle groups

Cool-down period
5 to 10 minutes
- Sitting or supine position:
  - muscle relaxation
  - concentration on specific body areas
  - controlled breathing
  - guided imagery

Modified from Lord SR, Ward JA, Williams P: Exercise effect on dynamic stability in older women: a randomized controlled trial, *Arch Phys Med Rehabil* 77:232-236, 1996.

Exercises to Improve Gait Velocity

Exercise Frequency
Three times a week for 12 weeks

Exercise Duration
60 to 70 minutes

Exercise Program
Flexibility exercises
Seated:
- Stretching with emphasis on upper extremities
- Pelvic tilts
- Chin tucks
Standing:
- Calf stretches
- Hamstring stretches
Supine:
- Hip abduction stretches
Prone:
- Spine extension stretches
Balance exercises
- Postural alignment exercises
- Anterior-posterior weight shifting
- Medial-lateral weight shifting
- Simple tai chi for 5 to 10 minutes

Resistance exercises (began week 3)
Seated:
- Knee extension:
  - 1 RM at 75%-80% 1 RM 10 R $\times$ 3
- Ankle dorsiflexion:
  - 20-25 R $\times$ 2 to fatigue
Sidelying:
- Hip abduction:
  - 10-12 R $\times$ 3 to fatigue
Prone:
- Knee flexion:
  - 12-15 R $\times$ 1
- Hip extension:
  - 12-15 R $\times$ 1
- Shoulder extension:
  - 15 R $\times$ 1 not performed to fatigue

Modified from Judge JO, Underwood M, Gennosa T: Exercise to improve gait velocity in older persons, *Arch Phys Med Rehabil* 74:400-406, 1993.
R, Repetitions; *RM,* repetition maximum.

ADULT FINE MOTOR EVALUATION

Fine motor skills refer to the ability of patients to perform smooth, coordinated, purposeful movements with their hands. These skills allow patients to participate in high-level tasks such as writing, coin handling, buttoning, and feeding. Fine motor-assessment tools allow therapists to objectify hand function and target treatment interventions to the restoration and/or compensation for fine motor deficits. Associated standards provide normative reference values for range of motion and dynamometry strength values. Specific dermatomal and myotomal standards provide pictorial descriptions of these key neurological data. Associated guidelines offer descriptions of grasp and pinch variations, fine motor training strategies, and compensatory techniques.

Fine Motor Assessments
Arthritis Impact Measurement Scale Dexterity Subset

The Arthritis Impact Measurement Scale (AIMS) Dexterity Subset provides a subjective assessment of patient dexterity. It determines the ability of patients with arthritis to perform five tasks, such as writing or opening food jars. The AIMS Dexterity Subset is a self- or therapist-administered tool. The higher number of negative responses denotes a higher impact of arthritis on hand function.

AIMS Dexterity Subset Form

Dexterity task	Yes	No
Can you easily write with a pen or pencil?		
Can you easily turn a key in a lock?		
Can you easily button articles of clothing?		
Can you easily tie a pair of shoes?		
Can you easily open a jar of food?		

From Meenan RF, Gertman PM, Mason JH: Measuring health status in arthritis: the arthritis impact measurement scales *Arth Rheum* 23(2):146-152, 1980.

Functional Life Activity Test

The Functional Life Activity Test (FLAT) assesses aspects of daily life that may be affected by limitations in hand movement. Specifically, it measures the amount of time required to complete 10 tasks, including unlocking doors and buttoning clothing The FLAT is a therapist-administered tool. The total score is the amount of time required to complete all tasks. Higher scores denote greater hand impairment.

FLAT Form

Task	Time (seconds)	Comments
Opening jar		
Opening carton		
Unlocking door		
Pouring		
Carrying laundry		
Carrying groceries		
Buttoning		
Unbuttoning		
Zipping		
Unzipping		

Modified from Rondinelli RD and others: A simulation of hand impairments: effects on upper extremity function and implications toward medical impairment rating and disability determination, *Arch Phys Med Rehabil* 78:1358-1363, 1997.

Grip Ability Test

The Grip Ability Test (GAT) measures hand function of patients who have rheumatoid arthritis. It specifically examines patient performance with three tasks: donning a flexigrip stocking, putting a paper clip on an envelope, and pouring water from a jug. The GAT is a therapist-administered tool. The total score is the amount of time required to complete all tasks. The maximum score is 180 seconds. Higher scores denote greater hand function deficits.

GAT Form

General instructions: All tasks start with the patient's hands on the table. If the patient has not been able to perform the task in 60 seconds, this will be the maximum score.

Task	Score

Item 1:
Put Flexigrip stocking over nondominant hand

Materials
25 cm of a Tubigrip elasticized tubular bandage, 7.5-cm width for women and 10-cm width for men

Instructions
Take the Flexigrip stocking on the table in front of you with your dominant hand, and pull it like a glove over your other hand until all fingertips, including the thumb, are shown under it. Start now.

Scoring
Seconds from "start now" until all fingertips are visible; correction factor $\times$ 1.8

Item 2:
Put paperclip on envelope

Materials
Metal paper clip 30 $\times$ 10 mm, letter envelope 11.5 $\times$ 16 cm

Instructions
Pick up the paper clip from the table. You are not allowed to pull it over the edge of the table. Put the paper clip anywhere on the envelope, and put the envelope back on the table. Start now.

Scoring
Seconds from "start now" until the envelope is back on the table

Item 3:
Pour water from jug

Materials
A 1-liter water jug with handle, filled with water; a cup, size 2 dl

Instructions
Take the water jug with your dominant hand, lift the jug, fill the cup with water, and put the jug back on the table. Start now.

Scoring
Seconds from "start now" until the water jug is back on the table; correction factor $\times$ 1.8

Modified from Dellhag B, Bjelle A: A grip ability test for use in rheumatology practice, *J Rheumatol* 22(8):1559-1565, 1995.

Jebsen Hand Function Test

The Jebsen Hand Function Test assesses hand function in adults. It evaluates prehension and manipulation skills with functional tasks such as writing and simulated feeding. The Jebsen Hand Function Test is a therapist-administered tool. The total score is the amount of time required to complete all tasks. Higher scores denote greater hand function impairment.

Jebsen Hand Function Test Form

Subtest 1: Writing

Procedure—The patient is given a black ball-point pen and four 8-by-11-inch sheets of unruled white paper fastened, one on top of the other, to a clip board. The sentence to be copied has 24 letters and is of third-grade reading difficulty.* The sentence is typed in all capital letters and centered on a 5-by-8-inch index card. The card is presented with the typed side face down on a bookstand. After the articles are arranged to the comfort of the patient (see Instructions), examiner turns the card over with an immediate command to begin. The patient is timed from the word "go" until the pen is lifted from the page at the end of the sentence. The item is repeated with the dominant hand writing a new sentence.

Instructions—"Do you require glasses for reading? If so, put them on. Take this pen in your left hand and arrange everything so that it is comfortable for you to write with your left hand. On the other side of this card (indicate) is a sentence. When I turn the card over and say 'Go,' write the sentence as quickly and as clearly as you can using your left hand. Write. Do not print. Do you understand? Ready? Go."

For Dominant Hand—"All right, now repeat the same thing, only this time using your right hand. I've given you a different sentence. Are you ready? Go."

Subtest 2: Card Turning (Simulated Page Turning)

Procedure—Five 3-by-5-inch index cards, ruled on one side only, are placed in a horizontal row

Subtest 2: Card Turning (Simulated Page Turning)—cont'd

2 inches apart on the desk in front of the patient. Each card is oriented vertically, 5 inches from the front edge of the desk. This distance is indicated on the side edge of the desk with a piece of tape. Timing occurs from the word "Go" until the last card is turned over. No accuracy of placement after turning is necessary. The item is repeated with the dominant hand.

Instructions—"Place your left hand on the table, please. When I say 'Go,' use your left hand to turn these cards over one at a time as quickly as you can, beginning with this one (indicate card to extreme right). You may turn them over in any way that you wish, and they need not be in a neat pattern when you finish. Do you understand? Ready? Go."

Dominant Hand—"Now the same thing with the right hand, beginning with this one (indicate extreme left card). Ready? Go."

Subtest 3: Small Common Objects

Procedure—An empty 1-pound coffee can is placed directly in front of the patient, 5 inches from the front edge of the desk. Two 1-inch paper clips (oriented vertically), two regular-sized bottle caps (each 1-inch in diameter, placed with the inside of the cap facing up), and two United States pennies are placed in a horizontal row to the left of the can. The paper clips are to the extreme left, and the pennies are nearest the can. The objects are 2 inches apart.

Timing occurs from the word "Go" until the sound of the last object striking the inside of the

Modified from Jebsen RH and others: An objective and standardized test of hand function, *Arch Phys Med Rehabil* 311–319 June 1969.
*Different sentences were used when subsequent tests were given to an individual. Available sentences were the following: (1) The old man seemed to be tired; (2) John saw the red truck coming; (3) whales live in the blue ocean; and (4) fish take air out of the water.

Subtest 3: Small Common Objects—cont'd

can is heard. The item is repeated with the dominant hand. The layout for the dominant hand is a mirror image of the one described, with the objects to the right of the can.

Instructions—"Place your left hand on the table, please. When I say 'Go,' use your left hand to pick up these objects one at a time and place them in the can as fast as you can, beginning with this one (indicate paper clip on the extreme left). Do you understand? Ready? Go."

Dominant Hand—"Now the same thing with the right hand, beginning here (indicate paper clip now on the extreme right). Ready? Go."

Subtest 4: Simulated Feeding

Procedure—Five kidney beans of approximately ⅜-inch length are placed on a board* clamped to the desk in front of the patient 5 inches from the front edge of the desk. The beans are oriented to the left of center, parallel to and touching the upright of the board 2 inches apart. An empty 1-pound coffee can is placed centrally in front of the board. A regular teaspoon is provided. Timing occurs from the word "Go" until the last bean is heard hitting the bottom of the can. The item is repeated with the dominant hand, the beans being placed to the right of center.

Instructions—"Take the teaspoon in your left hand, please. When I say 'Go,' use your left hand to pick up these beans one at a time with the teaspoon, and place them in the can as fast as you can beginning with this one (indicate bean on the extreme left). Do you understand? Ready? Go."

Dominant Hand—"Now the same thing with the right hand beginning here (indicate bean on the extreme right). Ready? Go."

Subtest 5: Checkers

Procedure—Four standard sized (1¼-inch diameter) red wooden checkers are placed in front of and touching a board* clamped to the desk in front of the subject, 5 inches from the front edge of the desk. The checkers are oriented two on each side of the center in a 0000 configuration. Timing occurs from the word "Go" until the fourth checker makes contact with the third checker. The fourth checker need not stay in place. The item is repeated with the dominant hand.

Instructions—"Place your left hand on the table, please. When I say 'Go,' use your left hand to stack these checkers on the board in front of you as fast as you can, like this, one on top of the other (demonstrate). You may begin with any checker. Do you understand? Ready? Go."

Dominant Hand—"Now the same thing with the right hand. Ready? Go."

Subtest 6: Large Light Objects

Procedure—Five empty No. 303 cans are placed in front of a board* clamped to the desk in front of the patient 5 inches from the front edge of the desk. The cans are spaced 2 inches apart with the open end of the can facing down. Timing occurs from the word "Go" until the fifth can has been released. The item is repeated with the dominant hand.

Instructions—"Place your left hand on the table, please. When I say 'Go,' use your left hand to stand these cans on the board in front of you, like this (demonstrate). Begin with this one (indicate can on extreme left). Do you understand? Ready? Go."

Dominant Hand—"Now the same thing with the right hand, beginning here (indicate extreme right can). Ready? Go."

*A wooden board 4½ inches long, 11¼ inches wide and ¾-inch thick was secured to the desk with a "C" clamp. The front edge (¾-inch thickness) of the board was marked at 4-inch intervals for easy reference when placing objects. A center piece of plywood, 20 inches long, 2 inches high, and ½-inch thick, was glued to the board 4⅜ inches from the right end and 6 inches from the front of the board (this is for a secretary-type desk with a right-sided knee hole). The front of the center upright should be marked at 2-inch intervals beginning 1-inch from each end for convenience in placing objects.

Continued

Box—cont'd

Subtest 7: Large Heavy Objects

Procedure—Five full (1-pound) No. 303 cans are placed in front of a board* clamped to the desk in front of the patient 5 inches from the front edge of the desk. The cans are spaced 2 inches apart. Timing occurs from the word "Go" until the fifth can has been released. The item is repeated with the dominant hand.

Instructions—"Now do the same thing with these heavier cans. Place your left hand on the

Subtest 7: Large Heavy Objects— cont'd

table. When I say 'Go,' use your left hand to stand these cans on the board as fast as you can. Begin here (indicate can on extreme left). Do you understand? Ready? Go."

Dominant Hand—"Now the same thing with your right hand, beginning here (indicate can on far right). Ready? Go."

Modified from Jebsen RH and others: An objective and standardized test of hand function, *Arch Phys Med Rehabil* 50:311–319 June 1969.

Sequential Occupational Dexterity Assessment

The Sequential Occupational Dexterity Assessment (SODA) measures bimanual dexterity in daily life. It assesses performance on a variety of hand tasks, including writing, squeezing toothpaste, and washing hands. The SODA is a therapist-administered tool. The total score ranges from 0 to 72 for single-hand performance. Higher scores denote greater bimanual hand dexterity.

SODA Form

Scoring Criteria
Task score = ability + difficulty score

Ability Scale
0 = unable
1 = able to perform the task in a different way
4 = able to perform the task as described

Difficulty Scale
0 = very difficult
1 = somewhat difficult
2 = not difficult

Task	Score
Writing a sentence	
Picking up an envelope	
Picking up coins	
Holding the receiver of a phone to one ear	
Unscrewing the cap of a tube of toothpaste	
Squeezing toothpaste onto a toothbrush	
Handling a spoon and knife	
Buttoning a blouse	
Unscrewing a large bottle	
Pouring water into a glass	
Washing hands	
Drying hands	
TOTAL SCORE	

Modified from van Lankveld W and others: Sequential occupational dexterity assessment: a new test to measure hand disability, *J Hand Ther* 9:27-32, 1996.

Timed Manual Performance—Doors

The Timed Manual Performance (TMP)—Doors is a shortened version of the TMP Test that measures manual performance. It consists of opening and/or closing three different types of fasteners attached to a plywood panel (Figure 3-30). The TMP—Doors is a therapist-administered tool. The total score is the amount of time required to complete all tasks. Higher scores denote greater manual performance impairment.

FIGURE 3-30 Timed manual performance (TMP) board—a plywood panel with nine doors. A, Cabinet lock. **B,** Door knob. **C,** Round knob. Manual performance is measured by timing subjects as they open and close the doors. (Modified from Gerrity MS, Gaylord S, Williams ME: Short versions of the timed manual performance test: development, reliability, and validity, *Med Care* 31(7):617-628, 1993.)

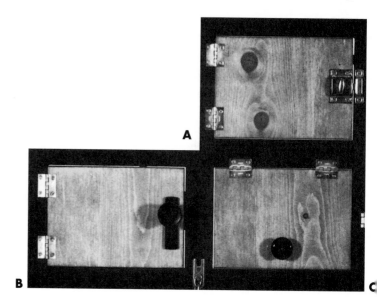

A

B

C

TMP—Doors Form

Task	Time (seconds)
Open round knob door	
Open and close door knob	
Open and close cabinet lock	

From Gerrity MS, Gaylord S, Williams ME: Short versions of the timed manual performance test: development, reliability, and validity, *Med Care* 31(7):617-628, 1993.

Timed Manual Performance—Table

The TMP—Table is a shortened version of the TMP Test that measures manual performance. It evaluates manipulation and prehension skills with three tasks: feeding, stacking checkers, and turning cards. The total score is the amount of time required to complete all tasks with the dominant and nondominant hand. Higher scores denote greater manual performance impairment.

TMP—Table Form

Task	Time (seconds) for dominant and nondominant hand
Simulated feeding	
Checkers stacking	
Card turning	

Modified from Gerrity MS, Gaylord S, Williams ME: Short versions of the time manual performance test: development, reliability, and validity, *Med Care* 31(7):617-628, 1993.

Normative Data Standards for Hand Function
Normative Data for Hand Function—Functional Range of Motion

	Thumb (degrees)		Fingers (degrees)		
Joint	MCP	IP	MCP	PIP	DIP
Range	10-32 ± 5	2-43 ± 5	33-73 ± 5	36-86 ± 5	20-61 ± 5
Average result	21	18	61	60	39
Median result	22	19	62	63	39

n: 35 right-handed males (26-28 years) without history of hand injury
Method: The subject was seated and measured with standard goniometric methods to record the
    maximum active ROM. This was then repeated with an electrogoniometer. Measurements were
    taken when the hand was in position to perform the following tasks: holding a telephone, holding a
    can, using a zipper, holding a toothbrush, turning a key, using a comb, printing with a pen, holding
    a fork, holding scissors, unscrewing a jar, and holding a hammer.

Modified from Hume MC and others: Functional range of motion of the joints of the hand, *J Hand Surg* 15A(2):240-243, 1990.
MCP, Metacarpophalangeal; *IP,* interphalangeal; *PIP,* proximal interphalangeal; *DIP,* distal interphalangeal; *ROM,* range of motion.

Normative Data for Hand Function—Female Finger and Hand Strength

Age	Hand grip (pounds)		Tip pinch (pounds)		Key pinch (pounds)		Palmer pinch (pounds)	
	Left	Right	Left	Right	Left	Right	Left	Right
20-24	61.0	70.4	10.5	11.1	16.2	17.6	16.3	17.2
25-29	63.5	74.5	11.3	11.9	16.6	17.7	17.0	17.7
30-34	68.0	78.7	11.7	12.6	17.8	18.7	18.1	19.3
35-39	66.3	74.1	11.9	11.6	16.0	16.6	17.1	17.5
40-44	62.3	70.4	11.1	11.5	15.8	16.7	16.6	17.0
45-49	56.0	62.2	12.1	13.2	16.6	17.6	17.5	17.9
50-54	57.3	65.8	11.4	12.5	16.1	16.7	16.4	17.3
55-59	47.3	57.3	10.4	11.7	14.7	15.7	15.4	16.0
60-64	45.7	55.1	9.9	10.1	14.1	15.5	14.3	14.8
65-69	41.0	49.6	10.5	10.6	14.3	15.0	13.7	14.2
70-74	41.5	49.6	9.8	10.1	13.8	14.5	14.0	14.4
75+	37.6	42.6	9.3	9.6	11.4	12.6	11.5	12.0

n: 318 females with no acute pain in upper extremities; 6 months status post hospitalization; normal
    lifestyle without health-related activities of daily living restrictions
Method: subject seated with shoulder in adduction, neutral rotation; 90 degrees elbow flexion, neutral
    forearm, 0-30 degrees wrist extension, and 0-15 degrees ulnar deviation; mean of three trials
Grip: adjustable Jamar Dynamometer
Pinch: B & L Pinch Gauge

Modified from Mathiowetz V and others: Grip and pinch strength: normative data for adults, *Arch Phys Med Rehab* 66:69-74, 1985.

Normative Data for Hand Function—Male Finger and Hand Strength

Age	Hand grip (pounds)		Tip pinch (pounds)		Key pinch (pounds)		Palmer pinch (pounds)	
	Left	Right	Left	Right	Left	Right	Left	Right
20-24	104.5	121.0	17.0	18.0	24.8	26.0	25.7	26.6
25-29	110.5	120.8	17.5	18.3	25.0	26.7	25.1	26.0
30-34	110.4	121.8	17.6	17.6	26.2	26.4	25.4	24.7
35-39	112.9	119.7	17.7	18.0	25.6	26.1	25.9	26.2
40-44	112.8	116.8	17.7	17.8	25.1	25.6	24.8	24.5
45-49	100.8	109.9	17.6	18.7	24.8	25.8	23.7	24.0
50-54	101.9	113.6	17.8	18.3	26.1	26.7	24.0	23.8
55-59	83.2	101.1	15.0	16.6	23.0	24.2	21.3	23.7
60-64	76.8	89.7	15.3	15.8	22.2	23.2	21.2	21.8
65-69	76.8	91.1	15.4	17.0	22.0	23.4	21.2	21.4
70-74	64.8	75.3	13.3	13.8	19.2	19.3	18.8	18.1
75+	55.0	65.7	13.9	14.0	19.1	20.5	18.3	18.7

n: 310 individuals with no acute pain in upper extremities; 6 months status post hospitalization; normal lifestyle without health-related activities of daily living restrictions
Method: subject seated with shoulder in adduction, neutral rotation; 90 degrees elbow flexion, neutral forearm, 0-30 degrees wrist extension, and 0-15 degrees ulnar deviation; mean of three trials
Grip: adjustable Jamar Dynamometer
Pinch: B & L Pinch Gauge

Modified from Mathiowetz V and others: Grip and pinch strength: normative data for adults, *Arch Phys Med Rehab* 66:69-74, 1985.

Normative Data for Hand Function—Finger Pinch Strength

Age	Female (kg)					Male (kg)				
	Chuck	Pulp 2	Pulp 3	Pulp 4	Pulp 5	Chuck	Pulp 2	Pulp 3	Pulp 4	Pulp 5
5-12	3.6	2.4	2.4	1.7	1.1	4.0	2.7	2.7	1.9	1.2
18-40	7.0	4.7	4.5	3.1	2.0	9.4	7.3	7.0	4.4	2.9
60-89	4.6	3.0	2.8	1.9	1.3	5.9	4.3	4.0	2.7	1.7

n: 94 females and 88 males able to perform all grips and pinches
Method: two repetitions recording peak torque; subject seated with 30 degrees shoulder flexion and 90 degrees elbow flexion

Modified from Imrhan SN: Trends in finger pinch strength in children, adults, and the elderly, *Human Factors* 31(6):689-701, 1989.

Normative Data for Hand Function—Finger Tapping Test

	Number of index finger taps per 10 seconds			
	Female		Male	
Age	Dominant	Nondominant	Dominant	Nondominant
16-24	49.5	45.6	52.9	48.2
25-39	49.0	44.6	52.7	48.7
40-54	47.0	43.5	54.3	48.9
55-70	45.7	40.4	53.5	48.3

n: 179 females and 179 males; no psychiatric history, polypharmacy, or neurological disorders
Method: mean of five trials

Modified from Ruff RM, Parker SB: Gender and age-specific changes in motor speed and eye-hand coordination in adults: normative values for the finger tapping and grooved pegboard, *Perceptual and Motor Skills* 76:1219-1230, 1993.

Hand Sensory Dermatome Distribution Standards

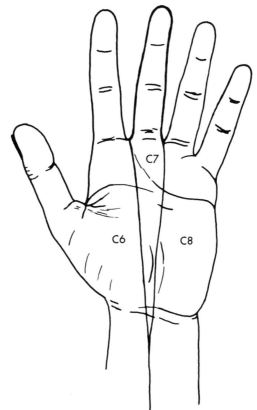

FIGURE 3-31 Sensory dermatomes by neurological level. (From Hunter JM, Mackin EJ, Callahan AD, eds: *Rehabilitation of the hand: surgery and therapy*, ed 4, St Louis, 1995, Mosby.)

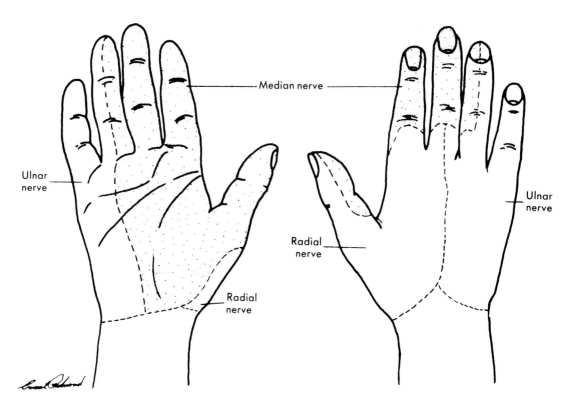

FIGURE 3-32 Sensory dermatomes by radial, median, and ulnar nerves. (From Hunter JM, Mackin EJ, Callahan AD, eds: *Rehabilitation of the hand: surgery and therapy,* ed 4, St Louis, 1995, Mosby.)

Grasp and Pinch Guidelines
The Six Most Commonly Used Hand-Finger Prehension Patterns

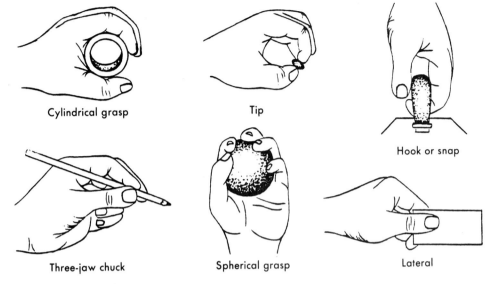

Cylindrical grasp

Tip

Hook or snap

Three-jaw chuck

Spherical grasp

Lateral

FIGURE 3-33 The six most commonly used hand-finger prehension patterns. (From Hunter JM, Mackin EJ, Callahan AD, eds: *Rehabilitation of the hand: surgery and therapy,* ed 4, St Louis, 1995, Mosby.)

Fine Motor Training Guidelines
Hand and Finger Function Exercises

Items	Exercises
Cards	• Shuffle cards. • Deal cards one by one. • Turn cards over one by one. • Cut the deck. • Play 52 pick-up.
Shoe laces or string	• Tie and untie knots. • Lace and unlace shoes. • Make bows. • Cut string with scissors.
Small items (e.g., coins, marbles, keys, buttons, seeds, beans, nuts, bolts, paper clips)	• Pick up small items one at a time with your hand. • Pick up small items one at a time with tweezers. • Grab a handful of small items and drop them one by one into a can. • Hold a small item in your hand and try and rotate it in as many directions as you can.

Continued

Table—cont'd

Items	Exercises
Paper	• Crumple and straighten a piece of paper in one hand. • Flip the crumpled piece of paper into the air using the fingertips. • Fold and unfold a piece of paper in one hand. • Tear a piece of paper into small strips. • Use scissors to cut a piece of paper into small strips. • Place a piece of paper into an envelope. • Open mail and retrieve items one by one from the envelope.
Household items	• Screw and unscrew wing nuts to and from bolts. • Use a screwdriver to screw and unscrew screws. • Open and close safety pins. • Staple paper together. • Use a staple remover to remove staples. • Use a flour sifter. • Open and close doors. • Use keys to open doors. • Turn lights on and off. • Open and close drawers.
Clothing	• Button and unbutton shirts. • Zip and unzip zippers. • Hook and unhook bra clasps. • Buckle and unbuckle belts. • Fold clothes. • Roll socks together. • Put mittens or gloves on, and then take them off.
Containers	• Screw and unscrew various size lids from containers. • Pour fluid from one container to another. • Pick up various size containers with one hand.
Writing implements	• Write with various implements (markers, pencils, pens, crayons). • Complete dot-to-dot drawings. • Trace pictures in a coloring book.

Table—cont'd

Items	Exercises
Crafts	• String beads. • Sew. • Use paint-by-number pictures. • Use woodwork. • Use macrame. • Use model kits. • Use needlepoint. • Use rug hooking. • Use origami.
Games	• Play dominoes. • Stack checkers. • Play Scrabble. • Play cribbage. • Play cards.
Dough	• Roll dough into a log shape. • Roll dough into a ball shape. • Cut dough with a knife. • Pull dough apart with both hands. • Pull dough apart with the thumb and each finger, one at a time. • Make a ring and put fingers through it. Spread the fingers apart to enlarge the ring. • Squeeze dough with one hand. • Squeeze dough between the thumb and each finger, one at a time. • Squeeze dough between each finger, one at a time. • Pinch dough with fingers. • Twist two strands of dough. • Braid three strands of dough. • Flatten dough with one hand. • Make finger and thumb prints in the dough.

Adult Population

Fisting Sequence Exercises

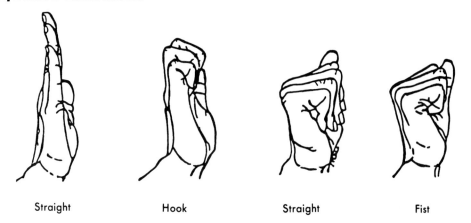

Straight   Hook   Straight   Fist

FIGURE 3-34 Positions for soft tendon gliding exercises. Hook fist, straight fist, and full fist. (From Hunter JM, Mackin EJ, Callahan AD, eds: *Rehabilitation of the hand: surgery and therapy,* ed 4, St Louis 1995, Mosby.)

Splinting Guidelines
Splinting Guidelines Form

Upper-limb orthoses are generally used to restore upper limb function by assisting or supporting weak muscles, substituting for paralyzed muscle, protecting painful or deformed parts, correcting (or minimizing) existing deformities or malalignment, permitting controlled directional movement, and allowing attachment of assistive devices (e.g., utensil holders). The prescribed upper-limb orthosis should be properly fitted so the patient can easily don and doff it and either rest the desired segment or perform the prescribed movement comfortably when wearing the orthosis. Also, the orthosis must be functionally as well as cosmetically acceptable to the patient. When the orthosis is removed, the skin should be unblemished 10 minutes afterwards. Most wrist and hand orthoses can adequately be held in place with a strap, whereas other upper-limb orthoses need to be suspended from the torso for ambulatory patients or suspended from the wheelchair for patients using wheelchairs. Suspension systems commonly used include hoops, shoulder caps, and harnesses.

Traditionally, upper-limb orthoses are classified into *static* (i.e., rigid; gives support without allowing movement) and *dynamic* (also called *functional;* i.e., allows certain degree of movement). Dynamic upper-limb orthoses improve upper limb functions through the use of joints, levers, pulleys, and external power sources (including rubber bands, springs, batteries, and cartridges of compressed gas). The traditional classification, however, can be confusing because static orthoses are often used to create movement; however, dynamic splints usually have components that restrict motion to create movement at another joint. Another way of classifying upper-limb orthoses is by the anatomical joint covered by the orthosis (e.g., FO [finger orthosis], TO [thumb orthosis], WHFO [wrist-hand-finger orthosis], WO [wrist orthosis], WHO [wrist-hand orthosis], EWHO [elbow-wrist-hand orthosis], EO [elbow orthosis], and SEWHO [shoulder-elbow-wrist-hand orthosis]). However, this anatomical classification does not indicate function. Therefore the following classification is used to combine function and anatomy (based on the classification of upper-limb orthoses of the New York University Prosthetic and Orthotics Faculty published in the *American Academy of*

Modified from Tan JC: *Practical manual of physical medicine and rehabilitation,* St Louis, 1998, Mosby.

Box—cont'd

Orthopedic Surgeons' Atlas of Orthotics: Biomechanical Principles and Application).
A. Wrist, Hand, and Finger Orthoses
  1. **Assistive and substitutive orthoses** are primarily used to enhance hand function in patients with residual strength (i.e., using assistive orthoses) or absent strength (i.e., using

substitutive orthoses). They are usually worn throughout the day (Figure 3-35).
  a. **Positional orthoses** are used to promote optimal wrist, hand, and finger positions for facilitation of active hand and finger grasp and prevention of joint contracture.

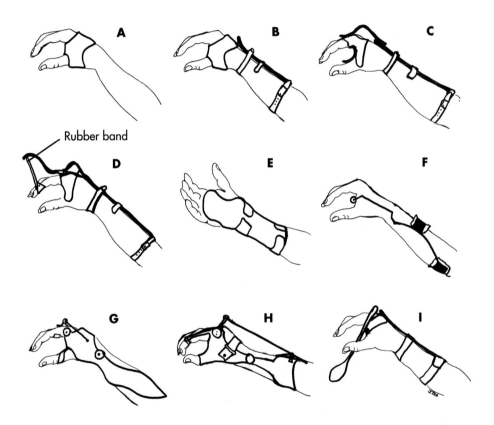

Rubber band

FIGURE 3-35 Assistive and substitutive wrist, hand, and finger orthoses. A through **F,** Positional orthoses. **A,** Basic (i.e., C-bar, short opponens) orthoses. **B,** Opponens orthoses with wrist control attachments (i.e., long opponens orthoses). **C,** Opponens orthoses with lumbrical bar. **D,** Opponens orthoses with finger extension assist assembly (using rubber bands). **E,** Volar wrist-flexion control orthoses (cock-up spling). **F,** Wire wrist-extension assist orthoses (Oppenheimer splint). **G** through **I,** Prehension orthoses. **G,** Finger-driven hand prehension orthoses. **H,** Wrist-driven prehension orthoses (tenodesis orthoses). **I,** Utensil holders (i.e., universal splints, activities of daily living [ADLs] splint). (From Tan JC: *Practical manual of physical medicine and rehabilitation,* St Louis, 1998, Mosby.)

Continued

Adult Population

Box—cont'd

(1) **Opponens orthoses and their variations** are primarily used to position the weak thumb in opposition to other fingers to improve hand function by facilitating a three-jaw chuck pinch.

(2) **Wrist control orthoses** are used to promote slight extension of the wrist or prevent wrist flexion, thus assisting weak grasp (i.e., via tenodesis effect).

b. **Prehension orthoses** are used to stabilize the thumb while substituting muscle strength from other parts of the body or from an external power source to provide hand grasping, holding, and releasing functions. They are used in patients with severe paralysis of the upper limb (e.g., spinal cord injury and polio). The prehension pattern may be a three-jaw chuck or a lateral grasp.

(1) **Hand prehension orthoses,** such as finger-driven hand prehension orthoses are FOs that provide prehension for the index and middle fingers through transmission of active flexion of one or more fingers. Active metacarpophalangeal (MCP) or interphalangeal (IP) flexion must be present in at least one finger of the hand.

(2) **Wrist-hand prehension orthoses** can be anatomically classified as WHFOs.

c. **Utensil holders** consist of a handcuff with a palmar pocket into which the utensil can be inserted. Most individuals with tetraplegia prefer them over the other complex orthoses.

2. **Protective orthoses** are used to protect the wrist, hand, and fingers from potential deformity or damage by restricting active function (e.g., to promote tissue healing) while maintaining a desired functional position. Most of them may be worn throughout the day and night to rest the joint (Figure 3-36).

a. **Digital stabilizers**

b. **Wrist-hand-finger stabilizers** are WHFOs that extend from two thirds of the distal forearm to the tips of the fingers and/or thumb (sometimes the thumb is left free). Wrist-hand-finger stabilizers are used to immobilize and promote tissue healing, to passively maintain ROM of the wrist and hand (often used at night) in patients with upper motor neuron (UMN) lesions, and to maintain stretch on MCP/IP collateral ligaments.

c. **Wrist-hand stabilizers**

d. **Tone-reduction orthoses** are used to reduce spastic flexor tone. They are typically worn 2 hours on and 2 hours off throughout the day. They can be hand-based WHOs or forearm-based WHFOs.

e. **Gloves** are worn circumferentially on the hand and wrist. If needed, the tips or whole fingers of the gloves may be cut off.

3. **Mobilization (corrective) orthoses** are used to increase passive ROM and alter joint alignment by stretching articular or musculotendinous contractures or adhesions. In general, a submaximal load is applied for long periods dynamically using traction or statically by holding the joint on low tension circumferentially. The most commonly used stretching method is dynamic elastic load, specifically rubber bands whose amount of force can be regulated by the rubber tension. Mobilization orthoses are worn for only a specific time during the day (Figure 3-37).

Modified from Tan JC: *Practical manual of physical medicine and rehabilitation,* St Louis, 1998, Mosby.

Box—cont'd

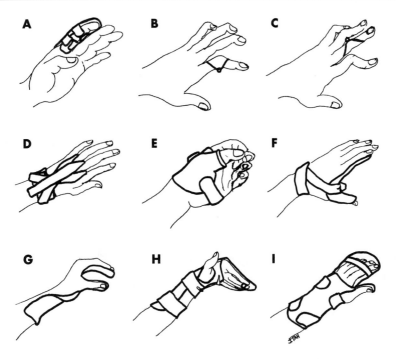

FIGURE 3-36 Protective wrist, hand, and finger orthoses. A, Interphalangeal (IP) stabilizer (static finger splints, finger gutter splint). **B,** Swan neck ring (proximal interphalangeal [PIP] or distal interphalangeal [DIP] extension-stop digital stabilizer). **C,** Boutonnière ring (PIP flexion-stop digital stabilizer). **D,** Finger web-space stabilizers (finger web spacers). **E,** Thumb carpometacarpal stabilizers (thumb posts). **F,** Thumb web-space stabilizer (thenar web spacers). **G,** Volar wrist-hand-finger stabilizers (resting hand splint). **H,** Dorsal blocking splint. **I,** Tone-reduction orthosis (Snook spling). (From Tan JC: *Practical manual of physical medicine and rehabilitation,* St Louis, 1998, Mosby.)

a. **Finger-mobilization orthoses**
b. **Thumb-mobilization orthoses**
c. **Wrist-mobilization orthoses** are WOs used to passively increase ROM. They can also be used to replace or assist

weak wrist extensors to enhance activities of daily living (ADLs). However, they should not be used on spastic muscles because they may further increase tone.

Continued

Box—cont'd

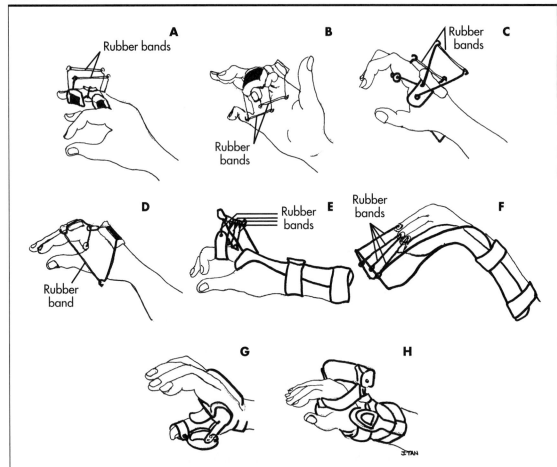

FIGURE 3-37   Mobilization (or corrective) wrist, hand, and finger orthoses.
A, Interphalangeal (IP) extension mobilization orthosis (reverse finger knuckle bender).
B, IP flexion mobilization orthosis (finger knuckle bender). **C,** Reverse metacarpophalangeal
(MCP) knuckle bender. **D,** MCP knuckle bender. **E,** Dynamic MCP extension splint with
dorsal outrigger. **F,** Dynamic MCP flexion splint with volsar outrigger and fingernail hooks.
G, Dynamic thumb IP extension splints. **H,** Wrist mobilization orthoses. (From Tan JC:
Practical manual of physical medicine and rehabilitation, St Louis, 1998, Mosby.)

ADULT NEUROLOGICAL EVALUATION

Patients and families encounter challenges daily as they attempt to deal with and
overcome the changes brought about by neurological conditions. Strategies and
techniques that were successful during their stays in hospitals and rehabilitation or
nursing centers may not adapt well to home situations. To effectively transition patients with neurological conditions to their homes, and ultimately their communi-
ties, home care therapists select appropriate evaluation tools. With these tools, ther-

apists pinpoint problem areas and implement effective treatment strategies. Neurological standards and guidelines further augment therapists' understanding of neurological diagnoses.

Brain Injury Assessments
Brunnstrom Stages

The Brunnstrom Stages describe the course of motor function recovery for patients with brain injuries. It consists of seven stages through which brain-injured individuals progress. Scores range from 1 to 7. Higher scores denote more normal motor function.

Brunnstrom Stages of Recovery after a Cerebrovascular Accident

Stage	Motor function
Stage 1	Immediately after the acute episode, flaccidity of the involved limbs is present, and no movement, on a reflex or a voluntary basis, can be initiated.
Stage 2	As recovery begins, the basic limb synergies or some of their components may appear as associated reactions or minimal voluntary movement responses may be present. Spasticity begins to develop and may be particularly evident in muscle groups that dominate synergy movement (e.g., elbow flexors, knee extensors).
Stage 3	The patient gains voluntary control of the movement synergies, although full range of all synergy components does not necessarily develop. Spasticity, which may become severe in some cases, reaches its peak. This stage in the recovery process may be thought of as semivoluntary in that the patient is able to initiate movement in the involved limbs on a volitional basis but is unable to control the form of the resulting movement, which will be the basic limb synergies.
Stage 4	Some movement combinations that do not follow the paths of the basic limb synergies are mastered, first with difficulty, then with increasing ease. Spasticity begins to decline, but the influence of spasticity on nonsynergistic movements is still readily observable.
Stage 5	If recovery continues, more difficult movement combinations are mastered as the basic limb synergies lose their dominance over motor acts. Spasticity continues to decline.
Stage 6	Individual joint movements become possible, and coordination approaches normalcy. As spasticity disappears, the patient becomes capable of a full spectrum of movement patterns.
Stage 7	Normal motor function is restored.

Modified from Swaner KA, LaVigne JM: *Brunnstrom's movement therapy in hemiplegia,* ed 2, New York, 1992, JB Lippincott.

Disability Rating Scale

The Disability Rating (DR) Scale provides quantitative information on the progress from coma to community of patients with severe brain injuries. It consists of eight items in four categories: (1) arousability, awareness, and responsivity; (2) cognitive ability for self-care activities; (3) dependence on others; and (4) psychosocial adaptability. Each item is scored, and the item scores are summed to achieve a total DR score. The total score ranges from 0 to 30. Higher scores denote increased disability.

Adult Population

Disability Rating Scale Form

Name _____ Date of Injury _____

Date of Birth _____ Age _____

Category	Item	Date of rating				
Arousability, awareness, and responsivity	Eye opening					
	Verbalization					
	Motor response					
Cognitive ability for self-care activities	Feeding					
	Toileting					
	Grooming					
Dependence on others	Level of functioning					
Psychosocial adaptability	Employability					
TOTAL						

Eye Opening

Spontaneous	0
Responsive to speech	1
Responsive to pain	2
None	3

Best Verbal Response

Oriented	0
Confused	1
Inappropriate	2
Incomprehensible	3
None	4

Best Motor Response

Obeying	0
Localizing	1
Withdrawing	2
Flexing	3
Extending	4
None	5

Modified from Rappaport M and others: Disability rating scale for severe head trauma: coma to community, *Arch Phys Med Rehabil* 63:118-123, 1982.

3ox—cont'd

Cognitive Ability for Feeding, Toileting, Grooming

(Does patient know how and when? Ignore motor disability.)

Complete	0
Partial	1
Minimal	2
None	3

Level of Functioning

Completely independent	0
Independent in special environment	1
Mildly dependent (a)	2
Moderately dependent (b)	3
Markedly dependent (c)	4
Totally dependent (d)	5

Level of Functioning—cont'd

(a) needs limited assistance (nonresident helper)
(b) needs moderate assistance (individual in home)
(c) needs assistance with all major activities at all times
(d) needs 24-hour nursing care

Employability

Not restricted	0
Competitive, selected jobs	1
Not competitive, sheltered workshop	2
Not employable	3

Disability Categories

Total disability rating score	Level of disability
0	None
1	Mild disability
2-3	Partial disability
4-6	Moderate disability
7-11	Moderately severe disability
12-16	Severe disability
17-21	Extremely severe disability
22-24	Vegetative state
25-29	Extreme vegetative state
30	Death

Adult Population

Glasgow Coma Scale

The Glasgow Coma Scale (GCS) assesses levels of consciousness in patients who have brain injuries. Three aspects of coma are observed and rated numerically: (1) eye opening, (2) best motor response, and (3) verbal response. The sum of the scores of these three aspects results in an overall coma score ranging from 3 to 15. Higher scores denote increased responsiveness.

GCS Form

Aspect	Score	Aspect	Score
Eye Opening (E)		**Verbal Response (V)**	
Spontaneous	4	Oriented response	5
Responsive to speech	3	Confused conversation	4
Responsive to pain	2	Inappropriate words	3
Nil	1	Incomprehensible sounds	2
		Nil	1
Best Motor Response (M)			
Obeys	6		
Localizes	5		
Withdraws	4		
Has abnormal flexion	3		
Has extensor response	2		
Nil	1		
COMA SCORE (E + M + V)			

Modified from Teasdale G, Jennett B: Assessment of coma and impaired consciousness. A practical scale, *Lancet* 2:81, 1974

Glasgow Outcome Scale

The Glasgow Outcome Scale (GOS) describes the degree of recovery in patient who have brain injuries. It indicates the degree of disability but does not analyze the factors contributing to the handicap. It consists of four categories into which patients are placed after assessment. Higher categories denote decreased disability.

GOS Form

Degree of disability	Degree of recovery
Persistent vegetative state	• Reduced responsiveness associated with wakefulness
	• Possibility of opening eyes, sucking, and yawning
	• Localized motor responses only
Severe disability	• Consciousness
(conscious but disabled)	• 24-hour dependency because of cognitive, behavioral, or physical disabilities
Moderate disability	• Independence in activities of daily living and
(disabled but independent)	in-home and community activities, but with disability
	• Possibility of memory deficits, personality changes, ataxia, cranial nerve deficits, hemiparesis, dysphagia, or acquired epilepsy
Good recovery	• Ability to resume normal life
	• Possibility of minor neurological and psychological deficits

Modified from Jennett B, Bond M: Assessment of outcome after severe brain damage, *Lancet* 3:480-484, 1975.

Rancho Los Amigos Scale of Cognitive Levels and Expected Behaviors*

The Rancho Los Amigos Scale of Cognitive Levels and Expected Behaviors describes cognitive function of patients who have brain injuries. It evaluates eight levels of cognitive functioning, which are grouped into four basic recovery phases with corresponding intervention strategies. Scores range from 1 to 8. Higher scores denote increased cognitive function.

Rancho Los Amigos Scale of Cognitive Levels and Expected Behaviors Form

	Level of cognitive function	Expected behavior	Recovery phase	Treatment approach
I	No response	Is completely unresponsive to any stimuli		
II	Generalized response	Reacts inconsistently and nonpurposefully to stimuli in nonspecific manner	Decreased response	Stimulation
III	Localized response	Reacts specifically but inconsistently to stimuli	Decreased response	Stimulation
IV	Confused-agitated response	Is in heightened state of activity with severely decreased ability to process information	Agitated response	Structure
V	Confused-inappropriate response	Appears alert and is able to respond to simple commands fairly consistently	Confused response	Structure
VI	Confused-appropriate response	Shows goal-directed behavior but depends on external input for direction	Confused response	Structure
VII	Automatic-appropriate response	Appears appropriate and oriented in hospital or home; goes through daily routine automatically, with minimal to absent confusion, and has shallow recall of actions	Automatic response	Community
VIII	Purposeful-appropriate response	Is alert and oriented, is able to recall and integrate past and recent events, and is aware of and responsive to culture	Automatic response	Community

Adult Population

*This section modified from Malkmus D and others: *Rehabilitation of the head-injured adult-comprehensive cognitive management,* Downey, CA, 1980, Professional Staff Association of Rancho Los Amigos Hospital; Phipps WJ and others: *Medical-surgical nursing: concepts and clinical practice,* ed 5, St Louis, 1995, Mosby.

Supervision Rating Scale

The Supervision Rating Scale (SRS) measures levels of assistance required for ADL. Points correspond to degrees of supervision ranked in order of intensity and duration. The total score ranges from 1 to 5. Higher scores denote greater independence with ADL.

SRS Form

Instructions: Circle the rating (numbers 1 through 13) that is closest to the amount of supervision the patient actually receives. *Supervision* means that someone is responsible for being with the patient.

Level 1: Independence
1. The patient lives alone or independently. Other individuals can live with the patient, but they cannot take responsibility for supervision (e.g., a child or older adult).
2. The patient is unsupervised overnight. The patient lives with one or more individuals who can be responsible for supervision (e.g., a spouse or roommate), but they are all sometimes absent overnight.

Level 2: Overnight Supervision
3. The patient is only supervised overnight. One or more supervising individuals are always present overnight, but they are all sometimes absent for the rest of the day.

Level 3: Part-Time Supervision
4. The patient is supervised overnight and part-time during waking hours, but he or she is allowed on independent outings. One or more supervising individuals are always present overnight and also during part of waking hours every day. However, the patient is sometimes allowed to leave the residence without being accompanied by someone who is responsible for supervision.
5. The patient is supervised overnight and part-time during waking hours, but he or she is unsupervised during working hours. Supervising individuals are all sometimes absent for enough time for them to work full-time outside the home.
6. The patient is supervised overnight and during most waking hours. Supervising

Level 3: Part-Time Supervision—cont'd
individuals are all sometimes absent for longer than 1 hour, but less than the time needed to hold a full-time job away from home.
7. The patient is supervised overnight and during almost all waking hours. Supervising individuals are all sometimes absent for shorter than 1 hour.

Level 4: Full-Time Indirect Supervision
8. The patient is under full-time indirect supervision. At least one supervising individual is always present, but he or she does not check on the patient more than once every 30 minutes.
9. This rating is the same as number 8, but it also requires overnight safety precautions (e.g., a deadbolt on outside door).

Level 5: Full-Time Direct Supervision
10. The patient is under full-time direct supervision. At least one supervising individual is always present, and he or she checks on the patient more than once every 30 minutes.
11. The patient lives in a setting in which others physically control the exits.
12. This rating is the same as number 11, but a supervising individual is also designated to provide full-time line-of-sight supervision (e.g., an escape watch or suicide watch).
13. The patient is physically restrained.

Modified from Boake C: Supervision rating scale: a measure of functional outcome from brain injury, *Arch Phys Med Rehabil* 77:765-772, 1996.

Cerebrovascular Accident Assessments
European Stroke Scale

The European Stroke Scale (ESS) evaluates levels of impairment resulting from middle cerebral artery strokes. It consists of 14 items scored on a weighted scale, with more emphasis placed on motor function. The total score ranges from 0 to 100. Higher scores denote fewer impairments.

ESS Form

Level of Consciousness
- Is alert, keenly responsive ☐ 10
- Is drowsy, but can be aroused by minor stimulation to obey, answer, or respond ☐ 8
- Requires repeated stimulation to attend, or is lethargic or obtunded, requiring strong or painful stimulation to make movements ☐ 6
- Cannot be roused by stimulation; does react purposefully to painful stimuli ☐ 4
- Cannot be roused by stimulation; does react with decerebration to painful stimuli ☐ 2
- Cannot be roused by stimulation; does not react to painful stimuli ☐ 0

Comprehension
Verbally give the patient the following commands:
1. Stick out your tongue.
2. Put your finger (of the unaffected side) on your nose.
3. Close your eyes.

Important: Do not demonstrate.

- Patient performs three commands ☐ 8
- Patient performs two or one command(s) ☐ 4
- Patient does not perform any command ☐ 0

Speech
The examiner makes conversation with the patient (how the patient is feeling, whether the patient slept well, amount of time the patient has been in the hospital etc.).

- Normal speech ☐ 8
- Slight word-finding difficulties; conversation possible ☐ 6
- Severe word-finding difficulties; conversation difficult ☐ 4
- Only yes or no answers ☐ 2
- Mute response ☐ 0

Visual Field
The examiner stands at arm's length and compares the patient's field of vision by advancing a moving finger from the periphery inward. The patient must fixate on the examiner's pupil (first with one eye closed and then with the other).

- Normal result ☐ 8
- Deficit ☐ 0

Modified from Hantson L and others: The European Stroke Scale, *Stroke* 25(11):2215-2219, 1994.

Continued

Adult Population

Box—cont'd

Gaze

The examiner steadies the patient's head and asks him or her to follow his finger. The examiner observes the resting eye position and subsequently the full range of movements by moving the index finger from the left to the right and vice versa.

- Normal result ☐ 8
- Median eye position; deviation to one side impossible ☐ 4
- Lateral eye position; return to midline possible ☐ 2
- Lateral eye position; return to midline impossible ☐ 0

Facial Movement

The examiner observes the patient as he or she talks and smiles, noting any asymmetrical elevation of one corner of the mouth or flattening of the nasolabial fold. Only the muscles in the lower half of the face are assessed.

- Normal result ☐ 8
- Paresis ☐ 4
- Paralysis ☐ 0

Arm (Maintaining Outstretched Position)

The examiner asks the patient to close the eyes and actively lifts the patient's arms into position so that they are outstretched at 45 degrees in relation to the horizontal plane, with both hands in mid-position so that the palms face each other. The examiner asks the patient to maintain this position for 5 seconds after the examiner withdraws the arms. Only the affected side is evaluated.

- Arm maintains position for 5 seconds ☐ 4
- Arm maintains position for 5 seconds, but affected hand pronates ☐ 3
- Arm drifts before 5 seconds pass and maintains a lower position ☐ 2
- Arm cannot maintain position but attempts to oppose gravity ☐ 1
- Arm falls ☐ 0

Arm (Raising)

The patient's arm is rested next to the leg with the hand in mid-position. The examiner asks the patient to raise the arm outstretched to 90 degrees.

- Normal result ☐ 4
- Straight arm; movement not full ☐ 3
- Flexed arm ☐ 2
- Trace movements ☐ 1
- No movement ☐ 0

Extension of the Wrist

The examiner tests the patient with the forearm supported and the hand unsupported, relaxed in pronation. The examiner asks the patient to extend the hand.

- Normal result (full isolated movement, no decrease in strength) ☐ 8
- Full isolated movement; reduced strength ☐ 6
- Movement (not isolated and/or full) ☐ 4
- Trace movements ☐ 2
- No movement ☐ 0

Modified from Hantson L and others: The European stroke scale, *Stroke* 25(11):2215-2219, 1994.

Box—cont'd

Fingers

The examiner asks the patient to form with both hands and as strongly as possible a pinch grip with the thumb and forefinger and to try to resist a weak pull. The examiner checks the strength of this grip by pulling the pinch with one finger.

- Equal strength is observed ☐ 8
- Reduced strength is observed on affected side ☐ 4
- Pinch grip is impossible on affected side ☐ 0

Leg (Maintaining Position)

The examiner actively lifts the patient's affected leg into position so that the thigh forms an angle of 90 degrees with the bed, with the shin parallel with the bed. The examiner asks the patient to close the eyes and maintain this position for 5 seconds without support.

- Leg maintains position for 5 seconds ☐ 4
- Leg drifts to intermediate position by the end of 5 seconds ☐ 2
- Leg drifts to bed within 5 seconds, but not immediately ☐ 1
- Leg falls to bed immediately ☐ 0

Leg (Flexing)

The patient is in the supine position with the legs outstretched. The examiner asks the patient to flex the hip and knee.

- Normal result ☐ 4
- Movement against resistance; reduced strength ☐ 3
- Movement against gravity ☐ 2
- Trace movements ☐ 1
- No movement ☐ 0

Dorsiflexion of the Foot

The examiner tests the patient with the leg outstretched. The examiner asks the patient to dorsiflex the foot.

- Normal result (outstretched leg, full movement, no decrease in strength) ☐ 8
- Outstretched leg; full movement; reduced strength ☐ 6
- Outstretched leg; movement not full, knee flexed, or foot in supination ☐ 4
- Trace movements ☐ 2
- No movement ☐ 0

Gait

- Result is normal ☐ 10
- Gait has abnormal aspect and/or distance/speed limited ☐ 8
- Patient can walk with aid ☐ 6
- Patient can walk with the physical assistance of one or more individuals ☐ 4
- Patient cannot walk, but can stand supported ☐ 2
- Patient cannot walk or stand ☐ 0

Fugl-Meyer Assessment

The Fugl-Meyer Assessment quantifies the physical performance of patients who have had cerebral vascular accidents. It measures motor recovery, balance, sensation, and joint range of motion. The total score ranges from 0 to 226. Higher score denote increased physical function.

Fugl-Meyer Assessment Form

Joint Motion and Pain

- Score the best of three trials.
- Do not facilitate movement.
- Test the wrist and hand independently of the arm.

Motion scoring criteria (maximum = 44)

0 = only a few degrees of motion
1 = decreased passive range of motion
2 = normal passive range of motion

Pain scoring criteria (maximum = 44)

0 = marked pain at end of range or pain through range
1 = some pain
2 = no pain

Sensation

Light touch scoring criteria (maximum = 8)

0 = anesthesia
1 = hyperaesthesia or dysaesthesia
2 = normal sensation

Proprioception scoring criteria (maximum = 16)

0 = no sensation
1 = correct answers to ¾ of questions, but considerable difference in sensation compared with unaffected side
2 = correct answers to all questions; little or no difference

Reflexes

Reflex scoring criteria (maximum = 8)

0 = no reflex activity can be elicited
2 = reflex activity can be elicited

Synergy

- For upper-extremity flexor synergy, instruct the patient to bring the forearm to the ear of the affected side with full forearm supination, elbow flexion, and shoulder abduction of at least 90 degrees.
- For upper-extremity extensor synergy, instruct the patient to reach the arm toward the unaffected knee with shoulder abduction and internal rotation.
- For lower-extremity flexor synergy, instruct the patient to fully flex the hip, knee, and ankle.
- For lower-extremity extensor synergy, instruct the patient to extend and abduct the leg against resistance.

Synergy scoring criteria

0 = detail not performed
1 = detail partly performed
2 = detail completely performed

Normal reflex scoring criteria

0 = at least two of the three phasic reflexes markedly hyperactive
1 = one reflex markedly hyperactive, or at least two reflexes lively
2 = no more than one reflex lively and no reflexes markedly hyperactive

Wrist scoring criteria (stability and flexion-extension)

0 = no dorsiflexion
1 = no dorsiflexion against resistance
2 = dorsiflexion against resistance

Wrist scoring criteria (circumduction)

0 = no circumduction
1 = jerky or incomplete circumduction
2 = complete circumduction

Modified from Fugl-Meyer AR and others: The post-stroke hemiplegic patient, *Scand J Rehab Med* 7:13-31, 1975.

3ox—cont'd

Hand

- For grasp A, instruct the patient to extend the metacarpophalangeal joints of the fingers and flex the proximal and distal interphalangeal joints.
- For grasp B, instruct the patient to perform pure thumb adduction with the first carpometacarpophalangeal and interphalangeal joints in neutral. Interpose a scrap of paper.
- For grasp C, instruct the patient to oppose the thumb against the second finger. Interpose a pencil.
- For grasp D, instruct the patient to grasp a cylindrical object (e.g., small can) with the volar surfaces of the first and second fingers against each other.
- For grasp E, instruct the patient to grasp a tennis ball.

Hand scoring criteria (mass flexion and extension)
0 = none
1 = some, but not full
2 = full
Hand scoring criteria (grasp A)
0 = cannot perform
1 = has weak grasp
2 = holds grasp against resistance
Hand scoring criteria (grasps B, C, D, and E)
0 = cannot perform
1 = holds object, but not against a tug
2 = holds object well against a tug

Coordination and Speed

- For the upper extremity, instruct the blindfolded patient to put the tip of the index finger to the nose five times as quickly as possible.
- For the lower extremity, instruct the patient in the supine position to bring the heel to the knee cap of the opposite leg five times as quickly as possible.

Tremor and dysmetria scoring criteria
0 = marked
1 = slight
2 = none
Speed scoring criteria
0 = at least 6 seconds slower than on the unaffected side
1 = 2-5 seconds slower than on the unaffected side
2 = less than 2 seconds different than the unaffected side

Balance

Sitting without support scoring criteria
0 = cannot maintain position without support
1 = maintains position for short time
2 = maintains position for 5 minutes
Parachute Reaction Scoring Criteria
0 = does not abduct shoulder or extend elbow to avoid falling
1 = has impaired reaction
2 = has normal reaction
Standing with support scoring criteria
0 = cannot stand
1 = stands with massive support
2 = stands at least 1 minute with slight support
Standing without support scoring criteria
0 = cannot stand without support
1 = stands for less than 1 minute or stands for longer time but sways
2 = has good standing balance for more than 1 minute
Standing on one leg scoring criteria
0 = cannot maintain position for more than a few seconds
1 = maintains position for 4-9 seconds
2 = maintains position for more than 10 seconds

Continued

Area and movement	Motion score	Pain score
Joint Motion and Pain		
Shoulder		
Flexion		
Abduction to 90 degrees		
External rotation		
Internal rotation		
Elbow		
Flexion		
Extension		
Forearm		
Pronation		
Supination		
Wrist		
Flexion		
Extension		
Fingers		
Flexion		
Extension		
Hip		
Flexion		
Abduction		
External rotation		
Internal rotation		
Knee		
Flexion		
Extension		
Ankle		
Dorsiflexion		
Plantar Flexion		
Foot		
Pronation		
Supination		
TOTAL JOINT MOTION AND PAIN SCORE (MAX = 88)		

Modified from Fugl-Meyer AR and others: The post-stroke hemiplegic patient, *Scand J Rehab Med* 7:13-31, 1975.

Area and movement	Score
Sensation	
Light touch	
Upper arm	
Palm of hand	
Thigh	
Sole of foot	
Proprioception	
Shoulder	
Elbow	
Wrist	
Thumb	
Hip	
Knee	
Ankle	
Toe	
TOTAL SENSATION SCORE (max = 24)	
Reflexes	
Triceps	
Biceps	
Patella	
Achilles	
TOTAL REFLEX SCORE (max = 8)	
Synergies	
Upper-extremity flexor	
Shoulder elevation	
Shoulder retraction	
Shoulder abduction at least 90 degrees	
Shoulder external rotation	
Elbow flexion	
Forearm pronation	
Upper-extremity extensor	
Shoulder adduction and internal rotation	
Elbow extension	
Forearm	
Lower-extremity flexor	
Hip flexion	
Knee flexion	
Ankle dorsiflexion	

Adult Population

Continued

Box—cont'd

Area and movement	Score
Synergies—cont'd	
Lower-extremity extensor	
Hip extension	
Hip adduction	
Knee extension	
Ankle plantarflexion	
TOTAL SYNERGY SCORE (max = 32)	
Mixing Synergies	
Upper extremity	
Hand to lumbar spine	
Shoulder flexion to 90 degrees with elbow extended	
Forearm pronation and supination with elbow flexed	
Lower extremity	
Knee flexion in sitting position	
Ankle dorsiflexion in sitting position	
TOTAL MIXING SYNERGIES SCORE (max = 10)	
Movement out of Synergy	
Upper extremity	
Shoulder abduction	
Shoulder flexion	
Forearm pronation and supination	
Lower extremity	
Knee flexion	
Ankle dorsiflexion	
TOTAL MOVEMENT OUT OF SYNERGYSCORE (max = 10)	
Normal Reflex	
Biceps	
Triceps	
Finger flexors	
Patella	
Knee flexor	
Achilles	
TOTAL NORMAL REFLEX SCORE (max = 4)	
Wrist	
Stability with elbow at 90 degrees	
Flexion and extension with elbow at 90 degrees	
Stability with elbow at 0 degrees	

Modified from Fugl-Meyer AR and others: The post-stroke hemiplegic patient, *Scand J Rehab Med* 7:13-31, 1975.

Box—cont'd

Area and movement	Score
Wrist—cont'd	
Flexion and extension with elbow at 0 degrees	
Circumduction	
TOTAL WRIST SCORE (max = 10)	
Hand	
Mass flexion	
Mass extension	
Grasp A	
Grasp B	
Grasp C	
Grasp D	
Grasp E	
TOTAL HAND SCORE (max = 14)	
Coordination and Speed	
Upper extremity	
Tremor	
Dysmetria	
Speed	
Lower extremity	
Tremor	
Dysmetria	
Speed	
TOTAL COORDINATION AND SPEED SCORE (max = 12)	
Balance	
Sitting position without support	
Parachute reaction, nonaffected side	
Parachute reaction, affected side	
Standing position with support	
Standing position without support	
Standing position on nonaffected leg	
Standing position on affected leg	
TOTAL BALANCE SCORE (max = 14)	
TOTAL FUGL-MEYER SCORE	

The National Institutes of Health Stroke Scale

The National Institutes of Health Stroke Scale (NIHSS) assesses acute cerebral infarcts. It consists of 13 items, including level of consciousness, motor response, and language. The total score ranges from 0 to 36. Higher scores denote poorer neurological function.

NIHSS Form

The NIDS t-PA Stroke Trial No. __ __ - __ __ __ - __ __ __

Patient's Date of Birth __ __ / __ __ / __ __

Hospital _____ (__ __ - __ __)

Date of Examination __ __ / __ __ / __ __

Interval: 1[ ] Baseline   2[ ] 12 hours post treatment   3[ ] 24-hours post onset of symptoms
± 20 minutes   4[ ] 7-10 days   5[ ] 3 months   6[ ] Other _____ (_____)

Time: __ __ : __ __ 1[ ] AM   2[ ] PM

Administer stroke scale items in the order listed. Record the performance in each category after each subscale examination. Do not go back and change scores. Follow the directions provided for each examination technique. Scores should reflect what the patient does, not what the clinician thinks the patient can do. The clinician should record answers while administering the examination and work quickly. Except where indicated, the patient should not be coached (i.e., repeated requests to patient to make a special effort).

If any item is left untested, a detailed explanation must be clearly written on the form. All untested items will be reviewed by the medical monitor and discussed with the examiner by telephone.

Instruction	Scale definition	Score
1a. LOC: The investigator must choose a response, even if a full evaluation is prevented by such obstacles as an endotracheal tube, language barrier, orotracheal trauma or bandages. A 3 is scored only if the patient makes no movement (other than reflexive posturing) in response to noxious stimulation.	0 = Is alert; keenly responsive 1 = Is not alert, but is arousable by minor stimulation to obey, answer, or respond 2 = Is not alert; requires repeated stimulation to attend, or is obtunded and requires strong or painful stimulation to make movements (not stereotyped) 3 = Responds only with reflex motor or autonomic effects, or is totally unresponsive, flaccid, and are flexic	_____
1b. LOC questions: The examiner asks the patient the month and his or her age. The answer must be correct; there is no partial credit for being close. Aphasic and stuporous patients who do not comprehend the questions score a 2. Patients unable to speak because of endotracheal intubation, orotracheal trauma, severe dysarthria from any cause, language barrier, or any other problem not secondary to aphasia are given a 1. Only the initial answer must be graded, and the examiner must not "help" the patient with verbal or nonverbal cues.	0 = Answers both questions correctly 1 = Answers one question correctly 2 = Answers neither question correctly	_____

Modified from Brott T and others: Measurement of acute cerebral infarction: a clinical examination scale, *Stroke* 20(7): 864-870, 1989.
LOC, Level of consciousness; CN, cranial nerve.

Form 5   The NIDS t-PA Stroke Trial No. __ __ - __ __ __ - __ __ __

Interval: 1[ ] Baseline   2[ ] hours post treatment   3[ ] 24-hours post onset of symptoms
           ± 20 minutes   4[ ] 7-10 days   5[ ] 3 months   6[ ] Other _____ (_____)

Instruction	Scale definition	Score
1c. LOC commands: The examiner asks the patient to open and close the eyes and then to grip and release the nonparetic hand. Another one-step command should be substituted if the hands cannot be used. Credit is given if an unequivocal attempt is made but not completed due to weakness. If the patient does not respond to the command, the examiner should demonstrate the task to the patient (pantomime) and score the result (i.e., follows none, one, or two commands). Patients with trauma, amputation, or other physical impediments should be given suitable one-step commands. Only the first attempt is scored.	0 = Performs both tasks correctly 1 = Performs one task correctly 2 = Performs neither task correctly	_____
2. Best gaze: Only horizontal eye movements are tested. Voluntary or reflexive (oculocephalic) eye movements are scored, but caloric testing is not done. If the patient has a conjugate deviation of the eyes that can be overcome by voluntary or reflexive activity, the score is 1. If a patient has an isolated peripheral nerve paresis (CN IIL, IV, or VI), the score is 1. Gaze is testable in all aphasic patients. Patients with ocular trauma, bandages, preexisting blindness, or other disorders of visual acuity or fields should be tested with reflexive movements and a choice made by the investigator. Establishing eye contact and then moving about the patient from side to side occasionally clarifies the presence of a partial gaze palsy.	0 = Normal result 1 = Partial gaze palsy; this score given when gaze is abnormal in one or both eyes, but where forced deviation or total gaze paresis are not present 2 = Forced deviation, or total gaze paresis not overcome by the oculocephalic maneuver	_____

Adult Population

Continued

Box—cont'd

Form 5   The NIDS t-PA Stroke Trial No. __ __ - __ __ __ __ - __ __ __

3 of 7

Interval: 1[ ] Baseline   2[ ] hours post treatment   3[ ] 24-hours post onset of symptoms
            ± 20 minutes   4[ ] 7-10 days   5[ ] 3 months   6[ ] Other _____ (_____)

Instruction	Scale definition	Score
3. Visual Fields: Visual Fields (upper and lower quadrants) are tested by confrontation, using finger counting or visual threat as appropriate. Patients must be encouraged, but if they look at the side of the moving fingers appropriately, this can be scored as normal. If there is unilateral blindness or enucleation, visual fields in the remaining eye are scored. A 1 should be scored only if a clear asymmetry, including quadrantanopia, is found. If the patient is blind from any cause, a 3 should be scored. Double simultaneous stimulation is performed at this point. If there is extinction, the patient receives a 1 and the results are used to answer question 11.	0 = No visual loss 1 = Partial hemianopia 2 = Complete hemianopia 3 = Bilateral hemianopia (blind, including cortical blindness)	_____
4. Facial palsy: The examiner should ask or use pantomime to encourage the patient to show teeth, raise eyebrows, or close eyes. Symmetry of grimace should be scored in response to noxious stimuli in the poorly responsive or noncomprehending patient. If facial trauma or bandages, or tracheal tube, tape, or other physical barriers obscure the face, these should be removed to the extent possible.	0 = Normal symmetrical movement 1 = Minor paralysis (flattened nasolabial fold, asymmetry on smiling) 2 = Partial paralysis (total or near total paralysis of lower face) 3 = Complete paralysis of one or both sides (absence of facial movement in the upper and lower face)	_____

Modified from Brott T and others: Measurement of acute cerebral infarction: a clinical examination scale, *Stroke* 20(7): 864-870, 1989.

Box—cont'd

Form 5   The NIDS t-PA Stroke Trial No. __ __ - __ __ __ - __ __ __

4 of 7

Interval: 1[ ] Baseline   2[ ] hours post treatment   3[ ] 24-hours post onset of symptoms
            ± 20 minutes   4[ ] 7-10 days   5[ ] 3 months   6[ ] Other _____ (_____)

Instruction	Scale definition	Score
5 & 6. Motor arm and leg: The limb is placed in the appropriate position: the arms should be extended (palms down) 90 degrees (if sitting) or 45 degrees (if supine) and the leg 30 degrees (always tested supine). Drift is scored if the arm falls before 10 seconds or the leg before 5 seconds. The aphasic patient is encouraged using urgency in the voice and pantomime, but not noxious stimulation. Each limb is tested in turn, beginning with the nonparetic arm. Only in the case of amputation or joint fusion at the shoulder or hip may the score be 9, and the examiner must clearly write the explanation for scoring as a 9.	0 = No drift; limb holds 90 (or 45) degrees for full 10 seconds 1 = Drift; limb holds 90 (or 45) degrees, but drifts down before full 10 seconds; does not hit bed or other support 2 = Some effort against gravity; limb cannot get to or maintain (if cued) 90 (or 45) degrees; drifts down to bed, but has some effort against gravity 3 = No effort against gravity; limb falls 4 = No movement 9 = Amputation, joint fusion; explain: _____	
	5a. Left arm	_____
	5b. Right arm	_____
	0 = No drift; leg holds 30-degrees position for full 5 seconds 1 = Drift; leg falls by the end of the 5-second period but does not hit bed 2 = Some effort against gravity; leg falls to bed by 5 seconds, but has some effort against gravity 3 = No effort against gravity; leg falls to bed immediately 4 = No movement 9 = Amputation, joint fusion; explain: _____	
	6a. Left leg	_____
	6b. Right leg	_____

Continued

Adult Population

Box—cont'd

Form 5   The NIDS t-PA Stroke Trial No. __ __ - __ __ __ __ - __ __ __

Interval: 1[ ] Baseline   2[ ] hours post treatment   3[ ] 24-hours post onset of symptoms
           ± 20 minutes   4[ ] 7-10 days   5[ ] 3 months   6[ ] Other _____ (_____)

Instruction	Scale definition	Score

7. Limb ataxia: This item is aimed at finding evidence of a unilateral cerebellar lesion. The examiner should test the patient with the eyes open. In case of visual defect, the examiner should ensure testing is done in the intact visual field. The finger-nose-finger and heel-shin tests are performed on both sides, and ataxia is scored only if present out of proportion to weakness. Ataxia is absent in the patient who cannot understand or is paralyzed. Only in the ease of amputation or joint fusion may the item be scored 9, and the examiner must clearly write the explanation for not scoring. In case of blindness, the patient should be tested by touching the nose from an extended arm position.	0 = Absent
	1 = Present in one limb
	2 = Present in two limbs
	
	If present; is ataxia in:
	  Right arm 1 = Yes 2 = No
	    9 = amputation or joint fusion;
	      explain: _____
	  Left arm 1 = Yes 2 = No
	    9 = amputation or joint fusion;
	      explain: _____
	  Right leg 1 = Yes 2 = No
	    9 = amputation or joint fusion;
	      explain: _____
	  Left leg 1 = Yes 2 = No
	    9 = amputation or joint fusion;
	      explain: _____
		_____
		
		_____
		
		_____
		
		_____
		
		_____

8. Sensation: Sensation or grimace to pin prick or withdrawal from noxious stimulus in the obtunded or aphasic patient is tested. Only sensory loss attributed to stroke is scored as abnormal, and the examiner should test as many body areas [arms (not hands), legs, trunk, and face] as needed to accurately check for hemisensory loss. A score of 2, "severe or total," should be given only when a severe or total loss of sensation can be clearly demonstrated. Stuporous and aphasic patients therefore probably score 1 or 0. The patient with brain-stem stroke who has bilateral loss of sensation is scored 2. If the patient does not respond and is quadriplegic, a 2 is scored. Patients in coma (item 1a = 3) are arbitrarily given a 2 on this item.	0 = Normal; no sensory loss 1 = Mild to moderate sensory loss; patient feels pin prick is less sharp or is dull on the affected side, or there is a loss of superficial pain with pin prick but patient is aware he or she is being touched 2 = Severe to total sensory loss; patient not aware of being touched in the face, arm, and leg	 _____

Modified from Brott T and others: Measurement of acute cerebral infarction: a clinical examination scale, *Stroke* 20(7): 864-870, 1989.

Form 5   The NIDS t-PA Stroke Trial No. __ __ - __ __ __ __ - __ __ __ __

Interval: 1[   ] Baseline   2[   ] hours post treatment   3[   ] 24-hours post onset of symptoms
            ± 20 minutes   4[   ] 7-10 days   5[   ] 3 months   6[   ] Other _____ (_____)

Instruction	Scale definition	Score
9. Best language: A great deal of information about comprehension is obtained during the preceding sections of the examination. The patient is asked to describe what is happening in the attached picture (Figure 3-38), to name the items on the attached naming sheet (Figure 3-39), and to read from the attached list of sentences (Figure 3-40). Comprehension is judged from responses here, as well as to all of the commands in the preceding general neurological examination. If visual loss interferes with the tests, the examiner should ask the patient to identify objects placed in the hand, repeat, and produce speech. The patient receiving intubation should be asked to write. The patient in a coma (question 1a = 3) arbitrarily scores 3 on this item. The examiner must choose a score for the patient with stupor or limited cooperation, but a score of 3 should be used only if the patient is mute and follows no one-step commands.	0 = No aphasia; normal 1 = Mild to moderate aphasia; some obvious loss of fluency or facility of comprehension, without significant limitation on ideas expressed or form of expression; reduction of speech and/or comprehension; however, makes conversation about provided material difficult or impossible (e.g., in conversation about provided materials, examiner can identify picture or naming card from patient's response) 2 = Severe aphasia; all communication through fragmentary expression; great need for inference, questioning, and guessing by the listener; range of information that can be exchanged limited; listener carries burden of communication; examiner unable to identify materials provided from patient response 3 = Mute, global aphasia; no useable speech or auditory comprehension	_____

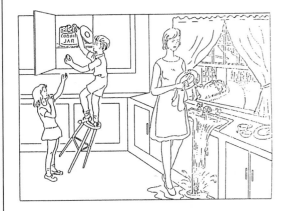

FIGURE 3-38 Best language appendix 1.

Continued

Box—cont'd

Form 5   The NIDS t-PA Stroke Trial No. __ __ - __ __ __ - __ __ __

Interval: 1[   ] Baseline   2[   ] hours post treatment   3[   ] 24-hours post onset of symptoms
            ± 20 minutes   4[   ] 7-10 days   5[   ] 3 months   6[   ] Other _____ (_____)

Instruction	Scale definition	Score
10. Dysarthria: If the patient is thought to be normal, an adequate sample of speech must be obtained by asking the patient to read or repeat words from the attached list (Figure 3-41). If the patient has severe aphasia, the clarity of articulation of spontaneous speech can be rated. Only if the patient is intubated or has other physical barriers to producing speech, may the item be scored 9. In addition, the examiner must clearly write an explanation for not scoring. The patient must not be told the reason he or she is being tested.	0 = Normal 1 = Mild to moderate; patient slurs at least some words and, at worst, can be understood with some difficulty 2 = Severe; patient's speech so slurred as to be unintelligible in the absence of or out of proportion to any dysphasia, or is mute/anarthric 9 = Intubation or other physical barrier; explain: _____	_____

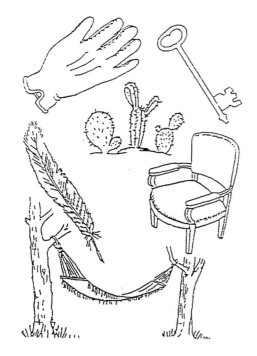

FIGURE 3-39 Best language appendix 2.

> You know how.
>
> Down to earth.
>
> I got home from work.
>
> Near the table in the dining room.
>
> They heard him speak on the radio last night.

FIGURE 3-40 Best language appendix 3.

Modified from Brott T and others: Measurement of acute cerebral infarction: a clinical examination scale, *Stroke* 20(7): 864-870, 1989.

Box—cont'd

Form 5   The NIDS t-PA Stroke Trial No. __ __ - __ __ __ - __ __ __

Interval: 1[   ] Baseline   2[   ] hours post treatment   3[   ] 24-hours post onset of symptoms
            ± 20 minutes   4[   ] 7-10 days   5[   ] 3 months   6[   ] Other _____ (_____)

Instruction	Scale definition	Score
11. Extinction and inattention (formerly neglect): Sufficient information to identify neglect may be obtained during the prior testing. If the patient has a severe visual loss preventing visual double simultaneous stimulation, and the cutaneous stimuli are normal, the score is normal. If the patient has aphasia but does appear to attend to both sides, the score is normal. The presence of visual spatial neglect or anosagnosia may also be taken as evidence of abnormality. Because the abnormality is scored only if present, the item is never untested.	0 = No abnormality 1 = Visual, tactile, auditory, spatial, or personal inattention or extinction to bilateral simultaneous stimulation in one of the sensory modalities 2 = Profound hemi-inattention or hemi-inattention to more than one modality; does not recognize own hand or orients to only one side of space	_____

FIGURE 3-41 Best language appendix 4.

MAMA

TIP-TOP

FIFTY-FIVE

THANKS

HUCKLEBERRY

BASEBALL PLAYER

Continued

Adult Population

Box—cont'd

Form 5	The NIDS t-PA Stroke Trial No. __ __ - __ __ __ - __ __ __

Interval: 1[ ] Baseline 2[ ] hours post treatment 3[ ] 24-hours post onset of symptoms
± 20 minutes 4[ ] 7-10 days 5[ ] 3 months 6[ ] Other _____ (_____)

Instruction	Scale definition	Score
Additional Item (Not Part of the NIH Stroke Scale Score)		
A. Distal motor function: The examiner holds the patient's hand up at the forearm and asks the patient to extend his or her fingers as much as possible. If the patient cannot or does not extend the fingers, the examiner places the fingers in full extension and observes for any flexion movement for 5 seconds. Only the patient's first attempts are graded. Repetition of the instructions or of the testing is prohibited.	0 = Normal (no flexion after 5 seconds) 1 = At least some extension after 5 seconds, but not full extension; any movement of the fingers that is not commanded not scored 2 = No voluntary extension after 5 seconds; movements of the fingers at another time not scored a. Left arm b. Right arm	_____ _____
12. _____ Individual Administering Scale	(__ __ __) Code	

Modified from Brott T and others: Measurement of acute cerebral infarction: a clinical examination scale, *Stroke* 20(7): 864-870, 1989.

Wisconsin Gait Scale

The Wisconsin Gait Scale (WGS) quantifies hemiplegic gait quality. In the WGS, 14 observable variables measure clinically relevant gait components. The total score ranges from 14 to 45. Higher scores denote poorer gait quality.

WGS Form

Observe the patient walking toward and away from the observer, and from the side.

Stance Phase Affected Leg

1. Use of a hand-held gait aid*
   1 = No gait aid
   2 = Minimal gait aid use   A gait aid is used optionally with minimal weight transferred on to it. There is a narrow base of support.
   3 = Minimal gait aid, wide base   A gait aid is used minimally. The legs of a quad cane may be rocked as weight is transferred forward. The distance between the unaffected foot to the cane is greater than the distance between the affected and unaffected foot (wide support base).
   4 = Marked use   Weight is transferred through the aid. There is a narrow base of support.
   5 = Marked use, wide base   Weight is transferred through the aid. There is a wide support base.

2. Stance time on impaired side
   1 = Equal   An equal amount of time is spent on the affected leg compared with the unaffected leg during single leg stance.
   2 = Unequal   The patient remains on the affected leg for a shorter time compared with the unaffected leg during single leg stance.
   3 = Extremely brief   The patient spends the least amount of time on the affected leg necessary to accomplish advancing the unaffected leg.

3. Step length of unaffected side
   1 = Steps through   The heel of the unaffected foot clearly advances beyond the toe of the affected foot.
   2 = Foot does not clear   The heel of the unaffected foot does not advance beyond the toe of the affected foot.
   3 = Steps to   The unaffected foot is placed behind or up to, but not beyond, the affected foot.

4. Weight shift to the affected side, with or without a gait aid*
   1 = Full shift   The patient's head and trunk shift laterally over the affected foot during single stance.
   2 = Decreased shift   The patient's head and trunk cross midline, but not over the affected foot.
   3 = Extremely limited shift   The patient's head and trunk do not cross midline. There is a minimal weight shift in the direction of the affected side.

5. Stance width (measure distance between feet prior to toe off of affected foot)
   1 = Normal   There is up to one shoe width between the feet.
   2 = Moderate   There is up to two shoe widths between the feet.
   3 = Wide   There are greater than two shoe widths between the feet.

Adult Population

Modified from Rodriquez AA and others: Gait training efficacy using a home-based practice model in chronic hemiplegia, *Arch Phys Med Rehabil* 77:801-805, 1996.

*Items 1 and 4 are weighted by ⅔ and ¾, respectively, before adding individual items for a total score.

Continued

Box—cont'd

Toe Off Affected Leg

6. Guardedness (pause prior to advancing affected leg)
   1 = No hesitation   There is good forward momentum with no hesitancy noted.
   2 = Slight hesitation   There is slight pause prior to toe off.
   3 = Marked hesitation   The patient pauses prior to toe off.
7. Hip extension of affected side (observe gluteal crease from behind patient)
   1 = Equal extension   The hips equally extend during push-off. The patient maintains erect posture during toe off.
   2 = Slight flexion   The hip extends at least to neutral, but less than the unaffected side.
   3 = Marked flexion   There is forward trunk and hip flexion at toe off.

Swing Phase Affected Leg

8. External rotation during initial swing
   1 = Same as unimpaired leg
   2 = Increased rotation   The patient externally rotates the leg <45 degrees, but more than the uninvolved side.
   3 = Marked rotation   The patient externally rotates the leg >45 degrees.
9. Circumduction at mid-swing (observe path of affected heel)
   1 = None   The affected foot adducts no more than the unaffected foot during swing.
   2 = Moderate   The affected foot adducts up to one shoe width during swing.
   3 = Marked   The affected foot circumducts more than one shoe width during swing.
10. Hip hiking at mid-swing
    1 = None   The pelvis slightly dips during the swing phase.
    2 = Elevation   The pelvis is elevated during the swing phase.
    3 = Vaulting   There is little true hip flexion. The patient contracts the lateral trunk muscles and elevates the hip during the swing phase.
11. Knee flexion from toe off to mid-swing
    1 = Normal   The affected knee flexes equally to the unaffected side.
    2 = Some   The affected knee flexes, but less than the unaffected knee.
    3 = Minimal   The minimal flexion is noted in the affected knee (flexion barely seen).
    4 = None   The knee remains in extension throughout the swing phase.
12. Toe clearance
    1 = Normal clearance   The toe clears the floor throughout the swing phase.
    2 = Slight drag   The toe drags slightly at the beginning of the swing phase.
    3 = Marked drag   The toe drags during the majority of the swing phase.
13. Pelvic rotation at terminal swing
    1 = Forward   The pelvis is rotated forward to prepare for the heel strike.
    2 = Neutral   The posture is erect with the pelvis in neutral rotation.
    3 = Retracted   The pelvis has marked lag behind the unaffected pelvis.

Heel Strike Affected Leg

14. Initial foot contact
    1 = Heel strike   The heel makes initial contact with the floor.
    2 = Flat foot   The foot lands with weight distributed over the entire foot.
    3 = No contact of heel   The foot lands on the lateral border of the foot or toes.

Modified from Rodriquez AA and others: Gait training efficacy using a home-based practice model in chronic hemiplegia, *Arch Phys Med Rehabil* 77:801-805, 1996.

Multiple Sclerosis Assessments
Ambulation Index

The Ambulation Index quantifies changes in the gait of patients who have multiple sclerosis. It assesses dependence, endurance, and speed of ambulation. The total score ranges from 0 to 9. Higher scores denote decreased ambulation skills.

Ambulation Index Form

Score	Changes in gait
0	• Is asymptomatic • Is fully active
1	• Walks normally but reports fatigue that interferes with athletic or other demanding activities
2	• Has abnormal gait or episodic imbalance • Has a gait disorder noticed by family and friends • Is able to walk 25 feet (8 meters) in 10 seconds or less
3	• Walks independently • Is able to walk 25 feet in 20 seconds or less
4	• Requires unilateral support (cane or single crutch) to walk • Walks 25 feet in 20 seconds or less
5	• Requires bilateral support (e.g., canes, crutches, or walker) • Walks 25 feet in 20 seconds or less OR • Requires unilateral support but needs more than 20 seconds to walk 25 feet
6	• Requires bilateral support and more than 20 seconds to walk 25 feet • May use wheelchair* on occasion
7	• Is limited to several steps walking with bilateral support • Is unable to walk 25 feet • May use wheelchair* for most activities
8	• Is restricted to wheelchair • Is able to transfer self independently
9	• Is restricted to wheelchair • Is unable to transfer self independently

Modified from British and Dutch Multiple Sclerosis Azathioprine Trial Group: Double-masked trial of azathioprine in multiple sclerosis, *Lancet* 2:179-183, 1988.

*The use of a wheelchair may be determined by lifestyle and motivation. It is expected that patients in Grade 7 will use a wheelchair more frequently than those in Grades 5 or 6. However, assignment of a grade in the range of 5 to 7 is determined by the patient's ability to walk a given distance, and not by the extent to which the patient uses a wheelchair.

Environmental Status Scale

The Environmental Status Scale (ESS) assesses social handicaps resulting from multiple sclerosis. It consists of seven items, including working ability and potential for rehabilitation. The total score ranges from 0 to 30. Higher scores denote increased social handicap.

ESS Form

Name: _____ Address: _____ Zip Code: _____

Date of birth: _____ Occupation: _____ Gender: _____

1. *Marital status:* ☐
    1. Married
    2. Single
    3. Divorced
    4. Widowed
    5. Separated

Preschool children: ☐
Children under education: ☐

Occupation of spouse:
Full time: ☐
Part time: ☐

2. *Residence:* ☐
    1. Owns residence
    2. Rents residence
    3. Lives in housing for handicapped
    4. Lives in nursing home
    5. Lives with patients or family

0 No need
1 Need covered
☐ 2. Need *not* covered
9 Unknown

Multilevel house: ☐
    0. Lives entirely on street level
    1. Lives on street level but with some steps
    2. Lives on higher level with elevator
    3. Lives on higher level without elevator

0 No need
1 Need covered
☐ 2 Need *not* covered
9 Unknown

3. *Working ability:* ☐
    0. Normal ability
    1. Nearly, but restricted functions (e.g., transferred to less demanding position)
    2. Reduced capacity (e.g., half time or greater)
    3. Reduced capacity (e.g., less than half time)
    4. Sheltered work
    5. No working capacity

Because of the following:
Dismissal: ☐
Resignation of the job: ☐
Physical handicap: ☐   0 No
Fatigue: ☐   1 Yes
    9 Unknown

4. *Potential for rehabilitation:* ☐
    0 No   Age: ☐   0 No
    1 Yes   Mentation: ☐   1 Yes
    9 Unknown   Motivation: ☐   9 Unknown
    Physical handicap: ☐

☐
    1. Unskilled worker
    2. Employee
    3. Skilled worker
    4. Professional and academic individual
    5. Self-employed individual
    9. Unknown

Modified from Mellerup E and others: The socio-economic scale, *Acta Neurol Scand* 64(Suppl 87):130-138, 1981.

5. *Economic support on account of impaired ability to work:* ☐

   0. There are no MS-related pension or financial problems.

   1. There are some economic disadvantages resultant from MS, but the patient is able to absorb them without any financial assistance.

   2. The patient has a moderately modified lifestyle because of *reduced income* resultant from MS and may receive some financial support or potential pension.

   3. The patient has a lifestyle moderately modified by financial status and depends on financial aid to cover some but not all costs or partial pension and supplementary support.

   4. There is major alteration of lifestyle that consistently requires additional financial assistance to cover subsistence and medical costs. The patient receives a full pension and supplementary support.

   5. The family has a continuing deficit budget causing frequent applications for additional financial assistance or a full pension plus supplementary support.

   0 No need
   1 Need covered ———
   2 Need *not* covered   ☐
   9 Unknown

   Lives free with the following:
   Relatives: ☐   0 No
   Public support: ☐   1 Yes
   Own resources: ☐   9 Unknown

6. *Transportation:* ☐

   0. The patient is able to use all public and private transportation without adaptation.

   1. In general the patient is independent for mobility, not requiring the help of another individual, but may have limited access to some public transportation or require minor adaptation to private transportation.

   2. Independent mobility is severely registered, but independent transportation is possible and/or some public transportation only with the help of another individual.

   3. The patient cannot manage public transportation, but requires independent transportation only with major adaptation or the help from another individual.

   4. The patient has no independent mobility and requires special transportation, but not an ambulance (e.g., transportation, in or with a wheelchair).

   5. The patient requires ambulance transportation.

   0 No need
   ☐   1 Need covered
   2 Need *not* covered ———
   9 Unknown

   0 No
   1 Yes
   9 Unknown

   Insufficiency of social laws: ☐
   Physician's inertness: ☐
   Unawareness of family: ☐
   Denial by the social service: ☐

Adult Population

MS, Multiple sclerosis.

Continued

Box—cont'd

7. *Activity of daily living:*

   Aid of individuals: ☐
   0. None
   1. Minor help; relatives involved but personal independence
   2. Major help; relatives involved but some personal independence ☐
   3. Outside help at least once a week (homeaid, nurse, etc.)
   4. Outside help almost daily (homeaid, nurse, etc.)
   5. Daycenter, special housing; total assistance

   0 No need
   1 Need covered
   2 Need *not* covered
   9 Unknown

   Modification of the home: ☐
   0. No change in facilities necessary
   1. Minor modification (maximum $500)
   2. Moderate modification (maximum costs $2,000) ☐
   3. Major modification (maximum costs $10,000)
   4. Additional rebuilding (>$10,000)
   5. Unsuitable home; alternative needed

   0 No need
   1 Need covered
   2 Need *not* covered
   9 Unknown

   Mechanical aids:

	Indoor	Outdoor	
Common manual wheelchair:	☐	☐	0 No need
Electrical wheelchair:	☐	☐	☐ 1 Need covered
Other electrical transportation:	☐	☐	2 Need *not* covered
			9 Unknown

   Other mechanical aids:

			Own payment	Public payment
Bed-lift:	☐	0 No need	☐	☐
Alarm systems:	☐	1 Need covered	☐	☐
Aids for impaired vision:	☐	2 Need *not* covered	☐	☐
Hospital bed:	☐	9 Unknown	☐	☐
Telephone:	☐		☐	☐
Staircase elevator:	☐		☐	☐

   Other aids:
   Large amount:
   Small amount:

8. *Ability of leisure activity:* ☐

   Use of leisure time:
   0 Fully able
   1 Moderately able
   2 Practically unable ──────────┐
            Lack of financial
              resources: ☐ 0 No
            Physical handicap: ☐ 1 Yes
            Fatigue: ☐ 9 Unknown

Modified from Mellerup E and others: The socio-economic scale, *Acta Neurol Scand* 64(Suppl 87):130-138, 1981.

3ox—cont'd

9. *Maintenance of physical therapy:*

☐ 0 Annual appraisal; no treatment   0 No need
     1 Semiannual appraisal; minimal   ☐   1 Need covered
       treatment   2 Need *not* covered
     2 Quarterly appraisal
     3 Monthly appraisal
     4 Weekly appraisal   1 Periodic
     5 Daily appraisal   ☐   2 Permanent
            9 Unknown

Established: At home: ☐   0 No
          In clinics: ☐   1 Yes

10. *Hospitalization:* ☐   0 Never   *Medical care:* ☐   0 Never
            1 Seldom   1 Seldom
            2 Occasional   2 Occasional
            3 Often (several times a year)   3 Often
            4 Permanent or long-term   4 Unknown
            9 Unknown

11. *Medication:* ☐   0 No medication
            1 Short-term medication
            2 Long-term medication
            3 Permanent medication
            9 Unknown

                        Type of medicine: _____

Adult Population

Expanded Disability Status Scale

The Expanded Disability Status Scale (EDSS) measures maximal functioning of patients who have multiple sclerosis based on neurological evaluation. It involves eight functional groups called *Functional Systems* (FS), which are given numerical grades that can be compared over time. The FS are not additive—each FS score can only be compared with itself. The FS scores are then used to obtain a grade on the EDSS. The total score ranges from 0 to 10. Higher grades denote increased disability.

0 = Has normal neurologic examination (all grade 0 in FSs; cerebral grade 1 acceptable)

1.0 = Has no disability; shows minimal signs in one FS (i.e., grade 1 excluding cerebral grade 1).

1.5 = Has no disability; shows minimal signs in more than one FS (more than one grade 1 excluding cerebral grade 1)

2.0 = Has minimal disability in one FS (one FS grade 2, others 0 or 1)

2.5 = Has minimal disability in two FSs (two FSs grade 2, others 0 or 1)

3.0 = Has moderate disability in one FS (one FS grade 3, others 0 or 1), or mild disability in three or four FSs (three or four FSs grade 2, others 0 or 1), though fully ambulatory

3.5 = Is fully ambulatory but with moderate disability in one FS (one grade 3) and one or two FSs grade 2; or two FSs grade 3; or five FSs grade 2 (others 0 or 1)

4.0 = Is fully ambulatory without aid; is self-sufficient; is up and about 12 hours a day despite relatively severe disability consisting of one FS grade 4 (others 0 or 1), or combinations of lesser grades exceeding limits of previous steps; is able to walk without aid or rest for 500 m

4.5 = Is fully ambulatory without aid; is up and about much of the day; is able to work a full day; may otherwise have some limitation of full activity or require minimal assistance; is characterized by relatively severe disability, usually consisting of one FS grade 4 (others 0 or 1) or combinations of lesser grades exceeding limits of previous steps; is able to walk without aid or rest for 300 m

5.0 = Is ambulatory without aid or rest for about 200 m; has disability severe enough to impair full daily activities, such as working a full day without special provisions (usual FS equivalents are one grade 5 alone, others 0 or 1; or combinations of lesser grades usually exceeding specifications for step 4.0)

5.5 = Is ambulatory without aid or rest for about 100 m; has disability severe enough to preclude full daily activities (usual FS equivalents are one grade 5 alone, others 0 or 1; or combinations of lesser grades usually exceeding those for step 4.0)

6.0 = Requires intermittent or unilateral constant assistance (e.g., cane, crutch, or brace) to walk about 100 m with or without resting (usual FS equivalents are combinations with more than two FSs grade 3 +)

6.5 = Requires constant bilateral assistance (e.g., canes, crutches, or braces) to walk about 20 m without resting (usual FS equivalents are combinations with more than two FSs grade 3 +)

7.0 = Is unable to walk beyond about 5 m, even with aid; is essentially restricted to wheelchair; wheels self in standard wheelchair and transfers alone; is up and about in wheelchair 12 hours a day (usual FS equivalents are combinations with more than one FS grade 4 +; rarely, pyramidal grade 5 alone)

7.5 = Is unable to take more than a few steps; is restricted to wheelchair; may need aid in transfer; wheels self but cannot carry on in standard wheelchair a full day; may require motorized wheelchair (usual FS equivalents are combinations with more than one FS grade 4 +)

8.0 = Is essentially restricted to bed or chair or perambulated in wheelchair, but may be out of bed much of the day; retains many self-care functions; generally has effective use of arms (usual FS equivalents are combinations, generally grade 4 + in several systems)

8.5 = Is essentially restricted to bed much of the day; has some effective use of arm(s); retains some self-care functions (usual FS equivalents are combinations, generally 4+ in several systems)

9.0 = Is helpless bed patient; can communicate and eat (usual FS equivalents are combinations, mostly grade 4+)

Modified from Kurtzke JF: Rating neurologic impairment in multiple sclerosis: an expanded disability status scale (EDSS) *Neurology* 33:1444-1452, 1983.
FS, Functional system.

9.5 = Is totally helpless bed patient; is unable to communicate effectively or eat/swallow (usual FS equivalents are combinations, almost all grade 4+)

10.0 = Experiences death due to MS

Functional Systems

Pyramidal functions

0. Normal functions
1. Abnormal signs without disability
2. Minimal disability
3. Mild or moderate paraparesis or hemiparesis; severe monoparesis
4. Marked paraparesis or hemiparesis, moderate quadriparesis, or monoplegia
5. Paraplegia, hemiplegia, or marked quadriparesis
6. Quadriplegia
V. Unknown

Cerebellar functions

0. Normal functions
1. Abnormal signs without disability
2. Mild ataxia
3. Moderate truncal or limb ataxia
4. Severe ataxia, all limbs
5. Inability to perform coordinated movements due to ataxia
V. Unknown
X. Weakness (grade 3 or more on pyramidal) interference with testing (used throughout after each number)

Brain-stem functions

0. Normal functions
1. Signs only
2. Moderate nystagmus or other mild disability
3. Severe nystagmus, marked extraocular weakness, or moderate disability of other cranial nerves
4. Marked dysarthria or other marked disability
5. Inability to swallow or speak
V. Unknown

Sensory functions (revised 1982)

0. Normal functions
1. Vibration or figure-writing decrease only, in one or two limbs
2. Mild decrease in touch, pain, or position sense, and/or moderate decrease in vibration

Functional Systems—cont'd

Sensory functions (revised 1982)—cont'd

in one or two limbs; or vibratory (with or without figure writing) decrease alone in three or four limbs

3. Moderate decrease in touch, pain, or position sense, and/or essentially lost vibration in one or two limbs; or mild decrease in touch or pain and/or moderate decrease in all proprioceptive tests in three or four limbs
4. Marked decrease in touch, pain, or loss of proprioception, alone or combined, in one or two limbs; or moderate decrease in touch or pain and/or severe proprioceptive decrease in more than two limbs
5. Loss (essentially) of sensation in one or two limbs; or moderate decrease in touch or pain and/or loss of proprioception for most of the body below the head
6. Loss (essentially) of sensation below the head
V. Unknown

Bowel and bladder functions (revised 1982)

0. Normal functions
1. Mild urinary hesitancy, urgency, or retention
2. Moderate hesitancy, urgency, retention of bowel or bladder, or rare urinary incontinence
3. Frequent urinary incontinence
4. Requirement of almost constant catheterization
5. Loss of bladder function
6. Loss of bowel and bladder function
V. Unknown

Visual (or optic) functions

0. Normal functions
1. Scotoma with visual acuity (corrected) better than 20/30
2. Worse eye with scotoma with maximal visual acuity (corrected) of 20/30 to 20/59
3. Worse eye with large scotoma, or moderate decrease in fields, but with maximal visual acuity (corrected) of 20/60 to 20/99
4. Worse eye with marked decrease of fields and maximal visual acuity (corrected) of 20/100 to 20/200; grade 3 plus maximal acuity of better eye of 20/60 or less

Adult Population

MS, Multiple sclerosis.

Continued

Box—cont'd

Functional Systems—cont'd

Visual (or optic) functions—cont'd

5. Worse eye with maximal visual acuity (corrected) less than 20/200; grade 4 plus maximal acuity of better eye of 20/60 or less
6. Grade 5 plus maximal visual acuity of better eye of 20/60 or less

V. Unknown

X. Addition to grades 0 to 6 for presence of temporal pallor

Cerebral (or mental) functions

0. Normal functions
1. Mood alteration only (does not affect DSS score)

Functional Systems—cont'd

Cerebral (or mental) functions—cont'd

2. Mild decrease in mentation
3. Moderate decrease in mentation
4. Marked decrease in mentation (chronic brain syndrome—moderate)
5. Dementia or chronic brain syndrome—severe or incompetent

V. Unknown

Other functions

0. None
1. Any other neurological findings attributed to MS (specify)

V. Unknown

Modified from Kurtzke JF: Rating neurologic impairment in multiple sclerosis: an expanded disability status scale (EDSS), *Neurology* 33:1444-1452, 1983.

Incapacity Status Scale

The Incapacity Status Scale (ISS) assesses disability in ADL. The total score ranges from 0 to 64. Higher scores denote increased disability.

ISS Form

Activities of daily living	Score

1. Stair climbing; ability to ascend and descend a flight of stairs of about 12 steps
  0 = is normal
  1 = has some difficulty but performs without aid
  2 = needs canes, braces, prostheses, or banister to perform
  3 = needs human assistance to perform
  4 = is unable to perform; includes mechanical lifts	

2. Ambulation; ability to walk on level ground or indoors for about 50 m without rest
  0 = is normal
  1 = has some difficulty but performs without aid
  2 = needs canes, braces, or prostheses to perform
  3 = needs human assistance or manual wheelchair, which patient uses to enter, leave, and maneuver without aid
  4 = is unable to perform; includes perambulation in a wheelchair and motorized wheelchair	

Modified from Granger CV: Assessment of functional status: a model for multiple sclerosis, *Acta Neurol Scand* 64 (Suppl 87):40-47, 1981.

Table—cont'd

Activities of daily living	Score
3. Chair or bed transfer; ability to enter and leave regular chair and/or bed; includes wheelchair transfers as indicated 0 = is normal 1 = has some difficulty but performs without aid 2 = needs adaptive or assistive devices such as trapeze, sling, bars, lift, or sliding board to perform 3 = requires human aid to perform 4 = must be lifted or moved almost completely by another individual 4. Toilet transfer; ability to seat self and arise from fixed toilet, as well as maintain position 0 = is normal 1 = has some difficulty but performs without aid 2 = needs adaptive or assistive devices such as bars or trapeze to accomplish 3 = requires human aid to accomplish transfer or positioning 4 = must be lifted, moved, or held almost completely by another individual 5. Bowel function 0 = is normal 1 = has bowel retention not requiring more than occasional enemas or suppositories (self-administered) 2 = has bowel retention requiring regular enemas or suppositories (self-administered) to induce evacuation; cleanses self 3 = has bowel retention requiring enemas or suppositories administered by another; needs assistance in cleansing; has occasional incontinence; tends colostomy by self 4 = has frequent soiling due to incontinence or a poorly maintained ostomy device, or an ostomy that the patient cannot maintain without assistance 6. Bladder function 0 = is normal 1 = has occasional hesitance or urgency 2 = has frequent hesitance, urgency or retention; uses indwelling or external catheter applied and maintained by self 3 = has occasional incontinence; uses indwelling or external catheter applied and maintained by others; maintains ileostomy or suprapubic cystostomy by self 4 = has frequent incontinence; uses ostomy device that patient cannot maintain without assistance 7. Bathing 0 = is normal 1 = has some difficulty with washing and drying self, though performed without aid whether in tub or shower or by sponge bathing, whichever is usual for the patient 2 = needs assistive devices (trapezes, slings, lifts, shower, or tub bars) to bathe self; needs to bathe self outside tub or shower if that is the patient's usual method 3 = needs human assistance in bathing parts of body or in entry, exit, or positioning in tub or shower 4 = has bathing performed by others (aside from face and hands)	

Adult Population

Continued

Table—cont'd

Activities of daily living	Score

8. Dressing
   0 = is normal
   1 = has some difficulty clothing self completely in standard garments, but accomplishes by self
   2 = requires specially adapted clothing (e.g., special closures, elastic-laced shoes, front-closing garments) or devices (e.g., long shoe horns, zipper extenders) to dress self
   3 = needs human aid to accomplish; performs considerable portion by self
   4 = needs almost complete assistance; is unable to dress self
9. Grooming; care of teeth or dentures and hair; shaving or application of cosmetics
   0 = is normal
   1 = has some difficulty but performs all tasks without aid
   2 = needs adaptive devices (e.g., electric razors or toothbrushes, special combs or brushes, arm rests or slings) but performs without aid
   3 = needs human aid to perform some of the tasks
   4 = has almost all tasks performed by another individual
10. Feeding; ingestion, mastication, swallowing of solids and liquids, and manipulation of the appropriate utensils
    0 = is normal
    1 = has some difficulty but performs without aid
    2 = needs adaptive devices (e.g., special feeding utensils, straws) or special preparation (e.g., portions precut or minced, bread buttered) to feed self
    3 = needs human aid in delivery of food; has dysphagia, preventing solid diet; maintains and uses esophagostomy or gastrostomy by self; performs tube-feeding by self
    4 = is unable to feed self or manage ostomies
11. Vision
    0 = is normal
    1 = requires lenses or has mild corrected visual acuity deficit (better than 20/50 both eyes); is able to read standard newspaper print
    2 = has corrected acuity about 20/50 or worse in the better eye; requires magnifying lenses or large print for reading; has one eye grade 4 and the other grade 0 or 1
    3 = has corrected acuity about 20/100 or worse in the better eye; is essentially unable to read; has one eye grade 4 and the other grade 2
    4 = has legal blindness; has corrected acuity 20/200 or worse in both eyes
12. Speech and hearing; verbal output and input for interpersonal communication purposes
    0 = is normal; has no subjective hearing loss; has articulation and language appropriate to the culture
    1 = has impaired hearing or articulation, not interfering with communication
    2 = has deafness sufficient to require hearing aid and/or dysarthria interfering with communication
    3 = has severe deafness compensated for by sign language or lip reading facility and/or severe dysarthria compensated for by sign language or self-written communication
    4 = has severe deafness and/or dysarthria without effective compensation

Modified from Granger CV: Assessment of functional status: a model for multiple sclerosis, *Acta Neurol Scand* 64 (Suppl 87):40-47, 1981.14. Societal role; primarily refers to patient's ordinary occupation, including housewife or student as applicable, as it may be modified by the impairment or disability

Table—cont'd

Activities of daily living	Score

13. Physical problems; presence of general medical, neurological, and/or orthopedic disorders, including multiple sclerosis
  0 = has no significant disorder
  1 = has disorder(s) not requiring active care; may be on maintenance medication; does not require monitoring more often than every 3 months
  2 = has disorder(s) requiring occasional monitoring by physician or nurse
  3 = has disorder(s) requiring regular attention (at least weekly) by physician or nurse
  4 = has disorder(s) requiring daily attention by physician or nurse; is usually in hospital	

14. Societal role; primarily refers to patient's ordinary occupation, including housewife or student as applicable, as it may be modified by the impairment or disability
  0 = has no impairment
  1 = performs usual role and tasks despite some difficulty with their performance
  2 = has impairments that require modification of usual role and tasks in nature, frequency, or duration
  3 = has impairments that preclude usual role and tasks; is unemployable outside sheltered workshop or unique skills; generally depends on assistance (public, private, or family) to maintain situation in usual household
  4 = requires long-term institutional care or its equivalent if maintained at home by intensive nursing, whether societal or familial	

15. Fatigability; a sense of overwhelming weakness or lassitude that dramatically alters baseline motor and coordination (occasionally visual or sensory) functions; possibly transient or persistent for hours or even days, occurring at varying frequency; a common complaint in multiple sclerosis
  0 = has no fatigability
  1 = has fatigability, but it does not notably interfere with baseline physical function; has fatigability causing intermittent and generally transient impairment of baseline physical function
  2 = has fatigability causing intermittent transient loss or frequent moderate impairment of baseline physical function
  3 = has fatigability that generally prevents prolonged or sustained physical function
  4 = has fatigability that generally prevents prolonged or sustained physical function	

16. Psychic (mood and mentation) function
  0 = is normal
  1 = has mild mood or behavior disturbance not interfering with usual function
  2 = has moderate mood or behavior disturbance (e.g., depression, anxiety) and/or mild mentation impairment with some interference with usual function
  3 = has severe mood or behavior disturbance (e.g., depression, euphoria, anxiety), moderate mentation impairment, and/or mild active psychotic reaction
  4 = has severe mentation impairment or psychosis ("mentation impairment" includes mental retardation as well as "organic brain syndrome" or "dementia")	

TOTAL ISS SCORE	

Minimal Record of Disability

The Minimal Record of Disability (MRD) assesses the neurological status of patients who have multiple sclerosis. It consists of four parts: the FS, EDSS, ISS, and ESS. The four tools together express an overall score of patients' neurological function. Higher scores denote greater degrees of impairment.

Parkinson's Disease Assessments

Hoehn and Yahr Parkinson's Disease Scale

The Hoehn and Yahr Parkinson's Disease Scale is a practical classification system for the types of parkinsonism, as well as a scale for grading severity. The total score ranges from 1 to 5. Higher scores denote increased disease involvement.

Hoehn and Yahr Parkinson's Disease Scale Form

Classifications

Primary parkinsonism	• The disease is idiopathic.
Secondary parkinsonism	• The disease is a fragment of a more diffuse disease of systems not ordinarily involved in the classical syndrome.
Indeterminate parkinsonism	• The disease is associated with other neurological disease, and there is no indication whether this association is causatively and pathologically determined or merely coincidental.

Stage	Level of clinical disability
I	• Unilateral involvement only • Minimal or no functional impairment
II	• Bilateral or midline involvement • Involvement without impairment of balance
III	• First sign of impaired righting reflexes • Unsteadiness when turning • Impaired reaction when pushed from standing equilibrium with the feet together and eyes closed • Restriction (somewhat) in activities • Possibility of some work potential, depending on the type of employment
IV	• Fully developed, disabling disease • Ability to walk and stand unassisted
V	• Confinement to bed or wheelchair unless aided

Modified from Hoehn MM, Yahr MD: Parkinsonism: onset, progression, and mortality, *Neurology* 17:427-442, 1967.

Severity of Tremor Clinical Rating Scale

The Severity of Tremor Clinical Rating Scale assesses tremor in patients who have Parkinson's disease. It grades four types of tremor on five body areas. Scores range from 0 to 10 for each tremor type on each body area. A score of 0 denotes no tremor, a score of 1 to 3 denotes mild tremors, a score of 4 to 6 denotes moderate tremors, a score of 7 to 9 indicates severe tremors, and a score of 10 denotes extremely severe tremors.

Tremor Severity Rating Scale Form

Tremor type	Score
Resting Head Tremor Patient lies flat on couch with head supported by pillows	
Postural Head Tremor Patient sits without head support	
Postural Lower-Extremity Tremor (Right) Patient sits with leg extended	
Resting Lower-Extremity Tremor (Right) Patient places foot on the floor	
Postural Lower-Extremity Tremor (Left) Patient sits with leg extended	
Resting Lower-Extremity Tremor (Left) Patient places foot on the floor	
Postural Upper-Extremity Tremor (Right) Patient stretches out arms with hands pronated and fingers spread	
Resting Upper-Extremity Tremor (Right) Patient relaxes arms and places them in lap	
Postural Upper-Extremity Tremor (Left) Patient stretches out arms with hands pronated and fingers spread	
Resting Upper-Extremity Tremor (Left) Patient relaxes arms and places them in lap	
Kinetic Tremor Patient performs finger-to-nose test	
Intention Tremor Patient reaches index finger toward target	
Vocal Tremor Patient says own name, address, and birthday, as well as holds a note by singing "aah"	

Adult Population

Modified from Bain PG and others: Assessing tremor severity, *J Neurol Neurosurg Psychiatry* 56:868-873, 1993.

Unified Parkinson's Disease Rating Scale

The Unified Parkinson's Disease Rating Scale (UPDRS) quantifies the type, number and severity of extrapyramidal signs in patients who have Parkinson's disease. The items are summed to represent a total score. The UPDRS also includes a Modified Hoehn and Yahr Staging Scale and the Schwab and England Activities of Daily Living Scale. The total score ranges from 0 to 162. Higher scores denote more disease involvement.

UPDRS Form

I Mentation, Behavior, and Mood

1. Intellectual impairment:
   0 = No impairment
   1 = Mild impairment; consistent forgetfulness with partial recollection of events and no other difficulties
   2 = Moderate memory loss, with disorientation and moderate difficulty handling complex problems; mild but definite impairment of functions at home with need of occasional prompting
   3 = Severe memory loss with disorientation for time and often place; severe impairment in handling problems
   4 = Severe memory loss with orientation preserved to individual only; inability to make judgments or solve problems; requirement of much help with personal care; inability to be left alone
2. Thought disorder (due to dementia or drug intoxication):
   0 = No disorder
   1 = Vivid dreaming
   2 = Benign hallucinations with insight retained
   3 = Occasional to frequent hallucinations or delusions; no insight; possibility of interference with daily activities
   4 = Persistent hallucinations, delusions, or florid psychosis; inability to care for self
3. Depression:
   0 = No depression
   1 = Periods of sadness or guilt greater than normal, never sustained for days or weeks
   2 = Sustained depression (1 week or more)
   3 = Sustained depression with vegetative symptoms (insomnia, anorexia, weight loss, loss of interest)
   4 = Sustained depression with vegetative symptoms and suicidal thoughts or intent
4. Motivation and initiative:
   0 = Normal motivation and initiative
   1 = Less assertiveness than usual; more passivity
   2 = Loss of initiative or disinterest in elective (nonroutine) activities
   3 = Loss of initiative or disinterest in day-to-day (routine) activities
   4 = Withdrawal; complete loss of motivation

Modified from Fahn S and others, eds: *Recent developments in Parkinson's disease,* vol 2, Florham Park, NH, 1987, Macmillan.

Box—cont'd

II Activities of Daily Living (Determine for On/Off)

5. Speech:
   0 = Normal speech
   1 = Mildly affected speech; no difficulty being understood
   2 = Moderately affected speech; occasional requests to repeat statements
   3 = Severely affected speech; frequent requests to repeat statements
   4 = Unintelligibility most of the time
6. Salivation:
   0 = Normal salivation
   1 = Slight but definite excess of saliva in mouth; possibility of night-time drooling
   2 = Moderately excessive saliva; possibility of minimal drooling
   3 = Marked excess of saliva with some drooling
   4 = Marked drooling, requiring constant tissue or handkerchief
7. Swallowing:
   0 = Normal swallowing
   1 = Rare choking
   2 = Occasional choking
   3 = Requirement of soft food
   4 = Requirement of nasogastric tube or gastronomy feeding
8. Handwriting:
   0 = Normal handwriting
   1 = Slightly slow or small handwriting
   2 = Moderately slow or small handwriting; all words legible
   3 = Severely affected handwriting; not all words legible
   4 = Majority of words not legible
9. Cutting food and handling utensils:
   0 = Normal ability
   1 = Somewhat slow and clumsy ability, but no help needed
   2 = Ability to cut most foods, although clumsy and slow; requirement of some help
   3 = Requirement of food being cut by someone, but ability to feed slowly
   4 = Requirement to be fed
10. Dressing:
    0 = Normal ability
    1 = Somewhat slow ability, but no help needed
    2 = Occasional assistance with buttoning, getting arms in sleeves
    3 = Requirement of considerable help, but ability to do some tasks alone
    4 = Helpless patient
11. Hygiene:
    0 = Normal hygiene
    1 = Slowness (somewhat), but no help needed
    2 = Requirement of help to shower or bathe; extreme slowness in hygienic care
    3 = Requirement of assistance for washing, brushing teeth, combing hair, and going to bathroom
    4 = Foley catheter or other mechanical aids

Adult Population

Continued

II Activities of Daily Living (Determine for On/Off)—cont'd

12. Turning in bed and adjusting bed clothes:
    0 = Normal ability
    1 = Slowness and clumsiness (somewhat), but no help needed
    2 = Ability to turn alone or adjust sheets, but with great difficulty
    3 = Ability to initiate, but not turn or adjust sheets alone
    4 = Helpless patient
13. Falling (unrelated to freezing):
    0 = No falling
    1 = Rare falling
    2 = Occasional falling, less than once per day
    3 = Falling on average of once daily
    4 = Falling more than once daily
14. Freezing when walking:
    0 = No freezing when walking
    1 = Rare freezing when walking; possibility of start hesitation
    2 = Occasional freezing when walking
    3 = Frequent freezing; occasional falling from freezing
    4 = Frequent falling from freezing
15. Walking:
    0 = Normal walking
    1 = Mild difficulty; may not swing arms or may tend to drag leg
    2 = Moderate difficulty, but requires little or no assistance
    3 = Severe disturbance of walking, requiring assistance
    4 = Inability to walk at all, even with assistance
16. Tremor:
    0 = Absent tremor
    1 = Slight and infrequent tremor
    2 = Moderate tremor, bothersome to patient
    3 = Severe tremor, interfering with many activities
    4 = Marked tremor, interfering with most activities
17. Sensory complaints related to parkinsonism:
    0 = No complaints
    1 = Occasional numbness, tingling, or mild aching
    2 = Frequent numbness, tingling, or aching (not distressing)
    3 = Frequent painful sensations
    4 = Excruciating pain

III Motor Examination

18. Speech:
    0 = Normal speech
    1 = Slight loss of expression, diction, and/or volume
    2 = Monotone, slurred but understandable, moderately impaired speech
    3 = Marked impairment (difficult to understand)
    4 = Unintelligible

Modified from Fahn S and others, eds: *Recent developments in Parkinson's disease,* vol 2, Florham Park, NH, 1987, Macmillan.

III Motor Examination—cont'd

19. Facial expression:
    0 = Normal expression
    1 = Minimal hypomimia (could be normal "poker face")
    2 = Slight but definitely abnormal diminution of facial expression
    3 = Moderate hypomimia; lips parted some of the time
    4 = Masked or fixed facies with severe or complete loss of facial expression; lips parted ¼ inch or more
20. Tremor at rest:
    0 = Absent tremor
    1 = Slight and infrequent tremor
    2 = Mild tremor in amplitude and persistence, or moderate in amplitude but only intermittently present
    3 = Moderate tremor in amplitude and present most of the time
    4 = Marked tremor in amplitude and present most of the time
21. Action or postural tremor of hands:
    0 = Absent tremor
    1 = Slight tremor (present with action)
    2 = Moderate tremor in amplitude (present with action)
    3 = Moderate tremor in amplitude with posture holding as well as action
    4 = Marked tremor in amplitude (interferes with feeding)
22. Rigidity (judged on passive movement of major joints with patient relaxed in sitting position; cogwheeling to be ignored):
    0 = Absent rigidity
    1 = Slight rigidity (or detectable only when activated by mirror or other movements)
    2 = Mild to moderate rigidity
    3 = Marked rigidity (but full range of motion easily achieved)
    4 = Severe rigidity (range of motion achieved with difficulty)
23. Finger taps (patient taps thumb with index finger in rapid succession with widest amplitude possible, each hand separately):
    0 = Normal finger taps
    1 = Mild slowing and/or reduction in amplitude
    2 = Moderate impairment; definite and early fatigue; possibility of occasional arrests in movement
    3 = Severe impairment; frequent hesitation in initiating movements or arrests in ongoing movement
    4 = Extreme impairment (barely able to perform the task)
24. Hand movements (patient opens and closes hands in rapid succession with widest amplitude possible, each hand separately):
    0 = Normal movements
    1 = Mild slowing and/or reduction in amplitude
    2 = Moderate impairment; definite and early fatigue; possibility of occasional arrests in movement
    3 = Severe impairment; frequent hesitation in initiating movements or arrests in ongoing movement
    4 = Extreme impairment (barely able to perform the task)
25. Rapid alternating movements of hands (pronation-supination movements of hands, vertically or horizontally, with as large an amplitude as possible, both hands simultaneously):
    0 = Normal movements
    1 = Mild slowing and/or reduction in amplitude
    2 = Moderate impairment; definite and early fatigue; possibility of occasional arrests in movement
    3 = Severe impairment; frequent hesitation in initiating movements or arrests in ongoing movement
    4 = Extreme impairment (barely able to perform the task)

Adult Population

Continued

III Motor Examination—cont'd

26. Leg agility (patient taps heel on ground in rapid succession, picking up entire leg; amplitude should be about 3 inches):
    0 = Normal agility
    1 = Mild slowing and/or reduction in amplitude
    2 = Moderate impairment; definite and early fatigue; possibility of occasional arrests in movement
    3 = Severe impairment; frequent hesitation in initiating movements or arrests in ongoing movement
    4 = Extreme impairment (barely able to perform the task)

27. Arising from chair (patient attempts to rise from a straight-backed wood or metal chair, with arms folded across chest):
    0 = Normal ability
    1 = Slowness (or may need more than one attempt)
    2 = Ability to push self up from arms of seat
    3 = Tendency to fall back (may have to try more than one time), but ability to get up without help
    4 = Inability to rise without help

28. Posture:
    0 = Erect (normal) posture
    1 = Not quite erect, slightly stooped posture (could be normal for older adult)
    2 = Moderately stooped posture (definitely abnormal, can be slightly leaning to one side)
    3 = Severely stooped posture with kyphosis (can be moderately leaning to one side)
    4 = Marked flexion with extreme abnormality of posture

29. Gait:
    0 = Normal gait
    1 = Slow walking, possibly shuffling with short steps, but not festination or propulsion
    2 = Difficulty in walking, but requiring little or no assistance; possibility of some festination, short steps, or propulsion
    3 = Severe disturbance of gait, requiring assistance
    4 = Inability to walk, even with assistance

30. Postural stability (response to sudden posterior displacement produced by pull on shoulders while patient erect with eyes open and feet slightly apart; patient is prepared):
    0 = Normal stability
    1 = Retropulsion, but recovering unaided
    2 = Absence of postural response (would fall if not caught by examiner)
    3 = Extreme instability; tendency to lose balance spontaneously
    4 = Inability to stand without assistance

31. Body bradykinesia and hypokinesia (combining slowness, hesitancy, decreased arm swing, small amplitude, and poverty of movement in general):
    0 = No bradykinesia or hypokinesia
    1 = Minimal slowness, giving movement a deliberate character (could be normal for some individuals); possibly reduced amplitude
    2 = Mild degree of slowness and poverty of movement, which is definitely abnormal; alternatively, some reduced amplitude
    3 = Moderate slowness; poverty or small amplitude of movement
    4 = Marked slowness; poverty or small amplitude of movement

Modified from Fahn S and others, eds: *Recent developments in Parkinson's disease*, vol 2, Florham Park, NH, 1987, Macmillan.

IV Complications of Therapy (in the Past Week)

A Dyskinesias

32. Duration: What proportion of the waking day are dyskinesias present (historical information)?

    0 = None
    1 = 1%-25% of day
    2 = 26%-50% of day
    3 = 51%-75% of day
    4 = 76%-100% of day

33. Disability: How disabling are the dyskinesias (historical information; may be modified by office examination)?

    0 = Not disabling
    1 = Mildly disabling
    2 = Moderately disabling
    3 = Severely disabling
    4 = Completely disabling

34. Painful dyskinesias: How painful are the dyskinesias?

    0 = No painful dyskinesias
    1 = Slightly painful dyskinesias
    2 = Moderately painful dyskinesias
    3 = Severely painful dyskinesias
    4 = Markedly painful dyskinesias

35. Presence of early-morning dystonia (historical information):

    0 = No
    1 = Yes

B Clinical fluctuations

36. Are any "off" periods predictable as to the timing after a dose of medication?

    0 = No
    1 = Yes

37. Are any "off" periods unpredictable as to the timing after a dose of medication?

    0 = No
    1 = Yes

38. Do any of the "off" periods come on suddenly (e.g., over a few seconds)?

    0 = No
    1 = Yes

39. What proportion of the waking day is the patient "off" on average?

    0 = None
    1 = 1%-25% of day
    2 = 26%-50% of day
    3 = 51%-75% of day
    4 = 76%-100% of day

C Other complications

40. Does the patient have anorexia, nausea, or vomiting?

    0 = No
    1 = Yes

41. Does the patient have any sleep disturbances (e.g., insomnia or hypersomnolence)?

    0 = No
    1 = Yes

42. Does the patient have symptomatic orthostatis?

    0 = No
    1 = Yes

Record the patient's blood pressure, pulse, and weight on the scoring form.

Adult Population

Continued

Box—cont'd

V Modified Hoehn and Yahr Staging Scale

Stage 0 = No signs of disease
Stage 1 = Unilateral disease
Stage 1.5 = Unilateral plus axial involvement
Stage 2 = Bilateral disease, without impairment of balance
Stage 2.5 = Mild bilateral disease, with recovery on pull test
Stage 3 = Mild to moderate bilateral disease; some postural instability; physical independence
Stage 4 = Severe disability (still able to walk or stand unassisted)
Stage 5 = Wheelchair bound or bedridden patient, unless aided

VI Schwab and England Activities of Daily Living Scale

100% Is completely independent; is able to do all chores without slowness, difficulty, or impairment; is essentially normal; is unaware of any difficulty

90% Is completely independent; is able to do all chores with some degree of slowness, difficulty, and impairment; may take twice as long; is beginning to be aware of difficulty

80% Is completely independent in most chores; takes twice as long; is conscious of difficulty and slowness

70% Is not completely independent; has more difficulty with some chores (three to four times as long in some); must spend a large part of the day with chores

60% Has some dependency; can do most chores, but exceedingly slowly and with much effort; makes errors; finds some chores impossible

50% Is more dependent; has difficulty with everything

40% Is very dependent; can assist with all chores, but can do few alone

30% With effort, now and then does a few chores alone or begins alone; requires much help

20% Does nothing alone; can be a slight help with some chores; is a severe invalid

10% Is totally dependent and helpless; is a complete invalid

0% Is in a state in which vegetative functions such as swallowing, bladder, and bowel functions are not functioning; is bedridden

Modified from Fahn S and others, eds: *Recent developments in Parkinson's disease,* vol 2, Florham Park, NH, 1987, Macmillan.

Spinal Cord Injury Assessments
American Spinal Injury Association Neurological Examination

The American Spinal Injury Association (ASIA) Neurological Examination systematically assesses myotomes and dermatomes to determine cord segments affected by spinal cord injuries. It consists of a sensory form (Figure 3-42) and a motor form (Figure 3-43), which determine neurological levels and completeness of cord injuries. The sensory form tests 28 dermatomes bilaterally for pin prick and light touch. External anal sphincter sensation is graded "yes" or "no" and is imperative for determining the level of the injury's completeness. The motor form tests 10 myotomes bilaterally using manual muscle test grades. Voluntary anal sphincter contraction is also noted to determine the completeness of spinal cord injury. The total score ranges from 0 to 324. Higher scores denote more normal sensation and motor function.

SENSORY
KEY SENSORY POINTS

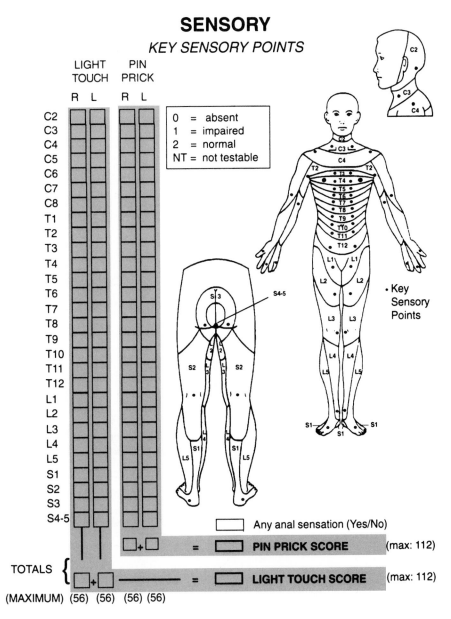

LIGHT TOUCH PIN PRICK

R L R L

	0	=	absent
	1	=	impaired
	2	=	normal
	NT	=	not testable

C2
C3
C4
C5
C6
C7
C8
T1
T2
T3
T4
T5
T6
T7
T8
T9
T10
T11
T12
L1
L2
L3
L4
L5
S1
S2
S3
S4-5

• Key Sensory Points

☐ Any anal sensation (Yes/No)

☐ + ☐ = ☐ **PIN PRICK SCORE** (max: 112)

TOTALS { ☐ + ☐ ———— = ☐ **LIGHT TOUCH SCORE** (max: 112)

(MAXIMUM) (56) (56) (56) (56)

FIGURE 3-42 American Spinal Injury Association (ASIA) sensory form. (Courtesy American Spinal Injury Association International, Atlanta, Ga.)

Adult Population

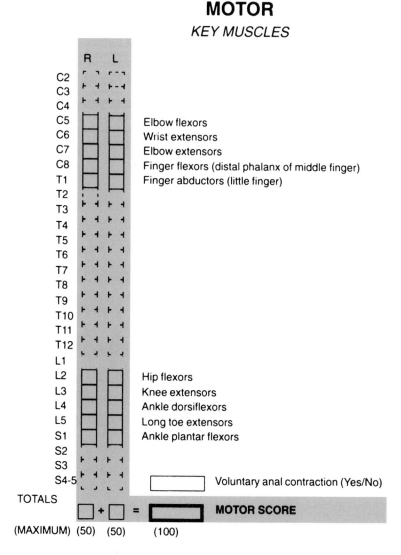

FIGURE 3-43 American Spinal Injury Association (ASIA) motor form. (Courtesy American Spinal Injury Association International, Atlanta, Ga.)

Craig Handicap Assessment and Reporting Technique

The Craig Handicap Assessment and Reporting Technique (CHART) measures handicaps in patients who have spinal cord injuries. It includes five areas of handicap: physical independence, mobility, occupation, social integration, and economic self-sufficiency. The maximum score for each area is 100. The total score ranges from 0 to 500. Higher scores denote increased handicap.

CHART Form

Items and questions	Score

Physical Independence Scale

How many hours in a typical 24-hour day do you have someone with you to provide assistance? (hours paid/hours unpaid)

Not including any regular care as previously reported, how many hours in a typical month do you occasionally have assistance with tasks such as grocery shopping, laundry, or housekeeping, or infrequent medical needs such as catheter changes?

Who takes responsibility for instructing and directing your attendants and/or caregivers? (self/others)

Total physical independence score

100 − (Total number of hours × 4)

100 − (Total number of hours × 3) if respondent takes primary responsibility for instructing and directing caregivers

Mobility Scale

On a typical day, how many hours are you out of bed?

In a typical week, how many days do you get out of your house and go somewhere?

In the last year, how many nights have you spent away from your home (excluding hospitalizations)? (none/1 to 2/3 to 4/5 or more)

Can you enter and exit your home without any assistance from someone? (yes/no)

In your home, do you have independent access to your sleeping area, kitchen, bathroom, telephone, and television (or radio)? (yes/no)

Can you use your transportation independently? (yes/no)

Does your transportation allow you to get to all the places you would like to go? (yes/no)

Does your transportation let you get out whenever you want? (yes/no)

Can you use your transportation with little or no advance notice? (yes/no)

Total mobility score

(Number of hours per day out of bed × 2) + (Number of days per week out of the house × 5)

Award up to 10 points for questions pertaining to home accessibility.

Award up to 20 points for spending nights away from home and independence in transportation.

Occupation Scale

How many hours per week do you spend working in a job for which you get paid?

How many hours per week do you spend in school working toward a degree or in an accredited technical training program?

How many hours per week do you spend in active homemaking, including parenting, housekeeping, and food preparation?

How many hours per week do you spend in home maintenance activities such as yard work, house repairs, or home improvement?

How many hours per week do you spend in ongoing volunteer work for an organization?

Modified from Whiteneck GG and others: Quantifying handicap: a new measure of long-term rehabilitation outcomes, *Arch Phys Med Rehabil* 73:519-526, 1992.

Continued

Adult Population

Items and questions	Score

Occupation Scale—cont'd

How many hours per week do you spend in recreational activities such as sports, exercise, playing cards, or going to movies? Please do not include time spent watching television or listening to the radio.

How many hours per week do you spend in other self-improvement activities such as hobbies or leisure reading? Please do not include time spent watching television or listening to the radio.

Total occupation score

Number of hours per week spent in working, schooling, homemaking, or performing home maintenance × 2) + (Number of hours spent each week in volunteer work, recreation, and other self-improvement activities) The maximum score is 100.

Social Integration Scale

Do you live alone or with any of the following: a spouse or significant other, children (how many), other relatives (how many), roommate (how many), or attendant (how many)?

If you do not live with a spouse or significant other, are you involved in a romantic relationship? (yes/no)

How many relatives (not in your household) do you visit, phone, or write at least once a month?

How many business or organizational associates do you visit, phone, or write at least once a month?

How many friends (nonrelatives contacted outside business or organizational settings) do you visit, phone, or write at least once a month?

With how many strangers have you initiated a conversation in the last month (e.g., to ask information or place an order)? (none/1 to 2/3 to 5/6 or more)

Total social integration score

Award up to 30 points based on household composition and romantic involvement.

Award points for the number of friends, relatives, and business associates with whom regular contact is maintained.

Award points for frequency of initiating conversations with strangers or acquaintances.

Economic Self-Sufficiency Scale

Approximately what was the combined annual income of all family members in your household last year? (Consider all sources, including wages and earnings, disability benefits, pensions and retirement income, income from court settlements, investments and trust funds, child support and alimony, contributions from relatives, and any other source.)

Approximately how much did you pay last year for medical care expenses? (Consider any amounts paid by yourself or family members in your household and not reimbursed by insurance or benefits.)

Total economic self-sufficiency score

Compare the total income to governmental poverty scales. Score 100 points if the total income is twice the poverty level.

TOTAL CHART SCORE

Modified from Whiteneck GG and others: Quantifying handicap: a new measure of long-term rehabilitation outcomes, *Arch Phys Med Rehabil* 73:519-526, 1992.

Spinal Cord Independence Measure

The Spinal Cord Independence Measure (SCIM) assesses functional changes in patients who have spinal cord injuries. It evaluates three areas of function: self-care, respiration and sphincter management, and mobility. The total score ranges from 0 to 100. Higher scores denote increased independence.

SCIM Form

Function	Score
Self-Care	
1. Feeding (cutting, opening containers, bringing food to mouth, holding cup with fluid)	
0 = needs parenteral, gastrostomy, or fully assisted oral feeding	
1 = eats cut food using several adaptive devices for hand and dishes	
2 = eats cut food using only one adaptive device for hand; is unable to hold cup	
3 = eats food without adaptive device; holds cup	
4 = eats cut food without adaptive devices; needs a little assistance (e.g., to open containers)	
5 = is independent in all tasks without any adaptive device	
2. Bathing (soaping, manipulating water tap, washing)	
0 = requires total assistance	
1 = soaps only small part of body with or without adaptive devices	
2 = soaps with adaptive devices; cannot reach distant parts of the body or cannot operate a tap	
3 = soaps without adaptive devices; needs a little assistance to reach distant parts of body	
4 = washes independently with adaptive devices or in specific environmental setting	
5 = washes independently without adaptive devices	
3. Dressing (preparing clothes, dressing upper and lower body, undressing)	
0 = requires total assistance	
1 = dresses upper body partially (e.g., without buttoning) in special setting (e.g., back support)	
2 = is independent in dressing and undressing upper body; needs much assistance for lower body	
3 = requires little assistance in dressing upper or lower body	
4 = dresses and undresses independently, but requires adaptive devices and/or special setting	
5 = dresses and undresses independently, without adaptive devices	
4. Grooming (washing hands and face, brushing teeth, combing hair, shaving, applying makeup)	
0 = requires total assistance	
1 = performs only one task (e.g., washing hands and face)	
2 = performs some tasks using adaptive devices; needs help to put on or take off devices	
3 = performs some tasks using adaptive devices; puts on or takes off devices independently	
4 = performs all tasks with adaptive devices or most tasks without devices	
5 = is independent in all tasks without adaptive devices	

Modified from Catz A and others: SCIM-spinal cord independence measure: a new disability scale for patients with spinal cord lesions, *Spinal Cord* 35:850-856, 1997.

Continued

Adult Population

Function	Score

Respiration and Sphincter Management

5. Respiration
   - 0 = requires assisted ventilation
   - 2 = requires tracheal tube and partially assisted ventilation
   - 4 = breathes independently but requires much assistance in tracheal tube management
   - 6 = breathes independently and requires little assistance in tracheal tube management
   - 8 = breathes without tracheal tube, but sometimes requires mechanical assistance for breathing
   - 10 = breathes independently without any device

6. Sphincter management—bladder
   - 0 = has indwelling catheter
   - 5 = receives assisted intermittent catheterization or no catheterization; has residual urine volume >100 cc
   - 10 = receives intermittent self-catheterization
   - 15 = does not require catheterization; has residual urine volume <100 cc

7. Sphincter management—bowel
   - 0 = experiences irregularity, improper timing, or extremely low frequency (less than once in 3 days) of bowel movements
   - 5 = experiences regular bowel movements with proper timing, but with assistance (e.g., for applying suppository)
   - 10 = experiences regular bowel movements with proper timing, without assistance

8. Use of toilet (perineal hygiene, clothes adjustment before and after, use of napkins or diapers)
   - 0 = requires total assistance
   - 1 = undresses lower body; needs assistance in all the remaining tasks
   - 2 = undresses lower body and partially cleans self (after); needs assistance in adjusting clothes and/or diapers
   - 3 = undresses and cleans self (after); needs assistance in adjusting clothes and/or diapers
   - 4 = is independent in all tasks but needs adaptive devices or special setting (e.g., grab-bars)
   - 5 = is independent without adaptive devices or special setting

Mobility (Room and Toilet)

9. Mobility in bed and action to prevent pressure sores
   - 0 = requires total assistance
   - 1 = has partial mobility (turns to one side only)
   - 2 = turns to both sides in bed but does not fully release pressure
   - 3 = releases pressure when lying only
   - 4 = turns in bed and sits up without assistance
   - 5 = is independent in bed mobility; performs push-ups in sitting position without full body elevation
   - 6 = performs push-ups in sitting position⁻

10. Transfer: bed-wheelchair (locking wheelchair, lifting footrests, removing and adjusting armrest, transferring, lifting feet)
    - 0 = requires total assistance
    - 1 = needs partial assistance and/or supervision
    - 2 = is independent

Modified from Catz A and others: SCIM-spinal cord independence measure: a new disability scale for patients with spinal cord lesions, *Spinal Cord* 35:850-856, 1997.

Function	Score

Mobility (Room and Toilet)—cont'd

11. Transfers: wheelchair-toilet-tub (if uses toilet wheelchair—transfers to and from; if uses regular wheelchair—locking wheelchair, lifting footrests, removing and adjusting armrests, transferring, lifting feet)
    0 = requires total assistance
    1 = needs partial assistance and/or supervision, or adaptive device (e.g., grab-bars)
    2 = is independent

Mobility (Indoors and Outdoors)

12. Mobility indoors (short distances)
    0 = requires total assistance
    1 = needs electrical wheelchair or partial assistance to operate manual wheelchair
    2 = moves independently in manual wheelchair
    3 = walks with a walking frame
    4 = walks with crutches
    5 = walks with two canes
    6 = walks with one cane
    7 = needs leg orthosis only
    8 = walks without aids
13. Mobility for moderate distances (10-100 m)
    0 = requires total assistance
    1 = needs electrical wheelchair or partial assistance to operate manual wheelchair
    2 = moves independently in manual wheelchair
    3 = walks with a walking frame
    4 = walks with crutches
    5 = walks with two canes
    6 = walks with one cane
    7 = needs leg orthosis only
    8 = walks without aids
14. Mobility outdoors (more than 100 m)
    0 = requires total assistance
    1 = needs electrical wheelchair or partial assistance to operate manual wheelchair
    2 = moves independently in manual wheelchair
    3 = walks with a walking frame
    4 = walks with crutches
    5 = walks with two canes
    6 = walks with one cane
    7 = needs leg orthosis only
    8 = walks without aids
15. Stair management
    0 = is unable to climb or descend stairs
    1 = climbs one or two steps only in a training setup
    2 = climbs and descends at least three steps with support or supervision of another individual
    3 = climbs and descends at least three steps with support of handrail, crutch, and/or cane
    4 = climbs and descends at least three steps without support or supervision

Adult Population

Continued

Table—cont'd

Function	Score
Mobility (Room and Toilet)—cont'd	
16. Transfers: wheelchair-car (approaching car, locking wheelchair, removing armrests and footrests, transferring to and from car, bringing wheelchair into and out of car) 0 = requires total assistance 1 = needs partial assistance, supervision, and/or adaptive devices 2 = is independent without adaptive devices	
TOTAL SCIM SCORE	

Modified from Catz A and others: SCIM-spinal cord independence measure: a new disability scale for patients with spinal cord lesions, *Spinal Cord* 35:850-856, 1997.

Vestibular Assessments
Hallpike-Dix Maneuver

The Hallpike-Dix Maneuver tests for benign paroxysmal positional vertigo. The patient turns the head to one side and is moved from sitting into the supine position with the heads hanging over the end of the table (Figure 3-44). The therapist observes the patient for nystagmus and notes complaints of vertigo. The direction of nystagmus aids in identifying canal involvement.

FIGURE 3-44 Hallpike-Dix maneuver. (From Herdman SJ: Treatment of benign positional vertigo, *Phys Ther* 70:381–388, 1990.)

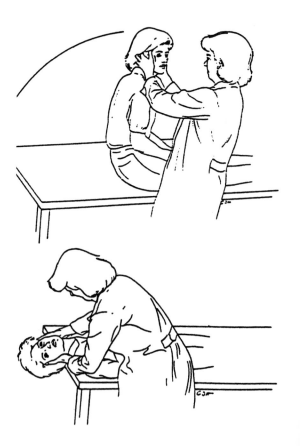

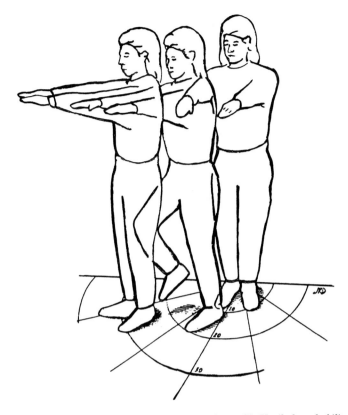

FIGURE 3-45 Fukuda's stepping test. (From Herdman SJ: *Vestibular rehabilitation,* Philadelphia, 1996, FA Davis.)

Fukuda's Stepping Test

Fukuda's Stepping Test assesses balance in patients who have suspected vestibular deficits. The patient marches in place first with the eyes open and then with the eyes closed (Figure 3-45). The therapist records the forward progression of the patient and the degree and direction of turning. Patients without vestibular impairments move forward less than 50 cm and turn less than 30 degrees after 50 steps. Patients with unilateral vestibular deficits tend to turn more than 30 degrees.

Vestibular System Evaluation

The Vestibular System Evaluation analyzes motion sensitivity response to activities. It consists of 16 rapid changes in body position scored for intensity and duration. These scores derive a motion sensitivity quotient (MSQ). The total score ranges from 0 to 100. Higher scores denote increased symptoms.

Vestibular System Evaluation

University of Michigan Vestibular Testing Center Habituation Training

Name:_____ Mrn:_____ Age:_____ Gender:_____

Date:_____

	Intensity	Duration	Score
Baseline Symptoms			
1. Sitting → Supine			
2. Supine → Left side			
3. →→ Right side			
4. Supine → Sitting			
5. Left Hallpike			
6. →→ Sitting			
7. Right Hallpike			
8. →→ Sitting			
9. Sitting → Nose to left knee			
10. Sitting → Erect left			
11. Sitting → Nose to right knee			
12. Sitting → Erect right			
13. Sitting → Head rotation			
14. Sitting → Head flexion and extension			
15. Standing → Turn to right			
16. Standing → Turn to left			

Intensity: Scale from 0 to 5 (0 = No SX; 5 = Severe SX)

Duration: Scale from 0 to 3 (5–10 sec = 1 point; 11–30 sec = 2 points; ≥30 sec = 3 points)

Motion Sensitivity Quotient: $\dfrac{\text{\# Positions} \times \text{Score}}{2048} \times 100 =$ _____   TOTAL

Modified from Smith-Wheelock M and others: Physical therapy program for vestibular rehabilitation, *Am Jl Otol* 12(3):218-225, 1991.

SX, Symptoms.

Cerebrovascular Accident Standards
Common Stroke Syndromes

Anatomic distribution	Stroke syndromes
Common Carotid Artery	Frequent resemblance to MCA, but can be asymptomatic if circle of Willis is competent
Internal Carotid Artery	Frequent resemblance to MCA, but can be asymptomatic if circle of Willis is competent
Middle Cerebral Artery (MCA)	
Main stem	Contralateral hemiplegia
	Contralateral hemianopia
	Contralateral hemianesthesia
	Head and eye turning toward lesion
	Dysphagia
	Uninhibited neurogenic bladder
	Dominant hemisphere:
	Global aphasia
	Apraxia
	Nondominant hemisphere:
	Aprosody and affective agnosia
	Visuospatial deficit
	Neglect syndrome
Upper division	Contralateral hemiplegia; leg more spared
	Contralateral hemianopia
	Contralateral hemianesthesia
	Head and eye turning toward lesion
	Dysphagia
	Uninhibited neurogenic bladder
	Dominant hemisphere:
	Broca (motor) aphasia
	Apraxia
	Nondominant hemisphere:
	Aprosody and affective agnosia
	Visuospatial deficit
	Neglect syndrome
Lower division	Contralateral hemianopia
	Dominant hemisphere:
	Wernicke aphasia
	Nondominant hemisphere:
	Affective agnosia
Anterior Cerebral Artery (ACA)	
Proximal (precommunal) segment (A1)	Possibly asymptomatic segment if circle of Willis is competent, but if both ACA arise from the same stem:
	Profound abulia (akinetic mutism)
	Bilateral pyramidal signs
	Paraplegia

Adult Population

Modified from Gillen G, Burkhardt A: *Stroke rehabilitation: a function-based approach,* St Louis, 1998, Mosby.

Table—cont'd

Anatomic distribution	Stroke syndromes
Anterior Cerebral Artery (ACA)—cont'd	
Postcommunal segment (A2)	Contralateral hemiplegia; arm more spared
	Contralateral hemianesthesia
	Head and eye turning toward lesion
	Grasp reflex, sucking reflex, gegenhalten
	Disconnection apraxia
	Abulia
	Gait apraxia
	Urinary incontinence
Anterior choroidal artery	Contralateral hemiplegia
	Hemianesthesia
	Homonymous hemianopsia
Posterior Cerebral Artery (PCA)	
Proximal (precommunal) segment (P1)	Thalamic syndrome:
	Choreoathetosis
	Spontaneous pain and dysesthesias
	Sensory loss (all modalities)
	Intention tremor
	Mild hemiparesis
	Thalamoperforate syndrome:
	Crossed cerebellar ataxia
	Ipsilateral third nerve palsy
	Weber's syndrome:
	Contralateral hemiplegia
	Ipsilateral third nerve palsy
	Contralateral hemiplegia
	Paralysis of vertical eye movement
	Contralateral action tremor
Postcommunal segment (P2)	Homonymous hemianopsia
	Cortical blindness
	Visual agnosia
	Prosopagnosia
	Dyschromatopsia
	Alexia without agraphia
	Memory deficits
	Complex hallucinations

Modified from Gillen G, Burkhardt A: *Stroke rehabilitation: a function-based approach,* St Louis, 1998, Mosby.

Table—cont'd

Anatomic distribution	Stroke syndromes
Vertebrobasilar Syndromes	
Superior cerebellar artery	Ipsilateral cerebellar ataxia
	Nausea and vomiting
	Dysarthria
	Contralateral loss of pain and temperature sensation
	Partial deafness
	Horner's syndrome
	Ipsilateral ataxic tremor
Anterior inferior cerebellar artery	Ipsilateral deafness
	Ipsilateral facial weakness
	Nausea and vomiting
	Vertigo
	Nystagmus
	Tinnitus
	Cerebellar ataxia
	Paresis of conjugate lateral gaze
	Contralateral loss of pain and temperature sensation
Medial basal midbrain (Weber's)	Contralateral hemiplegia
	Ipsilateral third nerve palsy
Tegmentum of midbrain (Benedikt's)	Ipsilateral third nerve palsy
	Contralateral loss of pain and temperature sensation
	Contralateral loss of joint position sensation
	Contralateral ataxia
	Contralateral chorea
Bilateral basal pons (locked in)	Bilateral hemiplegia
	Bilateral cranial nerve palsy (upward gaze spared)
Lateral pons (Millard-Gubler)	Ipsilateral sixth nerve palsy
	Ipsilateral facial weakness
	Contralateral hemiplegia
Lateral medulla (Wallenberg's)	Ipsilateral hemiataxia
	Ipsilateral loss of facial pain and sensation
	Contralateral loss of body pain and temperature sensation
	Nystagmus
	Ipsilateral Horner's syndrome
	Dysphagia and dysphonia

Cerebral Artery Dysfunction: Cortical

Artery	Location	Possible impairments
Middle cerebral artery: upper trunk	Lateral aspect of frontal and parietal lobe	Dysfunction of either hemisphere: Contralateral hemiplegia, especially of the face and the upper extremity Contralateral hemisensory loss Visual field impairment Poor contralateral conjugate gaze Ideational apraxia Lack of judgment Perseveration Field dependency Impaired organization of behavior Depression Lability Apathy Dysfunction of right hemisphere: Left unilateral body neglect Left unilateral visual neglect Anosognosia Visuospatial impairment Left unilateral motor apraxia Dysfunction of left hemisphere: Bilateral motor apraxia Broca's aphasia Frustration
Middle cerebral artery: lower trunk	Lateral aspect of right temporal and occipital lobes	Dysfunction of either hemisphere: Contralateral visual field defect Behavioral abnormalities Dysfunction of right hemisphere: Visuospatial dysfunction Dysfunction of left hemisphere Wernicke's aphasia
Middle cerebral artery: upper and lower trunks	Lateral aspect of the involved hemisphere	Impairments related to upper and lower trunk dysfunction as listed in the previous two sections

Modified from Gillen G, Burkhardt A: *Stroke rehabilitation: a function-based approach,* St Louis, 1998, Mosby.

Table—cont'd

Artery	Location	Possible impairments
Anterior cerebral artery	Medial and superior aspects of frontal and parietal lobes	Contralateral hemiparesis (greatest in foot) Contralateral hemisensory loss (greatest in foot) Left unilateral apraxia Inertia of speech or mutism Behavioral disturbances
Internal carotid artery	Combination of middle cerebral artery distribution and anterior cerebral artery	Impairments related to dysfunction of middle and anterior cerebral arteries as listed previously
Anterior choroidal artery, a branch of the internal carotid artery	Globus pallidus, lateral geniculate body, posterior limb of the internal capsule, medial temporal lobe	Hemiparesis of face, arm, and leg Hemisensory loss Hemianopsia

Posterior cerebral artery	Medial and inferior aspects of right temporal and occipital lobes, posterior corpus callosum, and penetrating arteries to midbrain and thalamus	Dysfunction of either side:
		  Homonymous hemianopsia
		  Visual agnosia (visual object agnosia, prosopagnosia, color agnosia)
		  Memory impairment
		  Occasional contralateral numbness
		Dysfunction of right side:
		  Cortical blindness
		  Visuospatial impairment
		  Impaired left-right discrimination
		Dysfunction of left side:
		  Finger agnosia
		  Anomia
		  Agraphia
		  Acalculia
		  Alexia

Adult Population

Continued

Table—cont'd

Artery	Location	Possible impairments
Basilar artery proximal	Pons	Quadriparesis Bilateral asymmetrical weakness Bulbar or pseudobulbar paralysis (bilateral paralysis of face, palate, pharynx, neck, or tongue) Paralysis of eye abductors Nystagmus Ptosis Cranial nerve abnormalities Diplopia Dizziness Occipital headache Coma
Basilar artery distal	Midbrain, thalamus, and caudate nucleus	Papillary abnormalities Abnormal eye movements Altered level of alertness Coma Memory loss Agitation Hallucinations
Vertebral artery	Lateral medulla and cerebellum	Dizziness Vomiting Nystagmus Pain in ipsilateral eye and face Numbness in face Clumsiness of ipsilateral limbs Hypotonia of ipsilateral limbs Tachycardia Gait ataxia
Systemic hypoperfusion	Watershed region on lateral side of hemisphere, hippocampus, and surrounding structures in medial temporal lobe	Coma Dizziness Confusion Decreased concentration Agitation Memory impairment Visual abnormalities due to disconnection from frontal eye fields Simultanognosia Impaired eye movements Weakness of shoulder and arm Gait ataxia

Modified from Gillen G, Burkhardt A: *Stroke rehabilitation: a function-based approach,* St Louis, 1998, Mosby.

Cerebral Artery Dysfunction: Noncortical

Location	Possible impairments
Anterolateral thalamus, either side	• Minor contralateral motor abnormalities • Long latency period • Slowness Right side: • Visual neglect Left side: • Aphasia
Lateral thalamus	• Contralateral hemisensory symptoms • Contralateral limb ataxia
Bilateral thalamus	• Memory impairment • Behavioral abnormalities • Hypersomnolence
Internal capsule or basis pontis	• Pure motor stroke
Posterior thalamus	• Numbness or decreased sensibility of face and arm • Choreic movements • Impaired eye movements • Hypersomnolence • Decreased consciousness • Decreased alertness Right side: • Visual neglect • Anosognosia • Visuospatial abnormalities Left side: • Aphasia • Jargon aphasia • Good comprehension of speech • Paraphasia • Anomia
Caudate	• Dysarthria • Apathy • Restlessness • Agitation • Confusion • Delirium • Lack of initiative • Poor memory • Contralateral hemiparesis • Ipsilateral conjugate deviation of the eyes

Modified from Gillen G, Burkhardt A: *Stroke rehabilitation: a function-based approach,* St Louis, 1998, Mosby.

Continued

Table—cont'd

Location	Possible impairments
Putamen	• Contralateral hemiparesis • Contralateral hemisensory loss • Decreased consciousness • Ipsilateral conjugate gaze • Motor impersistence Right side: • Visuospatial impairment Left side: • Aphasia
Pons	• Quadriplegia • Coma • Impaired eye movement
Cerebellum	• Ipsilateral limb ataxia • Gait ataxia • Vomiting • Impaired eye movements

Modified from Gillen G, Burkhardt A: *Stroke rehabilitation: a function-based approach*, St Louis, 1998, Mosby.

Language Disorders

Language change	Definition	Example
Asyndetic expression	A language disorder manifested by a juxtaposition of elements or meanings without adequate linkage	A patient, when asked the name of the President, responds, "White House."
Metonymic speech	The use of imprecise terms or words with approximate meaning	"I have eaten three meals" becomes "I have had three menus."
Echolalia	The purposeless repetition of a word or phrase just stated by another individual	The therapist says, "Turn on the lights," and the patient responds, "The lights, the lights, the lights, the lights."
Neologisms	A private word or phrase coined by the speaker that has special meaning to the speaker and cannot be understood by others	A patient responds to a question by saying, "Ethuel tanigram."
Clang associations	The repetition of words or phrases that have a similar sound but no other relationship	The nurse says, "What would you like to eat?" The patient's response is "Eat, feet, meet, beat."
Word salad	The linking of ordinary words and phrases in a meaningless, illogical, disconnected manner	A patient, pacing the hallway, says, "Vanilla reason lopsided can go left and right he is."

Modified from Stanhope M, Knollmueller RN: *Handbook of community and home health nursing*, ed 2, St Louis, 1996, Mosby.

Types of Aphasia

Type	Definition	Site of lesion	Clinical manifestations	Patient awareness
Wernicke's	Type of fluent aphasia	Wernicke's area of left hemisphere	Speech is fluent with normal and rapid rate; grammar and rhythm are in tact, but with little content to speech. Paraphasias, neologisms, and verbal nonwords occur	Is not aware of mistake
Anomic	Type of fluent aphasia	Area of angular gyrus	Speech is fluent, but patient cannot name objects or places; may define or describe what he or she is trying to name	Is aware
Conduction	Type of fluent aphasia	Arcuate fasciculus	Speech is characterized by literal paraphasia, but comprehension is intact	Is aware
Fluent	Impairment of ability to comprehend spoken language or written language			
Nonfluent	Loss of ability to express one's thoughts in speech or writing (motor, Broca's, expressive)	Motor cortex at Broca's area	Problems occur in selecting, organizing, and initiating motor speech patterns. Speech is halting, with effort to produce each word. Vocabulary is limited. Speech is telegraphic—omission of small grammatical words	Knows what he or she wishes to say and comprehends disability. Is often frustrated
Global	Type that occurs with extensive left damage and involves several speech areas. Few intact language skills	Several sites	Speech is nonfluent, comprehension is poor, ability is limited to name objects or repeat words	Cannot comprehend world around him or her

Modified from Stanhope M, Knollmueller RN: *Handbook of community and home health nursing,* ed 2, St Louis, 1996, Mosby.

Adult Population

Brain Injury Standards
Reflexes and Reactions Glossary
Reflexes

Asymmetrical tonic neck reflex (ATNR). Passive head rotation in the supine position produces extension of the arm and leg on the face side and flexion of the arm and leg on the back of the head side.

Babinski. Stroking the lateral sole of the foot from the heel to the ball of the foot produces splaying of toes and dorsiflexion of the hallux.

Bite. Oral stimulation produces swift biting action.

Chewing. Mouth stimulation produces repetitive chewing motions.

Crossed extension. Firm pressure to the ball of the foot or noxious stimulus of the extended leg produces extension and adduction of the opposite leg.

Flexor withdrawal. Noxious stimuli to the bottom of the foot produces uncontrolled flexion of the lower extremity.

Gag. Stimulation of the posterior pharynx produces a gag response.

Galant. Sweeping the paravertebral area between the twelfth rib and the iliac crest with the fingernail in the prone position produces trunk curvature to the same side.

Glabellar. Tapping briskly on the bridge of the nose produces eye closure.

Jaw jerk. Striking the lower jaw when it hangs open passively produces closure of the mouth.

Moro. Dropping the head from a semi-flexed position produces upper-extremity abduction and extension followed by upper-extremity flexion and adduction, lower-extremity extension and adduction, and crying.

Palmar grasp. Pressure on the palmar surface of the hand produces full finger flexion.

Pharyngeal. Stimulation of the posterior pharynx produces a gag response.

Placing. The top of the foot touching a hard object produces lifting of the leg.

Plantar grasp. Pressure on the ball of the foot produces toe flexion.

Positive support. Bouncing on the soles of the feet produces increased lower extremity extension tone and partial weightbearing.

Rooting. Touching beside the mouth produces head turning to that side and sucking.

Startle. A loud noise produces upper-extremity abduction and extension followed by upper-extremity flexion and adduction stepping. The sole of the foot touching a hard surface produces reciprocal flexion and extension of the leg.

Sucking. Stimulation of the oral area produces sucking movements.

Symmetrical tonic neck reflex (STNR). Neck flexion in the quadruped position produces upper-extremity flexion and lower-extremity extension.

Tonic labyrinthine. A change in the position of the head or body in space produces extension of the extremities in the supine position and flexion of the extremities in the prone position.

Tonic lumbar. Rotation to the right produces left upper-extremity and right lower-extremity extension, as well as right upper-extremity and left lower-extremity flexion. Rotation to the left produces left upper-extremity and right lower-extremity flexion, as well as right upper-extremity and left lower-extremity extension.

Traction. Pulling on the upper extremities produces neck flexion, elbow flexion and attempts at pull to sit.

Reactions

Amphibian. Lifting of the pelvis on one side in the prone position produces arm and leg flexion on the same side.

Associated. Performance of an action (e.g., squeezing a ball) produces mirroring on the opposite side and/or increased muscle tone in other parts of the body.

Body righting. Restoration or maintenance of normal postural relationships of the head, trunk, and extremities occurs during activity.

Equilibrium. Automatic, compensatory movements adapt the body to changes in the center of gravity and to changes in the position of the extremities in relation to the trunk.

Head righting. Restoration of the normal position of the head in space occurs.

Protective extension. A sudden loss of balance produces immediate upper-extremity extension, finger abduction, and finger extension.

Tone glossary

Decerebrate rigidity. Abnormal posture characterized by exaggerated extension of all extremities.

Decorticate rigidity. Abnormal posture characterized by exaggerated upper-extremity flexion and lower-extremity extension.

Dystonia. Abnormal involuntary movement or posture involving contraction of a group of muscles.

Extensor synergy, lower extremity. Hip extension, hip adduction, hip internal rotation, knee extension, ankle plantarflexion, and toe plantarflexion.

Extensor synergy, upper extremity. Shoulder protraction, shoulder internal rotation, shoulder adduction, elbow extension, and forearm pronation.

Flexor synergy, lower extremity. Hip flexion, hip abduction, hip external rotation, knee flexion, ankle dorsiflexion, ankle inversion, and toe dorsiflexion.

Flexor synergy, upper extremity. Shoulder retraction and/or elevation, shoulder external rotation, shoulder abduction, elbow flexion, and forearm supination.

Hypertonicity. Increased resistance to passive stretch.

Hypotonicity. Decreased resistance to passive stretch; inability to hold posture against gravity.

Rigidity. Resistance to passive range of motion affecting muscles on both sides of the joint.

Spastic diplegia. An increase in postural tone, primarily in the lower extremities and pelvis.

Spastic quadriplegia. An increase in postural tone in all four extremities.

Spasticity. Velocity-dependent increase in postural tone.

Synergy. A fixed set of muscle contractions with a predictable sequence and timing of contraction.

Adult Population

Hypotonicity Versus Hypertonicity

	Hypotonicity	Hypertonicity
1. Characteristics	Low tone, floppiness, "rag doll"	High tone, spasticity, or rigidity
2. Distribution	Generalized, symmetrical distribution	Generalized, often asymmetrical distribution
3. Range of motion	Excessiveness, joint hyperextensibility	Range of motion that is limited to midranges
4. Risk for contractures and deformities	Risk of dislocation (jaw, hip, atlantoaxial joint)	Risks for contractures (flexor), dislocations (hip), and deformities (scoliosis, kyphosis)
5. Deep tendon reflexes	Hypoactivity	Hyperactivity
6. Integration of primitive reflexes	Hyporeflexivity; sometimes delayed integration	Often delayed reflexes
7. Achievement of motor milestones	Delayed achievement (amount of delay correlates with severity of hypotonicity)	Delayed achievement (amount of delay correlates with severity of hypertonicity)
8. Influence of body position	Tone remaining the same	Tone fluctuating with changes in body position
9. Consistency of muscles	Soft, doughy consistency	Hard, rocklike consistency
10. Respiratory problems	Shallow breathing; choking secondary to decreased pharyngeal tone	Decreased thoracic mobility; limited inspiration and expiration
11. Speech problems	Shallow breathing; little sustained phonation	Dysarthria secondary to hypertonicity in oral muscles
12. Feeding problems	Hypoactive gag reflex; open mouth and protruding tongue; incoordination of swallowing	Hyperactive gag reflex; tongue thrust; bite reflex; rooting reflex

Modified from Umphred DA: *Neurological rehabilitation,* ed 3, St Louis, 1995, Mosby.

Characteristics of Seizures

Etiology	Characteristics	Clinical signs	Aura	Postictal period
Grand Mal Is most common type	Is generalized, characterized by loss of consciousness for several minutes	Aura Cry Loss of consciousness Fall Tonic-clonic movements Incontinence	Present Flashing lights Smells Spots before eyes Dizziness	Present Need for sleep for 1 to 2 hrs Headache common
Petit Mal Usually occurs during childhood and adolescence Frequency decreases as child gets older	Involves sudden impairment in or loss of consciousness with little or no tonic-clonic movement Occurs without warning Has tendency to appear a few hours after arising or when individual is quiet	Sudden vacant facial expression with eyes focused straight ahead All motor activity ceasing, except perhaps for slight symmetrical twitching about eyelids Possible loss of muscle tone Return of consciousness	None	None

Psychomotor
Occurs at any age
	Involves sudden change in awareness associated with complex distortion of feeling and thinking, as well as partially coordinated motor activity
	Is longer than petit mal
		Behavior as if partially conscious
		Often intoxicated appearance
		Antisocial acts such as exposing self or carrying out violent acts
		Autonomic complaints:
		  Chest pain
		  Respiratory distress
		  Tachycardia
		  Gastrointestinal distress
		  Urinary incontinence
			Present
			Complex hallucinations or illusions
				Present
				Confusion
				Amnesia
				Need for sleep

Continued

Modified from Stanhope M, Knollmueller RN: *Handbook of community and home health nursing*, ed 2, St Louis, 1996, Mosby.

Adult Population

Table—cont'd

Etiology	Characteristics	Clinical signs	Aura	Postictal period
Jacksonian, or Focal				
Occurs almost entirely in patients with structural brain disease	Depends on site of focus May or may not be progressive	Typical starting point is hand, foot, or face Possibility that it ends in grand mal seizure	Present Numbness Tingling Crawling feeling	Present
Myoclonic				
May antedate grand mal by months or years	May be extremely mild or may cause rapid, forceful movements	Sudden involuntary contraction of muscle group, usually in extremities or trunk No loss of consciousness	None	None
Akinetic				
Is uncommon	Involves peculiar generalized tonelessness	Individual in flaccid state Unconsciousness for 1 or 2 min	Rarely present	None

Modified from Stanhope M, Knollmueller RN: *Handbook of community and home health nursing*, ed 2, St Louis, 1996, Mosby.

Parkinson's Disease Standards
Parkinson's Disease Glossary

Akathisia. Extreme restlessness.

Akinesia. State of immobility.

Basal ganglia. Portion of the brain composed of the caudate nuclei, the putamen, and the globus pallidus responsible for initiation and control of movement and posture, as well as for sensory integration.

Blepharospasm. Spasmodic walking pattern.

Bradykinesia. Slowness of movement.

Bradyphrenia. Slowing of thought processes.

Cogwheel rigidity. Jerky, ratchetlike response to passive movement.

Dysarthria. Impaired speech.

Dysphagia. Impaired swallowing.

Dystonia. Involuntary movements with sustained contraction at the end of the movement.

Festination. Progressive increase in gait speed with shortened stride length.

Glabellar reflex. Tapping the bridge of the nose between the eyes, producing eye blink.

Hypokinesia. State of decreased range, speed, and amplitude of automatic movements.

Hypophonia. Decreased volume of speech.

Intention tremor. Involuntary oscillation of a body part that becomes more pronounced at the end of a goal-directed movement.

Kinetic tremor. Involuntary oscillation of a body part that is present during any form of movement.

Kyphosis. Increased flexion of the thoracic spine.

Leadpipe rigidity. Constant, uniform resistance to passive movement.

Masklike facies. Lack of facial expression and infrequent blinking.

Micrographia. Small writing.

Mutism. Inability to speak.

Pill-rolling tremor. Resting tremor of the hand.

Postural tremor. Involuntary oscillation of a body part that occurs when the limb is maintained against gravity.

Resting tremor. Involuntary oscillation of a body part that is present when muscles are not voluntarily activated and the body part is completely supported.

Retropulsion. Backward acceleration.

Rigidity. Increased resistance to passive motion.

Sialorrhea. Impairment of saliva management.

Simian posture. Flexed posture of the trunk and limbs.

Tremor. Involuntary oscillation of a body part occurring at a rate of 3 to 6 cycles per second.

Adult Population

Signs of Parkinson's Disease

Tremor	Retropulsion	Dysarthria
Rigidity	Shuffling gait	Hypophonia
Bradykinesia	Kyphosis	Sialorrhea
Postural instability	Scoliosis	Dystonia
Masklike facies	Flexion contractures	Muscle atrophy
Festination	Dysphagia	Bradyphrenia

Characteristics of Parkinson's Disease

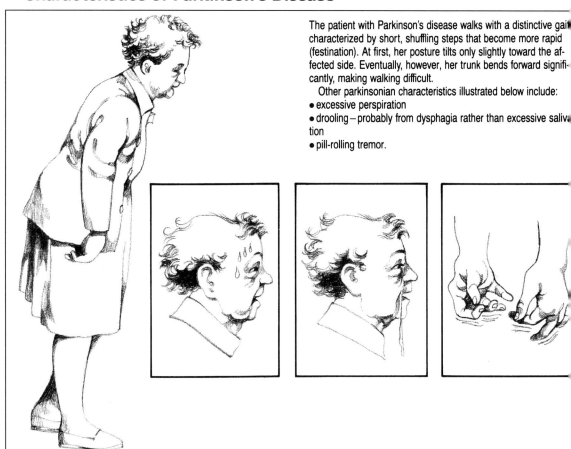

The patient with Parkinson's disease walks with a distinctive gait characterized by short, shuffling steps that become more rapid (festination). At first, her posture tilts only slightly toward the affected side. Eventually, however, her trunk bends forward significantly, making walking difficult.

Other parkinsonian characteristics illustrated below include:
- excessive perspiration
- drooling—probably from dysphagia rather than excessive salivation
- pill-rolling tremor.

FIGURE 3-46 Characteristics of Parkinson's disease. (From Lewis JA, editor: *Illustrated manual of nursing practice,* ed 2, Springhouse, Pa, 1994, Springhouse.)

Spinal Cord Injury Standards
Deep Tendon Reflexes

	Root level	Muscle	Peripheral nerve
Upper quarter:	C5-6	Biceps	Musculocutaneous
	C5-6	Brachioradialis	Radial
	C-7	Triceps	Radial
Lower quarter:	L3-4	Quadriceps	Femoral
	S1	Gastrocnemius	Sciatic (tibial)

The degree of reflex activity is graded on a 0-to-4 scale. Grades are awarded based on a predicted response and comparison of responses between body halves.

0 = no reflex response
1 = minimal response
2 = moderate response   } normal range
3 = brisk, strong response
4 = clonus

Modified from O'Sullivan SB, Schmitz TJ: *Physical rehabilitation and treatment,* ed 3, Philadelphia, 1988, FA Davis.

Dermatomes

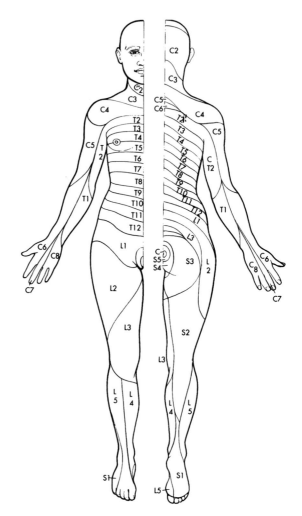

FIGURE 3-47 Dermatomal distribution of spinal nerves. (From Nicholas JA, Hershman EB: *The lower extremity & spine in sports medicine,* ed 2, St Louis, Mo, 1995, Mosby.)

Myotomes

Level	Action to be tested	Muscle
Upper Quarter Myotomes		
C-5	Shoulder abduction	Deltoid
C-5, C-6	Elbow flexion	Biceps
C-7	Elbow extension	Triceps
C-8	Ulnar deviation	Flexor carpi ulnaris
		Extensor carpi ulnaris
T-1	Digit abduction/adduction	Interossei
Lower Quarter Myotomes		
L-2, L-3	Hip flexion	Iliopsoas
L-3, L-4	Knee extension	Quadriceps
L-5	Ankle dorsiflexion	Anterior tibialis
	Extension of great toe	Extensor hallicus longus
S-1	Plantarflexion	Gastrocnemius

Modified from O'Sullivan SB, Schmitz TJ: *Physical rehabilitation and treatment,* ed 3, Philadelphia, 1988, FA Davis.

Nerve Root Origins of the Lower Extremity

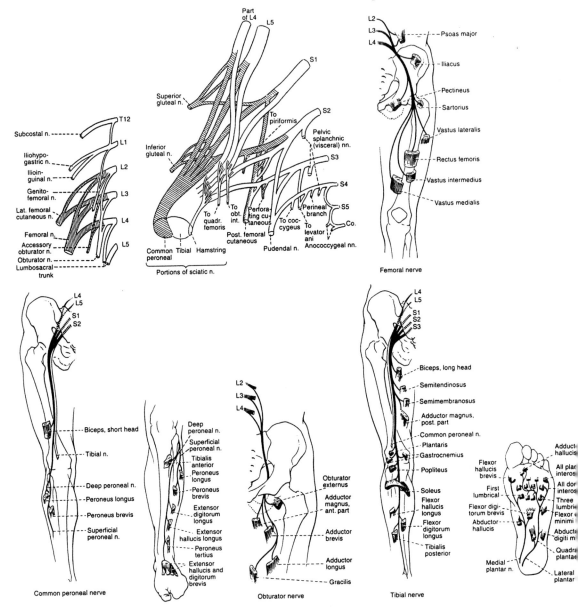

FIGURE 3-48 Lower extremity nerve root origins. (From Jenkins DB: *Hollinshead's functional anatomy of the limbs and back*, ed 6, Philadelphia, 1991, WB Saunders.)

Nerve Root Origins of the Upper Extremity

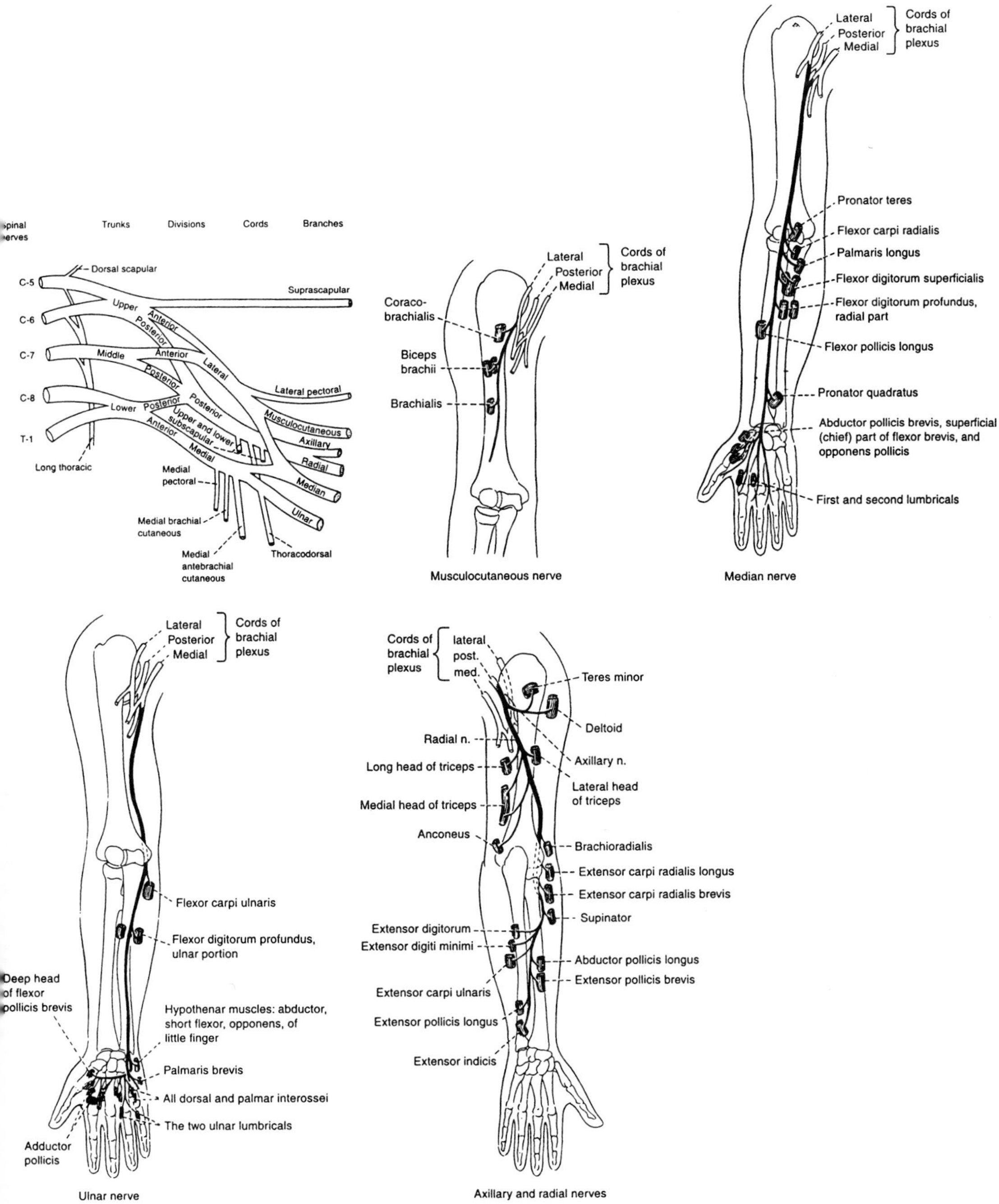

FIGURE 3-49 Upper extremity nerve root origins. (From Jenkins DB: *Hollinshead's functional anatomy of the limbs and back,* ed 6, Philadelphia, 1991, WB Saunders.)

Neurological Interventions Guidelines
Comparison of Neurological Interventions

	Premise	Aim	Techniques
Bobath	• The problem is not lack of power, but lack of ability to perform normal movements.	• To change abnormal movements into normal movements	• Reflex-inhibiting patterns to facilitate more normal movement
Brunnstrom	• Recovery of function follows an established pattern through various stages.	• To facilitate stages of spasticity development and the patient's ability to overcome tone	• Primitive reflexes • Associated reactions • Muscle strengthening • Coordination exercises
Carr and Shepherd	• Activities become better organized and more effective when practiced. • Balance preservation must be trained. • True learning occurs when tasks can be performed without thinking.	• To find the missing component to a task, practice the missing component, combine it with the whole task and practice, and then transfer it to another task involving the same component	• Repetition • Manual guidance through activities • Gradual decrease of assistance by the therapist
Proprioceptive neuromuscular facilitation	• Normal neuromuscular mechanisms become integrated and efficient without awareness. • Deficient neuromuscular mechanisms are unable to meet the demands of life. • Deficiency appears as weakness, incoordination, joint immobility, muscle spasm, and spasticity. • Neuromuscular mechanisms are facilitated by placing specific demands on patients.	• To promote response of neuromuscular mechanisms by stimulating the proprioceptors	• Maximal resistance • Manual contacts • Stretch • Traction • Approximation • Timing

Tone Inhibition and Facilitation Guidelines
Tone Inhibition and Facilitation Techniques

Inhibitory Techniques
- Maintained pressure
- Maintained touch
- Maximal loading
- Neutral warmth (15-20 minutes)
- Prolonged ice (15-20 minutes)
- Prolonged stretch
- Slow rocking
- Slow rolling
- Slow spinning
- Slow stroking

Facilitory Techniques
- Bone pounding
- Bounding
- Fast brushing
- Fast rocking
- Fast rolling
- Fast spinning
- Inverted labyrinthine position
- Joint compression
- Maintained ice (3-5 seconds)
- Maintained stretch (3-5 seconds)
- Oscillation
- Quick ice (1-3 strokes)
- Quick stretch
- Quick, light stroke
- Slapping
- Swinging
- Tapping
- Tendon tapping
- Traction
- Vibration
- Weight bearing

Spinal Cord Injury Guidelines
Prediction of Function from Level of Spinal Cord Injuries

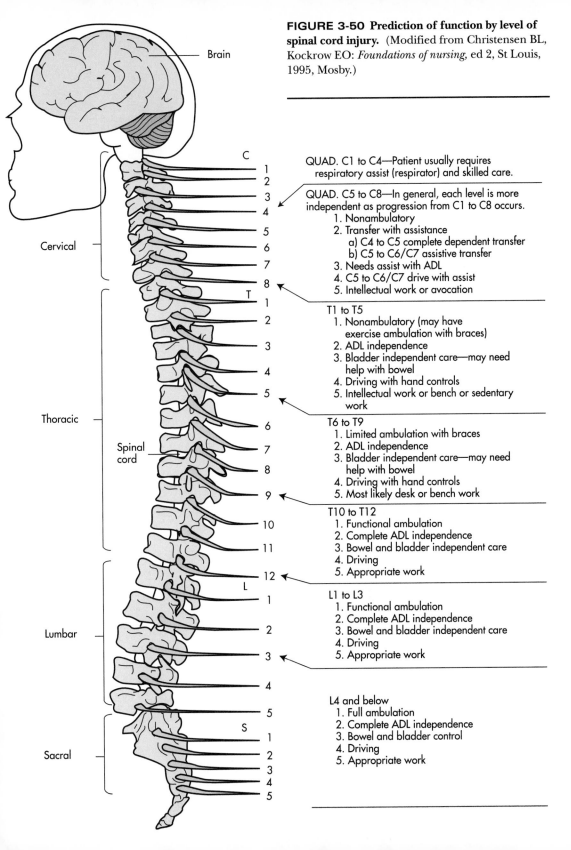

FIGURE 3-50 Prediction of function by level of spinal cord injury. (Modified from Christensen BL, Kockrow EO: *Foundations of nursing,* ed 2, St Louis, 1995, Mosby.)

Brain

C

QUAD. C1 to C4—Patient usually requires respiratory assist (respirator) and skilled care.

QUAD. C5 to C8—In general, each level is more independent as progression from C1 to C8 occurs.
1. Nonambulatory
2. Transfer with assistance
   a) C4 to C5 complete dependent transfer
   b) C5 to C6/C7 assistive transfer
3. Needs assist with ADL
4. C5 to C6/C7 drive with assist
5. Intellectual work or avocation

Cervical

T

T1 to T5
1. Nonambulatory (may have exercise ambulation with braces)
2. ADL independence
3. Bladder independent care—may need help with bowel
4. Driving with hand controls
5. Intellectual work or bench or sedentary work

Thoracic

Spinal cord

T6 to T9
1. Limited ambulation with braces
2. ADL independence
3. Bladder independent care—may need help with bowel
4. Driving with hand controls
5. Most likely desk or bench work

T10 to T12
1. Functional ambulation
2. Complete ADL independence
3. Bowel and bladder independent care
4. Driving
5. Appropriate work

L

L1 to L3
1. Functional ambulation
2. Complete ADL independence
3. Bowel and bladder independent care
4. Driving
5. Appropriate work

Lumbar

L4 and below
1. Full ambulation
2. Complete ADL independence
3. Bowel and bladder control
4. Driving
5. Appropriate work

Sacral

S

Adult Population

Functional Outcomes of Complete Spinal Cord Lesions

Functional skills	Level of assistance required (by SCI level groups)			
	High tetraplegia (C1-C5)	Midlevel tetraplegia (C6)	Low tetraplegia (C7-C8)	Paraplegia
Bed Mobility				
• Rolling side to side • Rolling from the supine to the prone position • Moving from the supine to the sitting position • Scooting all directions	• Dependence (C1-C4) • Moderate to maximal assistance (C5) • Ability to verbally direct all	• Minimal assistance to modified independence with equipment • Ability to verbally direct all	• Independence with all	• Independence
Transfers				
• Bed • Car • Toilet • Bath equipment • Floor • Upright wheelchair	• Dependence (C1-C4) • Maximal assistance with level sliding board transfers (C5) • Ability to verbally direct all	• Minimal assistance to modified independence for sliding board transfers • Dependence with wheelchair loading in car • Dependence with floor transfers and uprighting wheelchair • Ability to verbally direct all	• Modified independence to independence with level surface transfer (sliding board or depression) • Moderate assistance to modified independence with car transfer • Maximal to moderate assistance with floor transfers and uprighting wheelchair • Ability to verbally direct all	• Independence with level surface and care transfers (depression) • Minimal assistance to independence with floor transfer and uprighting wheelchair • Ability to verbally direct all

Weight Shifts

- Pressure relief
- Repositioning in wheelchair

• Setup to modified independence with power recline/tilt weight shift • Dependence with manual recline/tilt/lean weight shift • Ability to verbally direct all	• Modified independence with power recline/tilt weight shift • Minimal assistance to modified independence with side to side/forward lean weight shift • Ability to verbally direct all	• Modified independence with side to side forward lean, or depression weight shift • Ability to verbally direct all	• Modified independence with depression weight shift

Wheelchair Mobility

- Smooth surfaces
- Up and down ramps
- Up and down curbs
- Rough terrain
- Up and down steps (manual wheelchair only)

• Supervision and setup to modified independence on smooth, ramp, and rough terrain with power wheelchair • Modified independence with manual wheelchair on smooth surface in forward direction (C5) • Maximal assistance to dependence with manual wheelchair in all other situations (C5) • Ability to verbally direct all	• Modified independence in smooth, ramp, and rough terrain with power wheelchair • Dependence to maximal assistance up and down curb with power wheelchair • Modified independence on smooth surfaces with manual wheelchair • Moderate to minimal assistance on ramps and rough terrain with manual wheelchair • Maximal to moderate assistance up and down curbs with manual wheelchair • Dependence up and down steps with manual wheelchair • Ability to verbally direct all	• Modified independence on smooth, ramp, and rough terrain with power wheelchair • Dependence to maximal assistance up and down curb with power wheelchair • Modified independence on smooth surfaces and up and down ramps with manual wheelchair • Minimal assistance to modified independence on rough terrain • Moderate to minimal assistance up and down curbs with manual wheelchair • Dependence to maximal assistance up and down steps with manual wheelchair • Ability to verbally direct all	• Minimal assistance to modified independence up and down 6-inch curbs with manual wheelchair • Modified independence with descending steps with manual wheelchair • Maximal to minimal assistance to ascend steps with manual wheelchair • Ability to verbally direct all

Adult Population

Continued

Modified from Umphred DA: *Neurological rehabilitation,* ed 3, St Louis, 1995, Mosby.
SCI, Spinal cord injury.

Table—cont'd

Functional skills	Level of assistance required (by SCI level groups)			
	High tetraplegia (C1-C5)	Midlevel tetraplegia (C6)	Low tetraplegia (C7-C8)	Paraplegia
Wheelchair Management • Wheel locks • Armrests • Footrests and legrests • Safety strap(s) • Cushion adjustment • Antitip levers • Wheelchair maintenance	• Dependence with all • Ability to verbally direct all	• Requirement of some assistance • Ability to verbally direct all	• Possible requirement of assistance with cushion adjustment, antitip levers, and wheelchair maintenance • Ability to verbally direct all	• Independence with all
Gait • Donning and doffing orthoses • Sitting and standing • Smooth surfaces • Up and down ramps • Up and down curbs • Up and down steps • Rough terrain • Safe falling	• Not applicable	• Not applicable	• Not applicable	• Abilities range from following: • exercise only with KAFOs • household ambulation with KAFOs • limited community ambulation with KAFOs or AFOs • functional community ambulation with or without orthoses
ROM/ Positioning • PROM to trunk, legs, and arms • Pad and position in bed	• Dependence • Ability to verbally direct all	• Moderate assistance to modified independence with all	• Minimal assistance to modified independence with all	• Independence

Feeding

• Drinking • Finger feeding • Utensil feeding	• Dependence (C1-C4) • Minimal assistance with adaptive equipment (C5) • Ability to verbally direct all	• Modified independence with adaptive equipment	• Modified independence with adaptive equipment (C7)	• Independence

Grooming

• Face • Teeth • Hair • Makeup • Shaving face	• Dependence (C1-C4) • Minimal assistance with adaptive equipment for face, teeth, makeup, and shaving (C5) • Maximal to moderate assistance for hair grooming (C5) • Ability to verbally direct all	• Modified independence with adaptive equipment	• Modified independence	• Independence

Dressing

• Dressing and undressing (in bed and wheelchair) • Upper body and lower body (in bed and wheelchair)	• Dependence • Ability to verbally direct all	• Modified independence for upper body in bed or wheelchair • Minimal assistance with lower body dressing in bed • Moderate assistance with lower body undressing in bed • Ability to verbally direct all	• Modified independence for upper and lower body dressing and undressing in bed • Minimal assistance with lower body dressing and undressing in wheelchair (C7) • Modified independence for upper and lower body dressing and undressing in wheelchair (C8) • Ability to verbally direct all	• Modified independence

Adult Population

Continued

Modified from Umphred DA: *Neurological rehabilitation*, ed 3, St Louis, 1995, Mosby.
ROM, Range of motion; *KAFO,* knee-ankle-foot orthosis; *AFO,* ankle-foot orthosis.

Table—cont'd

Functional skills	Level of assistance required (by SCI level groups)			
	High tetraplegia (C1-C5)	Midlevel tetraplegia (C6)	Low tetraplegia (C7-C8)	Paraplegia
Bathing • Bathing and drying off • Upper body and lower body	• Dependence • Ability to verbally direct all	• Minimal assistance for upper body bathing and drying • Moderate assistance for lower body bathing and drying • Use of shower or tub chair • Ability to verbally direct all	• Modified independence with all with shower or tub chair	• Modified independence with all on tub bench or tub bottom cushion
Bowel and Bladder Programs • Intermittent catheterization • Leg bag care • Condom application • Clean up • In bed and wheelchair (bladder) • Feminine hygiene • Bowel program	• Dependence • Ability to verbally direct all	• Bladder: • minimal assistance for male in bed or wheelchair • moderate assistance for female in bed • Bowel: • moderate assistance with use of equipment • Ability to verbally direct all	• Bladder: • modified independence for male in bed or wheelchair • modified independence for female in bed; moderate assistance for female in wheelchair • Bowel: • minimal assistance to modified independence with use of equipment • Ability to verbally direct all	• Bladder: • modified independence for male and female • Bowel: • modified independence for male and female

Communication

• Verbal communication • Page turning • Keyboard • Writing • Telephone	• Setup modified independence using equipment for verbal communication (C1-C3) • Independent verbal communication (C4-C5) • Setup to modified independence with equipment for nonverbal communication • Ability to verbally direct all	• Independence for verbal communication • Setup to modified independence for nonverbal communication • Ability to verbally direct all	• Independence for verbal communication • Modified independence to independence for nonverbal communication	• Independence

Home Management

• Meal preparation • Environmental control	• Dependence to maximal assistance with meal preparation • Setup to modified independence with environmental control unit	• Moderate to minimal assistance with meal preparation • Modified independence with environmental control unit	• Minimal assistance to modified independence with meal preparation • Modified independence with environmental control unit	• Independence

Adult Population

Modified from Umphred DA: *Neurological rehabilitation*, ed 3, St Louis, 1995, Mosby.

Continued

Orthotics Correlated with Spinal Cord Injury Level

Injury level	Muscles present	Orthoses	Goals	Bracing recommended
Above T2	Partial upper-extremity function	Standing frames RGOs	Standing ?? Exercise amb.	No
T2 to T6	Complete upper-extremity function	Standing frames RGOs KAFOs with spreader bar	Standing ? Exercise amb.	No
T7 to T10	Partial function of trunk muscles	RGOs KAFOs with spreader bar	Standing Exercise amb.	No
T11 to T12	Almost complete function of trunk	RGOs KAFOs with spreader bar	Exercise amb.	Sometimes
L1	Complete function of trunk	RGOs KAFOs with spreader bar	Exercise amb. Sometimes household	Usually
L2	Hip flexors	KAFOs	Exercise amb. Household amb.	Usually
L3	Quadriceps	Combination KAFO/AFO Bilateral AFOs	Household amb. Community amb.	Yes
L4 and below	Quadriceps Partial hamstrings Partial ankle Partial hips	AFOs UCBL	Community amb.	Yes

Modified from Umphred DA: *Neurological rehabilitation,* ed 3, St Louis, 1995, Mosby.
RGO, Reciprocating gait orthosis; *KAFO,* knee-ankle-foot orthosis; *AFO,* ankle-foot orthosis; *UCBL,*University of California biomechanics laboratory insert; *amb.,* ambulation.

Aphasia Guidelines
Communication with Patients Who Have Aphasia

- Explain situations, treatments, and anything else that is pertinent to the patient because he or she may understand; the sounds of normal speech tend to be rehabilitative even if the words are not understood. Talk as if the patient understands.
- Avoid patronizing and childish phrases.
- The aphasic client may be especially sensitive to feelings of annoyance; remain calm and patient.
- Speak slowly, ask one question at a time, and wait for a response.
- Ask questions in a way that can be answered with a nod or the blink of an eye; if the patient cannot verbally respond, instruct him or her in nonverbal responses.
- Speak of things familiar and of interest to patient.
- Use visual cues, objects, pictures, and gestures, as well as words.
- Organize the environment to be as predictable as possible.
- Encourage articulation even if words convey no meaning.
- Show interest in the patient as an individual.

Modified from Stanhope M, Knollmueller RN: *Handbook of community and home health nursing,* ed 2, St Louis, 1996, Mosby.

Vestibular Guidelines
Vestibular Glossary

Anterior vestibular artery. Blood supply for the anterior and horizontal canals of the utricle.

Benign paroxysmal positional vertigo (BPPV). Condition characterized by brief episodes of vertigo as a result of inappropriate excitation of one or more of the semicircular canals.

Bone labyrinth. Area of the vestibular system comprised of the three semicircular canals and the vestibule or central chamber.

Brandt-Daroff habituation exercises. Treatment techniques for benign paroxysmal positional vertigo due to cupulolithiasis affecting the posterior semicircular canal.

Canalithiasis. Floating of debris in the endolymph of the semicircular canals.

Canalith repositioning maneuver. Treatment technique for benign paroxysmal positional vertigo for canalithiasis affecting the posterior, anterior, and horizontal semicircular canals.

Cupule. Gelatinous membrane that covers the crista.

Cupulolithiasis. Adherence of debris to the cupula of a semicircular canal.

Hallpike-Dix position. A test for benign paroxysmal positional vertigo in which patients are positioned in the supine position with cervical rotation and extension.

Liberatory maneuver. A treatment technique for benign paroxysmal positional vertigo for cupulolithiasis or canalithiasis affecting the posterior and horizontal semicircular canals.

Macula. Consists of hair cells enclosed by a gelatinous mass topped by calcium salt crystals.

Membranous labyrinth. An area of the vestibular system containing the sensory organs—membranous portions of the three semicircular canals, the utricle, and the saccule.

Nystagmus. Nonvoluntary, rhythmic oscillation of the eyes.

Oscillopsia. Illusionary back-and-forth movement of the environment implying bilateral vestibular function loss.

Otoconia. Calcium carbonate crystals that are more dense than the surrounding fluid, allowing them to displace hairs in response to movement.

Posterior vestibular artery. Blood supply for the posterior canal of the saccule.

Saccule. An otolithic organ that responds to head position relative to gravity and linear acceleration and deceleration.

Semicircular canal. Part of the vestibular apparatus that responds to movements of the head, exerts influences on the limbs and eye muscles, and assists in equilibrium responses and orientation in space.

Utricle. An otolithic organ that responds to head position relative to gravity and linear acceleration and deceleration.

Vertigo. An illusion of movement specific to vestibular system disease.

Vestibular paresis. Loss of vestibular hair cells or vestibular neurons, resulting in decreased vestibular system response to head movement.

Vestibulo-ocular reflex (VOR). A reflex generating eye movements that allow clear vision when the head is in motion.

Vestibulospinal reflex (VSR). A reflex generating compensatory body movement to maintain head and postural stability.

Adult Population

Identification of Canal Involvement

Canal	Eye muscle (excited)	Right Hallpike-Dix position	Reversal phase	Return to sitting position
Right posterior	Ipsilateral superior oblique, contralateral inferior rectus	Upbeat, counterclockwise	Down and clockwise	Down and clockwise
Right anterior	Ipsilateral superior rectus, contralateral inferior oblique	Downbeat, counterclockwise	Up and clockwise	Up and clockwise
Left anterior	Ipsilateral superior rectus, contralateral inferior oblique	Downbeat, clockwise	Up and counterclockwise	Up and counterclockwise
Right horizontal	Ipsilateral medial rectus, contralateral lateral rectus	Horizontal*	Horizontal	Horizontal
Left horizontal	Ipsilateral medial rectus, contralateral lateral rectus	Horizontal*	Horizontal	Horizontal

Modified from Herdman SJ: Advances in the treatment of vestibular disorders, *Phys Ther* 77(6): 602-618, 1997.

NOTE: The direction of fast-phase eye movement of nystagmus is generated by excitation of different canals (1) when the patient is moved into the right Hallpike-Dix position, (2) during the reversal phase, and (3) after the patient returns to the sitting position. *Clockwise* and *counterclockwise* refer to the direction of movement of the superior pole of the eye.

*Ageotropic if cupulolithiasis, geotropic if canalithiasis; Hallpike-Dix is not the best provoking position; the affected side is determined by the intensity of symptoms.

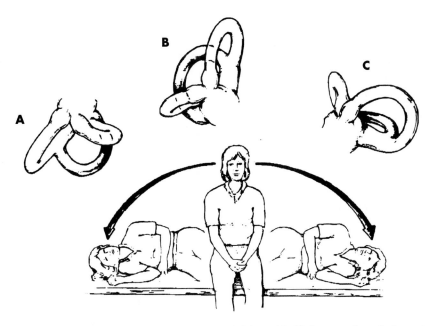

FIGURE 3-51 **Brandt-Daroff habituation.** **A,** Sidelying with 45 degrees of cervical rotation. **B,** Sitting. **C,** Opposite sidelying with 45 degrees of cervical rotation to opposite side. (Modified from Brandt T, Daroff RB: Physical therapy for benign paroxysmal positional vertigo, *Arch Otolaryngol* 106:484, 1980.)

Brandt-Daroff Habituation Exercises

Brandt-Daroff Habituation Exercises (Figure 3-51) are treatment techniques for benign paroxysmal positional vertigo due to cupulolithiasis affecting the posterior semicircular canal. The therapist should position the patient in the sitting position. The patient rapidly moves into the sidelying position with 45 degrees of cervical rotation and remains in this position until 30 seconds after vertigo stops. The patient then sits up and remains sitting until 30 seconds after vertigo stops. The patient moves quickly into the opposite sidelying position with 45 degrees of cervical rotation upward and remains in this position for 30 seconds before sitting up. The patient repeats this until vertigo is absent or 5 to 20 times as tolerated.

Canalith Repositioning Maneuver

The canalith repositioning maneuver (Figure 3-52) is a treatment technique for benign paroxysmal positional vertigo due to canalithiasis affecting the posterior, anterior, and horizontal semicircular canals. The therapist should position the patient in the sitting position with 45 degrees of cervical rotation toward the affected side. The therapist should then quickly move the patient into the Hallpike-Dix position with the affected ear down. The patient stays in this position for 2 minutes, then rotates the head to the opposite direction while maintaining neck extension. The patient then moves to the sidelying position with 45 degrees of cervical rotation and maintains this position for 2 minutes before returning to the sitting position. The patient repeats this process until nystagmus is absent after returning to the sitting position.

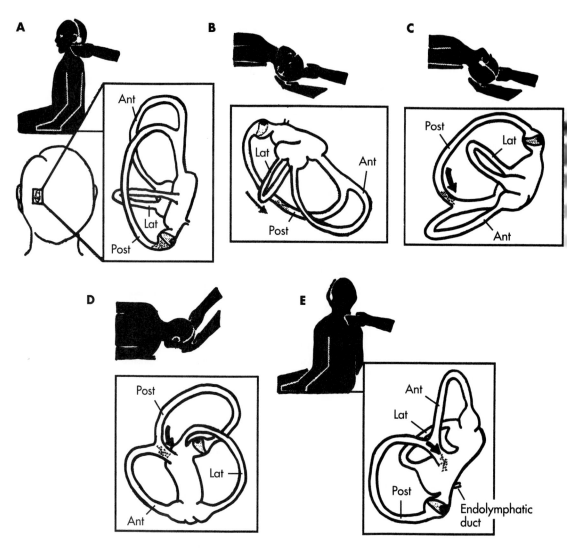

FIGURE 3-52 Positions through which head is moved during Epley canalith repositioning maneuver for treatment of left posterior canal benign paroxysmal positional vertigo (BPPV). Motion of debris within posterior canal during each head position is shown. **A,** Patient is seated upright on examination table in a position that allows head to be hyperextended below table when brought backward. Patient's head is turned 45 degrees toward left shoulder. Examiner stand behind patient. **B,** Patient's head is lowered into left Dixon-Hallpike position, resulting in debris movement within long arm of posterior canal away from ampulla of canal. Ampullofugal deflection of cupula is produced and nystagmus characteristic of posterior canal BPPV is elicited. **C,** Head is moved approximately 90 degrees in right Dix-Hallpike position, resulting in passage of debris into area of common crus. **D,** Head is moved another 90 degrees so that patient's nose points downward toward floor, resulting in debris being pulled into area of common crus closest to vestibule. **E,** Patient is returned to upright position, resulting in debris falling into vestibule. (Modified from Epley JM: The canalith repositioning procedure: for treatment of benign paroxysmal positional vertigo, *Otolaryngol Head Neck Surg* 107:401, 1992.)

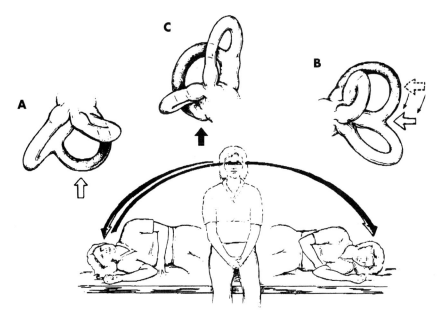

FIGURE 3-53 Liberatory maneuver. A, Sidelying with 45° of cervical rotation. **B,** Opposite sidelying maintaining 45° of cervical rotation. **C,** Sitting. (From Herdman SJ and others: Single treatment approaches to benign paroxysmal positional vertigo, *Arch Otolaryngol Head Neck Surg* 119:450, 1993.)

After this is achieved, the therapist immediately fits the patient with a soft collar and instructs him or her not to lie down or bend over for 48 hours and not to lie on the affected side for 5 days.

The Liberatory Maneuver

The liberatory maneuver (Figure 3-53) is a treatment technique for benign paroxysmal positional vertigo due to cupulolithiasis or canalithiasis affecting the posterior and horizontal semicircular canals. The therapist should position the patient in the sitting position. The therapist should then quickly move the patient into the sidelying position with 45 degrees of cervical rotation upward. The patient stays in this position for 2 minutes, then rapidly moves to the sitting position and over to the opposite sidelying position, maintaining the same head alignment. The patient should experience vertigo. If not, the therapist moves the patient's head abruptly to loosen debris. The patient stays in this position 2 minutes before slowly sitting up. If symptoms and nystagmus return after the patient has been sitting, the liberatory maneuver is repeated. The patient keeps the head upright for 48 hours and avoids symptom-provoking positions for 1 week.

ADULT INTEGUMENTARY EVALUATION

Often in home care, the integumentary system is primarily a nursing domain. Although nursing services play a major role in skin care, therapy services contribute to effective, comprehensive management of patients who have integumentary problems. Home care therapists use evaluation tools for objective goal setting and treatment planning. Integumentary standards and guidelines provide valuable information on numerous areas, such as wound measurement, positioning, and diabetic foot care.

Integumentary Assessments

Pressure Ulcer Assessments

Agency for Health Care Policy and Research Assessment Tool

The Agency for Health Care Policy and Research (AHCPR) Assessment Tool assesses pressure ulcers. It consists of pressure ulcer classifications, dimensions, appearances, and drainage characteristics. This tool is not scored numerically.

AHCPR Assessment Tool Form

Indicate ulcer sites:

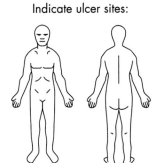

Anterior   Posterior

(Attach a color photo of the pressure ulcer[s] [optional])

Sample Pressure Ulcer Assessment Guide

Patient Name: _____ Date: _____ Time: _____

Ulcer 1:	Ulcer 2:
Site _____	Site _____
Stage _____	Stage _____
Size (cm):	Size (cm):
Length _____	Length _____
Width _____	Width _____
Depth _____	Depth _____

	No	Yes			No	Yes
Sinus tract	☐	☐		Sinus tract	☐	☐
Tunneling	☐	☐		Tunneling	☐	☐
Undermining	☐	☐		Undermining	☐	☐
Necrotic tissue:	☐	☐		Necrotic tissue:	☐	☐
Slough	☐	☐		Slough	☐	☐
Eschar	☐	☐		Eschar	☐	☐
Exudate:	☐	☐		Exudate:	☐	☐
Serous	☐	☐		Serous	☐	☐
Serosanguineous	☐	☐		Serosanguineous	☐	☐
Purulent	☐	☐		Purulent	☐	☐
Granulation	☐	☐		Granulation	☐	☐
Epithelialization	☐	☐		Epithelialization	☐	☐
Pain	☐	☐		Pain	☐	☐
Surrounding skin:						
Erythema	☐	☐		Erythema	☐	☐
Maceration	☐	☐		Maceration	☐	☐
Induration	☐	☐		Induration	☐	☐
Description of ulcer(s):						

Adult Population

Modified from Bergstrom N and others: *Treatment of pressure ulcers.* Clinical Practice Guideline, No. 15. Public Health Service, Agency for Health Care Policy and Research. AHCPR Publication No. 95-0652, Rockville, MD, December 1994, U.S. Department of Health and Human Services. *Continued*

Box—cont'd

Classification of pressure ulcers:

Stage I: Nonblanchable erythema of intact skin, the heralding lesion of skin ulceration. In individuals with darker skin, discoloration of the skin, warmth, edema, induration, or hardness may also be indicators.

Stage II: Partial thickness skin loss involving the epidermis, dermis, or both.

Stage III: Full thickness skin loss involving damage to or necrosis of subcutaneous tissue that may extend down to, but not through, underlying fascia. The ulcer appears clinically as a deep crater with or without undermining adjacent tissue.

Stage IV: Full thickness skin loss with extensive destruction, tissue necrosis, or damage to muscle, bone, or supporting structures (e.g., tendon or joint capsule).

Modified from Bergstrom N and others: *Treatment of pressure ulcers.* Clinical Practice Guideline, No. 15. Public Health Service Agency for Health Care Policy and Research. AHCPR Publication No. 95-0652, Rockville, Md, December 1994, U.S. Department of Health and Human Services.

Braden Scale

The Braden Scale identifies patients at risk for pressure ulcer development. It consists of six subscales graded from 1 to 3 or 4. The total score ranges from 6 to 23. Scores of 16 or less denote risk for development of pressure ulcers.

Braden Scale Form

Patient's Name _____ Evaluator's Name _____ Date of Assessment _____

	1	2	3	4
Sensory Perception Ability to respond meaningfully to pressure-related discomfort	1. Completely limited: Is unresponsive (does not moan, flinch, or grasp) to painful stimuli, due to diminished level of consciousness or sedation; OR has limited ability to feel pain over most of the body surface	2. Extremely limited: Responds only to painful stimuli; cannot communicate discomfort except by moaning or restlessness; OR has a sensory impairment that limits the ability to feel pain or discomfort over ½ of body	3. Slightly limited: Responds to verbal commands but cannot always communicate discomfort or need to be turned; OR has some sensory impairment that limits ability to feel pain or discomfort in one or two extremities	4. Not impaired: Responds to verbal commands; has no sensory deficit that would limit ability to feel or voice pain or discomfort
Moisture Degree to which skin is exposed to moisture	1. Constantly moist: Skin is kept moist almost constantly by perspiration, urine, etc. Dampness is detected every time the patient is moved or turned.	2. Moist: Skin is often but not always moist. Linen must be changed at least once a shift.	3. Occasionally moist: Skin is occasionally moist, requiring an extra linen change approximately once a day.	4. Rarely moist: Skin is usually dry. Linen requires changing only at routine intervals.
Activity Degree of physical activity	1. Bedfast: Is confined to bed	2. Chairfast: Is severely limited or unable to walk; cannot bear own weight and/or must be assisted into chair or wheelchair	3. Walks occasionally: Walks occasionally during day but for extremely short distances, with or without assistance; spends majority of each shift in bed or chair	4. Walks frequently: Walks outside the room at least twice a day and inside room at least once every 2 hours during waking hours
Mobility Ability to change and control body position	1. Completely immobile: Does not make even slight changes in body or extremity position without assistance	2. Extremely limited: Makes occasional slight changes in body or extremity position but is unable to make frequent or significant changes independently	3. Slightly limited: Makes frequent though slight changes in body or extremity position independently	4. No limitations: Makes major and frequent changes in position without assistance

TOTAL SCORE _____

Adult Population

Continued

Courtesy B Braden, N Bergstrom, 1988.

Box—cont'd

	1.	2.	3.	4.
Nutrition Usual food intake pattern	**Extremely poor:** Never eats a complete meal; rarely eats more than ⅓ of any food offered; eats two servings or less of protein (meat or dairy products) per day; takes fluids poorly; does not take a liquid dietary supplement; OR is NPO and/or maintained on clear liquids or intravenous tubes for more than 5 days	**Probably inadequate:** Rarely eats a complete meal and generally eats only about ½ of any food offered; protein intake includes only three servings of meat or dairy products per day; occasionally will take a dietary supplement; OR receives less than optimum amount of liquid diet or tube feeding	**Adequate:** Eats over half of most meals. Eats a total of four servings of protein (meat, dairy products) each day; occasionally will refuse a meal, but will usually take a supplement if offered; OR is on a tube feeding or TPN regimen, which probably meets most nutritional needs	**Excellent:** Eats most of every meal; never refuses a meal; usually eats a total of four or more servings of meat and dairy products; occasionally eats between meals; does not require supplementation.
Friction and Shear	**Problem:** The patient requires moderate to maximal assistance in moving. Complete lifting without sliding against sheets is impossible. The patient frequently slides down in bed or chair, requiring frequent repositioning with maximal assistance. Spasticity, contractures, or agitation leads to almost constant friction.	**Potential problem:** The patient moves feebly or requires minimal assistance. During a move, the skin probably slides to some extent against sheets, chair, restraints, or other devices. The patient maintains a relatively good position in chair or bed most of the time but occasionally slides down.	**No apparent problem:** The patient moves in bed and in chair independently and has sufficient muscle strength to lift up completely during the move. The patient maintains good position in bed or chair at all times.	
				TOTAL SCORE _____

Courtesy B Braden, N Bergstrom, 1988.
NPO, Nil per OS (nothing by mouth); *TPN*, total parenteral nutrition.

Norton Scale

The Norton Scale evaluates risk for pressure ulcer development. It assesses five conditions on a 4-point scale. The total score ranges from 5 to 20. Scores of 14 or less denote risk for pressure ulcer development, whereas scores under 12 indicate high risk.

Norton Scale Form

		Physical condition		Mental condition	Activity	Mobility	Incontinence	
		Good	4	Alert	4	Ambulant	4	Full	4	Never	4	TOTAL
		Fair	3	Apathetic 3	Walk/help	3	Slightly limited	3	Occasionally	3	SCORE
		Poor	2	Confused 2	Chairbound 2	Extremely limited 2	Usually/urine 2	
		Extremely bad 1	In stupor 1	Bed	1	Immobile	1	Doubly	1	
Name	Date							

Modified from Norton D and others: *An investigation of geriatric nursing problems in hospital,* Edinburgh, 1975, Churchill Livingstone.

Pressure Sore Status Tool

The Pressure Sore Status Tool evaluates wound healing characteristics, is sensitive to changes in wound status, and provides an objective method for quantifying wounds. As its name indicates, it is appropriate for use only with pressure ulcers, not wounds of other etiology. It consists of 15 items, 13 of which are scored on a modified Likert scale. The remaining 2 items, location and shape, are not scored. The total score ranges from 13 to 54. Higher scores denote poorer pressure ulcer quality.

Pressure Sore Status Tool Form

Instructions for Use

General guidelines

Fill out the attached rating sheet to assess a pressure sore's status after reading the definitions and methods of assessment described below. Evaluate once a week and whenever a change occurs in the wound. Rate according to each item by picking the response that best describes the wound and entering that score in the item score column for the appropriate date. When you have rated the pressure sore on all items, determine the total score by adding the 13 item scores. The *higher* the total score, the more severe the pressure sore status. Plot the total score on the Pressure Sore Status Continuum to determine the progress.

Specific instructions

1. Size: Use a ruler to measure the longest and widest aspect of the wound surface in centimeters; multiply the length by the width.
2. Depth: Pick the depth and thickness most appropriate to the wound using these additional descriptions:
   1 = tissues damaged but no break in skin surface
   2 = superficial, abrasion, blister, or shallow crater; even with, and/or elevated above, skin surface (e.g., hyperplasia)
   3 = deep crater with or without undermining of adjacent tissue
   4 = visualization of tissue layers not possible due to necrosis
   5 = supporting structures, including tendon and joint capsule
3. Edges: Use this guide:
Indistinct, diffuse	= unable to clearly distinguish wound outline
Attached	= even or flush with wound base; *no* sides or walls present; flat
Not attached	= sides or walls *are* present; floor or base of wound is deeper than edge
Rolled under, thickened	= soft to firm and flexible to touch
Hyperkeratotic	= callouslike tissue formation around wound and at edges
Fibrotic, scarred	= hard, rigid to touch
4. Undermining: Assess by inserting a cotton-tipped applicator under the wound edge. Advance it as far as it will go without using undue force. Raise the tip of the applicator so it may be seen or felt on the surface of the skin. Mark the surface with a pen. Measure the distance from the mark on the skin to the edge of the wound. Continue the process around the wound. Then use a transparent metric measuring guide with concentric circles divided into four (25%) pie-shaped quadrants to help determine the percentage of the wound involved.

Modified from Bates-Jensen BM: The pressure sore status tool: an outcome measure for pressure sores, *Top Geriatr Rehabil* 9(4):17-34, 1994.

5. Necrotic tissue type: Pick the type of necrotic tissue that is *predominant* in the wound according to color, consistency, and adherence using this guide:

White or gray nonviable tissue	=	white or gray skin surface; may appear prior to wound opening
Nonadherent, yellow slough	=	thin, mucinous substance; scattered throughout wound bed; easily separated from wound tissue
Loosely adherent, yellow slough	=	thick, stringy, clumps of debris; attached to wound tissue
Adherent, soft, black eschar	=	soggy tissue; strongly attached to tissue in center or base of wound
Firmly adherent, hard and black eschar	=	firm, crusty tissue; strongly attached to wound base *and* edges (like a hard scab)

6. Necrotic tissue amount: Use a transparent metric measuring guide with concentric circles divided into four (25%) pie-shaped quadrants to help determine the percentage of the wound involved.

7. Exudate type: Some dressings interact with wound drainage to produce a gel or trap liquid. Before assessing the exudate type, gently cleanse the wound with normal saline or water. Pick the exudate type that is *predominant* in the wound according to color and consistency, using this guide:

Bloody	=	thin, bright red
Serosanguineous	=	thin, watery pale red to pink
Serous	=	thin, watery, clear
Purulent	=	thin or thick, opaque tan to yellow
Foul purulent	=	thick, opaque yellow to green with offensive odor

8. Exudate amount: Use a transparent metric measuring guide with concentric circles divided into four (25%) pie-shaped quadrants to determine the percentage of dressing involved with exudate. Use this guide:

None	=	wound tissues dry
Scant	=	wound tissues moist; no measurable exudate
Small	=	wound tissues wet; moisture evenly distributed in wound; drainage involves $\leq 25\%$ dressing
Moderate	=	wound tissues saturated; drainage may or may not be evenly distributed in wound; drainage involves $>25\%$ to $\leq 75\%$ dressing
Large	=	wound tissues bathed in fluid; drainage freely expressed; may or may not be evenly distributed in wound; drainage involves $>75\%$ of dressing

9. Skin color surrounding wound: Assess tissues within 4 cm of wound edge. Dark-skinned individuals show the colors "bright red" and "dark red" as a deepening of normal ethnic skin color or a purple hue. As healing occurs in dark-skinned individuals, the new skin is pink and may never darken.

10. Peripheral tissue edema: Assess tissues within 4 cm of the wound edge. Nonpitting edema appears as skin that is shiny and taut. Identify pitting edema by firmly pressing a finger down into the tissues and waiting for 5 seconds; on release of pressure, tissues fail to resume the previous position and an indentation appears. Crepitus is accumulation of air or gas in tissues. Use a transparent metric measuring guide to determine how far edema extends beyond the wound.

11. Peripheral tissue induration: Assess tissues within 4 cm of the wound edge. Induration is abnormal firmness of tissues with margins. Assess by gently pinching the tissues. Induration results in an inability to pinch the tissues. Use a transparent metric measuring guide with concentric circles divided into four (25%) pie-shaped quadrants to determine the percentage of the wound and area involved.

12. Granulation tissue: Granulation tissue is the growth of small blood vessels and connective tissue to fill in full-thickness wounds. Tissue is healthy when bright, beefy red, shiny, and granular with a velvety appearance. Poor vascular supply appears as pale pink or balanced to dull, dusky red color.

13. Epithelialization: Epithelialization is the process of epidermal resurfacing and appears as pink or red skin. In partial-thickness wounds, it can occur throughout the wound bed, as well as from the wound edges. In full-thickness wounds it occurs from the edges only. Use a transparent metric measuring guide with concentric circles divided into four (25%) pie-shaped quadrants to help determine the percentage of the wound involved and to measure the distance the epithelial tissue extends into the wound.

Adult Population

Continued

Box—cont'd

Pressure Sore Status Tool   Name _____

Complete the rating sheet to assess the pressure sore status. Evaluate
each item by picking the response that best describes the wound and
entering the score in the item score column for the appropriate
date.

Location: Anatomic site. Circle, identify right (R) or left (L) and use
"X" to mark site on body diagrams:

_____ Sacrum and coccyx   _____ Lateral ankle
_____ Trochanter   _____ Medial ankle
_____ Ischial tuberosity   _____ Heel   Other site _____

Shape: Overall wound pattern; assess by observing perimeter and depth. Circle and *date* appropriate
description:

_____ Irregular   _____ Linear or elongated
_____ Round or oval   _____ Bowl or boat
_____ Square or rectangle   _____ Butterfly   Other shape _____

Item	Assessment	Date	Date	Date
		Score	Score	Score
1. Size	1 = Length × width <4 cm^2 2 = Length × width 4 to 16 cm^2 3 = Length × width 16.1 to 36 cm^2 4 = Length × width 36.1 to 80 cm^2 5 = Length × width >80 cm^2			
2. Depth	1 = Nonblanchable erythema on intact skin 2 = Partial-thickness skin loss involving epidermis and/or dermis 3 = Full-thickness skin loss involving damage or necrosis of subcutaneous tissue; may extend down to but not through underlying fascia; and/or mixed partial and full thickness and/or tissue layers obscured by granulation tissue 4 = Skin loss obscured by necrosis 5 = Full-thickness skin loss with extensive destruction, tissue necrosis or damage to muscle, bone or supporting structure			
3. Edges	1 = Indistinct, diffuse, none clearly visible 2 = Distinct, outline clearly visible, attached, even with wound base 3 = Well-defined, not attached to wound base 4 = Well-defined, not attached to base, rolled under, thickened 5 = Well-defined, fibrotic, scarred, or hyperkeratotic			

Modified from Bates-Jensen BM: The pressure sore status tool: an outcome measure for pressure sores, *Top Geriatr Rehabil*
9(4):17-34, 1994.

3ox—cont'd

Item	Assessment	Date	Date	Date
		Score	Score	Score
4. Undermining	1 = Undermining <2 cm in any area 2 = Undermining 2 to 4 cm involving <50% wound margins 3 = Undermining 2 to 4 cm involving >50% wound margins 4 = Undermining >4 cm in any area 5 = Tunneling and/or sinus tract formation			
5. Necrotic tissue type	1 = None visible 2 = White or grey nonviable tissue and/or nonadherent yellow slough 3 = Loosely adherent yellow slough 4 = Adherent, soft, black eschar 5 = Firmly adherent, hard, black eschar			
6. Necrotic tissue amount	1 = None visible 2 = <25% of wound bed covered 3 = 25% to 50% of wound covered 4 = >50% and <75% of wound covered 5 = 75% to 100% of wound covered			
7. Exudate type	1 = None or bloody 2 = Serosanguineous: thin, watery, pale red or pink 3 = Serous: thin, watery, clear 4 = Purulent: thin or thick, opaque, tan or yellow 5 = Foul purulent: thick, opaque, yellow or green with odor			
8. Exudate amount	1 = None 2 = Scant 3 = Small 4 = Moderate 5 = Large			
9. Skin color surrounding wound	1 = Pink or normal for ethnic group 2 = Bright red and/or blanches to touch 3 = White or grey pallor or hypopigmented 4 = Dark red or purple and/or nonblanchable 5 = Black or hyperpigmented			
10. Peripheral tissue edema	1 = Minimal swelling around wound 2 = Nonpitting edema extending <4 cm around wound 3 = Nonpitting edema extending ≥4 cm around wound 4 = Pitting edema extending <4 cm around wound 5 = Crepitus and/or pitting edema extending ≥4 cm			

Adult Population

Continued

Box—cont'd

Item	Assessment	Date	Date	Date
		Score	Score	Score
11. Peripheral tissue induration	1 = Minimal firmness around wound 2 = Induration <2 cm around wound 3 = Induration 2 to 4 cm extending <50% around wound 4 = Induration 2 to 4 cm extending ≥50% around wound 5 = Induration >4 cm in any area			
12. Granulation tissue	1 = Skin intact or partial thickness wound 2 = Bright, beefy red wound; 75% to 100% of wound filled and/or tissue overgrowth 3 = Bright, beefy red wound; <75% and >25% of wound filled 4 = Pink and/or dull, dusky red wound; and/or fills ≤25% of wound 5 = No granulation tissue present			
13. Epithelialization	1 = 100% wound covered; surface intact 2 = 75% to <100% wound covered and/or epithelial tissue extending >0.5 cm into wound bed 3 = 50% to <75% wound covered and/or epithelial tissue extending to <0.5 cm into wound bed 4 = 25% to <50% wound covered 5 = <25% wound covered			
TOTAL SCORE				
Signature				

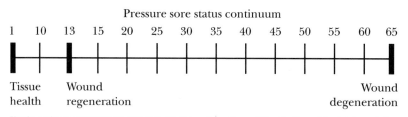

Pressure sore status continuum

1　10　13　15　20　25　30　35　40　45　50　55　60　65

Tissue health　Wound regeneration　　　　　　　　　　Wound degeneration

Plot the total score on the Pressure Sore Status Continuum by putting an "X" on the line and the date beneath the line. Plot multiple scores with their dates to see at a glance regeneration or degeneration of the wound.

Modified from Bates-Jensen BM: The pressure sore status tool: an outcome measure for pressure sores, *Top Geriatr Rehabil* 9(4):17-34, 1994.

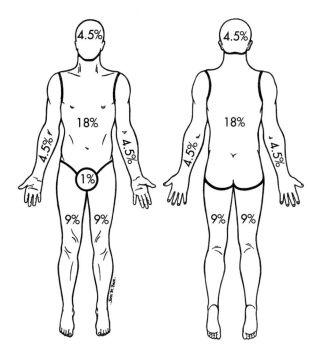

FIGURE 3-54 Rule of nines. (From Christensen BL, Kockrow EO: *Foundations of nursing*, ed 2, St Louis, 1995, Mosby.)

Burn Assessments

Rule of Nines

The Rule of Nines estimates the amount of skin surface affected by burns in adults (Figure 3-54). It consists of dividing the body surfaces into areas, then assigning each a numeric value divisible by nine. The total score ranges from 0% to 100%. Higher scores denote larger burns.

American Burn Association Severity Classification for Burn Injuries

The American Burn Association Severity Classification for Burn Injuries classifies burns in children and adults. It consists of three categories based on the location of the burn and the percentage of body area affected. The total score ranges from 1 to 3. Higher scores denote less severity of injury.

American Burn Association Severity Classification for Burn Injuries Form

Major Burn Injury

25% TBSA burn in adults <40 years old
20% TBSA burn in adults >40 years old
20% TBSA burn in children <10 years old
or

Burns involving the face, eyes, ears, hands, feet, and perineum likely to result in functional or cosmetic disability
or

High-voltage electrical burn injury
or

All burn injuries with concomitant inhalation injury or major trauma

Moderate Burn Injury

15%-25% TBSA burn in adults <40 years old
10%-20% TBSA burn in adults >40 years old
10%-20% TBSA burn in children <10 years old
with

Less than 10% TBSA full-thickness burn without cosmetic or functional risk to burn involving the face, eyes, ears, hands, feet, or perineum

Minor Burn Injury

<15% TBSA burn in adults <40 years old
<10% TBSA burn in adults >40 years old
<10% TBSA burn in children <10 years old
with

<2% TBSA full-thickness burn and no cosmetic or functional risk to the face, eyes, ears, hands, feet, or perineum

Modified from American Burn Association: Guidelines for service standards and severity classification in the treatment of burn injury, *Am Coll of Surg Bull* 69(10): 24-28, 1984.
TBSA, Total body surface area.

Numeric Scar Rating Scale

The Numeric Scar Rating Scale evaluates the appearance of scars. It assesses four scar characteristics. The total score ranges from −4 to 16. Higher scores denote poorer scar quality.

Numeric Scar Rating Scale Form

Circle one response on the scale. Do not mark between grid marks.

1. Burn scar surface

   −1----------0------------1----------------2----------------3--------------4

     smooth   normal   rough   rough   rough   rough

2. Burn scar border height

   −1----------0------------1----------------2----------------3--------------4

   depressed   normal   raised   raised   raised   raised

3. Burn scar thickness

   −1----------0------------1----------------2----------------3--------------4

     thinner   normal   thicker   thicker   thicker   thicker

4. Color differences between scar and adjacent normal skin

   −1----------0------------1----------------2----------------3--------------4

   hypopigmented normal hyperpigmented hyperpigmented hyperpigmented hyperpigmented

Modified from Yeong EK and others: Improved burn scar assessment with use of a new scar-rating scale, *J Burn Care Rehab* 18(4): 353-355, 1997.

Residual Limb Assessment
Houghton Questionnaire

The Houghton Questionnaire assesses rehabilitation of patients with lower-extremity amputations. It consists of four questions graded numerically. The total score ranges from 0 to 12. Scores of 9 or greater indicate satisfactory rehabilitation.

Houghton Questionnaire Form

Question	Score
1. Did patients use the limb to walk during . . .	
a. less than 25% of waking hours?	0
b. between 25% and 50% of waking hours?	1
c. more than 50% of waking hours?	2
d. all their waking hours?	3
2. Did patients use the limb to walk . . .	
a. just when visiting the physician or limb-fitting center?	0
b. at home but not to go outside?	1
c. outside the home on occasions?	2
d. inside and outside all the time?	3
3. When going outside wearing the limb, did patients . . .	
a. use a wheelchair?	0
b. use two crutches, two canes, or a walker?	1
c. use one cane?	2
d. use nothing?	3
4. When walking with the limb outside, did patients feel unstable when . . .	
a. walking on the flat surfaces?	No 1
b. walking on slopes?	No 1
c. walking on rough ground?	No 1
d. yes to any section	0
If the patient used a wheelchair outside, he or she score 0 for question 4.	
TOTAL SCORE	

Modified from Houghton A and others: Rehabilitation after lower limb amputation: a comparative study of above-knee, through-knee and Gritti-Stokes amputations, *Br J Surg* 76:622-624, 1989.

Skin Lesions Standards
Integumentary Glossary

Abscess. A collection of pus that forms because of infection and often causes destruction of tissue and inflammation.

Alginates. Absorbing dressings composed of seaweed.

Antibiotics. Substances that inhibit growth of or destroy microorganisms.

Antimicrobial. Destructive to or preventing the development of microorganisms.

Autolytic debridement. Process by which eschar self-digests via enzymes contained in wound fluid.

Bacteremia. Presence of bacteria in the blood.

Bactericidal. Destructive to bacteria.

Bacteriostatic. Inhibitory to the growth of bacteria.

Biosynthetics. Dressings composed of human- or animal-derived tissues.

Bottoming out. Condition that occurs when less than an inch of support material is felt between the support surface and the body segment at risk for pressure ulcers

Cellulitis. Inflammation of cellular or connective tissue.

Chemical debridement. Breakdown of necrotic tissue via topical application of enzymes.

Clean. Absence of foreign material.

Collagens. Dressings composed of the fibrous, insoluble protein collagen.

Composites. Single dressings that combine two or more distinct products.

Contaminated. Presence of microorganisms or foreign material.

Continuously moist saline gauze. Gauze dressings that are frequently remoistened to provide a constantly moist wound environment.

Cytotoxic. Destructive to cells.

Dakin's solution. Sodium hypochlorite.

Debridement. Removal of foreign material and/or necrotic tissue from wounds.

Decubitus ulcers. Skin lesions caused by unrelenting pressure, resulting in damage to underlying tissues.

Dehiscence. Separation of wound layers.

Dermis. The inner layer of the skin.

Dextranomers. Hydrophilic dextran-polymer beads that absorb wound drainage and debride devitalized tissue.

Disinfection. Elimination of pathogenic microorganisms.

Dressings. Materials applied to wounds for protection and absorbency.

Electrical stimulation. The use of electrical current to enhance wound healing.

Enzymatic debridement. See *chemical debridement.*

Epidermis. The outer layer of the skin.

Epithelialization. The wound-healing stage in which epithelial cells move across the surface of wounds.

Erythema. Redness.

Eschar. Thick, necrotic, devitalized tissue.

Exudates. Fluids expelled from tissues because of injuries or inflammation.

Fascia. Fibrous tissue that lies deep below the skin and encases muscles and various body organs.

Full thickness. Including the epidermis and the dermis.

Gauze. Cotton or synthetic fabric dressing.

Granulation. Process of wound healing in which beefy red tissue that contains blood vessels, collagen, fibroblasts, and inflammatory cells fills in the wound.

Healing. Restoration of anatomical and functional integrity.

Heterotopic bone formation. Complication of pressure ulcers in which bone growth occurs at abnormal sites.

Hydrocolloids. Adhesive, carbohydrate-based dressings that do not allow oxygen, water, or water vapor to pass through.

Hydrogels. Water-based, polymer-based dressings.

Hydrotherapy. The use of water for wound cleansing.

Hyperbaric oxygen. The use of oxygen at greater than atmospheric pressure.

Hypertrophic scarring. Scar formation that occurs when collagen synthesis exceeds collagen lysis.

Impregnated gauze. Gauze dressings that contain compounds to aid in wound healing.

Indurated. Hardened.

Infection. The presence of microorganisms in quantities of 10^5 or greater per gram of tissue.

Inflammatory response. The stage of wound healing in which destruction of tissues destroys, dilutes, and/or walls off injured tissue and injurious agents.

Irrigation. The use of a stream of fluid to clean wounds.

Ischemia. Lack of blood supply to tissues, resulting in tissue death.

Maceration. The process of softening a solid by wetting or soaking.

Mechanical debridement. Removal of foreign materials and/or devitalized tissues from wounds via physical forces.

Necrosis. Tissue death.

No-touch technique. Changing dressings without touching wounds or surfaces of dressings that contact wounds.

Pallor. Lack of color.

Pathogenic. Disease producing.

Phagocytosis. Ingestion and digestion of debris by white blood cells.

Pressure reduction. Lessening interface pressure, but not necessarily below capillary closing pressure.

Pressure relief. Lessening interface pressure below capillary closing pressure.

Pressure ulcers. See *decubitus ulcers*.

Primary intention healing. Closure and healing of sutured wounds.

Proteases. Protein-splitting enzymes.

Purulent drainage. Containing or forming pus.

Reactive hyperemia. Skin reddening as a result of blood returning to ischemic tissue.

Secondary intention healing. Closure and healing of wounds by formation of granulation tissue and epithelialization.

Semi-permeable films. Dressings composed of transparent polyurethane membranes that are waterproof and impermeable to bacteria, but permeable to water vapor.

Semi-permeable foams. Dressings that are hydrophilic on the wound side and hydrophobic on the other side.

Sepsis. Presence of pathogenic organisms in blood or tissues.

Sharp debridement. Removal of foreign materials and/or devitalized tissues from wounds via sharp instruments.

Sinus tracks. Cavities under wounds that encompass areas larger than visible surfaces of wounds and usually have narrow openings.

Slough. Devitalized tissues in the process of separating from viable tissues.

Stasis ulcers. Areas of skin breakdown associated with venous hypertension.

Tissue loads. Distributions of pressure, friction, and shear on tissues.

Topical antibiotics. Drugs applied to superficial surfaces that inhibit or kill microorganisms.

Topical antiseptics. Antimicrobials applied to skin or superficial tissues.

Tunneling. Cavities under the skin surface, but open at the skin level.

Undermining. Closed cavities under the skin surface open only at the skin surface.

Wet to dry saline gauze. Dressings consisting of saline-soaked gauze applied to wounds wet and removed dry.

Wound fillers. Pastes, gels, granules, powders, or beads that absorb exudate, debride wounds, and provide moist wound environments.

Pressure Ulcer Stages

Stage	Description
Stage I	Nonblanchable erythema of intact skin, the heralding lesion of skin ulceration. In individuals with darker skin, discoloration of the skin, warmth, edema, induration, or hardness may also be indicators.
Stage II	Partial thickness skin loss involving the epidermis, dermis, or both. The ulcer is superficial and appears clinically as an abrasion, a blister, or a shallow crater.
Stage III	Full thickness skin loss involving damage to or necrosis of subcutaneous tissue that may extend down to, but not through, underlying fascia. The ulcer appears clinically as a deep crater with or without undermining of adjacent tissue.
Stage IV	Full thickness skin loss with extensive destruction, tissue necrosis, or damage to muscle, bone, or supporting structures (e.g., tendon, joint capsule). Undermining and sinus tracts may also be associated with Stage IV ulcers.

Modified from Bergstrom N and others: *Treatment of pressure ulcers, clinical practice guideline*, No. 15. Rockville, MD, U.S. Department of Health and Human Services, Public Health Service, Agency for Health Care Policy and Research, AHCPR Publication No. 95-0652, December 1994.

Bony Prominences Vulnerable to Pressure

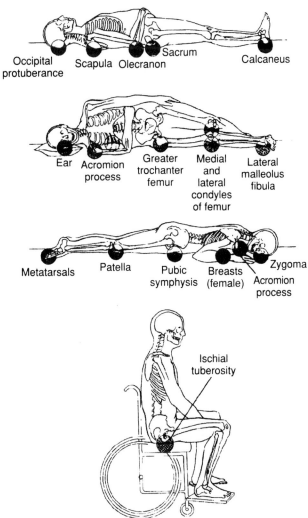

FIGURE 3-55 Bony prominences vulnerable to pressure. (From Forbes EJ, Fitzsimons VM: *The older adult: a process for wellness,* St Louis, 1981, Mosby.)

Types of Skin Lesions

Observed skin changes	Differentiation	Term	Example
Change in Color or Texture			
Spotting	Circumscription; flatness; color change	Macule	Freckle
Discoloration (red-purple)	Bleeding beneath the surface; injury to tissue	Contusion	Bruise
Soft whitening	Result of repeated wetting of skin	Maceration	Area between toes after soaking
Flaking	Dry cells of surface	Scale	Dandruff; psoriasis
Roughness from dried fluid	Dry exudate over lesions	Crust	*Eczema*; impetigo
Roughness from cells	Leathery thickening of outer skin layer	Lichenification	Callus on foot
Change in Shape			
Fluid-filled lesions	Clear fluid (less than 1 cm)	Vesicle	Blister; chickenpox
	Clear fluid (greater than 1 cm)	Bulla	Large blister; pemphigus
	Small, thick yellow fluid (pus)	Pustule	Acne
Solid mass, *cellular* growth	Less than 5 mm	Papule	Small mole; raised rash
	5 mm to 2 cm	Nodule	Enlarged lymph node
	Greater than 2 cm	Tumor	Benign or malignant tumor
	Excess connective tissue over scar	Keloid	Overgrown scar
Swelling of tissue	Generalized swelling; fluid between cells	Edema	Inflammation; swelling of feet
	Circumscribed surface edema; transient; some itching	Wheal ("hive")	Allergic reaction
Breaks in Skin Surfaces			
Oozing, scraped surface	Loss of superficial structure of skin	Abrasion	"Floor burn"; scrape
Scooped-out depression	Loss of deeper layers of skin	Ulcer	Decubitus or stasis ulcer
Superficial linear skin breaks	Scratch marks, frequently by fingernails	Excoriations	Scratches
Linear cracks or cleft	Slit or splitting of skin layers	Fissure	Athlete's foot
Jagged cut	Tearing of skin surface	Laceration	Accidental cut by blunt object
Linear cut, approximated edges	Cutting by sharp instrument	Incision	Knife cut
Vascular Lesions			
Small, flat, round, red-purple	Intradermal or submucous hemorrhage	Petechia	Bleeding tendency; vitamin C deficiency
Spiderlike, red, small	Dilation of capillaries, arterioles, or venules	Telangiectasis	Liver disease; vitamin B deficiency
Discolored, red-purple	Escape of blood into tissue	Ecchymosis	Trauma to blood vessels

Differences between Arterial, Diabetic, and Venous Ulcers

	Arterial	Diabetic	Venous
Location	• Lateral malleolus • Phalanges • Heels • Distal leg	• Bony prominences • Metatarsal heads • Plantar foot • Heel	• Medial malleolus • Bony prominences
Appearance	• Deepness • Even edges • Dryness • Grayness • Little granulation	• Deepness • Even edges • Drainage • Paleness • Little granulation	• Superficiality • Uneven edges • Drainage • Pinkness • Granulation
Pain	• Burning pain • Sharp pain • Acute pain	• No pain	• Moderate discomfort • Aching
Pulses	• Decreased or absent	• Normal	• Normal
Claudication	• Intermittent	• None	• None
Temperature	• Cool	• Warm or cold	• Warm
Other	• Skin atrophy • Extremity hair loss	• Peripheral neuropathy	• Extremity edema

Skin Lesion Measurement Guidelines
Measuring Wound Size
Length and width

- View wounds as clocks, with 12:00 being the patient's head.
- Measure the distance from 12:00 to 6:00 for length.
- Measure the distance from 9:00 to 3:00 for width.

Depth

- Insert a sterile, flexible, cotton-tipped applicator into the deepest part of the wound.
- Grab the applicator with the thumb and forefinger at the point level with the skin.
- Maintain the position of the thumb and forefinger as the applicator is withdrawn.
- Measure the distance from the thumb and forefinger to the tip of the applicator.

Adult Population

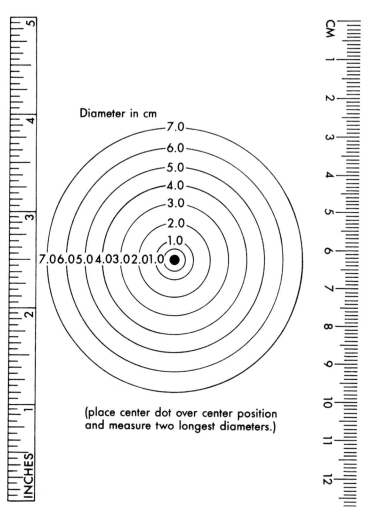

FIGURE 3-56 Transparent film. (From Stanhope M, Knollmueller RN: *Handbook of community and home health nursing: tools for assessment, intervention, and education,* ed 2, St Louis, 1996, Mosby.)

Tunnels

- Identify tunneling by inserting a sterile, flexible, cotton-tipped applicator into the wound and gently pushing outward beneath the wound border. Tunnels are present when the applicator meets no resistance.
- Document the locations of tunnels by viewing the wounds as clocks, with 12:00 being the patient's head.
- Gently insert a sterile, flexible, cotton-tipped applicator into the tunnel.
- Mark the applicator with the thumb and/or forefinger at the point level with the entrance to the tunnel.
- Maintain the position of the thumb and/or forefinger as the applicator is withdrawn.
- Measure the distance from the thumb and/or forefinger to the tip of the applicator.

Tracing Wounds

- Place sterilized, transparent film (Figure 3-56) over the surface of the wounds.
- Trace the outer perimeter of the wounds using a black felt-tipped pen.
- Wipe off the surface of the film that was in contact with the wound surface.
- Place the tracing in a sealed bag.
- Place clean, white paper over the sealed bag.
- Trace the outline of the wound onto the tracing paper.
- Retain the tracing paper in the medical record to use for future comparison.
- Dispose of the sealed bag containing the transparent film.

Positioning Guidelines
*Agency for Health Care Policy and Research (AHCPR) Guidelines for Pressure Ulcer Prevention and Treatment**

In bed

- Turn and reposition every 2 hours.
- Avoid positioning directly on bony prominences.
- Use pillows and foam wedges to prevent direct contact between bony prominences and to raise the heels off the bed.
- Maintain the head of the bed at the lowest degree of elevation.
- Limit the amount of time the head of the bed is elevated.
- Use pressure-reducing surfaces.
- Check for bottoming out beneath the mattress by placing your hand between the mattress and the bed. Less than 1 inch of support is inadequate.

Sitting

- Reposition every 15 minutes.
- Use pressure-reducing surfaces.
- Use pillows and foam wedges to prevent direct contact between bony prominences.

*This section modified from Bergstrom N and others: *Treatment of pressure ulcers,* Clinical Practice Guideline, No. 15, Rockville, MD, U.S. Department of Health and Human Services. Public Health Service, Agency for Health Care Policy and Research. AHCPR Publication No. 95-0652, December 1994.

Adult Population

Positioning Patients with Burns

Area of concern	Possible contracture development	Therapeutic position	Positioning strategy
Hip	• Internal rotation, flexion, and adduction	• Hip extension	• Pillows under buttocks in supine position • Trochanter rolls to maintain neutral rotation
Knee	• Flexion	• Knee extension	• Supine position with knees extended • Prone position with feet off end of bed • Sitting position with knees extended • Knee splints
Ankle	• Plantar flexion	• Neutral position	• Padded footboards • Ankle-positioning devices
Pectoral area	• Shoulder protraction	• Shoulder abduction and external rotation	• No pillows on bed
Chest	• Kyphosis	• Shoulder abduction and external rotation • Neutral hips	• No pillows under head or legs
Lateral trunk	• Scoliosis	• Affected arm abduction in supine position	• Pillows or towel rolls at sides
Anterior axilla	• Shoulder adduction and internal rotation	• Shoulder external rotation and 100 degrees abduction	• Arms suspended on IV poles, slings, or bedside tables
Posterior axilla	• Shoulder adduction and external rotation	• Shoulder flexion and 100 degrees abduction	• Arms suspended on IV poles, slings, or bedside tables
Elbow	• Flexion and pronation	• Elbow extension and supination	• Armboards • Elbow splints • Arm troughs
Anterior wrist	• Flexion	• 15 degrees extension	• Hand splints
Posterior wrist	• Extension	• 15 degrees flexion	• Hand splints
Fingers	• Extensor tendon adhesions • Loss of palmar grasp	• MCP flexion • IP flexion • Thumb abduction	• Hand splints
Anterior neck	• Flexion	• Extension	• No pillows • Towel rolls beneath shoulders
Posterior neck	• Extension	• Neutral position	• No pillows

IV, Intravenous; *MCP,* metacarpophalangeal; *IP,* interphalangeal.

Wound Dressing Guidelines
Wound Dressings

Types	Examples	Appropriate wounds	Absorptive properties	Debridement properties
Alginates	• Kaltostat • Sorbsan	• Stage 2-4 pressure ulcers • Partial-thickness wounds • Full-thickness wounds • Draining wounds • Tunneling wounds	• Yes	• Yes
Biosynthetics	• Biobrane	• Donor sites • Superficial and medium depth partial-thickness wounds	• No	• No
Collagens	• SkinTemp • Medifil	• Stage 3-4 pressure ulcers • Partial-thickness wounds • Full-thickness wounds • Burns • Donor sites • Venous ulcers • Surgical incisions	• Yes	• Yes
Composites	• Telfa adhesives • Tegaderm	• Stage 1-4 pressure ulcers • Partial-thickness wounds • Full-thickness wounds • Necrotic wounds • Draining wounds • Granulating wounds • Mixed wounds	• Yes	• Yes
Continuously moist saline gauze	• Nugauze • Steripad	• Stage 1-4 pressure ulcers • Partial-thickness wounds • Full-thickness wounds • Necrotic wounds • Draining wounds • Wounds with slough • Wounds with hard eschar • Tunneling wounds • Burns	• Yes	• No

Adult Population

Continued

Table—cont'd

Types	Examples	Appropriate wounds	Absorptive properties	Debridement properties
Hydrocolloids	• Tegasorb • Duoderm	• Stage 1-4 pressure ulcers • Partial-thickness wounds • Full-thickness wounds • Necrotic wounds • Draining wounds • Wounds with slough	• Yes	• Yes
Hydrogels	• Transorbent • CarraSorb	• Stage 1-4 pressure ulcers • Partial-thickness wounds • Full-thickness wounds • Necrotic wounds • Wounds with slough • Minor burns • Deep wounds	• Yes	• Yes
Impregnated gauze	• Xeroform • Mesalt	• Stage 1-4 pressure ulcers • Partial-thickness wounds • Full-thickness wounds • Necrotic wounds • Draining wounds • Wounds with slough • Wounds with hard eschar • Tunneling wounds • Burns	• No	• Yes
Semipermeable films	• Bioclusive • OpSite	• Stage 1 pressure ulcers • Partial-thickness wounds • Full-thickness wounds • Draining wounds • Wounds with slough • Burns	• No	• Yes

Table—cont'd

Types	Examples	Appropriate wounds	Absorptive properties	Debridement properties
Semipermeable foams	• Hydrasorb • Polyderm	• Stage 2-4 pressure ulcers • Partial-thickness wounds • Full-thickness wounds • Draining wounds • Wounds requiring packing	• Yes	• Yes
Wet to dry saline gauze	• Nugauze • Steripad	• Stage 1-4 pressure ulcers • Partial-thickness wounds • Full-thickness wounds • Necrotic wounds • Draining wounds • Wounds with slough • Wounds with hard eschar • Tunneling wounds • Burns	• Yes	• No
Wound fillers	• Hydragran • Bard absorptive dressing	• Stage 2-4 pressure ulcers • Partial-thickness wounds • Full-thickness wounds • Draining wounds • Wounds requiring packing	• Yes; depends on product	• Yes
Wraps	• Unna boot	• Stage 2-4 pressure ulcers	• No	• No

Topical Agents Guidelines
Topical Agents

Topical agents	Actions	Topical agents	Actions
Bacitracin	• Inhibits growth of microorganisms	Saline	• Moistens tissues without damaging cells
Dakin's solution	• Kills bacteria	Santyl	• Facilitates debridement
	• Facilitates debridement	Scarlet red	• Dries exudate
	• Cleans drainage		• Protects from environmental contamination
Debrisan	• Absorbs exudate		
Elase	• Facilitates debridement	Silvadene	• Inhibits microbial growth
Furacin	• Inhibits bacterial growth		• Soothes
	• Inhibits enzyme action	Silver nitrate	• Inhibits bacterial growth
Ganulex	• Stimulates blood flow		• Decreases pain
	• Facilitates debridement		• Decreases water loss
Garamycin	• Inhibits microbial growth		• Decreases odor
Neomycin	• Inhibits microbial growth	Sulfamylon	• Inhibits bacterial growth
Neosporin	• Inhibits growth of microorganisms		• Penetrates eschar
		Travase	• Facilitates debridement
Polysporin	• Inhibits growth of microorganisms	Xeroform	• Facilitates debridement
			• Protects donor sites
Proderm	• Stimulates blood flow		

Foot Care Guidelines
Guidelines for Foot Care for Patients with Diabetes

1. Inspect the feet daily for color changes, temperature changes, swelling, cuts, cracks, redness, blisters, or other signs of trauma; report changes immediately. (A mirror can be used to see the bottom of the feet.)
2. Wear well-fitting shoes and clean stockings when walking; never walk barefoot.
   a. Inspect the shoes, before putting them on, for foreign objects, nail points, or wrinkles.
   b. Ensure there is enough room in the shoes to allow the toes to wiggle easily.
   c. Break in new shoes gradually.
3. Bathe feet daily and dry them well, paying particular attention to the area between the toes.
4. Immediately after bathing, when the toenails are soft, cut (or have someone else cut) the nails straight across; smooth the cut nails with an emery board.
5. If the feet are dry, apply bland cream or petroleum jelly to the heels and feet (but not the toes).
6. Do not self-treat calluses, corns, or ingrown toenails; consult a podiatrist if these are present.
7. Ensure that the bath water is 30° to 32° C (84° to 90° F), and test it with a bath thermometer or elbow before immersing the feet.
8. Do not use heating pads and hot-water bottles; wear socks if the feet are cold.
9. Institute measures that increase circulation to the lower extremities, including the following:
   a. Avoid smoking.
   b. Avoid crossing legs when sitting.
   c. Protect extremities when exposed to cold.
   d. Avoid immersing feet in cold water.
   e. Use socks or stockings that do not apply pressure to the legs at specific sites.
   f. Institute an exercise regimen.
10. Do not walk or jog in the dark; have a light source.
11. Obtain proper shoes before jogging.

Modified from Stanhope M, Knollmueller RN: *Handbook of community and home health nursing,* ed 2, St Louis, 1996, Mosby.

Risk Categories and Associated Footwear Guidelines

	Clinical findings	Footwear changes
Category 0	Has protective sensation	Education on proper footwear
Category 1	Has lost protective sensation	Addition of soft insole to shoe of proper contour and fitting
Category 2	Has lost protective sensation and has foot deformity	Depth footwear or custom shoe for severe deformity, molded insoles
Category 3	Has lost protective sensation and has history of foot ulcer	Inspection of type and condition of footwear and insoles at every visit

Modified from Stanhope M, Knollmueller RN: *Handbook of community and home health nursing,* ed 2, St Louis, 1996, Mosby.

Residual Limb Management Guidelines
Bandaging the Residual Limb

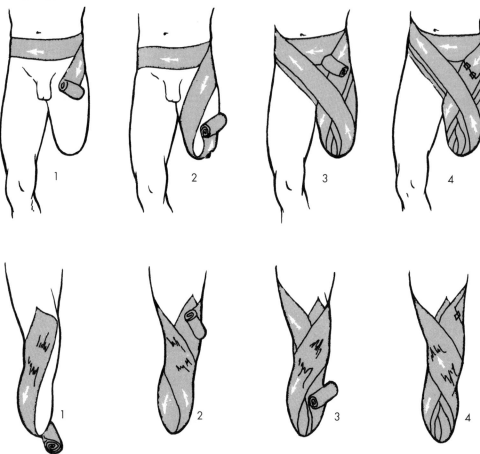

FIGURE 3-57 Bandaging the residual limb (From Christensen BL, Kockrow EO: *Foundations of nursing,* ed 2, St Louis, 1995, Mosby.)

ADULT CARDIOPULMONARY EVALUATION

With the advent of new technology and medical procedures, home care agencies provide more services for patients who previously would have required hospitalization. Many of these patients need effective management of cardiac and/or respiratory conditions. Home care therapists are integral components of this effective management of patients who have cardiopulmonary problems as primary or secondary diagnoses. To set the objective, form realistic goals, and implement safe and effective treatment interventions, therapists must understand not only various methods for assessing the cardiopulmonary status of patients, but also identify abnormalities that signal serious problems.

Cardiopulmonary Assessments
Metabolic Equivalent System

The metabolic equivalent (MET) system measures the amount of oxygen needed to perform activities. One MET is equal to 3.5 ml of oxygen per kilogram of body weight per minute and is about equivalent to the amount of oxygen necessary at rest. Total METs range from 1 to 10 or more. Higher METs denote increased oxygen requirements.

MET System Form

Metabolic equivalents	Activities	Metabolic equivalents	Activities
One MET	• Resting in bed • Sitting • Eating • Reading • Sewing • Watching television	**Two to three METs—cont'd**	• Fishing • Bowling • Golfing (with motorized cart) • Operating a motorboat • Riding horseback (at a walk)
One to two METs	• Dressing • Shaving • Brushing teeth • Washing at sink • Making a bed • Working at a desk • Driving a car • Playing cards • Knitting • Typing • Walking 1 mph on level surfaces	**Three to four METs**	• Performing general housework • Cleaning windows • Gardening (light) • Pushing a light power mower • Having sexual intercourse • Performing assembly-line work • Driving a large truck • Laying bricks • Plastering • Walking 3 mph • Bicycling 6 mph • Sailing • Golfing (with a hand cart) • Pitching horseshoes • Participating in archery • Playing badminton (doubles) • Riding horseback (at a slow trot) • Fly-fishing
Two to three METs	• Bathing in a tub • Cooking • Waxing a floor • Riding a power lawn mower • Playing a piano • Driving a small truck • Using hand tools • Repairing a car • Walking 2 mph on level surfaces • Bicycling 5 mph on level surfaces • Playing pool		

Adult Population

Continued

Table—cont'd

Metabolic equivalents	Activities	Metabolic equivalents	Activities
Four to five METs	• Performing heavy housework • Gardening (heavy) • Doing home repairs • Raking leaves • Painting • Doing masonry • Paperhanging • Doing calisthenics • Playing table tennis • Golfing (carrying bag) • Playing tennis (doubles) • Dancing • Swimming (slow)	**Six to seven METs**	• Shoveling snow • Splitting wood • Mowing lawn with a hand mower • Walking or jogging 5 mph • Bicycling 11 mph • Playing tennis (singles) • Water skiing • Skiing (light downhill)
Five to six METs	• Sawing softwood • Digging a garden • Shoveling light loads • Using heavy tools • Lifting 50 pounds • Walking 4 mph • Bicycling 10 mph • Skating • Fishing with waders • Hiking • Hunting • Square dancing • Riding horseback (at a brisk trot)	**Seven to eight METs**	• Sawing hardwood • Digging ditches • Lifting 80 pounds • Moving heavy furniture • Playing paddleball • Playing touch football • Swimming (backstroke) • Playing basketball • Playing ice hockey
		Eight to nine METs	• Lifting 100 pounds • Running 5.5 mph • Bicycling 13 mph • Swimming (breast stroke) • Playing handball (noncompetitive) • Skiing (cross-country) • Fencing
		Ten or more METs	• Running 6 mph or faster • Playing handball (competitive) • Playing squash (competitive) • Doing gymnastics • Playing football (contact)

The Simple Walk Test*

The Simple Walk Test evaluates exercise capacity. The patient walks 600 feet as rapidly as possible. The therapist times the duration of the walk and monitors the patient's pulse at the end of the walk. The therapist uses the peak heart rate during the walk test to determine the target heart rate when prescribing exercise.

The 6-Minute Walk Test**

The 6-Minute Walk Test assesses exercise capacity. The patient walks for 6 minutes as quickly as possible, and the therapist monitors the distance walked and the pulse rate. Longer distances denote improved exercise tolerance. The heart rate during the 6-Minute Walk Test assists in determining the target heart rate for exercise.

Borg Scale of Ratings of Perceived Exertion

The Borg Scale of Ratings of Perceived Exertion quantifies the patient's impressions of dyspnea at rest and during activities. The patient rates exertion levels from "very, very light" to "very, very hard." The total score ranges from 6 to 20. Higher scores denote perception of increased exertion.

Borg Scale of Ratings of Perceived Exertion Form

6	
7	Very, very light
8	
9	Very light
10	
11	Fairly light
12	
13	Somewhat light
14	
15	Hard
16	
17	Very hard
18	
19	Very, very hard
20	

From Borg GV: Psychophysical bases of perceived exertion, *Med Sci Sports Exercise* 14(5):377, 1982.

*Oh-Park M and others: A simple walk test to guide exercise programming of the elderly, *Am J Phys Med Rehabil* 76(3):208-212, 1997.
**Lipkin DP and others: Six minute walking test for assessing exercise capacity in chronic heart failure, *Br M J* 292:653-655, 1986.

Adult Population

Cardiopulmonary Standards
Cardiac Rhythms

ECG characteristics	Etiology	Treatment
Normal Sinus Rhythm (NSR, RSR, SR)		
P waves are present and regular. The QRS is constant and regular. Each P wave is followed by a QRS. The PR interval is 0.12 to 0.20. The QRS duration is 0.04 to 0.11. The ventricular rate is 60 to 100.	The impulse originates in the SA node and follows the normal conduction pathways for depolarization. The SA node readily responds to autonomic stimuli; *parasympathetic* (cholinergic) slows, whereas *sympathetic* (adrenergic) speeds the rate of discharge.	No treatment occurs. The significance of normal sinus rhythm is optimal cardiac output.
Sinus Arrest		
The underlying rhythm is sinus. Long "pauses" with no cardiac rhythm are noted. Three or more beats must be missing. The PR interval of the underlying rhythm is 0.12 to 0.20. P waves are followed by a QRS complex. The QRS duration is 0.04 to 0.11.	The SA node fails to initiate an impulse. Back-up pacemakers also fail to respond. Causes include the following: Sudden surge of parasympathetic activity: • Fear (rare) • Carotid sinus pressure • Pharyngeal stimulation Organic disease of the SA node and latent pacemaker: • Infarction • Sick sinus syndrome • Inflammation • Rheumatic process	Sinus arrest should be treated as an emergency. The patient status should be assessed. The source of vagal stimulus should be removed, if applicable. Atropine should be given. If it is an organic disease, the patient is a candidate for a permanent pacemaker. The significance of sinus arrest is *no* cardiac output during periods of arrest.

Modified from Irwin S, Tecklin J: *Cardiopulmonary physical therapy*, ed 3, St Louis, 1995, Mosby.
ECG, Electrocardiogram; *NSR*, normal sinus rhythm; *RSR*, regular sinus rhythm; *SR*, sinus rhythm; *SA*, sinoartrial.

Table—cont'd

ECG characteristics	Etiology	Treatment

SA Exit Block (SA Block)

The underlying rhythm is sinus. An occasional "pause" is noted. One whole complex is missing—P, QRS, T. The recorded rhythm should map out to exactly one missing cycle. The PR interval of the underlying rhythm is 0.12 to 0.20. P waves are always followed by QRS. The QRS duration is 0.04 to 0.11.

An impulse does not emerge from the SA node. The pause lasts for just one cycle or beat. Causes include the following:
- Increased vagal tone
- Carotid sinus sensitivity
- Acute infection (rare)
- Increased levels of digoxin (common), quinidine, salicylates
- Coronary artery disease

Potassium intoxication occurs.

The underlying cause should be treated, if possible. SA exit block is a rare phenomenon. The source of vagal stimulation should be removed (i.e., tight clothing around the neck). Digoxin or other drugs should be held. Atropine may be given. (rare) A permanent pacemaker may be considered (rare). The significance of SA exit block is that there is rarely any compromise to cardiac output.

Sinus with Premature Atrial Contractions (PACs)

The underlying rhythm is sinus. Normal complexes have one P wave configuration and one QRS configuration. The sinus PR intervals are 0.12 to 0.20. The QRS duration is 0.04 to 0.11. *Early beat occurs:* The P wave is present but with a different configuration. (The PR interval of the early beat differs from the sinus beats.) There may be multifocal PACs with variable P wave morphologies. The P wave of the early beat may be "buried" in the T wave. Often, a compensatory pause follows a PAC.

Ectopic or irritable focus in the atria (right or left) causes atrial firing. Causes include the following:
- Emotional stress
- Caffeine, nicotine
- Myocardial ischemia
- CAD
- Renal disease
- Rheumatic disease
- Hypoxemia
- Infection
- Hyperthyroidism

No intervention is required (if infrequent). Quinidine may be given. A small dose of beta blockers may be given. Digoxin may be given (if it is an organic disease). Frequent PACs may lead to SVT or atrial fibrillation. The significance of PACs is that it rarely compromises cardiac output.

CAD, Coronary artery disease; *SVT,* supraventricular tachycardia.

Continued

Adult Population

Table—cont'd

ECG characteristics	Etiology	Treatment

Wandering Atrial Pacemaker (WAPM)

The rhythm is not sinus in origin.

P waves are present, but vary in configuration.

The QRS follows each P wave.

PR intervals may vary; R to R varies.

Wandering rhythm most often appear in groups of one P wave configuration followed by three to four beats with a different P wave (type 1).

Each P wave may look different (type 2).

The QRS duration is 0.04 to 0.11.

The ventricular rate is less than 100.

Irritable foci initiate the impulse in the atria, but at a normal rate of discharge, and control wanders. This may be caused by increased vagal tone.

Control may also pass from the atria to the AV node.

Wandering rhythm occurs in the following:
• Advanced age
• Adolescence

Aberrancy may be abolished by increasing the heart rate.

WAPM generally requires no treatment.

The significance of WAPM is that it does not compromise cardiac output.

Nonconducted PACs (Blocked PACs)

The underlying rhythm is sinus.

Normal complexes have one P wave configuration and one QRS configuration.

Sinus PR intervals are 0.12 to 0.20.

The QRS duration is 0.04 to 0.11.

Early beat occurs:

The P wave is present, but with a different configuration.

There is no QRS.

The P wave may be buried in the T wave.

There is a compensatory pause.

A premature beat originates in the atria, but the impulse arrives when the ventricles are still refractory. Therefore the atria contract, but not the ventricles (absolute refractory period).

Blocked PACs occur as a benign process in the following patients:
• Patients with renal disease
• Patients with ischemic heart disease

Intervention is not required.

Rhythm occurs rarely.

The significance of blocked PACs is that there is generally no compromise to cardiac output.

Modified from Irwin S, Tecklin J: *Cardiopulmonary physical therapy,* ed 3, St Louis, 1995, Mosby.
AV, Atrioventricular.

Table—cont'd

ECG characteristics	Etiology	Treatment
Atrial Flutter (A. Flutter)		
The rhythm is not sinus in origin. P waves are present as "F" waves, or flutter waves that have a characteristic "sawtooth" pattern. There is AV block, and conduction ratios are recorded as 2:1, 3:1, and up to 8:1. The atrial firing rate is 250 to 350. The atrial wave often dominates the T wave. The QRS duration is 0.04 to 0.11.	The ectopic focus in the atria gains control, and the depolarization impulse originates there. The rate of discharge is rapid. Causes include the following: • Advanced age • CAD • Rheumatic heart disease • Hyperthyroidism • Constrictive pericarditis • Cor pulmonale • Infection • Hypoxemia • Exercise; stress • Myocardial infarction • Drug use (digoxin, epinephrine, quinidine) • Renal failure	Medications include the following: • Digoxin • Quinidine • Beta blockers • Calcium-channel blockers Cardioversion is 10 to 50 WS. Temporary atrial pacing is used to override the irritable focus. A. flutter may lead to atrial fibrillation. A. flutter occurs commonly. The significance of A. flutter is that there is usually no compromise to cardiac output except when it is too rapid or too slow.
Paroxysmal Atrial Tachycardia (PAT)		
The rhythm is not sinus in origin. The rapid rate rhythm is most often 160 to 250. P waves may be present but are often buried in the T wave and not visible. The QRS duration is 0.04 to 0.11, unless there is aberration. The rhythm starts and stops abruptly; it lasts less than 24 hours. ST elevation or depression is frequently noted. PAT is one of two forms of SVT.	PAT is a result of repetitive firing of a single atrial focus or circus reentry. Causes include the following: • Pulmonary emboli • Emotional factors • Overexertion • Hypokalemia • Caffeine, nicotine • Aspirin sensitivity • Rheumatic heart disease • Hyperventilation • Hypertension If PAT lasts longer than 24 hours, it is called *sustained atrial tachycardia.* Frequent PACs may induce PAT.	The underlying cause should be treated. If digoxin is toxic, digoxin use should be stopped. The carotid sinus should be massaged. The valsalva maneuver should be used. Gagging and coughing occur. Atrial pacing occurs (rare). Cardioversion occurs (rare). Medications include the following: • Digoxin • Verapamil • Quinidine • Pronestyl • Beta blocker Short bursts are fairly common. The significance of PAT is that, if the condition is prolonged, cardiac output is compromised, even with a healthy heart.

ST, Sinus tachycardia; *WS*, wave segment.

Adult Population

Continued

Table—cont'd

ECG characteristics	Etiology	Treatment
Atrial Fibrillation (A. fib)		
The rhythm is not sinus in origin. P waves are absent. "F" waves are absent and are replaced by a "wavy" or flat baseline. The atrial rate is 350 or more. The hallmark of this rhythm is *irregular.* The QRS duration is 0.04 to 0.11.	Ectopic focus in the atria gains control, and the depolarization impulse originates there. The rate of discharge is extremely rapid. The atria no longer contract. Causes include the following: • Rheumatic heart disease • Hypertension • Thyrotoxicosis • Stress, pain • CAD • Renal failure • Infection • Hypoglycemia • CHF • Pericarditis • Cardiomyopathy • Illegal drug use • Digoxin toxicity	Medications include the following: • Digoxin • Verapamil • Quinidine Cardioversion occurs (occasionally). The underlying cause should be treated. Mural thrombi may develop and lead to emboli; anticoagulants may be needed. About 30% of all patients with A-fib develop emboli— pulmonary or systemic. There is a common rhythm. The significance of A. fib is that cardiac output is generally intact. A compromise occurs if the rate is too fast or too slow.
Atrial Tachycardia with AV Block (PAT with Block)		
The rhythm is not sinus in origin. The P waves are present. The rhythm may be regular. P wave morphology is abnormal (focus is atrial). AV block exists. QRS may not follow a P wave. The ventricular rate is 75 to 200. *There are isoelectric intervals between the P waves.* The ventricular response may be regular or irregular. The QRS duration is 0.04 to 0.11.	The ectopic atrial focus has a slower discharge rate. A block is created when ventricles are unable to respond. Causes include the following: • Digoxin toxicity (50% to 70% of the patients with this rhythm) • Significant organic disease (cor pulmonale)	Digoxin should be discontinued, if toxic. If the patient is not taking digoxin, the drug should be given. After digitalization, the patient may require quinidine or pronestyl. For rapid rates, cardioversion may be done or verapamil may be used. Inderal may be used up to a total of 3 mg. PAT with block occurs rarely. The significance of PAT with block is that with block, the rate is generally in a normal range, so cardiac output is maintained.

Modified from Irwin S, Tecklin J: *Cardiopulmonary physical therapy,* ed 3, St Louis, 1995, Mosby.
CHF, Congestive heart failure.

Table—cont'd

ECG characteristics	Etiology	Treatment

Multifocal Atrial Tachycardia (MAT)

The rhythm is not sinus in origin.
P waves have variable morphology.
P waves may be followed by a QRS.
The PR interval varies.
The P to P interval varies.
The atrial rate is 100 to 250.
The QRS duration is generally 0.04 to 0.11.
The R to R interval varies.

Multiple irritable foci are in the atria at a moderate to rapid rate of discharge. Ventricles respond when possible, hence irregularity.
Causes include the following:
- Severe pulmonary disease with coexisting hypoxemia
- Hypokalemia
- Pulmonary hypertension
- Altered pH

There is usually no treatment.
The same treatment may be required as for PAT if the rate is extremely rapid.
MAT commonly occurs in patients with COPD.
The significance of MAT is that if the rate is too rapid, cardiac output may be compromised.

Junctional Rhythm*

The underlying rhythm is *not* sinus.
The QRS has a normal configuration and duration of 0.04 to 0.11.
The ventricular rate is 40 to 60.
The rhythm is *regular.*
There are three presentations.
Each QRS is preceded by an *inverted* P wave with a short PR interval (less than 0.12).
No P waves are present.
There is a retrograde P wave.

The impulse originates at the site of the AV junction (sinus node usurped).
Junctional rhythm is considered an escape rhythm.
Causes include the following:
- Sinus node disease
- Increased vagal tone
- Digoxin
- Inferior MI
- Possible normality on a temporary basis

The underlying cause should be treated, if possible.
The patient may need a pacemaker if cardiac output is compromised.
Atropine may be used, but isuprel is more effective.
Junctional rhythm occurs commonly.
The significance of junctional rhythm is that cardiac output usually is not compromised, except when the rate is less than 50.

Sinus Rhythm with Premature Junctional Contractions (PJCs)

The underlying rhythm is sinus in origin.
Normal complexes have one P wave configuration and one QRS configuration.
The sinus PR intervals are 0.12 to 0.20.
The QRS duration is 0.04 to 0.11.
Early beat occurs.
The early beat may have three presentations:
- Short PR interval (less than 0.12; inverted)
- Absent P wave
- Retrograde P wave

The AV node becomes irritated and initiates an impulse, thus causing an early beat.
Causes include the following:
- Carotid sinus pressure
- Digoxin on board
- CAD
- Rheumatic heart disease

Generally, no treatment is required.
Quinidine and pronestyl can be given.
PJCs is common with cardiac disease.
The significance of PJCs is that cardiac output generally is intact.

---

*Junctional rhythms with rates of 60 to 100 are referred to as *accelerated junctional rhythms.*
MI, Myocardial infarction; *COPD,* chronic obstructive pulmonary disease.

Continued

Adult Population

Table—cont'd

ECG characteristics	Etiology	Treatment
Junctional Tachycardia		
The underlying rhythm is *not* sinus.	An impulse arises in the AV junctional tissue with an accelerated rate of discharge.	The underlying cause should be treated.
The QRS has a normal configuration and duration of 0.04 to 0.11.	Junctional tachycardia may be paroxysmal or nonparoxysmal.	If junctional tachycardia is not digoxin toxic, junctional tachycardia should be digitalized.
The ventricular rate is 100 to 180.	Causes include the following:	Vagal stimulation should be done (cough, gag, ice water).
The rhythm is usually regular.	• *Paroxysmal:* hyperventilation, myocardial infarction, pulmonary emboli, rheumatic heart disease, hypertension, emotional factors, overexertion, caffeine, nicotine	Cardioversion should be done (if patient compromised).
There are three presentations. Each QRS is preceded by a P wave with a short PR interval (less than 0.12) that is *usually* inverted.		Verapamil and inderal should be given.
No P waves are present.		
A retrograde P wave is present.	• *Nonparoxysmal:* digoxin toxicity, after heart surgery, acute myocarditis	The significance of junctional tachycardia is that cardiac output is compromised when the rate is rapid.
Sinus Rhythm with Premature Ventricular Contractions (PVCs)		
The underlying rhythm is sinus (occasionally junctional or atrial).	Impulses arise from single or multiple foci in the ventricles or Purkinje fibers.	The therapist should know the patient—if chronic PVCs are present, they should be observed.
The PR interval is 0.12 to 0.20 for the sinus rhythm.	Causes include the following:	O_2 should be administered.
The QRS duration is 0.04 to 0.11 for the sinus rhythm.	• *Ischemia*	The underlying cause should be treated, if possible (give potassium supplements, hold digoxin).
An early beat occurs.	• Cardiac disease	
The early beat is wide and bizarre.	• Electrolyte imbalance (hypokalemia or hyperkalemia)	A lidocaine IV bolus and drip should be started.
The QRS duration of the early beat is greater than 0.11.	• Digoxin toxicity	A pronestyl IV bolus and drip should be started.
The P wave is absent.	• Quinidine or pronestyl toxicity	Oral antidysrhythmics should be given (quinidine, pronestyl, mexitil, enkaid, tambocor, tonocard, calan, amiodarone).
The ST segment often slopes in the opposite direction of the normal complexes.	• Caffeine, nicotine	
	• Stress, overexertion	
	• Acute MI	
PVCs are generally followed by a compensatory pause.	• Irritation from insertion of a pacer or hemodynamic catheter	PVCs may be benign.
If every other beat is a PVC, the rhythm is termed *bigeminal.*	• Overdistention of ventricular tissue (CHF, cardiomyopathy)	The significance of PVCs is that there is an increase in the number of PVCs and a positive cardiac history requires close monitoring: cardiac functioning may decrease.
If every third beat is a PVC, the rhythm is termed *trigeminal.*	• Chronic lung disease	

Modified from Irwin S, Tecklin J: *Cardiopulmonary physical therapy,* ed 3, St Louis, 1995, Mosby.

Table—cont'd

ECG characteristics	Etiology	Treatment

Sinus Rhythm with Premature Ventricular Contractions (PVCs)—cont'd

If every fourth beat is a PVC, the rhythm is termed *quadrigeminal.*

If PVC complexes differ in appearance, they are called *multifocal* or *multiformed.*

If each PVC looks alike, the term is *unifocal* or *uniformed.*

If three or more consecutive PVCs appear in a row at a rate above 100, they are called *V-tach,* a *salvo,* or a *triplet.*

If two PVCs appear in a row, they are called *couplets.*

If a PVC occurs at the same place in each cycle, it is called *fixed.*

If a PVC migrates in the cycle, it is called *nonfixed.*

If a PVC falls between two sinus beats that are separated by a normal R to R interval, the PVC is described as *interpolated.*

Ventricular Tachycardia (V-tach)

ECG characteristics	Etiology	Treatment
The underlying rhythm is not sinus. The ventricular rate is 100 to 250. The P wave is absent. The QRS is wide and bizarre.	Rapid firing occurs by a single ventricular focus with enhanced automaticity. Causes include the following: • Ischemia • Fresh (acute) MI • Electrolyte imbalance (hypokalemia or hyperkalemia) Cardiac disease occurs. CHF and cardiomyopathy occur. Irritation from intracardiac catheters occurs. Toxicities include digoxin, pronestyl, quinidine, and enkaid. Is idiopathic.	A lidocaine IV and bolus should be started. A pronestyl IV and bolus should be started. O_2 should be administered. Cardioversion and defibrillation should be done. Oral drugs should be given (quinidine, Pronestyl, mexitil, enkaid, tambocor, tonocard, amiodarone). The significance of V-tach is that V-tach with a rate less than 140 may allow for adequate cardiac output; higher rates compromise cardiac output and cause loss of consciousness.

ECG characteristics	Etiology	Treatment

Bidirectional V-tach

The underlying rhythm is not sinus.

The rhythm is ventricular in origin.

The ventricular rate is 100 to 250.

Ventricular complexes alternate in polarity, positive to negative.

The etiology may also be two ectopic foci in the ventricles.

Sometimes bidirectional V-tach is associated with digoxin toxicity—prognosis poor.

Treatment is conventional for V-tach (lidocaine, pronestyl).

Cardioversion should be done.

The significance of bidirectional V-tach is inadequate cardiac output, which may herald the impending loss of function.

V-Tach: Torsade de Pointes

The underlying rhythm is not sinus.

The rhythm is ventricular in origin.

The ventricular rate is 100 to 250.

Torsade de Pointes is called *twisting of the points.*

The polarity pattern swings from positive to negative.

Torsade de Pointes often converts to v-fib.

Class I antidysrhythmics may be dangerous (lidocaine, pronestyl).

Isuprel may be ordered.

Cardioversion should be done.

The significance of torsade de pointes is inadequate cardiac output, which may lead to no cardiac output.

Ventricular Fibrillation (v-fib)

The underlying rhythm is not sinus.

Essentially no QRS complexes are noted.

A bizarre, erratic electrical activity is noted.

Usually "fine" v-fib or "coarse" v-fib occurs.

Random, asynchronous ventricular electrical activity occurs.

V-fib results in the ventricular muscle merely quivering.

There is no cardiac output.

Causes include the following:
- Digoxin and quinidine toxicity
- Cardiac disease
- Acute MI
- Electrocution
- Hyperkalemia
- Hypothermia

This is considered a medical emergency.

CPR should be given.

Most importantly, defibrillation should be done as quickly as possible.

Epinephrine should be given.

Lidocaine, bretylol, or pronestyl should be given.

Oxygenation should be done.

The significance of V-fib is *no* cardiac output and no tissue perfusion.

Idioventricular Rhythm, or "Dying Heart"

The underlying rhythm is not sinus.

The rhythm is ventricular in origin. The QRS is wide and bizarre.

The ventricular rate is 20 to 40.

Complexes may be multifocal.

The impulse originates in the ventricles because of loss of other (primary) pacers.

There is a last-ditch effort to provide cardiac output.

This is an emergency that requires CPR.

Epinephrine should be given.

A temporary pacemaker may be attempted.

The significance of idioventricular rhythm is that cardiac output is compromised, with a highly unfavorable prognosis.

Modified from Irwin S, Tecklin J: *Cardiopulmonary physical therapy,* ed 3, St Louis, 1995, Mosby.
CPR, Cardiopulmonary resuscitation.

ECG characteristics	Etiology	Treatment

Accelerated Idioventricular Rhythm (AIR)

The underlying rhythm is not sinus.

The rhythm is ventricular in origin. The QRS duration is greater than 0.12.

The rhythm is generally regular.

The rate is 50 to 100.

The impulse originates in the ventricles; the rate is more controlled, and therefore adequate cardiac output occurs.

Often there is a reperfusion phenomenon.

AIR is considered benign; it generally does not lead to more lethal dysrhythmias.

Generally none; observe for v-tach

If the rate is too slow and the patient is symptomatic, the SA node should be stimulated with atropine.

The significance of AIR is that adequate cardiac output is generally provided.

Ventricular Standstill

The rhythm is initially sinus.

There is a sudden cessation of the QRS wave.

P waves are present and regular.

The lower pacemakers and conductile tissue fail. The SA node is intact. The impulse does not reach the ventricles.

Essentially no cardiac output occurs.

Causes include the following:
- Acute MI
- Ventricular rupture
- Possible occurrence with CHB

This is a medical emergency.

CPR should be given.

Epinephrine should be given.

Isuprel should be given.

A pacemaker should be inserted.

The significance of ventricular standstill is atrial contraction with no ventricular contraction, hence no cardiac output.

Cardiac Phenomenon: Electromechanical Dissociation (EMD) (or Pulseless Electrical Activity (PEA))

The underlying rhythm may appear to be junctional or sinus.

Criteria are met for these rhythms (i.e., rate and intervals as would be expected).

No palpable pulses or BP may be measured or recorded.

The conduction system remains intact.

The cardiac muscle is badly damaged and is unable to respond to the impulse.

There is no cardiac output.

Causes include the following:
- Acute MI
- Ventricular rupture
- Hypothermia
- Hypoxemia
- Acidosis
- Pulmonary emboli
- Cardiac tamponade
- Tension pneumothorax
- Sepsis

This is a medical emergency.

CPR should be given.

Epinephrine should be given.

Occasionally, isuprel should be given.

A pacemaker-aid (transcutaneous pacemaker) should be inserted.

The therapist must know the patient and practice sound assessment skills.

The significance of PEA is nonviable rhythm.

The condition is generally irreversible.

Adult Population

BP, Blood pressure; *CHB,* complete heart block.

Continued

Table—cont'd

ECG characteristics	Etiology	Treatment

Ventricular Fusion (Summation Beats)

The underlying rhythm is often sinus.

The PR interval is 0.12 to 0.20. The QRS duration is 0.04 to 0.11.

There will be PVCs.

There is a "fusion"; the beat takes on the appearance of the PVC and the normal beat.

Ventricles are partly activated by a descending atrial impulse and partly by an ascending ectopic ventricular focus.

This condition is seen most often when PVCs occur late in a cycle.

This condition is common with the following:
- Accelerated idioventricular rhythm
- Pacemakers: permanent and temporary

There is no treatment.

The condition is benign.

The significance of summation beats is that the cardiac output is intact.

Asystole

There is no underlying rhythm.

P, QRS, and T waves are absent.

asystole may occur abruptly.

All pacers fail to initiate an impulse.

There is no cardiac output.

Causes include the following:
- Conduction system failure
- Acute MI
- Ventricular rupture

This is a medical emergency.

CPR should be given.

Epinephrine should be given.

Isuprel should be given.

A pacemaker should be inserted.

The significance of asystole is no cardiac output.

Sinus Rhythm with First-Degree Heart Block (First-Degree AVB)

The underlying rhythm is sinus.

The QRS duration is 0.04 to 0.11.

The P wave is present and with normal configuration.

There is a P wave preceding every QRS.

The PR interval is *lengthened* and is greater than 0.20 (generally does not exceed 0.40).

The impulse from the SA node is delayed on the way to the AV tissue or in the AV tissue, and the AV conduction time is prolonged.

Causes include the following:
- CAD
- Rheumatic heart disease
- Myocardial infarction
- Digoxin
- Beta blockers

Usually no treatment is given.

Digoxin or beta blockers should be held if indicated.

First-degree AVB may lead to higher degree of block.

The significance of first-degree AVB is that the cardiac output is intact.

Modified from Irwin S, Tecklin J: *Cardiopulmonary physical therapy*, ed 3, St Louis, 1995, Mosby.
AVB, Atrioventricular block.

Table—cont'd

ECG characteristics	Etiology	Treatment

Second-Degree Heart Block, Type I (Mobitz I; Wenckebach)

The underlying rhythm is sinus, but there is intermittent AV block.

Initially a P wave precedes each QRS.

The QRS is normal in configuration, and the duration is 0.04 to 0.11.

The PR interval begins to *lengthen.*

As the PR interval increases, a *QRS is dropped* (P wave occurs, but no QRS).

This occurs in a repetitive cyclic manner.

Cycles vary (i.e., two Ps, one QRS drop, or three Ps, one QRS drop).

The pattern is characteristic and is referred to as *footprints of Wenckebach.*

The block occurs high in the AV junction.

Second-degree heart block, Type I is a benign, transient disturbance.

Second-degree heart block, Type I rarely progresses to higher forms of block.

Causes include the following:
• Inferior MI
• Rheumatic heart disease
• Digoxin toxicity
• Beta blockers
• CAD

No intervention is necessary if cardiac output is uncompromised.

Atropine or isuprel can be given.

Rarely a pacemaker is inserted.

The significance of second-degree heart block, Type I is transient rhythm; the cardiac output is most often intact.

Second-Degree Heart Block, Type II (Mobitz II)

There is an intermittent underlying sinus rhythm.

The ratio of P waves to QRS is altered; there may be two, three, or four P waves to every one QRS.

The atrial rate is regular, and the P to P interval can be measured.

The QRS rate is usually regular, and R to R intervals can be measured.

The QRS duration is 0.04 to 0.11.

Every time a P wave precedes a QRS, the PR interval remains the same.

The site of the block is usually below the bundle of His and is a periodic bilateral bundle branch block.

Second-degree heart block, Type II occurs with the following:
• MIs, especially those involving the LAD
• CAD
• Rheumatic heart disease
• Digoxin toxicity

With MI, a prophylactic pacemaker can be inserted.

If the patient is symptomatic, atropine should be given.

Second-degree heart block, Type II may progress to CHB.

The significance of second-degree heart block, Type II is adequate cardiac output if the ratio is 2:1. There is a potential for compromise if the ratio is 4:1 and the rhythm is continuous.

LAD, Left anterior descending artery.

Continued

Table—cont'd

ECG characteristics	Etiology	Treatment

Complete Heart Block (CHB); Third-Degree Heart Block

The underlying rhythm is not sinus. P waves are present, regular, and of uniform configuration, but have *no relationship with regard to the QRS.* QRS complexes are regular, and the R to R can be measured. The rate depends on the site of the latent pacemaker. The *junctional*-QRS is normal in appearance, and the duration is 0.04 to 0.11 (rate 40 to 60). The *ventricular*-QRS is wide. Occasionally bizarre, the QRS duration is greater than 0.12 (rate 20 to 40).	Complete block occurs in the conduction system in which no supraventricular impulses are conducted to the ventricles. Latent pacemakers respond (the AV node or the ventricles). Each system is independent (atria and ventricles). Causes include the following: • CAD • Rheumatic heart disease • Acute MI • Degenerative disease of the conduction system	The site of the block should be determined (junctional or ventricular). The patient's status should be assessed. Atropine or isuprel can be used. A pacemaker should be inserted. If the patient is unconscious, CPR should be initiated. The significance of third-degree heart block is that CHB with junctional escape is not usually compromised; CHB with ventricular escape may be a medical emergency.

Modified from Irwin S, Tecklin J: *Cardiopulmonary physical therapy,* ed 3, St Louis, 1995, Mosby.

Table—cont'd

ECG characteristics	Etiology	Treatment
Aberrant Ventricular Conduction (Aberrancy)		
The underlying rhythm is usually sinus. Usually a P wave is present. If there is a P wave, it is followed by a wide QRS (greater than 0.12). The initial QRS deflection is the same as for the normal beat. Many aberrant rhythms have an RSR pattern. Three forms exist.	Temporary abnormal intraventricular conduction of supraventricular impulses occurs. The impulse arrives early so that some portions of the bundle branches remain refractory; conduction is aberrant, through an abnormal pathway, or down the opposite branch. Impulse is not dependent on refractoriness; impulse is caused by anomalous conduction down the ventricles (Mahaim tract). Late aberrancy occurs (spontaneous depolarization of one fascicle).	No treatment is given. Aberrancy should be treated as PVCs. The condition is common and benign. The significance of aberrancy is that generally no compromise of cardiac output occurs.
Sinus Rhythm with Intraventricular Conduction Delay (IVCD)		
The underlying rhythm is sinus. The PR interval is 0.12 to 0.20. The QRS duration is greater than 0.11. The rhythm is regular.	Bundle branch block exists. Differentiation of right or left IVCD is not possible on a single lead system. 12-lead ECG confirms the origin of block. Causes include the following: • CAD • Post-MI • Benign	No treatment is given; only documentation is done. The condition is common. The significance of IVCD is that no compromise to cardiac output occurs.

Adult Population

Assessment of Chest Pain

Condition	Location	Quality	Severity
Angina	Occurs in retrosternal region; radiates to neck, jaw, epigastrium, shoulders, arms (left common)	Pressure, burning, squeezing, heaviness, indigestion	Moderate to severe
Intermediate syndrome or coronary insufficiency	Is same as angina	Same as angina	Increasingly severe
Myocardial infarction	Occurs in substernal region; may radiate like angina	Heaviness, pressure, burning, constriction	Severe, sometimes mild (in 25% of patients)
Pericarditis	Usually begins over sternum and may radiate to neck and down left upper extremity	Sharp, stabbing, knifelike pain	Moderate to severe
Dissecting aortic aneurysm	Occurs in anterior chest region; radiates to thoracic area of back; may be abdominal; pain shifts in chest	Tearing	Excruciating, tearing, knifelike
Mitral valve prolapse syndrome	Occurs in substernal region; sometimes radiates to the left arm, back, and jaw	Stabbing, sharp pain	Variable; generally mild but can become severe

Modified from Andreoli K and others: *Comprehensive cardiac care,* ed 6, St Louis, 1987, Mosby.

Course	Aggravating or relieving factors	Symptoms or signs
<10 min	Aggravated by exercise, cold weather, emotional stress, or after meals; relieved by rest or nitroglycerin; atypical (Prinzmetal's) angina may be unrelated to activity and caused by coronary artery spasm	S_4, paradoxical split S_2 during pain
>10 min	Same as angina, with gradually decreasing tolerance for exertion	Same as angina
Sudden onset, lasting longer than 15 min	Unrelieved	Shortness of breath, sweating, weakness, nausea, vomiting, severe anxiety
Many hours to days	Aggravated by deep breathing, rotating chest, or supine position; relieved by sitting up and leaning forward	Pericardial friction rub, syncope, cardiac tamponade, pulsus paradoxus (Kussmaul's sign)
Sudden onset, lasting for hours	Unrelated to anything	Lower blood pressure in one arm, absent pulses, paralysis, murmur of aortic insufficiency, pulsus paradoxus, stridor; myocardial infarction can occur
Paroxysmal episodes (may be prolonged)	Not related to exertion; not relieved by nitroglycerin or rest	Variable palpitations, dizziness, syncope, dyspnea, late systolic or pansystolic murmur

Continued

Table—cont'd

Condition	Location	Quality	Severity
Pulmonary embolism (many pulmonary emboli do not produce chest pain)	Occurs in substernal region ("anginal")	Deep, crushing pain; if pulmonary infection, may be pleuritic	Possibly absent, mild, or severe
Pulmonary hypertension	Occurs in substernal region	Pressure; oppressive feeling	Variable
Spontaneous pneumothorax	Occurs in unilateral region	Sharp, well localized pain	
Pneumonia with pleurisy	Is localized over area of consolidation	Pleuritic, well localized pain	Moderate
Gastrointestinal disorders	Occurs in lower substernal area, epigastric region, or right or left upper quadrant	Burning, coliclike aching	
Musculoskeletal disorders	Is variable	Aching	
Neurologic disorders (herpes zoster)	Is dermatomal in distribution		
Anxiety states	Is usually localized to a point	Sharp burning; commonly location of pain moves from place to place	Mild to moderate

P_2, Pulmonic second sound.

Course	Aggravating or relieving factors	Symptoms or signs
Sudden onset, lasting minutes to 1 hr	Aggravated (possibly) by breathing	Fever, tachypnea, tachycardia, hypotension, elevated jugular venous pressure, right ventricular lift, accentuated pulmonary valve (P_2) sound during S_2, occasional murmur of tricuspid insufficiency and right ventricular S_4; infarction usually in the presence of congestive heart failure; crackles, pleural rub, hemoptysis, and clinical phlebitis in minority of cases
	Aggravated by effort	Pain usually associated with dyspnea; right ventricular lift, accentuated P_2
Sudden onset, lasting many hours	Aggravated by painful breathing	Dyspnea, hyperresonance, and decreased breath and voice sounds over involved lung
	Aggravated by painful breathing	Dyspnea, cough, fever, dull-to-flat percussion, bronchial breathing, crackles, occasional pleural rub
	Precipitated by recumbency or meals	Nausea, regurgitation, food intolerance, melena, hematemesis, jaundice
Short or long duration Prolonged time	Aggravated by movement, history of muscle exertion	Tenderness to pressure or movement
Course unassociated with external events		Rash in area of discomfort with herpes
Variable course, usually extremely brief	Aggravated by situational anger	Sighing respirations, often chest wall tenderness

Differentiation of Angina from Nonanginal Discomfort

Stable angina	Nonanginal discomfort (chest wall pain)
1. Is relieved by nitroglycerin (30 seconds to 1 minute)	1. Nitroglycerin generally has no effect.
2. Comes on at the same heart rate and blood pressure and is relieved by rest (lasts only a few minutes)	2. It occurs any time and lasts for hours.
3. Is not palpable	3. Muscle and joint soreness occur, evoked by palpation or deep breaths.
4. Is associated with feelings of doom, cold sweats, shortness of breath	4. Minimal additional symptoms occur.
5. Is often seen with ST-segment depression	5. No ST-segment depression occurs.

Modified from Irwin S, Tecklin J: *Cardiopulmonary physical therapy*, ed 3, St Louis, 1995, Mosby.

Myocardial Infarction Pain Referral Sites

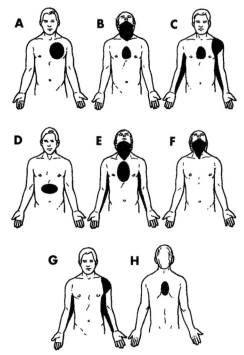

FIGURE 3-58 **Myocardial infarction pain referral sites. A,** Upper chest. **B,** Beneath sternum radiating to neck and jaw. **C,** Beneath sternum radiating down left arm. **D,** Epigastric. **E,** Epigastric radiating to neck, jaw, and arms. **F,** Neck and jaw. **G,** Left shoulder and inner aspect of both arms. **H,** Intrascapular. (From Christensen BL, Kockrow EO: *Foundations of nursing*, ed 2, St Louis, 1995, Mosby.)

Pitting Edema Scale

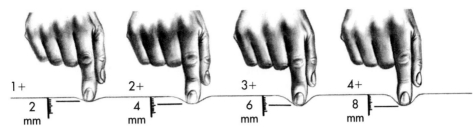

1+ 2 mm 2+ 4 mm 3+ 6 mm 4+ 8 mm

FIGURE 3-59 Pitting edema scale. (From Christensen BL, Kockrow EO: *Foundations of nursing,* ed 2, St Louis, 1995, Mosby.)

Percussion Sounds

Type of tone	Intensity	Pitch	Duration	Quality
Resonant	Loud	Low	Long	Hollow
Flat	Soft	High	Short	Extremely dull
Dull	Medium	Medium-high	Medium	Thudlike
Tympanic	Loud	High	Medium	Drumlike
Hyperresonant	Extremely loud	Extremely low	Longer	Booming

Modified from Seidel HM and others: *Mosby's physical examination handbook,* St Louis, 1995, Mosby.

Adult Population

Breathing Patterns

Pattern of breathing	Description
Apnea	Absence of ventilation
Fish-mouth	Apnea with concomitant mouth opening and closing (associated with neck extension and bradypnea)
Eupnea	Normal rate, normal depth, regular rhythm
Bradypnea	Slow rate, shallow or normal depth, regular rhythm (associated with drug overdose)
Tachypnea	Fast rate, shallow depth, regular rhythm (associated with restrictive lung disease)
Hyperpnea	Normal rate, increased depth, regular rhythm
Cheyne-Stokes (periodic)	Increasing then decreasing depth, interspersed period of apnea, somewhat regular rhythm (associated with critically ill patients)
Biot's	Slow rate, shallow depth, apneic periods, irregular rhythm (associated with central nervous system disorders such as meningitis)
Apneustic	Slow rate, deep inspiration followed by apnea, irregular rhythm (associated with brainstem disorders)
Prolonged expiration	Fast inspiration; slow and prolonged expiration, yet normal rate, depth, and regular rhythm (associated with obstructive lung disease)
Orthopnea	Difficulty breathing in postures other than erect
Hyperventilation	Fast rate, increased depth, regular rhythm (results in decreased arterial carbon dioxide, tension; called *Kussmaul breathing* in metabolic acidosis; also associated with central nervous system disorders such as encephalitis)
Psychogenic dyspnea	Normal rate, regular intervals of sighing (associated with anxiety)
Dyspnea	Rapid rate, shallow depth, regular rhythm (associated with accessory muscle activity)
Doorstop	Normal rate and rhythm (characterized by abrupt cessation of inspiration when restriction is encountered; associated with pleurisy)

Modified from Irwin S, Tecklin J: *Cardiopulmonary physical therapy,* ed 3, St Louis, 1995, Mosby.

Expected Breath Sounds

Sound	Characteristics	Findings
Vesicular	Heard over most of lung fields; low pitch; soft and short expirations; is accentuated in a thin person or a child and diminished in the overweight or extremely muscular patient	
Bronchovesicular	Heard over main bronchus area and over upper right posterior lung field; medium pitch; expiration equals inspiration	
Bronchial tracheal (tubular)	Heard only over trachea; high pitch; loud and long expirations, often somewhat longer than inspiration	

Modified from Seidel HM and others: *Mosby's physical examination handbook,* St Louis, 1995, Mosby.

Adventitious Breath Sounds

Fine crackles: high-pitched, discrete, discontinuous crackling sounds heard during the end of inspiration; not cleared by a cough

Medium crackles: lower, more moist sound heard during the mid-stage of inspiration; not cleared by a cough

Coarse crackles: loud, bubbly noise heard during inspiration; not cleared by a cough

Rhonchi (sonorous wheeze): loud, low, coarse sounds, such as a snore, most often heard continuously during inspiration or expiration; coughing may clear sound (usually means mucous accumulation in trachea or large bronchi)

Wheeze (sibilant wheeze): musical noise sounding like a squeak; most often heard continuously during inspiration or expiration; usually louder during expiration

Pleural friction rub: dry, rubbing, or grating sound, usually caused by inflammation of pleural surfaces; heard during inspiration or expiration; loudest over lower lateral anterior surface

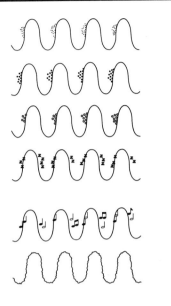

Modified from Seidel HM and others: *Mosby's physical examination handbook,* St Louis, 1995, Mosby.

Auscultation Guidelines
Auscultation Points

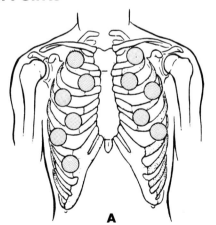
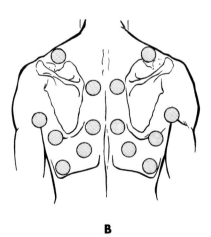

A **B**

FIGURE 3-60 Stethoscope placement points for auscultating the chest. A, Chest. **B,** Back. (From Buckingham EB: *A primer of clinical diagnosis,* ed 2, New York, 1979, Harper & Row.)

Documentation of Auscultated Sounds

Type of sound	Nomenclature	Interpretation
Breath sound	Normal	Normal, air-filled lung
	Decreased	Hyperinflation in chronic obstructive pulmonary disease
		Hypoinflation in acute lung disease (e.g., atelectasis, pneumothorax, pleural effusion)
	Absent	Pleural effusion
		Pneumothorax
		Severe hyperinflation
		Obesity
	Bronchial	Consolidation
		Atelectasis with adjacent patent airway
	Crackling	Secretions, if biphasic
		Deflation, if monophasic
	Wheezing	Diffuse airway obstruction, if polyphonic
		Localized stenosis, if monophobic
Voice sound	Normal	Normal, air-filled lung
	Decreased	Atelectasis
		Pleural effusion
		Pneumothorax
	Increased	Consolidation
		Pulmonary fibrosis
Extrapulmonary adventitious sounds	Crunching	Mediastinal emphysema
	Pleural rubbing	Pleural inflammation or reaction
	Pericardial rubbing	Pericardial inflammation

Modified from Irwin S, Tecklin J: *Cardiopulmonary physical therapy,* ed 3, St Louis, 1995, Mosby.

Pulse Oximetry

Steps	Rationale
1. Identify the patient who will benefit from pulse oximetry: a. Assess the patient's respiratory status: oxygen therapy, hemoglobin level. b. Review the patient's medical record for the physician's order.	Allows the therapist to monitor trends in the patient's level of oxygen; enables the nurse to use objective criteria to adjust nursing intervention to optimize oxygen saturation
c. Identify patients who may have oxygen desaturation with sleep, activity, and suctioning.	Identifies hypoxemia before signs and symptoms develop

2. Obtain equipment and place at bedside:
   a. Pulse oximeter
   b. Sensor probe

Type of sensor	Client's weight	
(1) Adhesive neonatal	Less than 3 kg (6.6 lb);	Ensures error-free data regarding oxygen saturation
(2) Adhesive infant	From 1 kg (2.2 lb) to 20 kg (44 lb)	
(3) Adhesive pediatric	From 10 kg (22 lb) to 50 kg (110 lb)	
(4) Adhesive adult	More than 30 kg (66 lb)	
(5) Adhesive adult nasal	More than 50 kg (110 lb)	
(6) Finger clip	More than 40 kg (88 lb)	

   c. Continuous printout (optional)

Steps	Rationale
3. Explain the purpose of the procedure to the patient and family.	Ensures patient and family understanding and increases compliance
4. Wash the hands.	Reduces transmission of microorganisms
5. Select an appropriate area to apply the sensor based on peripheral circulation and extremity temperature: a. Determine the adequacy of peripheral circulation by assessing capillary refill (toe and finger sites).	Peripheral vasoconstriction alters oxygen saturation
b. Do not use an adhesive adult nasal sensor if the patient has a large-bore nasogastric tube or nasoendotracheal tube (nose). c. Determine the use of vasoactive drugs.	Interferes with oxygen saturation readings because of poor peripheral circulation and excessive equipment or dressings
d. Align the photoelectron and light-emitting diode.	Permits transmission of light; alignment ensures accurate oxygen saturation readings

Modified from Potter PA: *Fundamentals of nursing: concepts, process, and practice*, St Louis, 1997, Mosby.

Continued

Table—cont'd

Steps	Rationale

6. Prepare the selected site:
  a. Remove nail polish and artificial nails.
  b. Remove earrings.
  c. Wash the selected site, wipe with alcohol, and air dry.
	Body oils, nail polish, and artificial nails interfere with transmission of light through nail, tissue, venous and arterial blood, and skin pigmentation

7. Attach a sensor probe to an appropriate site. Instruct the patient to breathe normally.	Prevents large fluctuations in minute ventilation and possible changes in oxygen saturation

8. Attach a pulse oximeter sensor to the patient cable.
  a. Turn the machine on.
  b. Listen for an audible beep.
	Senses with each pulse and indicates how well oximeter monitors pulse

9. Observe the waveform for a bar of light.	Light or waveform fluctuates with each pulsation and reflects pulse strength; poor light on small waveform usually indicates that signal is too weak to give accurate oxygen saturation reading
10. Ensure that the alarm limits for *both* high and low oxygen saturation and high and low pulse are set according to the physician's order and *turned on.*	Manufacturers preset limits, and adjustments can be made according to the patient's underlying physical condition, therapy, and risks Provides an audible and visual signal that high or low limits have been exceeded
11. Read the saturation level as ordered and while performing nursing interventions.	Documents oxygen saturation levels at rest, with activity such as ambulation, during procedure such as suctioning, and with changes in physical condition
12. Move a finger sensor every 4 hours and a spring-tension sensor every 2 hours.	Allows therapist to assess for and prevent impaired skin integrity caused by pressure from sensor
13. Record in the therapist's notes the patient's use of continuous pulse oximetry, and record the oxygen saturation.	Documents use of equipment for third-party payers; documents oxygen saturation
14. Correlate the oxygen saturation value with arterial blood gas measurements, if available.	Documents reliability of oximeter
15. Report the oxygen saturation and response to changes in therapy to the oncoming shift.	Provides oncoming therapist with baseline information and response to therapy

Modified from Potter PA: *Fundamentals of nursing: concepts, process, and practice,* St Louis, 1997, Mosby.

Postural Drainage Guidelines
Postural Drainage Positions

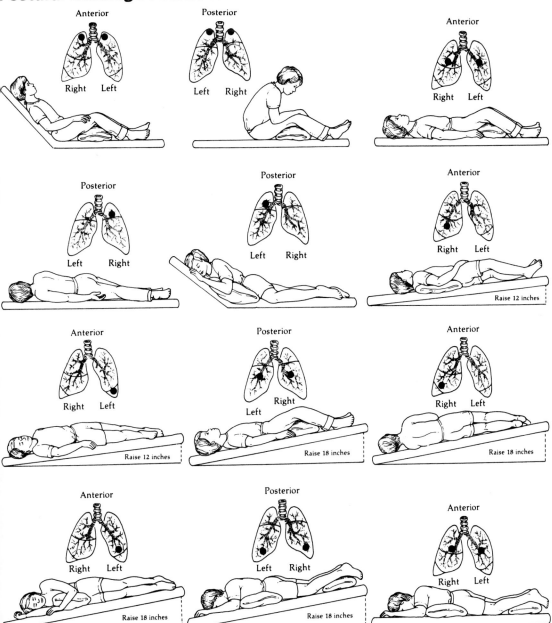

FIGURE 3-61 Postural drainage positions. (From Thompson J and others: *Mosby's clinical nursing,* ed 3, St Louis, 1993, Mosby.)

Objectives and Potential Outcomes of Position Changes

Objectives
Therapeutic objective
   Alleviate dyspnea
Physiological objectives
   Increase oxygenation
   Improve ventilation

Potential Outcomes
Prone
   Increased arterial oxygen tension in bilateral lung disease
Supine
   Decreased arterial oxygen tension in bilateral lung disease
Lateral
   Decreased arterial oxygen tension lying on the affected lung in unilateral lung disease
   Decreased arterial oxygen tension lying on the left side in bilateral lung disease
   Improved arterial oxygen tension lying on the unoperated side after thoracotomy (relative to the supine position)

Modified from Irwin S, Tecklin J: *Cardiopulmonary physical therapy,* ed 3, St Louis, 1995, Mosby.

Pulse Palpation Guidelines
Pulse Palpation Points

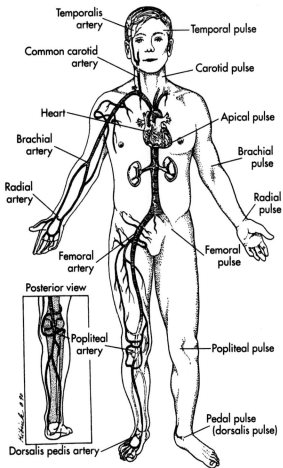

FIGURE 3-62 Pulse palpation points. (From Christensen BL, Kockrow EO: *Foundations of nursing,* ed 2, St Louis, 1995, Mosby.)

Arterial Pulse Abnormalities

Type	Description	Associated disorders
Alternating pulse (pulsus alternans)	Regular rate; amplitude varies from beat to beat with weak and strong beats	Left ventricular failure
Bigeminal pulse (pulsus bigeminus)	Two beats in rapid succession followed by longer interval; easily confused with alternating pulse	Regularly occurring ventricular premature beats
Bisferious pulse (pulsus bisferiens)	Two strong systolic peaks separated by a midsystolic dip	Aortic regurgitation alone or with stenosis
Bounding pulse	Increased pulse pressure; contour may have rapid rise, brief peak, rapid fall	Atherosclerosis, aortic regurgitation, patent ductus arteriosus, fever, anemia, hyperthyroidism, anxiety, exercise
Bradycardia	Rate less than 60 bpm	Hypothermia, hypothyroidism, drug intoxication, impaired cardiac conduction, excellent physical conditioning
Labile pulse	Normal rate when patient is resting but faster when standing or sitting	Not necessarily associated with disease; not a specific indicator of a problem
Paradoxical pulse (pulsus paradoxus)	Decreasing amplitude on inspiration	Chronic obstructive pulmonary disease, constrictive pericarditis, pericardial effusion
Pulsus differens	Unequal pulses between left and right extremities	Impaired circulation, usually from unilateral local obstruction
Tachycardia	Rate over 100 bpm	Fever, hyperthyroidism, anemia, shock, heart disease, anxiety, exercise
Trigeminal pulse (pulsus trigeminus)	Three beats followed by a pause	Often benign status, such as after exercise; cardiomyopathy; severe ventricular hypertrophy; severe aortic stenosis; dysfunctional right ventricle
Water-hammer pulse (Corrigan pulse)	Jerky pulse with full expansion followed by sudden collapse	Aortic regurgitation

Modified from Seidel HM and others: *Mosby's physical examination handbook*, St Louis, 1995, Mosby.

Target Heart Rate Guidelines
Calculating Target Heart Rate

Target heart rates allow therapists to quickly and easily determine appropriate demands placed on the cardiovascular systems of patients. Therapists calculate target heart rates by subtracting the patient's age from 220 and then multiplying the sum by 60% to 80%. The treatment focus is around the patient's achieving and maintaining, but not exceeding, this number.

Calculating Target Heart Rate Form

$$\frac{(220 - \text{Age}) \times 60 - 85}{100}$$

Age	60%	65%	70%	75%	80%
20	120	130	140	150	160
25	117	127	137	146	156
30	114	124	133	143	152
35	111	120	130	139	148
40	108	117	126	135	144
45	105	114	123	131	140
50	102	111	119	128	136
55	99	107	116	124	132
60	96	104	112	120	128
65	93	101	109	116	124
70	90	98	105	113	120
75	87	94	102	109	116
80	84	91	98	105	112
85	81	88	95	101	108
90	78	85	91	98	104
95	75	81	88	94	100
100	72	78	84	90	96

Adult Population

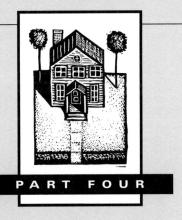

PART FOUR

Emergency Situations

WARNING SIGNS

CARDIOPULMONARY RESUSCITATION

FIRST AID

WARNING SIGNS

The provision of therapy in the home limits access to peer consultation when emergency situations arise. For example, when a patient is unusually short of breath and reports feeling ill, what should be done? Without other therapists, nurses, or physicians on hand, home care therapists must make independent and immediate clinical judgments. These clinical judgments include examining patients, gathering pertinent data, and assessing physical signs and symptoms to facilitate accurate and complete communication with agency supervisors and/or physicians. Warning signs offers therapists common signs and symptoms for an array of medical conditions encountered in home heath care. (NOTE: The warning signs are not all inclusive. Therapists should report any unusual signs to the physician or agency.)

Acute Renal Failure
Definition

A precipitous decline in kidney function.

Signs and Symptoms
- Altered consciousness (lethargy, somnolence)
- Altered mental status (poor concentration, confusion)
- Edema
- Generalized weakness
- Cramps
- Restless leg syndrome
- Distal sensorimotor neuropathy
- Anorexia
- Nausea
- Vomiting
- Decreased or absent urinary output
- Nocturia
- Yellow-tinged skin

Action
- Notify the physician of the patient's status.
- Notify the agency supervisor of the patient's status.
- Monitor vital signs and remain with the patient until directed further by the physician and agency supervisor.

Emergency Situations

Airway Obstruction—Complete

Definition

Full blockage of airways with complete absence of respiratory effort and gas exchange.

Signs and Symptoms

- Altered consciousness (unconsciousness)
- Absent respiration
- Cyanosis

Action

- Activate the emergency medical system.
- Initiate cardiopulmonary resuscitation (CPR) and continue CPR until directed further by emergency medical system personnel.
- Notify the physician of the patient's status.
- Notify the agency supervisor of the patient's status.

Airway Obstruction—Partial

Definition

Partial blockage of airways with compromised respiratory effort and gas exchange.

Signs and Symptoms

- Altered consciousness (lethargy, unconsciousness)
- Weak respiration
- Labored breathing
- Ineffective inspiratory effort with suprasternal, supraclavicular, and intercostal retractions
- Adventitious breath sounds (wheezing, stridor)
- Accessory muscle use with breathing
- Cough
- Poor voice quality, dysphonia, or aphonia
- Universal choking sign
- Cyanosis

Action

- Activate the emergency medical system.
- Assist the patient to the sitting position.
- Loosen clothing around the neck area.
- Monitor vital signs and be prepared to initiate CPR.
- Administer high-flow oxygen, if available, at 6 L/min through a nasal cannula.
- Encourage slow, deep breathing.
- Remain with the patient until directed further by emergency medical system personnel.
- Notify the physician of the patient's status.
- Notify the agency supervisor of the patient's status.

Anaphylactic Reaction
Definition

A catastrophic allergic reaction occurring minutes after parenteral (rarely oral) administration of drugs or nonhuman proteins, including foods, venoms, or sera.

Signs and Symptoms

- Altered consciousness (unconsciousness in later stages)
- Altered mental status (apprehension, uneasiness, anxiety, sense of impending doom, confusion)
- Headache
- Pain (back, pelvis, abdomen)
- Chest pressure
- Dysrhythmia
- Hypotension
- Choking sensation and/or throat tightness
- Cough
- Sneezing
- Dyspnea
- Bronchospasm
- Laryngeal edema
- Convulsions
- Light headedness or syncope
- Diarrhea
- Incontinence
- Generalized warmth and tingling of the face, mouth, upper chest, palms, soles, and/or site of exposure
- Hives
- Pupil dilation
- Ocular itch, tearing, and/or red eye

Action

- Activate the emergency medical system.
- Leave intact insect stingers imbedded in the patient.
- Administer epinephrine (following directions) if an anaphylactic kit is available.
- Position the patient in the supine position with the head slightly lower than the body.
- Monitor the vital signs and be prepared to initiate CPR.
- Remain with the patient until directed further by emergency medical system personnel.
- Notify the physician of the patient's status.
- Notify the agency supervisor of the patient's status.

Emergency Situations

Aspiration
Definition

Uptake of foreign material (e.g., food, fluid) into the airway.

Signs and Symptoms

- Altered consciousness (may be unconscious)
- Altered mental status
- Sudden onset of coughing, vomiting, choking, wheezing, and/or dyspnea, usu ally within 1 hour after the aspiration event, but possibly up to 6 hours after the aspiration event
- Fever
- Tachycardia
- Hypotension
- Tachypnea, leading to apnea
- Adventitious breath sounds (diffuse rales)
- Cyanosis

Action

- Activate the emergency medical system.
- Place the patient in a left lateral position with the head slightly lower than the body.
- Monitor the vital signs and be prepared to initiate CPR.
- Administer high-flow oxygen, if available, at 5 to 10 L per minute through a nasal cannula.
- Remain with the patient until directed further by emergency medical system personnel.
- Notify the physician of the patient's status.
- Notify the agency supervisor of the patient's status.

Asthma Attack
Definition

A lung disease with (1) airway obstruction or narrowing that is fully or incompletely reversible spontaneously or with treatment, (2) airway inflammation, and/or (3) air way hyperresponsiveness to a variety of stimuli.

Signs and Symptoms

- Altered mental status (anxiety, restlessness, agitation)
- Tachycardia
- Cough
- Sneezing
- Dyspnea
- Tachypnea
- Prolonged expiratory phase of breathing
- Flared nares
- Adventitious breath sounds (wheezing, rhonchi, rales)
- Yellow to green sputum
- Speaking difficulty
- Accessory muscle use with respiration
- Inability to lie in the supine position (prefers sitting)
- Syncope or near syncope
- Cyanosis
- Diaphoresis
- Barrel chest

Action

- Assist the patient to administer asthma medication, if available.
- Administer oxygen, if available, at 1 to 3 L per minute through a nasal cannula.
- Encourage coughing.
- Activate the emergency medical system if symptoms persist.
- Monitor the vital signs and be prepared to initiate CPR.
- Notify the physician of the patient's status.
- Notify the agency supervisor of the patient's status.
- Remain with the patient until directed further by emergency medical personnel and/or the physician and agency supervisor.

Cardiac Arrest

Definition

Cessation of heart function.

Signs and Symptoms

- Altered consciousness (unconsciousness)
- Absent pulse

Action

- Activate the emergency medical system.
- Initiate CPR and continue CPR until directed further by emergency medical system personnel.
- Notify the physician of the patient's status.
- Notify the agency supervisor of the patient's status.

Emergency Situations

Cerebrovascular Accident
Definition

An event marked by an abrupt onset of neurological deficits resulting from a disruption of regional blood flow to the brain.

Signs and Symptoms

- Altered consciousness (lethargy, unconsciousness)
- Altered mental status (disorientation, confusion)
- Headache
- Hypertension
- Hypoventilation
- Dyspnea, labored breathing
- Dysphagia
- Dysarthria
- Aphasia
- Unilateral weakness (bilateral weakness if bilateral disruption of blood flow is present)
- Ataxia
- Apraxia
- Unilateral sensory deficits (bilateral sensory deficits if bilateral disruption of blood flow is present)
- Vision deficits (diplopia, hemianopsia, mononuclear blindness)
- Neglect
- Dizziness and/or vertigo
- Vomiting
- Cyanosis

Action

- Activate the emergency medical system.
- Assist the patient to a resting position.
- Administer oxygen, if available, at 5 L per minute through a nasal cannula.
- Monitor the vital signs and be prepared to initiate CPR.
- Notify the physician of the patient's status.
- Notify the agency supervisor of the patient's status.
- Remain with the patient until directed further by emergency medical system personnel.

Chronic Obstructive Pulmonary Disease Exacerbation
Definition

A worsening of the respiratory syndrome consisting of emphysema, chronic bronchitis, and/or chronic airflow limitations.

Signs and Symptoms

- Altered consciousness (lethargy, stupor)
- Altered mental status (anxiety, restlessness, confusion)
- Dyspnea
- Tachypnea

- Adventitious breath sounds (wheezing, rhonchi)
- Hyperresonant lungs
- Purulent sputum
- Depressed diaphragm

Action

- Notify the physician of the patient's status.
- Notify the agency supervisor of the patient's status.
- Administer oxygen, if available and if directed by the physician, at 1 to 2 L per minute.
- Monitor the vital signs and remain with the patient until directed further by the physician and agency supervisor.

Congestive Heart Failure
Definition

Inability of the heart to pump oxygenated blood at a rate sufficient to satisfy organ demands.

Signs and Symptoms

- Altered consciousness (lethargy, stupor)
- Altered mental status (anxiety, confusion, agitation, apathy, depression)
- Tachycardia
- Dysrhythmia
- Jugular vein distension
- Dyspnea (initially with exertion, later at rest)
- Severe dyspnea and/or cough after periods of rest
- Tachypnea
- Adventitious breath sounds (moist rales, wheezing)
- Cough (productive with rust to brown color in advanced stages)
- Dependent peripheral edema
- Fatigue
- Generalized weakness
- Nausea
- Decreased appetite
- Weight loss
- Clammy skin
- Pallor to gray hue
- Cyanosis of lips and/or nail beds

Action

- Notify the physician of the patient's status.
- Notify the agency supervisor of the patient's status.
- Assist the patient to a resting position with the lower extremities elevated above the heart level.
- Administer high-flow oxygen, if available, and if directed by the physician, at 5 to 10 L per minute.
- Monitor the vital signs and remain with the patient until directed further by the physician and agency supervisor.

Emergency Situations

Deep Vein Thrombosis
Definition

A syndrome in which blood clots form in the deep veins of the lower extremities.

Signs and Symptoms

- Localized pain over clot site
- Localized tenderness over clot site
- Localized warmth at clot site
- Localized erythema at clot site
- Palpable vein
- Unilateral extremity edema (edema present bilaterally if clots occur bilaterally)
- Positive Homan's sign for lower-extremity deep vein thrombosis

Action

- Assist the patient to a resting position with suspected extremities elevated above the heart level.
- Notify the physician of the patient's status.
- Notify the agency supervisor of the patient's status.
- Monitor the vital signs and remain with the patient until directed further by the physician and agency supervisor.

Dehydration
Definition

A deficit of total body water, usually with associated electrolyte imbalance.

Signs and Symptoms

- Altered consciousness (lethargy, stupor)
- Altered mental status (irritability, confusion)
- Hypotension
- Orthostatic hypotension (present at 10% deficit)
- Supine hypotension (present at 15% deficit)
- Thirst
- Weakness
- Weight loss
- Decreased urine output
- Diminished sweating
- Soft, sunken eyes
- Dry mucous membranes (e.g., no tears)
- Poor skin turgor

Action

- Activate the emergency medical system.
- Notify the physician of the patient's status.
- Notify the agency supervisor of the patient's status.
- Monitor the vital signs and remain with the patient until directed further by the physician and agency supervisor.

Delirium
Definition

A condition marked by an acute, reversible change in cognitive status.

Signs and Symptoms

- Altered mental status (confusion, transient disorientation, memory deficit, language disturbance)
- Inability to focus, sustain, or shift attention
- Poor concentration
- Distractibility
- Hallucinations (visual, auditory)

Action

- Notify the physician of the patient's status.
- Notify the agency supervisor of the patient's status.
- Monitor the vital signs and remain with the patient until directed further by the physician and agency supervisor.

Depression
Definition

A psychiatric disorder marked by a depressed mood and at least three additional symptoms, including sleeping problems, decreased appetite, suicidal ideation, and lethargy.

Signs and Symptoms

- Altered mental status (preoccupation, restlessness, apathy, distractibility, tenseness)
- Altered mood (sadness, emptiness, worthlessness, inappropriate guilt, hopelessness, helplessness)
- Decreased interest in daily activities
- Recurrent thought of death
- Suicidal ideation
- Loss of appetite
- Change in weight by ±5% in 1 month
- Poorly defined organic symptoms (weakness, headache, general pain)
- Sleep disturbance (insomnia or hypersomnia)

Action

- Determine whether the patient expresses suicidal ideation.
- Notify the physician of the patient's status.
- Notify the agency supervisor of the patient's status.
- Remain with the patient until directed further by the physician and agency supervisor.

Emergency Situations

Hip Dislocation—Posterior
Definition
Dislocation of the prosthesis, usually from a fall or nonadherence to total hip replacement precautions, but possibly occurring with minimal provocation such a seated weight shifting.

Signs and Symptoms
- Hip pain
- Shortened, mildly flexed, internally rotated, and adducted lower extremity
- Palpable mass posterior to the hip
- Inability or difficulty flexing the knee
- Inability to bear full weight on the lower extremity
- Weakness of lateral hip muscles
- Impaired sensation of great toe, plantar aspect of foot, or lateral lower extremit

Action
- Activate the emergency medical system.
- Immobilize the patient by supporting the affected lower extremity in its deformed position (do not move) with pillows or blankets.
- Monitor the vital signs and be prepared to initiate CPR.
- Notify the physician of the patient's status.
- Notify the agency supervisor of the patient's status.
- Remain with the patient until directed further by emergency medical system personnel.

Shoulder Dislocation—Anterior
Definition
A displacement of the intact humerus, usually following a fall or blow to the abducted and externally rotated shoulder.

Signs and Symptoms
- Shoulder pain
- Shoulder muscle spasm
- Inability to abduct shoulder
- Loss of deltoid muscle mass
- Palpable head of humerus in the axilla
- Upper extremity held in guarded position
- Sensation loss over deltoid and lateral humerus

Action
- Activate the emergency medical system.
- Immobilize the upper extremity with a sling to maintain the arm in the guarded position.
- Notify the physician of the patient's status.
- Arrange transportation to the emergency room or other destination designated by the physician for the relocation procedure.

- Notify the agency of the patient's status.
- Remain with the patient until directed further by emergency medical system personnel, the physician, and/or the agency supervisor.

Dysrhythmia

Definition

A disturbance of normal cardiac rhythm.

Signs and Symptoms

- Altered consciousness if patient is hemodynamically unstable (lethargy, unconsciousness)
- Altered mental status if patient is hemodynamically unstable (disorientation, confusion)
- Chest pain if patient is hemodynamically unstable
- Altered heart rate (under 50 or above 120 beats/minute)
- Irregular heart rhythm
- Hypotension if patient is hemodynamically unstable
- Dyspnea if patient is hemodynamically unstable
- Adventitious breath sounds if patient is hemodynamically unstable (rales)
- Fatigue
- Syncope

Action

- Activate the emergency medical system if the patient is hemodynamically unstable.
- Monitor the vital signs closely and be prepared to initiate CPR.
- Notify the physician of the patient's status.
- Notify the agency supervisor of the patient's status.
- Remain with the patient until directed further by emergency medical system personnel or by the physician and agency supervisor.

Electrolyte Imbalance

Definition

Disturbance in the normal levels of electrolytes (primarily sodium, potassium, calcium) in the body, resulting in altered body fluid concentration.

Signs and Symptoms

- Altered consciousness (lethargy, somnolence, unconsciousness)
- Altered mental status (irritability, confusion, delirium, inattentiveness, apathy, poor concentration, depression, hallucinations, psychosis)
- Headache
- Tachycardia
- Orthostatic hypotension
- Weakness
- Muscle twitches or tremors
- Muscle cramps
- Hyporeflexive or hyperreflexive deep tendon reflexes
- Seizures
- Paresthesias
- Dehydration
- Thirst
- Dizziness
- Abdominal cramps
- Nausea
- Vomiting
- Anorexia
- Decreased urinary output
- Constipation
- Poor skin turgor

Action

- Activate the emergency medical system.
- Monitor the vital signs and be prepared to initiate CPR.
- Notify the physician of the patient's status.
- Notify the agency supervisor of the patient's status.
- Remain with the patient until directed further by emergency medical system personnel.

Fractures—Ankle
Definition

Fracture of the tibia, fibula, and/or calcaneous, usually by forces perpendicular to the normal motion of the joint, as with a fall.

Signs and Symptoms

- Ankle pain
- Bone tenderness
- Inability to bear full weight on the foot
- Limited ankle and foot range of motion
- Ankle and/or foot edema
- Joint deformity

Action

- Immobilize the ankle and foot.
- Assist the patient to the supine position with the lower extremities elevated above the heart level.
- Apply ice.
- Notify the physician of the patient's status.
- Arrange transportation to the emergency room or other destination designated by the physician for fracture care.
- Notify the agency supervisor of the patient's status.
- Remain with the patient until directed further by the physician and agency supervisor.

Fractures—Hip
Definition

Fracture of the proximal femur occurring from simple bone stress or a fall.

Signs and Symptoms

- Hip pain
- Groin pain
- Shortened and externally rotated lower extremity
- Joint deformity
- Inability to bear full weight on the limb

Action

- Activate the emergency medical system.
- Immobilize the patient by supporting the lower extremity in the deformed position (do not move in case of concurrent dislocation) with pillows or blankets.
- Apply ice.
- Monitor the vital signs and be prepared to initiate CPR.
- Notify the physician of the patient's status.
- Notify the agency supervisor of the patient's status.
- Remain with the patient until directed otherwise by emergency medical system personnel.

Emergency Situations

Fractures—Pelvis
Definition

Fracture of the pubis, ischium, and/or ileum after a fall or crushing injury, often accompanied by other life-threatening injuries such as hypovolemic shock.

Signs and Symptoms

- Pelvic pain
- Pain with fracture site palpation
- Pain with iliac crest compression and distraction
- Proximal displacement of hemipelvis
- Inability to bear full weight on affected side (if fracture is unilateral)
- Edema

Action

- Activate the emergency medical system.
- If the patient must change position, assist him or her with the log roll method.
- Monitor the vital signs and be prepared to initiate CPR.
- Notify the physician of the patient's status.
- Notify the agency supervisor of the patient's status.
- Remain with the patient until directed further by emergency medical system personnel.

Fractures—Rib
Definition

Fracture of the rib, usually resulting from a fall onto the side.

Signs and Symptoms

- Localized chest and/or rib pain
- Increased pain with deep breathing, sneezing, coughing, and trunk rotation
- Palpable rib pain
- Audible crepitus with movement
- Ecchymosis

Action

- Activate the emergency medical system (because of risk for pneumothorax).
- If the patient must change position, assist him or her with the log roll method to the opposite side of the injury or assist the patient to a sitting position.
- Instruct the patient in diaphragmatic and deep breathing.
- Monitor the vital signs for symptoms of pneumothorax.
- Notify the physician of the patient's status.
- Notify the agency supervisor of the patient's status.
- Remain with the patient until directed otherwise by emergency medical system personnel.

Fractures—Shoulder (Proximal Humerus)
Definition
Fracture of the proximal humerus, usually from a fall or blow to the abducted shoulder.

Signs and Symptoms
- Shoulder pain
- Affected arm held close to the body
- Shoulder tenderness
- Hematoma
- Edema
- Crepitus with movement
- Deformity

Action
- Immobilize the upper extremity with a sling to maintain the arm in the guarded position.
- Apply ice to the shoulder.
- Notify the physician of the patient's status.
- Arrange transportation to an emergency room or other destination designated by the physician for fracture care.
- Notify the agency supervisor of the patient's status.
- Remain with the patient until directed further by the physician and agency supervisor.

Fractures—Vertebral Compression
Definition
Fracture of the vertebral body, usually from a fall, but in the presence of osteoporosis, from minimal trauma or activity such as turning in bed.

Signs and Symptoms
- Spinal pain
- Pain increased with deep breathing, coughing, sneezing, trunk rotation, trunk flexion, palpation, and/or weight bearing
- Tachypnea to avoid deep respiration
- Accessory muscle use with respiration

Action
- Assist the patient to a comfortable resting position using the log roll method.
- Apply ice to the fracture site.
- Instruct the patient in diaphragmatic breathing.
- Monitor the vital signs.
- Notify the physician of the patient's status.
- Notify the agency supervisor of the patient's status.
- Remain with the patient until directed further by the physician and agency supervisor.

Emergency Situations

Gastrointestinal Bleeding with Evidence of Shock
Definition

Bleeding in the upper or lower gastrointestinal tract, causing hypovolemic shock.

Signs and Symptoms

- Altered mental status (agitation, restlessness, irritability, confusion)
- Chest pain
- Headache
- Tachycardia
- Orthostatic tachycardia
- Hypotension
- Orthostatic hypotension
- Dyspnea
- Fatigue
- Weakness
- Dizziness
- Syncope
- Numbness and/or tingling of extremities
- Insomnia
- Blood in vomit ("coffee ground vomit")
- Black stools secondary to blood content
- Pallor
- Cool, clammy skin

Action

- Activate the emergency medical system.
- Administer high-flow oxygen, if available, at 5 to 10 L per minute through a nasal cannula.
- Monitor the vital signs and be prepared to initiate CPR.
- Notify the physician of the patient's status.
- Notify the agency supervisor of the patient's status.
- Remain with the patient until directed further by emergency medical system personnel.

Gastrointestinal Bleeding without Evidence of Shock
Definition

Bleeding in the upper or lower gastrointestinal tract.

Signs and Symptoms

- Chest pain
- Tachycardia
- Hypotension
- Dyspnea
- Fatigue

- Weakness
- Dizziness
- Syncope
- Blood in vomit ("coffee ground vomit")
- Black stools secondary to blood content

Action

- Notify the physician of the patient's status.
- Notify the agency supervisor of the patient's status.
- Monitor the vital signs and remain with the patient until directed further by the physician and agency supervisor.

Heat Stroke

Definition

Loss of thermoregulatory control with hyperpyrexia (>105.8° F rectal temperature).

Signs and Symptoms

- Altered consciousness (lethargy, stupor, unconsciousness)
- Altered mental status (confusion, delirium, irrationality, irritability)
- Elevated body temperature
- Tachycardia
- Hypotension
- Tachypnea
- Seizures
- Vague complaints of malaise, fatigue, headache, dizziness, vertigo, and/or myalgia
- Paresthesias of hands and feet
- Visual disturbances
- Vomiting
- Diarrhea
- Hot, flushed skin turning to ashen gray
- Diaphoretic to dry skin

Action

- Activate the emergency medical system.
- Cool the patient down slowly. (Remove clothing, offer cool drinks, sprinkle with cool water, fan the patient, wipe with cool cloths, place ice on the patient—particularly the groin, posterior neck, and axilla—activate fans and air conditioning.)
- Administer oxygen, if available.
- Monitor the vital signs and be prepared to initiate CPR.
- Notify the physician of the patient's status.
- Notify the agency supervisor of the patient's status.
- Remain with the patient until directed further by emergency medical system personnel.

Emergency Situations

Hyperglycemia
Definition

A state of elevated blood glucose greater than 300 mg/dl.

Signs and Symptoms

- Altered consciousness (unconsciousness in severe hyperglycemia)
- Abdominal pain
- Weakness
- Dizziness
- Near syncope
- Blurred vision
- Thirst
- Weight loss
- Nausea
- Vomiting
- Polyuria

Action

- Activate the emergency medical system if the patient is unconscious.
- Determine the glucose level, if possible.
- Notify the physician of the patient's status.
- Notify the agency supervisor of the patient's status.
- Remain with the patient until directed further by emergency medical system personnel or the physician and agency supervisor.

Hypertensive Crisis
Definition

Acute elevation of blood pressure requiring a reduction in 1 hour to lower the risk of morbidity and mortality.

Mild to moderate hypertension. <200/120 mmHg and no acute symptoms.

Severe hypertension. >200/120 mmHg and no acute symptoms.

Accelerated (malignant) hypertension. >200/120 mmHg with significant end-organ damage.

Acute hypertensive crisis. >220/150 mmHg with symptoms noted in the following section.

Signs and Symptoms

- Headache
- Chest pain
- Elevated blood pressure
- Dyspnea
- Pulmonary edema
- Hemorrhagic stroke signs
- Retinal hemorrhage
- Blurred vision

Action

- Activate the emergency medical system with accelerated hypertension or hypertensive crisis signs and symptoms.
- Assist the patient to a sitting position.
- Monitor the vital signs and be prepared to initiate CPR.
- Notify the physician of the patient's status.
- Notify the agency supervisor of the patient's status.
- Remain with the patient until directed further by emergency medical system personnel.

Hypoglycemia
Definition

An abnormally low blood glucose level.
Moderate hypoglycemia. 30-50 mg/dl.
Severe hypoglycemia. <30 mg/dl.

Signs and Symptoms

- Altered consciousness (lethargy or unconsciousness in severe hypoglycemia)
- Altered mental status (anxiety, restlessness, nervousness, confusion, irritability)
- Mild hypothermia (90-95° F) in severe hypoglycemia
- Headache
- Tachycardia
- Normal ventilation to hypoventilation
- Weakness
- Ataxia (in severe hypoglycemia)
- Seizures (in severe hypoglycemia)
- Hunger
- Paresthesias of face and/or hands
- Visual disturbances
- Diaphoresis
- Clammy skin

Action

- Activate the emergency medical system if the patient is unconscious.
- Determine the glucose level, if possible.
- Administer 2 tablespoons of granulated sugar dissolved in water or fruit juice, or offer candy, sugar lumps, etc.
- Notify the physician of the patient's status.
- Notify the agency supervisor of the patient's status.
- Remain with the patient until directed further by emergency medical system personnel or the physician and agency supervisor.

Hypotension
Definition

Abnormally low blood pressure, usually less than 90 mmHg systolic blood pressure.

Signs and Symptoms

- Altered consciousness (lethargy, stupor)
- Low blood pressure
- Weakness
- Dizziness
- Syncope

Action

- Assist the patient to a resting position with the lower extremities elevated above the heart level.
- Monitor the vital signs and be prepared to activate an emergency medical system and/or initiate CPR.
- Notify the physician of the patient's status.
- Notify the agency supervisor of the patient's status.
- Remain with the patient until directed further by emergency medical system personnel or the physician and agency supervisor.

Hypothermia
Definition

A decrease in the body's core temperature attaining a point at which normal thermoregulatory mechanisms are overwhelmed.

Signs and Symptoms

- Altered consciousness (lethargy, stupor, unconsciousness)
- Altered mental status (impaired judgment, perseveration, flat affect, psychosis, apathy)
- Low body temperature (77-95° F) by rectal or tympanic thermometer
- Bradycardia (initially tachycardia)
- Dysrhythmia
- Hypotension
- Hypoventilation
- Adventitious breath sounds
- Edema
- Fatigue
- Weakness
- Ataxia
- Hyporeflexia to areflexia
- Increased muscle tone and/or rigidity
- Impaired coordination
- Shivering (absent in severe hypothermia)
- Dysarthria
- Erythema to pallor to cyanosis

Action

- Activate the emergency medical system if the temperature is below 91.4° F and/or the patient is unconscious.
- Avoid abrupt movement, jarring, handling, or turning of the patient secondary to myocardial irritability.
- Remove wet clothing.
- Avoid an extremity massage, which suppresses shivering and increases vasodilation too rapidly.
- Warm the patient slowly (e.g., by applying blankets and hot water bottles, turning on heating, offering warm drinks if the patient is conscious).
- Administer oxygen, if available.
- Monitor the vital signs and be prepared to initiate CPR.
- Notify the physician of the patient's status.
- Notify the agency supervisor of the patient's status.
- Remain with the patient until directed further by emergency medical system personnel or the physician and agency supervisor.

Myocardial Infarction
Definition

An abrupt blockage of a coronary artery.

Signs and Symptoms

- Altered mental status (anxiety, restlessness, apprehension)
- Retrosternal or substernal chest pain (squeezing, tight, oppressive, incapacitating, "heavy weight pushing on chest") lasting longer than 1 minute
- Pain radiation to left arm
- Pain radiation to jaw
- Elevated body temperature
- Altered heart rate (bradycardia to tachycardia)
- Altered blood pressure (hypotension or hypertension)
- Altered respiration (normal to tachypnea)
- Nausea
- Vomiting
- Diaphoresis
- Cool skin
- Pallor to cyanosis

Action

- Activate the emergency medical system.
- Direct the patient to take sublingual nitrates at the prescribed dose, if available.
- Assist the patient to a semireclining resting position.
- Administer oxygen, if available, at 2 to 5 L per minute through a nasal cannula.
- Monitor the vital signs and be prepared to initiate CPR.
- Repeat sublingual nitrates administration after 5 minutes at the prescribed dose if symptoms persist.
- Notify the physician of the patient's status.

Emergency Situations

- Notify the agency supervisor of the patient's status.
- Remain with the patient until directed further by emergency medical system personnel.

Myocardial Ischemia
Definition

A situation in which the cellular oxygen demands of the heart exceed the capacity of the coronary artery system to deliver oxygen.

Signs and Symptoms

- Retrosternal chest pain (pressure; squeezing, tight, "heavy weight pushing on chest"; burning; cramping) lasting less than 1 minute
- Pain radiation to neck, arm, and/or abdomen
- Nonradicular epigastrium, shoulder, mandible, back, and/or arm pain
- Pain after exertion and pain relief with rest
- Dyspnea
- Syncope or near syncope
- Nausea
- Vomiting
- Diaphoresis

Action

- Activate the emergency medical system.
- Direct the patient to take sublingual nitrates at the prescribed dose, if available.
- Assist the patient to a semireclining resting position.
- Administer oxygen, if available, at 2 to 5 L per minute through a nasal cannula.
- Monitor the vital signs and be prepared to initiate CPR.
- Repeat sublingual nitrates administration at the prescribed dose after 5 minutes if symptoms persist.
- Notify the physician of the patient's status.
- Notify the agency supervisor of the patient's status.
- Remain with the patient until directed further by emergency medical system personnel.

Orthostatic Hypotension
Definition

A greater than 10-mmHg drop in blood pressure with a change in position (e.g., supine to sitting, sitting to standing) secondary to failure of the baroreflex-mediated increase in peripheral vascular resistance because of deficient norepinephrine secretion.

Signs and Symptoms

- Greater than 10-mmHg drop in blood pressure with change in position
- Orthostatic tachycardia
- Weakness with change in position
- Dizziness with change in position
- Syncope or near syncope with change in position
- Vision dimming with change in position
- Diaphoresis with change in position

Action

- Assist the patient to a resting position with the lower extremities elevated above the heart level.
- Monitor for stabilization of the vital signs, and be prepared to activate the emergency medical system and/or initiate CPR.
- Notify the physician of the patient's status.
- Notify the agency supervisor of the patient's status.
- Remain with the patient until directed further by emergency medical system personnel or the physician and agency supervisor.

Pneumonia
Definition

An inflammation of the pulmonary parenchyma caused by bacteria, viruses, fungi, mycoplasmas, rickettsiae, or parasites.

Signs and Symptoms

- Altered consciousness (lethargy, stupor)
- Altered mental status (confusion, delirium)
- Fever
- Pleuritic chest pain
- Tachycardia
- Nonproductive cough progressing to purulent or rusty sputum
- Respiratory discomfort
- Dyspnea
- Tachypnea
- Adventitious breath sounds (coarse rales, noise, pleuritic friction rub)
- Dullness to percussion
- Malaise
- Shaking chills
- Splinting on the affected side
- Cyanosis

Action

- Notify the physician of the patient's status.
- Administer oxygen, if available and if directed by the physician, at 1 to 3 L per minute through a nasal cannula.
- Encourage the patient to cough.
- Encourage the patient to drink fluids.
- Notify the agency supervisor of the patient's status.
- Remain with the patient until directed further by the physician and agency supervisor.

Pneumothorax

Definition

The entry of air into the pleural space, causing partial or complete lung collapse.

Signs and Symptoms

- Altered consciousness (lethargy, unconsciousness)
- Altered mental status (agitation, restlessness)
- Chest pain
- Pain radiation to the shoulder
- Tachycardia
- Hypotension
- Distended jugular veins
- Cough
- Dyspnea
- Tachypnea
- Hyperresonant and tympanitic involved lung
- Decreased or absent breath sounds over involved lung
- Decreased chest mobility with respiration
- Lateral shift of trachea and/or mediastinum away from involved side
- Cyanosis

Action

- Activate the emergency medical system.
- Assist the patient to a resting position, sidelying on the injured side.
- Monitor the vital signs and be prepared to initiate CPR.
- Notify the physician of the patient's status.
- Notify the agency supervisor of the patient's status.
- Remain with the patient until directed further by emergency medical system personnel.

Postsurgical Infection
Definition

An inflammatory response noted at the surgical site as a result of abnormal levels of bacteria or viral agents.

Signs and Symptoms

- Fever
- Erythema of incision area
- Warmth of incision area
- Drainage

Action

- Notify the physician of the patient's status.
- Notify the agency supervisor of the patient's status.
- Keep the infected body part immobile.
- Elevate the infected body part above the heart level, unless contraindicated.
- Remain with the patient until directed further by the physician and agency supervisor.

Pulmonary Embolism
Definition

Obstruction of the pulmonary circulation by thrombus fragments entering through the right side of the heart.

Signs and Symptoms

- Altered mental status (anxiety, apprehension, restlessness)
- Sudden onset of pleuritic or retrosternal chest pain that may radiate to the neck or shoulder (some have only abdominal or back pain)
- Fever
- Tachycardia
- Hypotension
- Cough
- Dyspnea
- Tachypnea
- Adventitious breath sounds (wheezing, pleuritic friction rub, dullness at the base)
- Syncope
- Diaphoresis
- Cyanosis

Action

- Activate the emergency medical system.
- Administer high-flow oxygen, if available, at 5 to 10 L per minute through a nasal cannula.
- Monitor the vital signs and be prepared to initiate CPR.
- Notify the physician of the patient's status.

Emergency Situations

- Notify the agency supervisor of the patient's status.
- Remain with the patient until directed otherwise by emergency medical system personnel.

Seizure

Definition

Excessively disorganized discharge of cerebral neurons in random and unpredictable patterns.

Signs and Symptoms

- Altered consciousness (transient loss or impairment of consciousness, blank stare, stupor, unconsciousness)
- Altered mental status (confusion, affect changes, hallucinations, disturbed ideation, memory deficits, auras)
- Period of recuperative sleep
- Tachycardia
- Hypertension
- Repeated jerking of fingers, hands, eyelids, or face
- Muscle contractions, tremors, or atony
- Primitive, uncoordinated, purposeless activities (lip smacking, chewing, sucking)
- Spasmodic cry
- Localized numbness or tingling

Action

- Activate the emergency medical system.
- Assist the patient to a safe position, sidelying with the head slightly lower than the body.
- Protect the airway (e.g., remove dentures, gum, food).
- Clear the surrounding area of potentially hazardous objects.
- Pad the surrounding area, particularly around the head.
- Monitor the vital signs and be prepared to initiate CPR.
- Notify the physician of the patient's status.
- Notify the agency supervisor of the patient's status.
- Remain with the patient until directed further by emergency medical system personnel.

Shock
Definition

State of impaired tissue perfusion that occurs secondary to circulatory failure.

Cardiogenic Shock
Definition

Shock caused by poor myocardium contractile force and/or rhythm, resulting in poor cardiac output and ejection fraction.

Signs and Symptoms

- Altered consciousness (lethargy, stupor, somnolence, unconsciousness)
- Altered mental status (agitation, restlessness, anxiety, confusion)
- Chest pain
- Tachycardia (weak, thready pulse)
- Dysrhythmia
- Hypotension
- Jugular vein distension
- Tachypnea
- Adventitious breath sounds (rales)
- Decreased urinary output
- Diaphoresis
- Cool, clammy skin
- Peripheral cyanosis

Action

- Activate the emergency medical system.
- Assist the patient who does not have signs of respiratory distress or myocardial infarction to the physiological shock position, with the lower extremities elevated 30 degrees and the head elevated 15 to 30 degrees.
- Assist the patient who has signs of respiratory distress or myocardial infarction to the sitting position.
- Assist the unconscious patient or the patient who has oral hemorrhaging or is vomiting to the sidelying position, with the head slightly lower than the body.
- Administer high-flow oxygen, if available, at 5 to 10 L per minute through a nasal cannula.
- Monitor the vital signs and be prepared to initiate CPR.
- Notify the physician of the patient's status.
- Notify the agency supervisor of the patient's status.
- Remain with the patient until directed further by emergency medical system personnel.

Emergency Situations

Hypovolemic Shock

Definition

Shock caused by a reduction in the total blood volume (e.g., hemorrhage, burn, diarrhea, bowel obstruction).

Signs and Symptoms

- Altered consciousness (lethargy, stupor, unconsciousness)
- Altered mental status (anxiety, agitation, restlessness, confusion, progression to apathy)
- Tachycardia
- Orthostatic tachycardia
- Hypotension (systolic <90 mmHg)
- Orthostatic hypotension
- Tachypnea
- Thirst
- Poor capillary refill
- Cool, clammy skin
- Decreased urinary output

Action

- Activate the emergency medical system.
- Assist the patient who does not have signs of respiratory distress or myocardial infarction to the physiological shock position, with the lower extremities elevated 30 degrees and the head elevated 15 to 30 degrees.
- Assist the patient who has signs of respiratory distress or myocardial infarction to the sitting position.
- Assist the unconscious patient or the patient who has oral hemorrhaging or is vomiting to the sidelying position, with the head slightly lower than the body.
- Administer high-flow oxygen, if available, at 5 to 10 L per minute through a nasal cannula.
- Monitor the vital signs and be prepared to initiate CPR.
- Notify the physician of the patient's status.
- Notify the agency supervisor of the patient's status.
- Remain with the patient until directed further by emergency medical system personnel.

Vasogenic Shock
Definition

Shock caused by severe arterial and venous distension.

Signs and Symptoms
Early

- Altered consciousness (lethargy)
- Altered mental status (agitation, restlessness, confusion)
- Tachypnea
- Erythema
- Warm skin
- Fever (5%-10% of cases are hypothermic)

Late

- Altered consciousness (unconsciousness)
- Altered mental status (apathy)
- Hypotension
- Poor capillary refill
- Poor clotting (bruising)
- Decreased urinary output

Action

- Activate the emergency medical system.
- Administer high-flow oxygen, if available, at 5 to 10 L per minute through a nasal cannula.
- Monitor the vital signs and be prepared to initiate CPR.
- Notify the physician of the patient's status.
- Notify the agency supervisor of the patient's status.
- Remain with the patient until directed further by emergency medical system personnel.

Suicide Ideation
Definition

Patient verbalization of the desire to end his or her own life.

Signs and Symptoms

- Patient statements expressing the desire to be dead
- Verbalized hopelessness
- Verbalized helplessness
- Depressive symptoms (e.g., fatigue, loss of appetite)

Action

- Leave the home immediately if you feel in danger.
- Notify the physician of the patient's status.
- Notify the agency supervisor of the patient's status.

Emergency Situations

- Remove the means of suicide if the patient allows (e.g., if the patient plans to overdose on medications, remove medications).
- Remain with the patient until directed further by the physician and agency supervisor unless a threat to personal safety exists.

Transient Ischemic Attack

Definition

Transient focal neurological deficits resulting from anterior or posterior circulation occlusion, with deficit resolution within 24 hours.

Signs and Symptoms

- Altered consciousness (lethargy)
- Altered mental status (disorientation, confusion)
- Headache
- Hypertension
- Hypoventilation
- Dyspnea and/or labored breathing
- Dysphagia
- Dysarthria
- Aphasia
- Unilateral weakness (bilateral weakness if bilateral disruption of blood flow is present)
- Ataxia
- Apraxia
- Unilateral sensory deficits (bilateral sensory deficits if bilateral disruption of blood flow is present)
- Vision deficits (diplopia, hemianopsia, mononuclear blindness)
- Neglect
- Dizziness and/or vertigo
- Vomiting
- Cyanosis

Action

- Activate the emergency medical system.
- Assist the patient to a resting position.
- Administer oxygen, if available, at 5 L per minute through a nasal cannula.
- Monitor the vital signs and be prepared to initiate CPR.
- Notify the physician of the patient's status.
- Notify the agency supervisor of the patient's status.
- Remain with the patient until directed further by emergency medical system personnel.

Urinary Tract Infection

Definition

Abnormally high levels of microorganisms in the urinary tract.

Signs and Symptoms

- Low-grade fever
- Fatigue
- Dysuria
- Increased urinary frequency
- Increased urinary urgency
- Burning with urination
- Chills
- Nausea
- Vomiting

Action

- Notify the physician of the patient's status.
- Notify the agency supervisor of the patient's status.
- Encourage the patient to drink noncaffeinated fluids.
- Remain with the patient until directed further by the physician and agency supervisor.

CARDIOPULMONARY RESUSCITATION

CPR procedures provide quick references for the implementation of life saving actions.

Cardiopulmonary Resuscitation Procedures

The following procedures are based on and follow the American Heart Association guidelines (1997) for basic life support. Home care therapists should obtain recertification in basic life support procedures at least every 1 to 2 years to stay abreast of guideline changes.

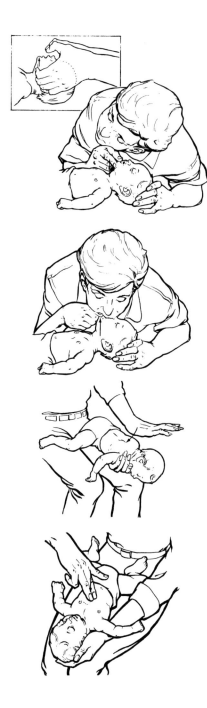

Gently tap or shake the infant. If the infant does not respond, shout for help.

NOTE: The use of latex gloves and a mouth barrier with a one-way valve (for rescue breathing) is recommended.

1. Open the airway and check breathing.

Lay the infant on his or her back. If you must roll the infant on the back, keep (support) the head and neck in a straight line. Tilt the head back gently (not too far), and lift the chin slightly. Make sure the mouth is clear and the tongue is not blocking the airway. Listen, look, and feel for breath (3-4 sec.). If the infant is not breathing, or you are in doubt, start rescue breathing. If you suspect neck or back injury, pull open the jaw without moving the head using the jaw-thrust maneuver (see inset).

2. Give two slow breaths.

Cover the infant's nose and mouth with your mouth. Give two slow, *very gentle* breaths (puffs) of 1 to 1½ seconds each. Allow the chest to rise and fall between breaths. NOTE: *Watch the chest.* If the chest does not rise and fall after two breaths, retilt the head, pull the chin up, and try again. If the airway is blocked, go to picture #3. If the chest does rise and fall, *check the brachial pulse,* as in picture #6.

3. If something is in the airway, use back blows.

Place the infant face down over your forearm, resting the arm on your thigh as shown, with the infant's head lower than the chest. Support the infant's head by holding the jaw with your hand. Give five quick, firm back blows between the shoulders with the heel of your hand. If this does not work, go to #4.

4. If the airway is still blocked, use chest thrusts.

Turn the infant over, still holding (supporting) the head lower than the chest. Place two or three fingers one finger width below the nipple line and give five downward thrusts. Open the infant's mouth by grasping the tongue and lower jaw between the thumb and fingers, and lifting. Only if you see the object, gently sweep the index finger (hooking motion) deeply into the mouth at the base of the tongue to remove the foreign object from the throat.

Modified from Manhoff D, Vogel S: *Mosby's emergency medical treatment: infants, children, adults,* St Louis, 1996, Mosby.

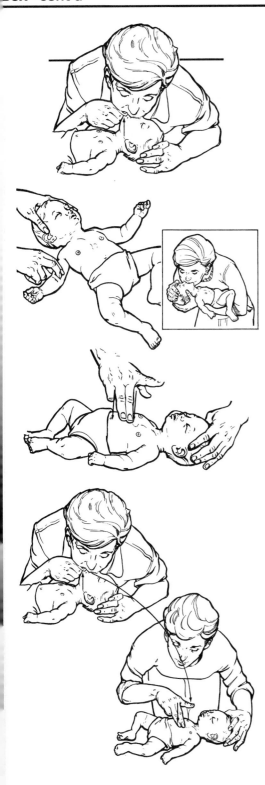

5. Repeat two slow breaths.

Tilt the head back, lift the chin, cover the infant's nose and mouth with your mouth, and give two slow, *very gentle* breaths (puffs). Watch the chest rise and fall. Repeat #3, #4, and #5, if necessary. Check for the brachial pulse.

6. Check for the brachial pulse.

With the thumb on the outside of the arm, press the middle and index fingers gently into the inside of the upper arm (see picture). Feel for a pulse 3 to 4 seconds. *If there is no pulse,* start chest compressions (#7), along with rescue breathing. If the infant has a pulse, but is not breathing, continue one breath every 3 seconds for 1 minute (20 breaths/puffs). **Activate the emergency medical system.** (If you do not suspect a neck or back injury take infant with you while you call.) Recheck the breathing and pulse and continue one breath every 3 seconds until the infant breathes on his or her own or emergency medical personnel arrive.

7. Place the middle and ring fingers on the midsternum. Push down on the chest ½ to 1 inch (1.25 to 2.5 cm) five times.

Push down on the chest five times (rate of 100/min.). Let the chest relax completely between downstrokes, without removing your fingers from the chest.

8. Give one slow breath.

Tilt the head back. Lift the chin. Cover the infant's nose and mouth with your mouth. Give one slow, *very gentle* breath (puff). Make sure the chest rises and falls.

9. Continue five chest compressions and then one breath for 20 cycles. Activate the emergency medical system.

Alternate five compressions and one breath for 20 cycles (1 minute). (If you do not suspect a neck or back injury, take infant with you.) Recheck the breathing and pulse (3 to 4 sec.). If there is a pulse but no breathing, give one breath (puff) every 3 seconds. If there is no pulse, continue five chest compressions and then one breath (puff). Continue this until the infant breathes on his or her own or emergency medical personnel arrive. Recheck the breathing pulse at least every 5 minutes. NOTE: Allow the chest to rise and fall between breaths, and let the chest relax completely between downstrokes.

Emergency Situations

Infant Foreign Body Airway Obstruction Removal

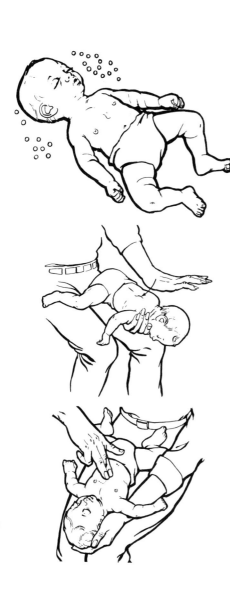

Do nothing if the infant is coughing, breathing, or "talking." Do not shake the infant or hold upside down.

NOTE: The use of latex gloves and mouth barrier with one-way valve (for rescue breathing) is recommended.

1. Recognize choking.

Use this procedure if you have seen or strongly suspect the infant is choking on an object and if breathing is becoming more difficult. Lips may appear blue.

2. If something is in the airway, use back blows.

Place the infant face down over your forearm, resting the arm on your thigh (as shown), with the infant's head lower than the chest. Support the infant's head by holding the jaw with your hand. Give five *quick, firm* back blows between the shoulders with the heel of your hand (if water or vomit comes up, clear the mouth). If this does not work, go to #3.

3. If the airway is still blocked, use chest thrusts.

Turn the infant over, still holding (supporting) the head lower than the chest. Place two or three fingers one finger width below the nipple line, and give five downward thrusts. Open the infant's mouth by grasping the tongue and lower jaw between the thumb and fingers, and lifting. Only if you see the object, gently sweep the index finger (hooking motion) deeply into the mouth at the base of the tongue to remove the foreign body from the throat. Repeat #2 and #3 until the obstruction is gone or the infant becomes unconscious.

If the infant becomes unconscious, shout for help and begin rescue breathing.

Modified from Manhoff D, Vogel S: *Mosby's emergency medical treatment: infants, children, adults,* St Louis, 1996, Mosby.

3ox—cont'd

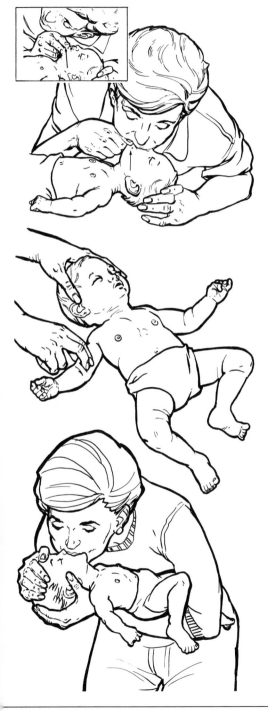

4. Open the airway and check the breathing. Give two slow breaths.

Lay the infant on his or her back. Tilt the head back gently (not too far), and lift the chin slightly. Look, listen, and feel for breath (3-4 sec.). Cover the infant's nose and mouth with your mouth. Give two slow, *very gentle* breaths (puffs) of 1 to 1½ seconds each. Allow the chest to rise and fall between breaths. NOTE: If the chest does not rise and fall after two breaths, retilt the head, lift the chin up, and try again. If the airway is still blocked, repeat #2, #3, and #4 until successful. When the airway is clear, check for a pulse (#5).

5. Check for the brachial pulse.

With the thumb on the outside of the arm, press the middle and index fingers gently into the inside of the upper arm (see picture). Feel for the pulse 3 to 4 seconds. *If there is no pulse,* start chest compressions (p. 555, #7), along with rescue breathing. If the infant has a pulse but is not breathing, go to #6.

6. Give one breath every 3 seconds for 1 minute.

Continue mouth-to-mouth/nose breathing, one breath every 3 seconds for 1 minute (20 breaths/puffs). **Activate the evergency medical system.** Recheck the breathing and pulse (3-4 sec.). Continue giving one breath every 3 seconds (20/min). Recheck the breathing/pulse at least every few minutes until the baby breathes on his or her own or emergency medical personnel arrive. NOTE: If you do not suspect head or neck injury, carry the infant to the phone (support the head and neck, as in the picture) while you continue rescue breathing.

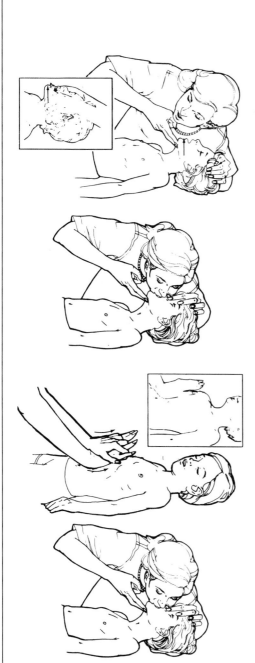

Gently tap or shake the child. Ask, "Are You OK?" If the child does not respond, shout for help.
NOTE: The use of latex gloves and a mouth barrier with a one-way valve (for rescue breathing) is recommended.

1. Open the airway and check for breathing.

Lay the child on his or her back. If you must roll the child on the back, keep (support) the head and neck in a straight line. Tilt the head back gently, lift the chin slightly. If you suspect a neck or back injury, pull open the jaw without moving the head using the jaw-thrust maneuver (see inset). Look, listen, and feel for breath (3 to 4 sec.). If the child is not breathing, or you are in doubt, start rescue breathing (#2). If the child is breathing, place the child on the side (unless head, neck, or back injury).

2. Give two slow breaths.

Pinch the nose. Cover the child's mouth with yours. Give two slow, *gentle* breaths (1 to 1½ sec. each) into the child's mouth. Allow the chest to rise and fall between breaths. NOTE: *Watch the chest.* If the chest does not rise and fall after two breaths, retilt the head, lift the chin up, and try again. If the airway is blocked, go to picture #3. If the chest does rise and fall, *check the pulse,* as in picture #5.

3. If something is in the airway, do the following:

Straddle the child's thighs. Place the heel of one hand just above the navel, but well below the xyphoid process. Place your other hand directly on top of your first hand with the fingers pointing to the head. Press upward into the abdomen with up to five quick thrusts. Open the mouth by grasping the tongue and lower jaw between the thumb and finger and lifting. Only if you see the object, gently sweep the index finger (hooking motion) deeply into the mouth at the base of the tongue to remove it from the throat.

4. Repeat two slow breaths.

Tilt the head back. Lift the chin. Pinch the nose. Cover the child's mouth with yours and give two slow, *gentle* breaths. Watch the chest rise and fall. Repeat #3 and #4 if necessary.

Modified from Manhoff D, Vogel S: *Mosby's emergency medical treatment: infants, children, adults,* St Louis, 1996, Mosby.

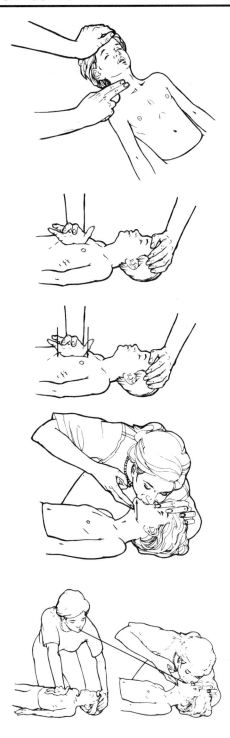

5. Check for the carotid pulse.

Press two or three fingers into the neck just to the side of the Adam's apple. Feel for a pulse 3 to 4 seconds. *If there is no pulse,* start chest compressions immediately (#6), along with rescue breathing. If the child has a pulse, but is not breathing, continue one breath every 3 seconds for 1 minute (20 breaths). **Activate the emergency medical system.** Return to the child, and recheck the breathing and pulse (3-4 sec.). Continue one breath every 3 seconds until the child breathes on his or her own or emergency medical personnel arrive. Roll the child onto the side if breathing resumes (unless head, neck, or back injury is suspected).

6. Place the heel of the hand 1 to 2 cm above the xyphoid process.

Follow the rib cage to where it meets in the center of the lower part of the chest. Place the entire heel of the hand 1 to 2 cm above the xyphoid process.

7. Push down on the chest 1 to 1½ inches (2.5 to 3.8 cm) for an older child and ¾ to 1½ inches (2 to 4 cm) for a toddler or preschooler five times.

Straighten your arm, lock the elbow, and push straight down on the chest five times (a rate of 100 per minute). Let the chest relax completely between downstrokes, without removing the hand from the chest.

8. Give one breath.

Tilt the head back. Lift the chin. Pinch the nose. Give one slow, gentle breath.

9. Continue with five chest compressions and then one breath for 20 cycles (1 minute).

Alternate five compressions and one breath for 20 cycles (1 minute). Quickly return to the child. Recheck the pulse and breathing (3 to 4 sec.). If there is a pulse but no breathing, give one breath every 3 seconds (20 per minute). If there is no pulse, continue five chest compressions and then one breath until the child breathes on his or her own or emergency medical personnel arrive. Recheck the breathing and pulse at least every 5 minutes. NOTE: Allow the chest to rise and fall between breaths, and let the chest relax completely between downstrokes. Roll the child onto the side if breathing resumes (unless head, neck, or back injury is suspected).

Emergency Situations

Child Foreign Body Airway Obstruction Removal (Heimlich Maneuver)

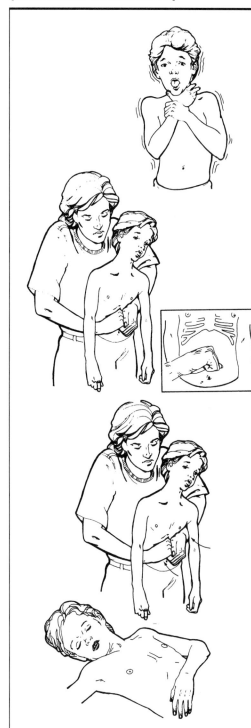

Ask, "Are you choking?"
NOTE: The use of latex gloves and a mouth barrier with a one-way valve (for rescue breathing) is recommended.

1. Recognize choking.
The child is unable to speak, breathe, or cough. *Do nothing* if the child is coughing, talking, or breathing. *Do not* slap the child on the back or turn upside down. *Do not* probe the throat with your fingers.

2. Stand behind the child with your arms wrapped around the waist.
Wrap your arms around the child's waist from behind. Make a fist and place the thumb side against the stomach just above the navel but well below the xyphoid process as pictured. Grasp the fist with your other hand.

3. Press the fist upward into the child's abdomen with up to five quick, upward thrusts.
Give up to five upward thrusts. Check the child. Repeat giving five upward thrusts, and check the child until the obstruction is cleared or the child becomes unconscious. For a small child, use less force.

If the child becomes unconscious, shout for help. Go to #4.

4. Lay the child on his or her back and check the airway.
Only if the child is unconscious, open the mouth by grasping the tongue and lower jaw between the thumb and fingers, and lifting. Only if you see the object, gently sweep the index finger (hooking motion) deeply into the mouth at the base of the tongue to remove it from the throat.

Modified from Manhoff D, Vogel S: *Mosby's emergency medical treatment: infants, children, adults,* St Louis, 1996, Mosby.

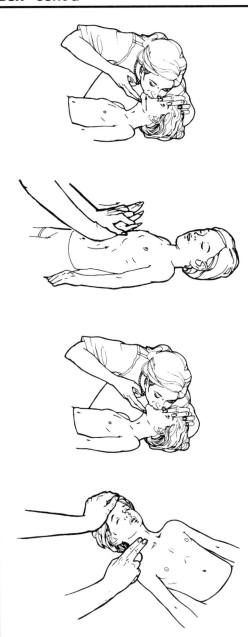

5. Give two slow breaths.

Tilt the head back gently, and lift the chin slightly. Pinch the nose. Cover the child's mouth with yours and give two slow, gentle breaths (1-1½ seconds each). Allow the chest to rise and fall between breaths. NOTE: If the chest does not rise and fall after two breaths, retilt the head, lift the chin up, and try again. If the airway is still blocked, go to #6.

6. Give up to five upward abdominal thrusts.

Straddle the child's thighs. Place the heel of one hand just above the navel, but well below the xyphoid process. Place your other hand directly on top of your first hand with the fingers pointing to the head. Press upward into the abdomen with up to five quick thrusts. Open the mouth by grasping the tongue and lower jaw between the thumb and fingers, and lifting. Only if you see the object, gently sweep the index finger (hooking motion) deeply into the mouth at the base of the tongue to remove the foreign body from the throat.

7. Repeat two slow breaths as above.

Repeat procedure #5. If the airway is still blocked (chest *does not* rise and fall), repeat #6. If the airway is clear (chest *does* rise and fall), go to #8.

8. Check for the carotid pulse.

Press two or three fingers into the neck just to the side of the Adam's apple. Feel for a pulse three or four seconds. If there is no pulse, start chest compressions (p. 559, #6) along with mouth-to-mouth breathing. If the child has a pulse, but is not breathing, continue one breath every 3 seconds for 1 minute (20 breaths).

Activate the emergency medical system and quickly return to child. Give one breath every 3 seconds until the child breathes on his or her own or emergency medical personnel arrive. Recheck the breathing and pulse every few minutes. Roll the child onto the side if breathing resumes (unless head, neck, or back injury is suspected).

Emergency Situations

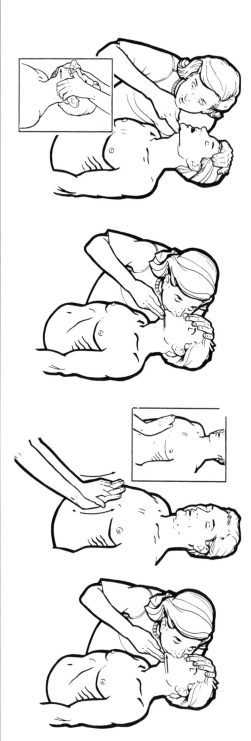

Gently tap or shake the individual. Ask, "Are you OK?" If the individual does not respond, activate the emergency medical system immediately.

NOTE: The use of latex gloves and a mouth barrier with a one-way valve (for rescue breathing) is recommended.

1. Open the airway and check for breathing.

Lay the individual on his or her back. To roll the individual on the back, keep (support) the head and neck in a straight line. Tilt the head back gently, and lift the chin slightly. If you suspect neck or back injury, pull open the jaw without moving the head using the jaw-thrust maneuver (see inset). Look, listen, and feel for breath (3 to 5 sec.). If the individual is not breathing or you are in doubt, start rescue breathing (#2). If the individual is breathing, place on the side (unless head, neck, or back injury).

2. Give two slow breaths.

Pinch the nose. Cover the individual's mouth with yours. Give two slow, *full* breaths (1½ to 2 seconds each) into the individual's mouth. Allow the chest to rise and fall between breaths. NOTE: *Watch the chest.* If the chest does not rise and fall after two breaths, retilt the head, lift the chin up, and try again. If the airway is blocked, go to picture #3. If the chest does rise and fall, *check the pulse,* as in picture #5.

3. If something is in the airway, do the following:

Straddle the individual's thighs, and place the heel of one hand just above the navel, but well below the xyphoid process (see inset). Place your other hand directly on top of your first hand with the fingers pointing to the head. Press upward into the abdomen with up to five quick thrusts. Open the mouth by grasping the tongue and lower jaw between the thumb and fingers, and lifting. Gently sweep the index finger (hooking motion) deeply into the mouth at the base of the tongue to remove the foreign body from the throat.

4. Repeat two slow breaths.

Tilt the head back. Lift the chin. Pinch the nose. Cover the individual's mouth with yours and give two slow, *full* breaths. Watch the chest rise and fall. Repeat #3 and #4 as long as necessary.

Modified from Manhoff D, Vogel S: *Mosby's emergency medical treatment: infants, children, adults,* St Louis, 1996, Mosby.

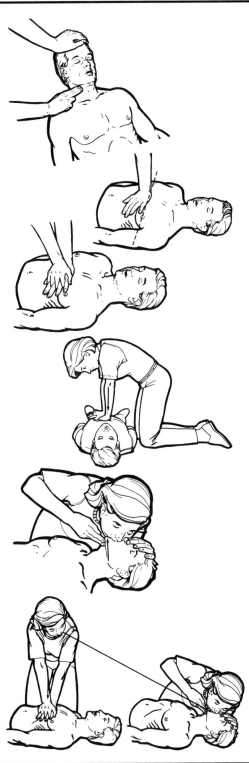

5. Check for a carotid pulse on the side of the neck.

Press two or three fingers into the neck just to the side of the Adam's apple. Feel for a pulse 5 to 10 seconds. *If there is no pulse,* start chest compressions (#6) along with mouth-to-mouth breathing. If the individual has a pulse, continue giving one breath every 5 seconds. NOTE: Recheck for breathing and a pulse every few minutes. Continue until the victim breathes on his or her own or an ambulance arrives.

6. Place the heel of the hand 1 to 2 cm above the xyphoid process. Place the other hand on top of the first hand.

Follow the rib cage to where it meets in the center of the lower part of the chest. Place the entire heel of the hand one or two finger widths above the lower tip of the breastbone, or draw an imaginary line between the nipples to find the mid-breastbone. Place the heel of the hand in the *middle* of the chest, *just below* the imaginary line.

7. Push down on the chest 1½ to 2 inches (3.8 to 5 cm) 15 times.

Straighten your arms, lock the elbows, and push straight down on the chest 15 times (rate of 80 to 100 per minute). Let the chest relax completely between downstrokes, without removing the hands from the chest.

8. Repeat two slow breaths.

Tilt the head back. Lift the chin. Pinch the nose. Cover the victim's mouth with yours and give two slow, full breaths.

9. Continue with 15 chest compressions and then two breaths.

Continue to alternate 15 compressions and two breaths for four cycles. Allow the chest to rise and fall between breaths, and let the chest relax completely between compressions. Recheck the carotid pulse and breathing. If there is a pulse but no breathing, give one breath every 5 seconds (12/min). If there is no pulse, continue alternating 15 chest compressions and two breaths. Recheck the breathing and pulse at least every few minutes. Continue until the individual breathes on his or her own or emergency medical personnel arrive. Roll the individual onto the side if breathing resumes (unless head, neck, or back injury is suspected).

Emergency Situations

Adult Foreign Body Airway Obstruction Removal (Heimlich Maneuver)

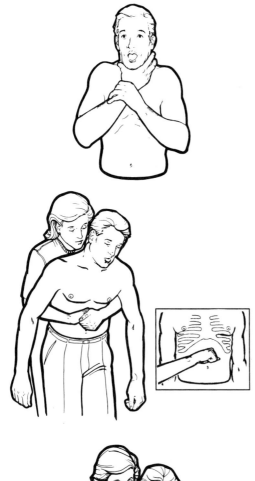

Ask, "Are you choking?"

NOTE: The use of latex gloves and a mouth barrier with a one-way valve (for rescue breathing) is recommended.

1. Recognize choking.

The individual is unable to speak, breathe, or cough. *Do nothing* if the individual is coughing, talking, or breathing. Do not slap the individual on the back. Do not probe the throat with your fingers.

2. Stand behind the individual with your arms wrapped around the waist.

Wrap your arms around the waist from behind. Make a fist and place the thumb side against the abdomen just above the navel but well below the xyphoid process as pictured. Grasp the fist with your other hand.

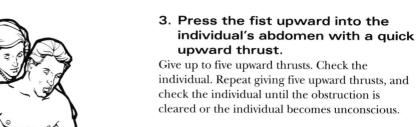

3. Press the fist upward into the individual's abdomen with a quick upward thrust.

Give up to five upward thrusts. Check the individual. Repeat giving five upward thrusts, and check the individual until the obstruction is cleared or the individual becomes unconscious.

If the individual becomes unconscious, activate the emergency medical system immediately.

Modified from Manhoff D, Vogel S: *Mosby's emergency medical treatment: infants, children, adults,* St Louis, 1996, Mosby.

3ox—cont'd

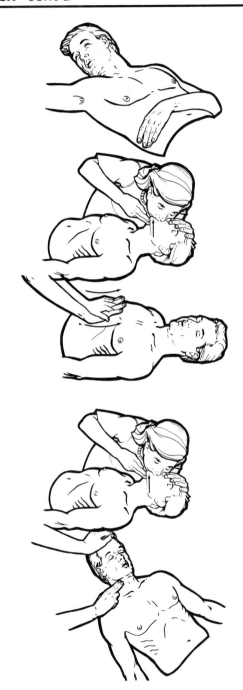

4. Lay the individual on his or her back and check the airway.

Only if the individual is unconscious, open the individual's mouth by grasping the tongue and lower jaw between the thumb and fingers, and lifting. Gently sweep the index finger deeply into the mouth at the base of the tongue to remove the object from the throat.

5. Give two slow breaths.

Tilt the head back gently, and lift the chin slightly. Pinch the nose. Cover the individual's mouth with yours and give two slow, full breaths (1½ to 2 seconds each). Allow the chest to rise and fall between breaths. NOTE: If the chest does not rise and fall, retilt the head, pull the chin up, and try again. If the airway is still blocked, go to #6.

6. Give up to five upward abdominal thrusts.

Straddle the individual's thighs, place the heel of one hand just above the navel, but well below the xyphoid process, and place your other hand directly on top of your first hand with the fingers pointing to the individual's head. Press upward into the abdomen with up to five quick thrusts. Open and clear the mouth (as in #4).

7. Repeat two slow breaths.

Tilt the head back. Lift the chin. Pinch the nose. Give two slow, full breaths. If the airway is still blocked, repeat #6. If the airway is clear, check for a pulse.

8. Check for the carotid pulse.

Press two or three fingers into the neck just to the side of the Adam's apple. Feel for a pulse 5 to 10 seconds. If there is no pulse, see p. 563, #6 and follow the instructions. If the victim has a pulse and is not breathing, continue giving one breath every 5 seconds. Recheck for breathing and a pulse at least every few minutes until the individual breathes on his or her own or emergency medical personnel arrive. Roll the individual onto the side if breathing resumes (unless head, neck, or back injury is suspected).

Cardiopulmonary Resuscitation Standards

Procedure	Adults (over 8 yrs)	Children (1-8 yrs)	Infants (under 1 yr)
Respiratory arrest inflation rate	Two initial breaths; then 12 per minute	Two initial breaths; then 20 per minute	Two initial breaths; then 20 per minute
Hand placement for chest compressions	Two to three fingers above the xyphoid process; use two hands	Two to three fingers above the xyphoid process; use one hand	Middle and ring fingers on the midsternum; use only two fingers
Depth of CPR chest compressions	1½ to 2 inches	1 to 1½ inches (older child) ¾ to 1½ inches (toddler or preschooler)	½ to 1 inch
Rate for CPR compressions	80 to 100 per minute	100 per minute	At least 100 per minute
Ratio of compressions to ventilations	15:2	5:1	5:1
Pulse monitoring site	Carotid pulse	Carotid pulse	Brachial pulse

Modified from Parcel GA, Rinear CE: *Basic emergency care of the sick and injured,* ed 4, St Louis, 1990, Mosby.
CPR, Cardiopulmonary resuscitation.

FIRST AID

First aid procedures provide quick references for the implementation of life and health saving actions. Therapists use these procedures while waiting for emergency medical system personnel to arrive.

First Aid Procedures
First aid assessment

Sign or symptom	What to look for
• State of consciousness	Alertness and orientation to time, individual, and place Drowsiness Semiconsciousness Unconsciousness
• Skin color	Red—increased blood flow to skin Pale—decreased blood flow Blue—insufficient oxygen
• Respiration	Rate—fast, slow, normal Depth—shallow, deep, normal Ease—labored, abnormal or gasping, normal
• Pulse	Rate—fast, slow, normal Strength—strong, weak, normal Regularity—regular, irregular (Check peripheral pulses below injury sites.)
• Pupils	Same—both dilated, constricted, or normal Unequal—one constricted, one dilated
• Pain	Location Type—sharp, dull, radiating Intensity—slight to severe Duration—all the time, intermittent, situational Onset—sudden, gradual (length of time)
• Ability to move	Paralysis—partial to complete, painful
• Numbness	Loss of sensation
• Swelling	Location and extent
• Deformity	Abnormal position or appearance
• Discharge(s) from body openings	Blood, mucus, or cerebrospinal fluid Note: color, consistency, and amount
• Nausea and/or vomiting	Note: amount, odor, color, and consistency
• Convulsions	Note: duration, number of seizures, and parts of the body initially involved, as well as the patient's condition afterward

Modified from Parcel GA, Rinear CE: *Basic emergency care of the sick and injured,* ed 4, St Louis, 1990, Mosby.

Control of Bleeding Standards
Purpose

The purpose is to slow and/or stop the loss of blood from open wounds.

Method

Direct pressure
- Wash the hands with soap and water.
- Apply gloves.
- Apply hard, firm, direct pressure over the wound site (Figure 4-1).

- Elevate the body part, unless contraindicated by musculoskeletal injuries (i.e. fracture) while maintaining pressure.
- Apply a pressure dressing and bandage to the wound while maintaining firm pressure.
- Apply ice (not effective with severe bleeding).

Pressure point

- Locate the pressure point most proximal to the wound (Figure 4-2).
- Apply direct pressure on the pressure point.
- Do not release the pressure point until the bleeding has stopped and/or you are directed by emergency medical system personnel.

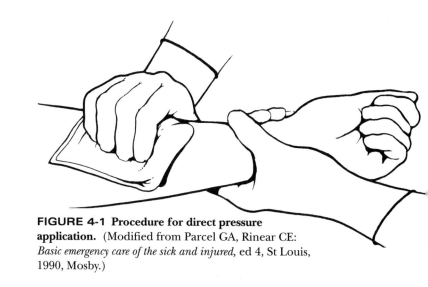

FIGURE 4-1 Procedure for direct pressure application. (Modified from Parcel GA, Rinear CE: *Basic emergency care of the sick and injured,* ed 4, St Louis, 1990, Mosby.)

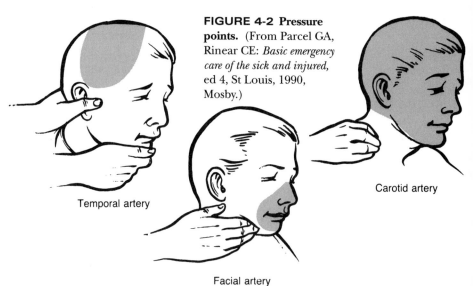

FIGURE 4-2 Pressure points. (From Parcel GA, Rinear CE: *Basic emergency care of the sick and injured,* ed 4, St Louis, 1990, Mosby.)

Temporal artery

Facial artery

Carotid artery

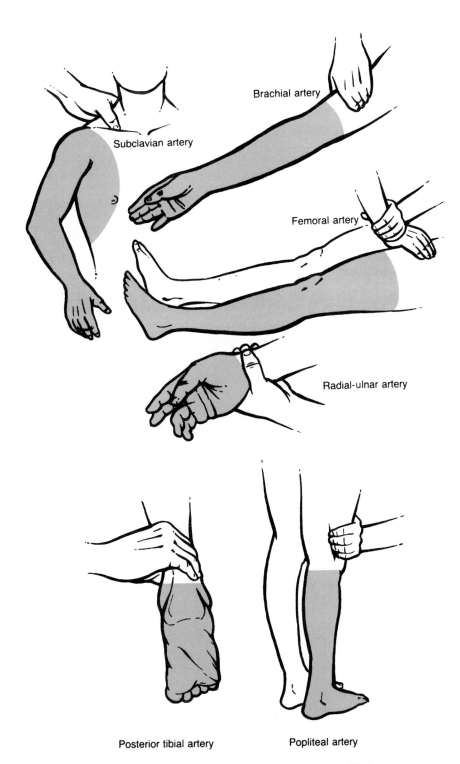

FIGURE 4-2, cont'd Pressure points. (From Parcel GA, Rinear CE: *Basic emergency care of the sick and injured,* ed 4, St Louis, 1990, Mosby.)

Tourniquet
- If the bleeding continues despite direct pressure and pressure point procedures, apply a tourniquet (Figure 4-3).

Wound Care Standards
Purpose

The purpose is to apply proper wound care that minimizes wound contamination and promotes healing.

Method

- Wash the hands with soap and water.
- Apply gloves.
- Control bleeding with direct pressure and pressure point procedures.
- Allow the wound to bleed slightly.
- Saturate gauze with water. (Use sterile gauze and sterile or saline water when possible.)
- Gently use the gauze to wipe debris and dirt from the wound.
- Flush the wound with water using saturated gauze and a clean water container or if possible, hold the affected body part under a gentle stream of water.
- Apply an antibiotic, if available, and if the patient is not allergic to the antibiotic cream.
- Cover the wound with sterile gauze and a bandage.
- Elevate the body part, unless contraindicated by musculoskeletal injuries (i.e., fracture).

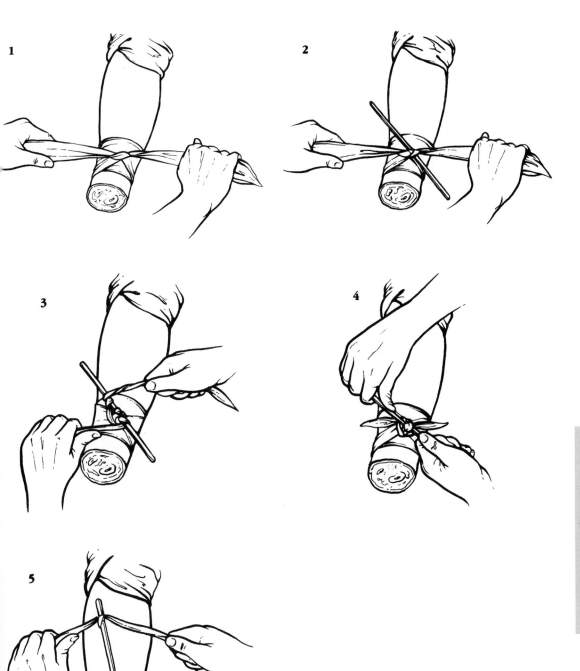

1

2

3

4

5

FIGURE 4-3 Procedure for application of a tourniquet. (From Parcel GA, Rinear CE: *Basic emergency care of the sick and injured,* ed 4, St Louis, 1990, Mosby.)

Internal Poisoning Standards
Purpose

The purpose is to minimize the risk of injury and/or death in poisoning episodes.

Method

Gather pertinent information about the poisoning.
- What poison was internalized?
- What is the dosage and potency of the poison?
- How was the poison internalized?
- When was the poison internalized?
- What has already been done for the patient?

Call the Poison Control Center.

Follow Poison Control Center instructions.

Burn Care Standards
Purpose

The purpose is to relieve pain and reduce the risk for infection.

Method

- Determine the depth of the burn.
- Determine the total body surface involvement (Figure 4-4).

Minor Burns

- Wash the hands with soap and water.
- Apply gloves.
- Immerse the burned area in cool water, or cover the area with an ice water dressing until the coldness becomes more uncomfortable than the burn pain.
- Remove the burned area from the cold water or ice water dressing.
- Cool the burned area again when the burn pain returns after a few minutes.
- Repeat this procedure three to four times, until the burn is no longer significantly painful.
- Apply a dry, sterile dressing and bandage.

Serious Burns

- Wash the hands with soap and water.
- Apply gloves.
- Assist the patient to a reclining position, and cover the patient with a clean sheet.
- Cover the burned area with dry, sterile dressing and a bandage.
- Immobilize the burned area.
- Remove constrictive clothing or jewelry.
- Monitor the vital signs and be prepared to initiate CPR.

Chemical Burns

- Flush the burned area with water in a shower or with a garden hose.
- Wash the hands with soap and water.
- Apply gloves.
- Remove clothing and jewelry while flushing the area.

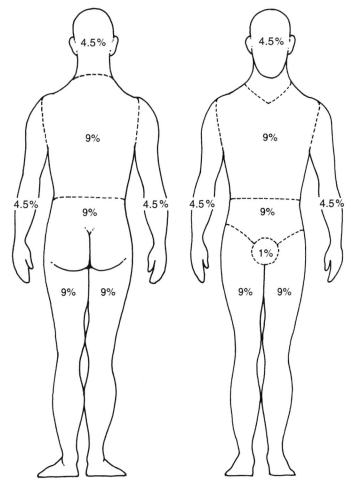

FIGURE 4-4 Classification of burns by body surface areas for adults. (From Parcel GA, Rinear CE: *Basic emergency care of the sick and injured,* ed 4, St Louis, 1990, Mosby.)

- Monitor the vital signs and be prepared to initiate CPR.
- Continue flushing the burned area.

Chemical Eye Burns

- Wash the hands with soap and water.
- Apply gloves.
- Hold the eyelids open with a gauze pad.
- Remove contact lenses.
- Tilt the patient's head to the injured side if only one eye is affected.
- Flush the eye(s) with water for 10 minutes for acid burns and 20 minutes for alkali burns (Figure 4-5).
- Direct the water from the inner corner to the outer corner of the eye.
- Cover the eye(s) with dry, sterile dressing and a bandage.

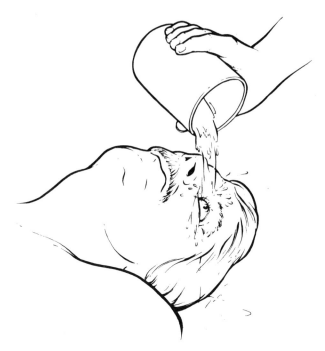

FIGURE 4-5 Eye flushing procedure. (From Parcel GA, Rinear CE: *Basic emergency care of the sick and injured,* ed 4, St Louis, 1990, Mosby.)

Fracture Care Standards
Purpose

The purpose is to minimize further displacement and injury to the fractured body part.

Method

- Immobilize above and below the fractured body part with a splint (Figure 4-6).
- Assist the patient to a resting position, keeping the fracture site immobilized. (Do not attempt to move someone with suspected vertebral fractures unless absolutely necessary.)
- Wash the hands with soap and water.
- Apply gloves.
- Control bleeding using direct pressure and pressure point procedures.
- Cover open fractures with a dry, sterile dressing and a bandage.
- Check the immobilized body part for ischemia.
- Pad areas of the splint that come into contact with the body.

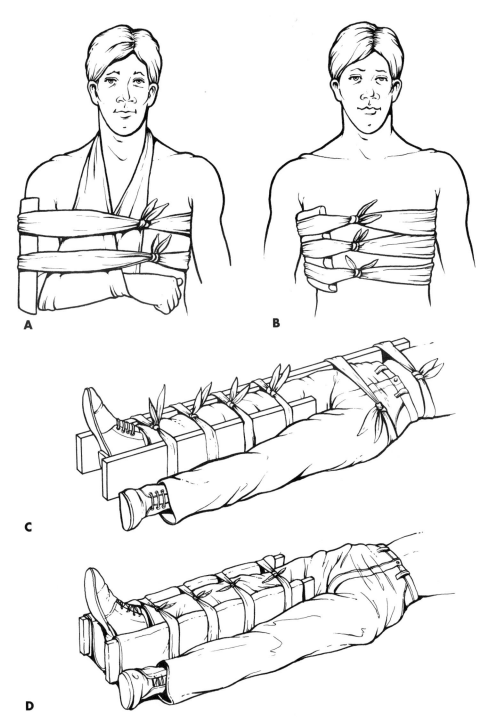

FIGURE 4-6 Immobilization of fracture. A, Upper arm. **B,** Ribs. **C,** Upper leg. **D,** Lower leg. (From Parcel GA, Rinear CE: *Basic emergency care of the sick and injured,* ed 4, St Louis, 1990, Mosby.)

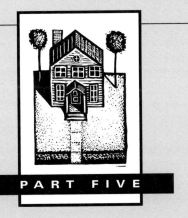

PART FIVE

Pharmacology

MEDICATION CLASSIFICATION

MEDICATION MANAGEMENT

MEDICATION CLASSIFICATION

As home care therapists assume roles of case managers, they need quick access to pharmacological information required to complete medication profiles and plans of care. Specifically, therapists require a basic understanding of drug actions and a user-friendly format for determining drug classification. The medication classification glossary defines drug classes. Although the mechanisms of most drugs are not fully understood, this glossary provides an overall summary of current knowledge. The medication indices assist therapists in accurately classifying drugs by generic and trade names.

Medication Classification Glossary

Adrenergic agents. Drugs that affect the sympathetic nervous system. Medication effects vary depending on the specific receptor sites targeted in the body. For example, agents stimulating lung beta$_2$-adrenergic receptors cause bronchodilation. The mechanism of drug action is direct stimulation or blockage of adrenergic receptors.

Adrenocorticosteroids. Drugs that imitate the endogenous hormone cortisol. Medication effects occur in multiple body systems, but the primary use is for their antiinflammatory effects. Other drug effects include alteration of protein and carbohydrate metabolism, redistribution of body fat, and balance of fluids and electrolytes. The mechanism of drug action is control of the rate of protein synthesis. (Protein synthesis may be accelerated or decelerated depending on the specific protein and body site.)

Anabolic steroids. Analogs of the endogenous hormone testosterone that enhance male secondary sexual characteristics. Medication effects vary and may include muscle hypertrophy, increased bone density, protein anabolism, and increased erythropoietin production. The mechanism of drug action is direct binding to receptor sites.

Analgesic agents. Drugs that decrease pain. Medication effects vary depending on the specific drug subclass (i.e., narcotics, nonsteroidal antiinflammatories). The mechanism of drug action varies by drug subclass and is not fully understood, but it may include binding to opiate receptors or inhibition of prostaglandin synthesis. (Prostaglandins are involved in peripheral pain mechanisms.)

Androgens. See *anabolic steroids.*

AntiAlzheimer's agents. Drugs that minimize or slow advancement of the symptoms of Alzheimer's disease. Medication effects include regulation of cerebral blood flow, which increases oxygen utilization of the brain. The mechanism of drug action is not fully understood but may include reversible binding to cholinesterase enzymes, which increases central nervous system acetylcholine levels or stabilization of ganglion metabolism, which optimizes oxygen utilization.

Antianginal agents. Drugs that minimize ischemic coronary artery episodes. Medication effects include reduction of preload and afterload, as well as dilatation of the coronary arteries. The mechanism of drug action is an increase in cyclic guanosine monophosphate, which relaxes vascular smooth muscle tone.

Antiarrhythmic agents. Drugs that correct rhythm disturbances such as atrial or ventricular tachycardia. Medication effects include conductivity alteration of the electrical pathways in the heart. The mechanism of drug action varies by the type of arrhythmia and antiarrhythmic subclass and is not fully understood. For example, some agents combine with fast sodium channels in their inactive states, inhibiting recovery after repolarization, which reduces the ventricular contraction rate.

Antiarthritic agents. Drugs that decrease the symptoms of arthritis. Medication effects include reduced inflammation and pain associated with osteoarthritis and rheumatoid arthritis. The mechanism of drug action varies by drug subclass and is not fully understood, but it includes inhibition of prostaglandin synthesis. (Prostaglandins are involved in peripheral pain mechanisms.)

Antibacterial agents. Drugs that combat infection and/or prevent the spread of infection. Medication effects include a decrease in the number of microorganisms. The mechanism of drug action varies by drug subclass and is not fully understood, but it includes blockage of bacterial production of essential metabolites and/or inhibition of bacterial cell wall synthesis.

Antibiotic agents. See *antibacterial agents.*

Anticholinergic agents. Drugs that decrease cholinergic effects in the body. Medication effects include decreased gastrointestinal motility, reduced stomach acid production, dry mouth, and promotion of urinary retention. The mechanism of drug action is blockage of acetylcholine receptor sites.

Anticoagulant agents. Drugs that retard blood coagulation. Medication effects include "thinning" the blood. The mechanism of drug action varies by drug subclass but includes blockage of specific steps of the clotting cascade.

Anticonvulsant agents. Drugs that decrease the incidence and/or severity of seizure activity in the brain. Medication effects include promotion of normal cell electroconductivity. The mechanism of drug action varies by drug subclass and is not fully understood, but it may include stabilization of neural membranes and/or reduced synaptic transmission.

Antidepressant agents. Drugs that improve mood. Medication effects include decreased feelings of anxiety and worthlessness, reduced cognitive disturbances, and decreased insomnia. The mechanism of drug action varies by drug subclass and is not fully understood, but it may include increased levels of certain neurochemicals (i.e., norepinephrine, serotonin), resulting in normalized neurochemistry.

Antidiarrheal agents. Drugs that inhibit gastrointestinal motility and propulsion. Medication effects include decreased fecal volume, increased fecal viscosity and density, and limited loss of fluids and electrolytes. The mechanism of drug action varies by drug subclass and is not fully understood, but it includes interference with cholinergic and noncholinergic mechanisms. These mechanisms stimulate circular and longitudinal gastrointestinal musculature, causing inhibition of peristaltic activity.

Antiemetic agents. Drugs that suppress nausea and vomiting. The mechanism of drug action varies by drug subclass and is not fully understood, but it may include increased central anticholinergic activity, inhibition of type three serotonergic receptors ($5\text{-}HT_3$), or blockage of dopamine receptors at the chemoreceptor trigger zone.

Antifungal agents. Drugs that combat the spread of fungal infections. Medication effects include fungal death and/or slowing of fungal growth. The mechanism of drug action varies by drug subclass and is not fully understood, but it includes disruption of fungal cell division or impairment of fungal cell membrane formation or function.

Antiglaucoma agents. Drugs that improve glaucoma. Medication effects include decreased aqueous production or increased aqueous outflow in the eye, which lower intraocular pressure. The mechanism of drug action varies by drug subclass and is not fully understood.

Antigout agents. Drugs that decrease the symptoms of gout. Medication effects include reduced pain, decreased inflammation, and less tenderness of affected joints. The mechanism of drug action is not fully understood, but it includes a decrease of uric acid in the body or stabilization and/or breakdown of urate crystals in affected joints.

Antihistamine agents. Drugs that modify immune responses to allergens. Medication effects range from decreased histamine response and drowsiness to reduced nausea and decreased vertigo symptoms. The mechanism of drug action is blockage of histamine$_1$ receptors.

Antihypertensive agents. Drugs that lower blood pressure (systolic and/or diastolic). Medication effects vary but may include lower peripheral vascular resistance, decreased pulse rate, and reduced intravascular volume. Drug subclasses include, but are not limited to, angiotensin converting enzyme inhibitors, beta-blockers, and calcium channel blockers, all of which have different mechanisms of action.

Antiinflammatory agents. Drugs that decrease the inflammatory response to injuries. Medication effects vary by drug subclass but include decreased edema, antipyresis, and reduced joint stiffness. The mechanism of drug action varies by drug subclass and is not fully understood, but it may include inhibition of cyclooxygenase. (Cyclooxygenase is responsible for prostaglandin production.)

Antimigraine agents. Drugs that decrease the intensity and/or duration of migraine headaches. Medication effects include vasoconstriction of the carotid vasculature. The mechanism of drug action varies by drug subclass and is not fully understood, but it includes stimulation of vascular serotonin receptors or alpha-adrenergic receptors, resulting in vasoconstriction.

Antinausea agents. See *antiemetic agents.*

Antineoplastic agents. Drugs that target cancerous cells. Drug classes include antitumor antibiotics, anthracene derivatives, alkylating agents, and antimetabolites. Medication effects vary by drug subclass but collectively diminish cancer cell replication. The mechanism of drug action varies by drug subclass and is not fully understood.

Antiosteoporosis agents. Drugs that reverse or limit progression of osteoporosis. Medication effects include inhibition of bone resorption and/or increased bone deposition. The mechanism of drug action varies by drug subclass and is not fully understood, but it may include triggering of osteoclast receptor sites, which inhibits resorption or decreased metabolic activity of the osteoclasts, slowing resorption.

AntiParkinson's agents. Drugs that reduce the symptoms of Parkinson's disease. Medication effects include decreased rigidity, tremor, and festination. The mechanism of drug action varies by drug subclass and is not fully understood, but it includes increased release of endogenous dopamine, supply of dopamine precursors, increased central anticholinergic effects, and direct stimulation of dopamine receptor sites.

Antipsychotic agents. Drugs that promote normalized mental function in patients who have psychiatric disorders. Medication effects include control of disorientation, hallucinations, emotional withdrawal, perceptual distortion, and hostility. The mechanism of drug action varies by drug subclass and is not fully understood, but it may include modulation of central nervous system neurotransmitters and/or reduced firing thresholds for central nervous system neurons.

Antipyretic agents. Drugs that reduce fever. The mechanism of drug action varies by drug subclass and is not fully understood, but it includes inhibition of prostaglandin synthesis and activation of the hypothalamus, resulting in lower body temperature in febrile patients.

Antirhinitis agents. Drugs that reduce inflammation of the nasal mucosa and include intranasal preparations containing antihistamines, steroids, or anticholinergics. Medication effects include minimization of the immune response to allergens and/or drying of nasal secretions. The mechanism of drug action varies by drug subclass. For example, anticholinergic properties result in drying of nasal secretions.

Antithrombotic agents. See *anticoagulant agents.*

Antiulcer agents. Drugs that prevent ulcer formation and enhance healing of existing ulcers. Medication effects include formation of a protective barrier over damaged gastrointestinal mucosa and reduced acidity of the upper gastrointestinal tract through a reduction in acid production or neutralization. The mechanism of drug action varies by drug subclass, but it may include formation of a viscous adhesive over damaged mucosal sites when exposed to acid, binding to histamine$_2$ receptors in parietal cells of the stomach, inhibition of hydrogen-potassium adenosine triphosphatase (ATPase) enzymes, or direct acid neutralization by the alkaline properties of the drug.

Antiviral agents. Drugs that combat viruses and/or prevent the spread of viruses. Medication effects include a decrease in the number of viral particles in the blood. The mechanism of action varies by drug subclass and is not fully understood, but collectively it causes inhibition of viral replication.

Anxiolytic agents. Drugs that decrease anxiety. Medication effects include decreased insomnia, apprehension, and tension. The mechanism of drug action varies by drug subclass and is not fully understood, but it may include potentiation of inhibitory activity of the neurotransmitter gamma-aminobutyric acid (GABA) or activity as a partial agonist of serotonin receptors.

Benign prostate hypertrophy agents. Drugs that decrease symptoms of benign prostate hypertrophy. Medication effects include improvement of daytime urinary frequency, urgency, hesitancy, and nocturia. The mechanism of drug action varies by drug subclass, but it includes inhibition of dihydrotestosterone (the primary androgen responsible for stimulation of prostatic growth) or blockage of alpha-adrenergic receptors located in the prostate capsule, prostate adenoma, and bladder trigone.

Bronchodilators. Drugs that enhance airflow to the lungs. Medication effects include expansion of bronchial passageways, decreased airway resistance, and increased vital capacity. The mechanism of drug action varies by drug subclass, but it includes stimulation of beta$_2$-adrenergic receptors, which initiates a process leading to bronchial tree smooth muscle relaxation.

Cardiac glycosides. Drugs that increase cardiac output and/or correct atrial fibrillation. Medication effects vary but include increased cardiac output, enhanced systolic emptying, decreased diastolic heart size, decreased conduction velocity through the atrioventricular node, sympatholytic effect, and decreased vagal activity. The mechanism of drug action is not fully understood, but it may include inhibition of the sodium-potassium ATPase pump in myocardial cells and/or direct suppression of the atrioventricular node.

Central nervous system stimulants. Drugs that decrease the symptoms of narcolepsy and attention deficit disorder and facilitate weight loss in obesity. Drug effects include direct central nervous system and respiratory system stimulation. The mechanism of drug action varies by drug subclass and is not fully understood, but it may include increased serotonin, norepinephrine, and dopamine levels in the central nervous system.

Cold preparations. Drugs that decrease symptoms of the common cold. Medication effects vary depending on the specific drug combination, but they may include cough suppression, antihistamine action, and/or increased sputum production. The mechanism of drug action varies by drug subclass. For example, some agents (e.g., dextromethorphan) affect the cough center in the medulla, resulting in cough suppression.

Diuretics. Drugs that promote excretion of water from the body. Medication effects include alteration of sodium and/or potassium balance in the kidney collection ducts, which promotes fluid excretion. The mechanism of drug action varies by drug subclass and is not fully understood, but it may include inhibition of electrolyte reabsorption in the ascending portion of the loop of Henle, in the distal renal tubule, or in the cortical diluting segment of the nephron.

Electrolytes and fluids. Agents that restore and/or maintain electrolyte and fluid balance. The mechanism of drug action is direct replacement of electrolytes and fluids in patients with deficient or at-risk states.

Erectile dysfunction agents. Drugs that improve symptoms of male erectile dysfunction. Medication effects include increased arterial blood flow to the vascular areas of the penis and/or decreased venous outflow. The mechanism of drug action varies by drug subclass and is not fully understood, but it may include increased cellular concentrations of cyclic adenosine monophosphate (cAMP), initiating a cascade process resulting in decreased venous outflow.

Estrogens. Drugs that restore balance in patients with female hormonal deficiencies and/or establish artificial regulation of female sexual responses. Medication effects include menstrual cycle regulation, oral contraception, and postmenopausal hormone replacement. The mechanism of drug action is direct replacement of the endogenous hormone.

Gastrointestinal motility agents. Drugs that enhance movement of matter along the gastrointestinal tract. Medication effects include increased lower esophageal sphincter pressure; increased esophageal motility; accelerated gastric emptying and intestinal transit; coordination of gastric, pyloric, and duodenal motor activity; and increased colonic motility. The mechanism of drug action varies by drug subclass and is not fully understood, but it may include potentiation of cholinergic excitatory processes at the postganglionic neuromuscular junction of the abdomen.

Hemorrheologic agents. Drugs that promote blood flow and tissue oxygenation. Medication effects include increased erythrocyte flexibility and reduced blood viscosity, which collectively serve to facilitate blood flow. The mechanism of drug action is not fully understood.

Hyperthyroid agents. Drugs that regulate overactive thyroid glands. Medication effects include reversal of hyperthyroid symptoms (i.e., nervousness, fatigability, heat intolerance). The mechanism of action is interference with the oxidation of iodine via blockage of iodine in the thyroid gland, which inhibits synthesis of thyroxine and triiodothyronine.

Hypnotic agents. See *sedatives.*

Hypoglycemic agents. Drugs that regulate glucose. Medication effects include elevated insulin levels, increased insulin sensitivity, slowed absorption of carbohydrates, and modification of carbohydrate use. The mechanism of drug action varies by drug subclass and is not fully understood, but it may include direct supply of exogenous insulin, stimulation of the pancreas to supply more endogenous insulin, or inhibition of alpha-glucosidase enzymes in the intestine.

Hypolipidemic agents. Drugs that normalize levels of lipids and cholesterol in the blood. Medication effects include decreased serum concentrations of low-density lipoproteins, triglycerides, and total cholesterol, as well as increased serum concentrations of high-density lipoproteins. The mechanism of drug action varies by drug subclass and is not fully understood, but it may involve reduced hepatic uptake of free fatty acids, decreased release of free fatty acids from adipose tissue, binding of bile acids in the intestinal tract, and/or inhibition of cholesterol precursor production.

Hypothyroid agents. Drugs that compensate for underactive thyroid glands. Medication effects include reversal of hypothyroid symptoms (i.e., dry skin, cold intolerance, constipation, and weakness). The mechanism of action is direct replacement of thyroid hormones with exogenous thyroid hormones.

Intravenous fluids. See *electrolytes and fluids.*

Laxatives. Drugs that decrease constipation. Medication effects vary depending on drug subclass. For example, some agents increase moisture retention of stool, whereas others irritate the gastrointestinal mucosa, inducing peristaltic activity. The mechanism of drug action varies by drug subclass and is not fully understood.

Muscle relaxants. Drugs that reduce muscle spasm. Medication effects range from central nervous system depression, resulting in muscle relaxation, to suppression of cutaneous reflexes, which lowers muscle excitability. The mechanism of drug action varies by drug subclass and is not fully understood.

Nonsteroidal antiinflammatory agents. See *antiinflammatory agents*.

Nutritional additives. See *electrolytes and fluids*.

Nutritional supplements. Agents that replenish body supplies of essential nutrients such as B_{12}, thiamine, folate, and magnesium. Agent effects vary by supplement type. The mechanism of action is direct replacement of deficient nutrient stores.

Progestins. See *estrogens*.

Sedatives. Drugs that reduce anxiety and insomnia. Medication effects include central nervous system depression such as drowsiness, decreased motor activity, and hyporeflexia. The mechanism of drug action varies by drug subclass and is not fully understood, but it may include enhancement of the inhibitory neurotransmitter gamma-aminobutyric acid.

Stool softeners. See *laxatives*.

Tranquilizers. See *antipsychotic agents*.

Medication Index by Generic Name

Generic name	Trade name	Agent class
acarbose	Precose	Hypoglycemic agents
acebutolol	Sectral	Antihypertensive agents
acetaminophen	Tylenol	Analgesic agents Antipyretic agents
acetaminophen with codeine	Tylenol with Codeine	Analgesic agents Antipyretic agents
acyclovir	Zovirax	Antiviral agents
albuterol	Proventil Ventolin Volmax	Bronchodilators
alendronate	Fosamax	Antiosteoporosis agents
allopurinol	Zyloprim	Antigout agents
alprazolam	Xanax	Anxiolytic agents Sedative agents
alprostadil	MUSE	Erectile dysfunction agents
amantadine	Symmetrel	AntiParkinson's agents
amikacin	Amikin	Antibacterial agents
amiodarone	Cordarone	Antiarrhythmic agents
amitriptyline	Elavil	Antidepressant agents
amlodipine	Norvasc	Antihypertensive agents
amoxicillin	Amoxil Trimox	Antibacterial agents
amoxicillin/clavulanic acid	Augmentin	Antibacterial agents

Pharmacology

Continued

Generic name	Trade name	Agent class
amphotericin B	Abelcet Amphotec Fungizone	Antifungal agents
ampicillin	Omnipen	Antibacterial agents
ardeparin	Normiflo	Anticoagulant agents
aspirin	Bufferin	Analgesic agents
	Ecotrin	Antiarthritic agents Antiinflammatory agents
astemizole	Hismanal	Antihistamine agents
atenolol	Tenormin	Antihypertensive agents
atorvastatin	Lipitor	Hypolipidemic agents
azithromycin	Zithromax	Antibacterial agents
baclofen	Lioresal	Muscle relaxants
beclomethasone	Beclovent Beconase AQ Vancenase AQ Vanceril	Adrenocorticosteroids
benazepril	Lotensin	Antihypertensive agents
benztropine	Cogentin	AntiParkinson's agents Anticholinergic agents
betamethasone dipropionate/ clotrimazole	Lotrisone	Adrenocorticosteroids Antibacterial agents
bisacodyl	Dulcolax	Laxatives
bromocriptine	Parlodel	AntiParkinson's agents
budesonide	Rhinocort	Adrenocorticosteroids
bupropion	Wellbutrin Zyban	Antidepressant agents
buspirone	BuSpar	Anxiolytic agents
calcitonin	Calcimar Miacalcin	Antiosteoporosis agents
captopril	Capoten	Antihypertensive agents
carbamazepine	Tegretol	Anticonvulsant agents
carbidopa/levodopa	Sinemet Sinemet CR	AntiParkinson's agents
carbinoxamine maleate/ pseudoephedrine hydrochloride/ dextromethorphan hydrobromide	Cardec DM	Cold preparations
carisoprodol	Soma	Muscle relaxants
carvedilol	Coreg	Antihypertensive agents
cefaclor	Ceclor	Antibacterial agents
cefadroxil	Duricef	Antibacterial agents
cefazolin	Ancef Kefzol	Antibacterial agents
cefixime	Suprax	Antibacterial agents

Generic name	Trade name	Agent class
cefotaxime	Claforan	Antibacterial agents
cefotetan	Cefotan	Antibacterial agents
cefoxitin	Mefoxin	Antibacterial agents
cefpodoxime proxetil	Vantin	Antibacterial agents
cefprozil	Cefzil	Antibacterial agents
ceftazidime	Fortaz Tazicef	Antibacterial agents
ceftizoxime	Cefizox	Antibacterial agents
ceftriaxone	Rocephin	Antibacterial agents
cefuroxime	Ceftin Zinacef	Antibacterial agents
cephalexin	Keflet Keflex Keftab	Antibacterial agents
cephradine	Velosef	Antibacterial agents
cetirizine	Zyrtec	Antihistamine agents
chlorambucil	Leukeran	Antineoplastic agents
chlordiazepoxide	Librium	Anxiolytic agents Sedatives
chlorpromazine	Thorazine	Antipsychotic agents
cholestyramine resin	Questran Light	Hypolipidemic agents
cimetidine	Tagamet Tagamet HB	Antiulcer agents
ciprofloxacin	Cipro	Antibacterial agents
cisapride	Propulsid	Gastrointestinal motility agents
clarithromycin	Biaxin	Antibacterial agents
clomipramine	Anafranil	Antipsychotic agents Sedatives
clonazepam	Klonopin	Anticonvulsant agents
clonidine	Catapres Catapres TTS	Antihypertensive agents
clopidogrel	Plavix	Anticoagulant agents
clotrimazole	Lotrimin Mycelex	Antifungal agents
clozapine	Clozaril	Antipsychotic agents
codeine	Codeine	Analgesic agents
colchicine	Colchicine	Antigout agents
colestipol	Colestid	Hypolipidemic agents
cyclobenzaprine	Flexeril	Muscle relaxants
cyclophosphamide	Cytoxan	Antineoplastic agents
dalteparin	Fragmin	Anticoagulant agents
desipramine	Norpramin	Antidepressant agents
dextroamphetamine	Dexedrine	Central nervous system stimulants
dextromethorphan	Benylin Adult	Cold preparations

Generic name	Trade name	Agent class
diazepam	Valium	Anxiolytic agents Sedatives
diclofenac potassium	Cataflam	Analgesic agents Antiarthritic agents Antiinflammatory agents
diclofenac sodium	Voltaren Voltaren-XR	Analgesic agents Antiarthritic agents Antiinflammatory agents
dicyclomine	Bentyl	Anticholinergic agents
digoxin	Lanoxin	Cardiac glycosides
dihydroergotamine	D.H.E.-45 Migranal	Antimigraine agents
diltiazem	Cardizem CD Cardizem SR Dilacor XR Tiazac	Antihypertensive agents
diphenoxylate hydrochloride/ atropine sulfate	Lomotil	Antidiarrheal agents
disopyramide	Norpace	Antiarrhythmic agents
divalproex	Depakote	Anticonvulsant agents
docusate	Colace	Laxatives
docusate/casanthranol	Peri-Colace	Laxatives
dolasetron	Anzemet	Antiemetic agents
donepezil	Aricept	AntiAlzheimer's agents
dorzolamide	Trusopt	Antiglaucoma agents
doxazosin	Cardura	Antihypertensive agents Benign prostate hypertrophy agents
doxorubicin	Adriamycin	Antineoplastic agents
doxycycline	Doryx Monodox Vibra-Tabs Vibramycin	Antibacterial agents
enalapril	Vasotec	Antihypertensive agents
enoxaparin	Lovenox	Anticoagulant agents
ephedrine	Ectasule Efedron	Cold preparations
ergotamine/caffeine	Cafergot Wigraine	Antimigraine agents
erythromycin	E-Mycin Ery-Tab Eryc Ilotycin PCE	Antibacterial agents
estazolam	ProSom	Anxiolytic agents Sedatives

Generic name	Trade name	Agent class
estradiol	Estrace Oral	Estrogens
estrogens	Premarin	Estrogens
etidronate	Didronel	Antiosteoporosis agents
etodolac	Lodine	Analgesic agents Antiarthritic agents Antiinflammatory agents
famotidine	Pepcid	Antiulcer agents
felbamate	Felbatol	Anticonvulsant agents
felodipine	Plendil	Antihypertensive agents
fenofibrate	TriCor	Hypolipidemic agents
finasteride	Proscar	Benign prostate hypertrophy agents
fluconazole	Diflucan	Antifungal agents
fluoxetine	Prozac	Antidepressant agents
fluphenazine	Prolixin	Antipsychotic agents
fluticasone	Flonase Flovent	Antirhinitis agents Adrenocorticosteroids
fluvastatin	Lescol	Hypolipidemic agents
fluvoxamine	Luvox	Antidepressant agents Antipsychotic agents
fosinopril	Monopril	Antihypertensive agents
fosphenytoin	Cerebyx	Anticonvulsant agents
furosemide	Lasix	Diuretic agents
ganciclovir	Cytovene	Antiviral agents
gemfibrozil	Lopid	Hypolipidemic agents
glimepiride	Amaryl	Hypoglycemic agents
glipizide	Glucotrol Glucotrol XL	Hypoglycemic agents
glyburide	Diaβeta Micronase	Hypoglycemic agents
glycopyrrolate	Robinul	Anticholinergic agents
granisetron	Kytril	Antiemetic agents
guaifenesin	Humbid LA Organidin	Cold preparations
guaifenesin with codeine	Brontex Robitussin AC	Cold preparations
guaifenesin/ pseudoephedrine	Robitussin PE	Cold preparations
haloperidal	Haldol	Antipsychotic agents
heparin	Heparin	Anticoagulant agents
hydralazine	Apresoline	Antihypertensive agents
hydrochlorothiazide	HydroDIURIL Microzide Oretic	Diuretic agents
hydrocodone with acetaminophen	Vicodin Vicodin ES	Analgesic agents

Generic name	Trade name	Agent class
hydrocodone/ chlorpheniramine	Tussionex	Cold preparations
hydrocortisone	Westcort	Adrenocorticosteroids
hydromorphone	Dilaudid	Analgesic agents
hydroxyzine	Atarax Vistaril	Anxiolytic agents Sedatives
ibuprofen	Advil Motrin Nuprin	Analgesic agents Antiarthritic agents Antiinflammatory agents
imipramine	Tofranil	Antidepressant agents
indinavir	Crixivan	Antiviral agents
indomethacin	Indocin	Analgesic agents Antiarthritic agents Antigout agents Antiinflammatory agents
insulin	Humulin N Humulin R Humulin 70/30	Hypoglycemic agents
ipratropium	Atrovent	bronchodilators
irbesartan	Avapro	antihypertensive agents
isosorbide dinitrate	Dilatrate-SR Isordil Sorbitrate	antianginal agents
isosorbide mononitrate	Imdur Ismo Monoket	Antianginal agents
isradipine	DynaCirc DynaCirc CR	Antihypertensive agents
itraconazole	Sporonox	Antifungal agents
ketoconazole	Nizoral Cream	Antifungal agents
ketoprofen	Actron Orudis Orudis KT Oruvail	Analgesic agents Antiarthritic agents Antiinflammatory agents
ketorolac	Acular Toradol	Analgesic agents Antiarthritic agents Antigout agents Antiinflammatory agents
labetalol	Normodyne Trandate	Antihypertensive agents
lactulose	Chronulac	Laxatives
lamivudine	Epivir	Antiviral agents
lamotrigine	Lamictal	Anticonvulsant agents
lansoprazole	Prevacid	Antiulcer agents
latanoprost	Xalatan	Antiglaucoma agents
levodopa	Larodopa	AntiParkinson's agents
levofloxacin	Levaquin	Antibacterial agents

Generic name	Trade name	Agent class
levonorgestrel/ethinyl estradiol	Triphasil-28	Estrogens Progestins
levothyroxine	Levothroid Levoxyl Synthroid	Hypothyroid agents
lisinopril	Prinivil Zestril	Antihypertensive agents
lithium	Lithobid	Antidepressant agents Antipsychotic agents
loperamide	Imodium	Antidiarrheal agents
loracarbef	Lorabid	Antibacterial agents
loratidine	Claritin	Antihistamine agents
lorazepam	Ativan	Anxiolytic agents Sedatives
losartan	Cozaar	Antihypertensive agents
lovastatin	Mevacor	Hypolipidemic agents
medroxyprogesterone	Cycrin Depo-Provera Prempro Provera	Progestins
melphalan	Alkeran	Antineoplastic agents
meperidine	Demerol	Analgesic agents
metformin	Glucophage	Hypoglycemic agents
methocarbamol	Robaxin	Muscle relaxants
methylphenidate	Ritalin	Central nervous system stimulants
methylprednisolone	Medrol	Adrenocorticosteroids
methysergide	Sansert	Antimigraine agents
metoclopramide	Reglan	Gastrointestinal motility agents Antiemetic agents
metoprolol	Lopressor Toprol-XL	Antihypertensive agents
metronidazole	Flagyl	Antibacterial agents
mexiletine	Mexitil	Antiarrhythmic agents
mezlocillin	Mezlin	Antibacterial agents
minocycline	Minocin	Antibacterial agents
mometasone	Nasonex	Adrenocorticosteroids
morphine	Kadian MS Contin MSIR Oramorph SR Roxanol	Analgesic agents
mupirocin	Bactroban	Antibacterial agents
nabumetone	Relafen	Analgesic agents Antiarthritic agents Antiinflammatory agents

Pharmacology

Continued

Table—cont'd

Generic name	Trade name	Agent class
naproxen	Aleve Anaprox Naprosyn	Analgesic agents Antiarthritic agents Antiinflammatory agents
naratriptan	Amerge	Antimigraine agents
nefazodone	Serzone	Antidepressant agents
neomycin/polymyxin/ hydrocortisone	Neomycin/Polymyxin/ Hydrocortisone	Antibacterial agents
niacin	Niaspan Nicolar	Hypolidemic agents
nicardipine	Cardene Cardene SR	Antihypertensive agents
nifedipine	Adalat Adalat CC Procardia Procardia XL	Antihypertensive agents
nitrofurantoin	Macrobid Macrodantin	Antibacterial agents
nitroglycerin	Nitro-Dur Nitrostat	Antianginal agents
nizatidine	Axid	Antiulcer agents
nortriptyline	Pamelor	Antidepressant agents
ofloxacin	Floxin	Antibacterial agents
olanzapine	Zyprexa	Antipsychotic agents
omeprazole	Prilosec	Antiulcer agents
oxaprozin	Daypro	Analgesic agents Antiarthritic agents Antiinflammatory agents
oxazepam	Serax	Anxiolytic agents Sedatives
oxycodone with acetaminophen	Percocet Tylox	Analgesic agents
paroxetine	Paxil	Antidepressant agents
pemoline	Cylert	Central nervous system stimulants
penicillin V	Pen•Vee K Veetids	Antibacterial agents
pentoxifylline	Trental	Hemorrheologic agents
pergolide	Permax	AntiParkinson's agents
phenobarbital	Phenobarbital	Anticonvulsant agents
phentermine	Adipex-P Fastin Ionamin	Central nervous system stimulants

Table—cont'd

Generic name	Trade name	Agent class
phenylpropanolamine hydrochloride/ guaifenesin	Contuss-XT	Cold preparations
phenytoin	Dilantin	Anticonvulsant agents
pilocarpine	Isopto Carpine Pilocar	Antiglaucoma agents
piperacillin	Pipracil	Antibacterial agents
piroxicam	Feldene	Analgesic agents Antiarthritic agents Antiinflammatory agents
potassium chloride	K-Dur K-Lor K-Tab Micro-K Slow-K	Electrolytes and fluids
pravastatin	Pravachol	Hypolipidemic agents
prednisolone	Prelone	Adrenocorticosteroids
prednisone	Deltasone	Adrenocorticosteroids
primidone	Mysoline	Anticonvulsant agents
probenecid	Probenecid	Antigout agents
procainamide	Procanabid	Antiarrhythmic agents
prochlorperazine	Compazine	Antiemetic agents
promethazine	Phenergan	Antiemetic agents
promethazine with codeine	Phenergan with Codeine	Analgesic agents
propafenone	Rythmol	Antiarrhythmic agents
propoxyphene	Darvon	Analgesic agents
propoxyphene with acetaminophen	Darvocet-N 100 Propacet 100	Analgesic agents
psyllium	Metamucil	Laxatives
quetiapine	Seroquel	Antipsychotic agents
quinapril	Accupril	Antihypertensive agents
quinidine gluconate	Quinaglute	Antiarrhythmic agents
quinidine polygalacturonate	Cardioquin	Antiarrhythmic agents
quinidine sulfate	Quinidex	Antiarrhythmic agents
ramipril	Altace	Antihypertensive agents
ranitidine	Zantac	Antiulcer agents
repaglinide	Prandin	Hypoglycemic agents
risedronate	Actonel	Antiosteoporosis agents
risperidone	Risperdal	Antipsychotic agents
ritonavir	Norvir	Antiviral agents
salmeterol	Serevent	Bronchodilators

Pharmacology

Continued

Table—cont'd

Generic name	Trade Name	Agent class
salsalate	Disalcid	Analgesic agents Antiarthritic agents Antiinflammatory agents
selegiline	Eldepryl	AntiParkinson's agents
senna	Senokot	Laxatives
sertraline	Zoloft	Antidepressant agents
sildenafil	Viagra	Erectile dysfunction agents
simvastatin	Zocor	Hypolipidemic agents
sorbitol	Sorbitol	Laxatives
spironolactone	Aldactone	Diuretic agents
sucralfate	Carafate	Antiulcer agents
sulfamethoxazole/ trimethoprim	Bactrim Bactrim DS Septra Septra DS	Antibacterial agents
sulindac	Clinoril	Analgesic agents Antiarthritic agents Antiinflammatory agents
sumatriptan	Imitrex	Antimigraine agents
tacrine	Cognex	AntiAlzheimer's agents
tamsulosin	Flomax	Benign prostate hypertrophy agents
temazepam	Restoril	Sedatives
terazosin	Hytrin	Antihypertensive agents Benign prostate hypertrophy agents
terbinafine	Lamisil	Antifungal agents
terconazole	Terazol 3 Terazol 7	Antifungal agents
testosterone	Androderm Depo-Testosterone Testoderm	Anabolic steroids
tetracycline	Sumycin	Antibacterial agents

Table—cont'd

Generic name	Trade name	Agent class
theophylline	Slo-bid Theo-Dur	Bronchodilators
thioridazine	Mellaril	Antipsychotic agents
thiothixene	Navane	Antipsychotic agents
ticlopidine	Ticlid	Anticoagulant agents
tiludronate	Skelid	Antiosteoporosis agents
timolol	Timoptic Blocadren	Antiglaucoma agents Antihypertensive agents
tobramycin	Tobrex	Antibacterial agents
tramadol	Ultram	Analgesic agents
triamcinolone	Azmacort	Adrenocorticosteroids
triamterene/ hydrochlorothiazide	Dyazide Maxzide	Diuretic agents
triazolam	Halcion	Anxiolytic agents Sedatives
trifluoperazine	Stelazine	Antipsychotic agents
trihexyphenidyl	Artane	AntiParkinson's agents
trimethoprim/polymyxin B	Polytrim	Antibacterial agents
troglitazone	Rezulin	Hypoglycemic agents
valproic acid	Depacon	Anticonvulsant agents
venlafaxine	Effexor	Antidepressant agents
verapamil	Calan Calan SR Isoptin Isoptin SR Verelan	Antihypertensive agents
warfarin	Coumadin	Anticoagulant agents
zalcitabine	Hivid	Antiviral agents
zidovudine	Retrovir	Antiviral agents
zolmitriptan	Zomig	Antimigraine agents
zolpidem	Ambien	Sedatives

Medication Index By Trade Name

Trade name	Generic name	Agent class
Abelcet	amphotericin B	Antifungal agents
Accupril	quinapril	Antihypertensive agents
Actonel	risedronate	Antiosteoporosis agents
Actron	ketoprofen	Analgesic agents Antiarthritic agents Antiinflammatory agents
Acular	ketorolac	Analgesic agents Antiarthritic agents Antigout agents Antiinflammatory agents
Adalat	nifedipine	Antihypertensive agents
Adalat CC	nifedipine	Antihypertensive agents
Adipex-P	phentermine	Central nervous system stimulants
Adriamycin	doxorubicin	Antineoplastic agents
Advil	ibuprofen	Analgesic agents Antiarthritic agents Antiinflammatory agents
Aldactone	spironolactone	Diuretic agents
Aleve	naproxen	Analgesic agents Antiarthritic agents Antiinflammatory agents
Alkeran	melphalan	Antineoplastic agents
Altace	ramipril	Antihypertensive agents
Amaryl	glimepiride	Hypoglycemic agents
Ambien	zolpidem	Sedatives
Amerge	naratriptan	Antimigraine agents
Amikin	amikacin	Antibacterial agents
Amoxil	amoxicillin	Antibacterial agents
Amphotec	amphotericin B	Antifungal agents
Anafranil	clomipramine	Antipsychotic agents Sedatives
Anaprox	naproxen	Analgesic agents Antiarthritic agents Antiinflammatory agents
Ancef	cefazolin	Antibacterial agents
Androderm	testosterone	Anabolic steroids
Anzemet	dolasetron	Antiemetic agents
Apresoline	hydralazine	Antihypertensive agents
Aricept	donepezil	AntiAlzheimer's agents
Artane	trihexyphenidyl	AntiParkinson's agents
Atarax	hydroxyzine	Anxiolytic agents Sedatives
Ativan	lorazepam	Anxiolytic agents Sedatives
Atrovent	ipratropium	Bronchodilators

Trade name	Generic name	Agent class
Augmentin	amoxicillin/clavulanic acid	Antibacterial agents
Avapro	irbesartan	Antihypertensive agents
Axid	nizatidine	Antiulcer agents
Azmacort	triamcinolone	Adrenocorticosteroids
Bactrim	sulfamethoxazole/ trimethoprim	Antibacterial agents
Bactrim DS	sulfamethoxazole/ trimethoprim	Antibacterial agents
Bactroban	mupirocin	Antibacterial agents
Beclovent	beclomethasone	Adrenocorticosteroids
Beconase AQ	beclomethasone	Adrenocorticosteroids
Bentyl	dicyclomine	Anticholinergic agents
Benylin Adult	dextromethorphan	Cold preparations
Biaxin	clarithromycin	Antibacterial agents
Blocadren	timolol	Antihypertensive agents
Brontex	guaifenesin with codeine	Cold preparations
Bufferin	aspirin	Analgesic agents Antiarthritic agents Antiinflammatory agents
BuSpar	buspirone	Anxiolytic agents
Cafergot	ergotamine/caffeine	Antimigraine agents
Calan	verapamil	Antihypertensive agents
Calan SR	verapamil	Antihypertensive agents
Calcimar	calcitonin	Antiosteoporosis agents
Capoten	captopril	Antihypertensive agents
Carafate	sucralfate	Antiulcer agents
Cardec DM	carbinoxamine maleate/ pseudoephedrine hydrochloride/ dextromethorphan hydrobromide	Cold preparations
Cardene	nicardipine	Antihypertensive agents
Cardene SR	nicardipine	Antihypertensive agents
Cardioquin	quinidine polygalacturonate	Antiarrhythmic agents
Cardizem	diltiazem	Antihypertensive agents
Cardizem CD	diltiazem	Antihypertensive agents
Cardizem SR	diltiazem	Antihypertensive agents
Cardura	doxazosin	Antihypertensive agents Benign prostate hypertrophy agents
Cataflam	diclofenac potassium	Analgesic agents Antiarthritic agents Antiinflammatory agents
Catapres	clonidine	Antihypertensive agents
Catapres TTS	clonidine	Antihypertensive agents

Trade name	Generic name	Agent class
Ceclor	cefaclor	Antibacterial agents
Cefizox	ceftizoxime	Antibacterial agents
Cefotan	cefotetan	Antibacterial agents
Ceftin	cefuroxime	Antibacterial agents
Cefzil	cefprozil	Antibacterial agents
Cerebyx	fosphenytoin	Anticonvulsant agents
Chronulac	lactulose	Laxatives
Cipro	ciprofloxacin	Antibacterial agents
Claritin	loratidine	Antihistamine agents
Clinoril	sulindac	Analgesic agents Antiarthritic agents Antiinflammatory agents
Clozaril	clozapine	Antipsychotic agents
Codeine	codeine	Analgesic agents
Cogentin	benztropine	AntiParkinson's agents Anticholinergic agents
Cognex	tacrine	AntiAlzheimer's agents
Colace	docusate	Laxatives
Colchicine	colchicine	Antigout agents
Colestid	colestipol	Hypolipidemic agents
Compazine	prochlorperazine	Antiemetic agents
Contuss-XT	phenylpropanolamine hydrochloride/ guaifenesin	Cold preparations
Cordarone	amiodarone	Antiarrhythmic agents
Coreg	carvedilol	Antihypertensive agents
Coumadin	warfarin	Anticoagulant agents
Cozaar	losartan	Antihypertensive agents
Crixivan	indinavir	Antiviral agents
Cycrin	medroxyprogesterone	Progestins
Cylert	pemoline	Central nervous system stimulants
Cytovene	ganciclovir	Antiviral agents
Cytoxan	cyclophosphamide	Antineoplastic agents
Darvocet-N 100	propoxyphene with acetaminophen	Analgesic agents
Darvon	propoxyphene	Analgesic agents
Daypro	oxaprozin	Analgesic agents Antiarthritic agents Antiinflammatory agents
Deltasone	prednisone	Adrenocorticosteroids
Demerol	meperidine	Analgesic agents
Depacon	valproic acid	Anticonvulsant agents
Depakote	divalproex	Anticonvulsant agents
Depo-Provera	medroxyprogesterone	Progestins

Trade name	Generic name	Agent class
Depo-Testosterone	testosterone	Anabolic steroids
Dexedrine	dextroamphetamine	Central nervous system stimulants
D.H.E-45	dihydroergotamine	Antimigraine agents
Diaβeta	glyburide	Hypoglycemic agents
Didronel	etidronate	Antiosteoporosis agents
Diflucan	fluconazole	Antifungal agents
Dilacor XR	diltiazem	Antihypertensive agents
Dilantin	phenytoin	Anticonvulsant agents
Dilatrate-SR	isosorbide dinitrate	Antianginal agents
Dilaudid	hydromorphone	Analgesic agents
Disalcid	salsalate	Analgesic agents Antiarthritic agents Antiinflammatory agents
Dulcolax	biscodyl	Laxatives
Doryx	doxycycline	Antibacterial agents
Duricef	cefadroxil	Antibacterial agents
Dyazide	triamterene/ hydrochlorothiazide	Diuretic agents
DynaCirc	isradipine	Antihypertensive agents
DynaCirc CR	isradipine	Antihypertensive agents
Ecotrin	aspirin	Analgesic agents Antiarthritic agents Antiinflammatory agents
Ectasule	ephedrine	Cold preparations
Efedron	ephedrine	Cold preparations
Effexor	venlafaxine	Antidepressant agents
Elavil	amitriptyline	Antidepressant agents
Eldepryl	selegiline	AntiParkinson's agents
E-Mycin	erythromycin	Antibacterial agents
Epivir	lamivudine	Antiviral agents
Eryc	erythromycin	Antibacterial agents
Ery-Tab	erythromycin	Antibacterial agents
Estrace Oral	estradiol	Estrogens
Fastin	phentermine	Central nervous system stimulants
Felbatol	felbamate	Anticonvulsant agents
Feldene	piroxicam	Analgesic agents Antiarthritic agents Antiinflammatory agents
Flagyl	metronidazole	Antibacterial agents
Flexeril	cyclobenzaprine	Muscle relaxants
Flomax	tamsulosin	Benign prostate hypertrophy agents

Pharmacology

Continued

Table—cont'd

Trade name	Generic name	Agent class
Flonase	fluticasone	Antirhinitis agents Adrenocorticosteroids
Flovent	fluticasone	Antirhinitis agents Adrenocorticosteroids
Floxin	ofloxacin	Antibacterial agents
Fortaz	ceftazidime	Antibacterial agents
Fosamax	alendronate	Antiosteoporosis agents
Fragmin	dalteparin	Anticoagulant agents
Fungizone	amphotericin B	Antifungal agents
Glucophage	metformin	Hypoglycemic agents
Glucotrol	glipizide	Hypoglycemic agents
Glucotrol XL	glipizide	Hypoglycemic agents
Halcion	triazolam	Anxiolytic agents Sedatives
Haldol	haloperidal	Antipsychotic agents
Heparin	heparin	Anticoagulant agents
Hismanal	Astemizole	Antihistamine agents
Hivid	zalcitabine	Antiviral agents
Humbid LA	guaifenesin	Cold preparations
Humulin 70/30	insulin	Hypoglycemic agents
Humulin N	insulin	Hypoglycemic agents
Humulin R	insulin	Hypoglycemic agents
HydroDIURIL	hydrochlorothiazide	Diuretic agents
Hytrin	terazosin	Antihypertensive agents Benign prostate hypertrophy agents
Ilotycin	erythromycin	Antibacterial agents
Imdur	isosorbide mononitrate	Antianginal agents
Imitrex	sumatriptan	Antimigraine agents
Imodium	loperamide	Antidiarrheal agents
Indocin	indomethacin	Analgesic agents Antiarthritic agents Antigout agents Antiinflammatory agents
Ionamin	phentermine	Central nervous system stimulants
Ismo	isosorbide mononitrate	Antianginal agents
Isoptin	verapamil	Antihypertensive agents
Isoptin SR	verapamil	Antihypertensive agents
Isopto Carpine	pilocarpine	Antiglaucoma agents
Isordil	isosorbide dinitrate	Antianginal agents
Kadian	morphine	Analgesic agents
K-Dur	potassium chloride	Electrolytes and fluids
Keflet	cephalexin	Antibacterial agents
Keflex	cephalexin	Antibacterial agents

Table—cont'd

Trade name	Generic name	Agent class
Keftab	cephalexin	Antibacterial agents
Kefzol	cefazolin	Antibacterial agents
Klonopin	clonazepam	Anticonvulsant agents
K-Lor	potassium chloride	Electrolytes and fluids
K-Tab	potassium chloride	Electrolytes and fluids
Kytril	granisetron	Antiemetic agents
Lamictal	lamotrigine	Anticonvulsant agents
Lamisil	terbinafine	Antifungal agents
Lanoxin	digoxin	Cardiac glycosides
Larodopa	levodopa	AntiParkinson's agents
Lasix	furosemide	Diuretic agents
Lescol	fluvastatin	Hypolipidemic agents
Leukeran	chlorambucil	Antineoplastic agents
Levaquin	levofloxacin	Antibacterial agents
Levothroid	levothyroxine	Hypothyroid agents
Levoxyl	levothyroxine	Hypothyroid agents
Librium	chlordiazepoxide	Anxiolytic agents Sedatives
Lioresal	baclofen	Muscle relaxants
Lipitor	atorvastatin	Hypolipidemic agents
Lithobid	lithium	Antidepressant agents Antipsychotic agents
Lodine	etodolac	Analgesic agents Antiarthritic agents Antiinflammatory agents
Lomotil	diphenoxylate hydrochloride/ atropine sulfate	Antidiarrheal agents
Lopid	gemfibrozil	Hypolipidemic agents
Lopressor	metoprolol	Antihypertensive agents
Lorabid	loracarbef	Antibacterial agents
Lotensin	benazepril	Antihypertensive agents
Lotrimin	clotrimazole	Antifungal agents
Lotrisone	betamethasone dipropionate/ clotrimazole	Adrenocorticosteroids Antibacterial agents
Lovenox	enoxaparin	Anticoagulant agents
Luvox	fluvoxamine	Antidepressant agents Antipsychotic agents
Macrobid	nitrofurantoin	Antibacterial agents
Macrodantin	nitrofurantoin	Antibacterial agents
Maxzide	triamterene/ hydrochlorothiazide	Diuretic agents
Medrol	methylprednisolone	Adrenocorticosteroids
Mefoxin	cefoxitin	Antibacterial agents
Mellaril	thioridazine	Antipsychotic agents
Metamucil	psyllium	Laxatives

Continued

Trade name	Generic name	Agent class
Mevacor	lovastatin	Hypolipidemic agents
Mexitil	mexiletine	Antiarrhythmic agents
Mezlin	mezlocillin	Antibacterial agents
Miacalcin	calcitonin	Antiosteoporosis agents
Micro-K	potassium chloride	Electrolytes and fluids
Micronase	glyburide	Hypoglycemic agents
Microzide	hydrochlorothiazide	Diuretic agents
Migranal	dihydroergotamine	Antimigraine agents
Minocin	minocycline	Antibacterial agents
Monodox	doxycycline	Antibacterial agents
Monoket	isosorbide mononitrate	Antianginal agents
Monopril	fosinopril	Antihypertensive agents
Motrin	ibuprofen	Analgesic agents Antiarthritic agents Antiinflammatory agents
MS Contin	morphine	Analgesic agents
MSIR	morphine	Analgesic agents
MUSE	alprostadil	Erectile dysfunction agents
Mycelex	clotrimazole	Antifungal agents
Mysoline	primidone	Anticonvulsant agents
Naprosyn	naproxen	Analgesic agents Antiarthritic agents Antiinflammatory agents
Nasonex	mometasone	Adrenocorticosteroids
Navane	thiothixene	Antipsychotic agents
Neomycin/Polymyxin/ Hydrocortisone	neomycin/polymyxin/ hydrocortisone	Antibacterial agents
Niaspan	niacin	Hypolidemic agents
Nicolar	niacin	Hypolidemic agents
Nitro-Dur	nitroglycerin	Antianginal agents
Nitrostat	nitroglycerin	Antianginal agents
Nizoral Cream	ketoconazole	Antifungal agents
Normiflo	ardeparin	Anticoagulant agents
Normodyne	labetalol	Antihypertensive agents
Norpace	disopyramide	Antiarrhythmic agents
Norpramin	desipramine	Antidepressant agents
Norvasc	amlodipine	Antihypertensive agents
Norvir	ritonavir	Antiviral agents
Nuprin	ibuprofen	Analgesic agents Antiarthritic agents Antiinflammatory agents
Omnipen	ampicillin	Antibacterial agents
Oramorph SR	morphine	Analgesic agents
Oretic	hydrochlorothiazide	Diuretic agents
Organidin	guaifenesin	Cold preparations

Trade name	Generic name	Agent class
Orudis	ketoprofen	Analgesic agents Antiarthritic agents Antiinflammatory agents
Orudis KT	ketoprofen	Analgesic agents Antiarthritic agents Antiinflammatory agents
Oruvail	ketoprofen	Analgesic agents Antiarthritic agents Antiinflammatory agents
Pamelor	nortriptyline	Antidepressant agents
Parlodel	bromocriptine	AntiParkinson's agents
Paxil	paroxetine	Antidepressant agents
PCE	erythromycin	Antibacterial agents
Pen•Vee K	penicillin V	Antibacterial agents
Pepcid	famotidine	Antiulcer agents
Percocet	oxycodone with acetaminophen	Analgesic agents
Peri-Colace	docusate/casanthranol	Laxatives
Permax	pergolide	AntiParkinson's agents
Phenergan	promethazine	Antiemetic agents
Phenergan with Codeine	promethazine with codeine	Analgesic agents
Phenobarbital	phenobarbital	Anticonvulsant agents
Pilocar	pilocarpine	Antiglaucoma agents
Pipracil	piperacillin	Antibacterial agents
Plavix	clopidogrel	Anticoagulant agents
Plendil	felodipine	Antihypertensive agents
Polytrim	trimethoprim/polymyxin B	Antibacterial agents
Prandin	repaglinide	Hypoglycemic agents
Pravachol	pravastatin	Hypolipidemic agents
Precose	acarbose	Hypoglycemic agents
Prelone	prednisolone	Adrenocorticosteroids
Premarin	estrogens	Estrogens
Prempro	medroxyprogesterone	Progestins
Prevacid	lansoprozole	Antiulcer agents
Prilosec	omeprazole	Antiulcer agents
Prinivil	lisinopril	Antihypertensive agents
Probenecid	probenecid	Antigout agents
Procanabid	procainamide	Antiarrhythmic agents
Procardia	nifedipine	Antihypertensive agents
Procardia XL	nifedipine	Antihypertensive agents
Prolixin	fluphenazine	Antipsychotic agents
Propacet 100	propoxyphene with acetaminophen	Analgesic agents
Propulsid	cisapride	Gastrointestinal motility agents

Pharmacology

Continued

Trade name	Generic name	Agent class
Proscar	finasteride	Benign prostate hypertrophy agents
ProSom	estazolam	Anxiolytic agents Sedatives
Proventil	albuterol	Bronchodilators
Provera	medroxyprogesterone	Progestins
Prozac	fluoxetine	Antidepressant agents
Questran Light	cholestyramine	Hypolipidemic agents
Quinaglute	quinidine gluconate	Antiarrhythmic agents
Quinidex	quinidine sulfate	Antiarrhythmic agents
Reglan	metoclopramide	Gastrointestinal motility agents Antiemetic agents
Relafen	nabumetone	Analgesic agents Antiarthritic agents Antiinflammatory agents
Restoril	temazepam	Sedatives
Retrovir	zidovudine	Antiviral agents
Rezulin	troglitazone	Hypoglycemic agents
Rhinocort	budesonide	Adrenocorticosteroids
Risperdal	risperidone	Antipsychotic agents
Ritalin	methylphenidate	Central nervous system stimulants
Robaxin	methocarbamol	Muscle relaxants
Robinul	glycopyrrolate	Anticholinergic agents
Robitussin AC	guaifenesin with codeine	Cold preparations
Robitussin PE	guaifenesin/ pseudoephedrine	Cold preparations
Rocephin	ceftriaxone	Antibacterial agents
Roxanol	morphine	Analgesic agents
Rythmol	propafenone	Antiarrhythmic agents
Sansert	methysergide	Antimigraine agents
Sectral	acebutolol	Antihypertensive agents
Senokot	senna	Laxatives
Septra	sulfamethoxazole/ trimethoprim	Antibacterial agents
Septra DS	sulfamethoxazole/ trimethoprim	Antibacterial agents
Serax	oxazepam	Anxiolytic agents Sedatives
Serevent	salmeterol	Bronchodilators
Seroquel	quetiapine	Antipsychotic agents
Serzone	nefazodone	Antidepressant agents
Sinemet	carbidopa/levodopa	AntiParkinson's agents
Sinemet CR	carbidopa/levodopa	AntiParkinson's agents
Skelid	tiludronate	Antiosteoporosis agents

Table—cont'd

Trade name	Generic name	Agent class
Slo-bid	theophylline	Bronchodilators
Slow-K	potassium chloride	Electrolytes and fluids
Soma	carisoprodol	Muscle relaxants
Sorbitol	sorbitol	Laxatives
Sorbitrate	isosorbide dinitrate	Antianginal agents
Sporonox	itraconazole	Antifungal agents
Stelazine	trifluoperazine	Antipsychotic agents
Sumycin	tetracycline	Antibacterial agents
Suprax	cefixime	Antibacterial agents
Symmetrel	amantadine	AntiParkinson's agents
Synthroid	levothyroxine	Hypothyroid agents
Tagamet	cimetidine	Antiulcer agents
Tagamet HB	cimetidine	Antiulcer agents
Tazicef	ceftazidime	Antibacterial agents
Tegretol	carbamazepine	Anticonvulsant agents
Tenormin	atenolol	Antihypertensive agents
Terazol 3	terconazole	Antifungal agents
Terazol 7	terconazole	Antifungal agents
Testoderm	testosterone	Anabolic steroids
Theo-Dur	theophylline	Bronchodilators
Thorazine	chlorpromazine	Antipsychotic agents
Tiazac	diltiazem	Antihypertensive agents
Ticlid	ticlopidine	Anticoagulant agents
Timoptic	timolol	Antiglaucoma agents
Tobrex	tobramycin	Antibacterial agents
Tofranil	imipramine	Antidepressant agents
Toprol-XL	metoprolol	Antihypertensive agents
Toradol	ketorolac	Analgesic agents Antiarthritic agents Antigout agents Antiinflammatory agents
Trandate	labetalol	Antihypertensive agents
Trental	pentoxifylline	Hemorrheologic agents
TriCor	fenofibrate	Hypolipidemic agents
Trimox	amoxicillin	Antibacterial agents
Triphasil-28	levonorgestrel/ethinyl estradiol	Estrogens Progestins
Trusopt	dorzolamide	Antiglaucoma agents
Tussionex	hydrocodone/ chlorpheniramine	Cold preparations
Tylenol	acetaminophen	Analgesic agents Antipyretic agents
Tylenol with codeine	acetaminophen with codeine	Analgesic agents Antipyretic agents

Continued

Trade name	Generic name	Agent class
Tylox	oxycodone with acetaminophen	Analgesic agents
Ultram	tramadol	Analgesic agents
Valium	diazepam	Anxiolytic agents Sedatives
Vancenase AQ	beclomethasone	Adrenocorticosteroids
Vanceril	beclomethasone	Adrenocorticosteroids
Vantin	cefpodoxime proxetil	Antibacterial agents
Vasotec	enalapril	Antihypertensive agents
Veetids	penicillin V	Antibacterial agents
Velosef	cephradine	Antibacterial agents
Ventolin	albuterol	Bronchodilators
Verelan	verapamil	Antihypertensive agents
Viagra	sildenafil	Erectile dysfunction agents
Vibramycin	doxycycline	Antibacterial agents
Vibra-Tabs	doxycycline	Antibacterial agents
Vicodin	hydrocodone with acetaminophen	Analgesic agents
Vicodin ES	hydrocodone with acetaminophen	Analgesic agents
Vistaril	hydroxyzine	Anxiolytic agents Sedatives
Volmax	albuterol	Bronchodilators
Voltaren	diclofenac sodium	Analgesic agents Antiarthritic agents Antiinflammatory agents
Voltaren-XR	diclofenac sodium	Analgesic agents Antiarthritic agents Antiinflammatory agents
Wellbutrin	bupropion	Antidepressant agents
Westcort	hydrocortisone	Adrenocorticosteroids
Wigraine	ergotamine/caffeine	Antimigraine agents
Xalatan	latanoprost	Antiglaucoma agents
Xanax	alprazolam	Anxiolytic agents Sedatives
Zantac	ranitidine	Antiulcer agents
Zestril	lisinopril	Antihypertensive agents
Zinacef	cefotaxime	Antibacterial agents
Zithromax	azithromycin	Antibacterial agents
Zocor	simvastatin	Hypolipidemic agents
Zoloft	sertraline	Antidepressant agents
Zomig	zolmitriptan	Antimigraine agents
Zovirax	acyclovir	Antiviral agents
Zyban	bupropion	Antidepressant agents
Zyloprim	allopurinol	Antigout agents
Zyprexa	olanzapine	Antipsychotic agents
Zyrtec	cetirizine	Antihistamine agents

MEDICATION MANAGEMENT

In addition to drug classification duties required of case managers, home care therapists must also have a working knowledge of the way various medications may affect patient response to therapy. Adverse drug reaction guidelines list potential responses the patient may experience with drugs. Adverse drug reactions are listed by class, and special notes draw attention to more specific adverse drug reactions therapists may encounter. Adverse drug reaction guidelines point out reactions that may occur secondary to medication use. The guidelines are not all inclusive but detail notable reactions. Drug interaction guidelines highlight possible problems with certain medication combinations of drug class to drug subclass or subclass to subclass. Medication effects guidelines provide general information on the way some drug classes affect functional performance. For example, some medications have therapeutic windows, during which functional performance is optimal. Other drugs may limit exercise tolerance and patient participation with therapy programs. Medication effects guidelines consolidate such information for select medications and drug classes for immediate access in the home. Finally, therapeutic monitoring guidelines offer a quick reference of therapeutic levels for specific medications.

Medication Management Glossary

Adverse drug reactions. Responses to drugs that are noxious and/or unintended and occurring at doses normally used in humans for prophylaxis, diagnosis, therapy of disease, or the modification of physiological function.

Common adverse drug reactions. Adverse drug reactions that are found collectively in a drug class or subclass. *Common* does not indicate a high frequency or incidence of adverse reactions, but simply means that these reactions may be generalized to the whole drug class or subclass.

Critical drug interactions. Drug interactions that have a high degree of severity (i.e., potentially life threatening in some cases) and well-documented history of occurrences.

Drug interactions. Reactions in which one drug alters the concentration of a second drug or potentiates the effect of a second drug.

Therapeutic concentrations. Ranges of serum drug concentration that produce desirable pharmacological effects without unwanted adverse drug reactions.

Therapeutic monitoring. A process by which therapeutic drug concentrations are attained and maintained through assessment, modification, and reassessment.

Adverse Drug Reaction Guidelines*

Adrenergics
Common adverse reactions**

- Altered mental status (excitability, hyperactivity, irritability, nervousness)
- Insomnia
- Headache
- Dizziness
- Chest pain and/or angina
- Arrhythmias
- Hypertension or hypotension
- Muscle weakness
- Muscle cramping
- Tremor

Adrenocorticosteroids
Common adverse reactions

- Altered mental status (anxiety, depression, euphoria, restlessness)
- Insomnia
- Myalgia
- Headache
- **Vertigo**
- **Hypertension**
- Edema
- **Muscle wasting, weakness**
- **Osteoporosis**
- **Seizures**
- Gastrointestinal upset
- Nausea
- Vomiting
- Diarrhea or constipation
- Decreased rate of wound healing
- Increased susceptibility to infection
- Masked signs of infection
- Decreased glucose tolerance
- **Amenorrhea or dysmenorrhea**

Special considerations

- The likelihood of adverse reactions varies because dosing varies greatly depending on the indication for drug use.
- All drugs in this class have the potential to cause adrenal suppression with prolonged use. Therefore abrupt discontinuation of the drug may cause adrenal insufficiency (i.e., myalgia, malaise, weakness, anorexia).

---

*Bolded adverse drug reactions consist of those with relatively rare incidence, usually <1%
**See "Medication Management Glossary" for the definition of common adverse drug reactions.

Anabolic Steroids
Common adverse reactions

- Altered mental status (anxiety, depression)
- Headache
- Arthralgia
- Muscle cramping
- Muscle spasms
- Edema
- Hypercalcemia
- Paresthesias
- Nausea
- Jaundice
- Hepatitis
- Gynecomastia
- Male pattern baldness
- Acne
- Hypersensitivity reactions
- Amenorrhea or dysmenorrhea
- Oligospermia
- Priapism

Special considerations

Potential for abuse with anabolic steroids

Analgesic Agents
Common adverse reactions

Adverse drug reactions vary from drug subclass to drug subclass.

Special considerations

Nonsteroidal antiinflammatory analgesic agents (i.e., ibuprofen, naproxen)
- Somnolence
- Headache
- Tinnitus
- Hearing loss
- Abdominal pain
- Heartburn
- Gastrointestinal mucosal irritation
- Gastrointestinal bleeding
- Nausea
- Vomiting
- Dyspepsia
- **Dysuria**
- **Hematuria**
- **Hepatitis**
- Rash
- Platelet inhibition
- **Blood dyscrasias (agranulocytosis, leukopenia, neutropenia, thrombocytopenia)**

Narcotic analgesic agents (i.e., codeine, morphine, meperidine)
- Potential for abuse with narcotic analgesic agents
- Altered mental status (agitation, **delirium,** dysphoria, euphoria, hallucinations, mental clouding, nervousness, restlessness)
- Sedation
- **Insomnia**
- Dizziness
- Faintness
- Respiratory depression
- Muscle weakness
- **Seizures**
- Nausea
- Vomiting
- Constipation
- Urinary retention
- Oliguria

AntiAlzheimer's Agents
Common adverse reactions

- Insomnia
- Myalgia
- Fatigue
- Muscle cramping
- Ataxia
- Seizures
- Nausea
- Vomiting
- Diarrhea
- Anorexia

Special considerations

tacrine
- Jaundice
- Elevated liver function tests

Antianginal Agents
Common adverse reactions

- Headache
- Dizziness
- Tachycardia or bradycardia
- Orthostatic hypotension
- Hypotension
- Dyspepsia
- Rash
- Flushing

Special considerations

- acetaminophen—Premedication with acetaminophen may limit the severity and incidence of headache.
- Topical preparations—Rotation of topical administration sites minimizes the incidence of local skin reaction.

Antiarrhythmic Agents
Common adverse reactions

- Exacerbated arrhythmias
- Dyspepsia

Special considerations

disopyramide
- Hypotension
- Lupuslike symptoms
- Blurred vision
- Constipation
- Urinary retention
- Dry mouth

mexiletine
- Nervousness
- Dizziness
- Blurred vision
- Tremor
- Ataxia
- Hepatotoxicity

procainamide
- Hypotension
- Lupuslike symptoms
- Rash

propafenone
- Headache
- Dizziness
- Blurred vision
- Dry mouth
- Constipation

Antiarthritic Agents

Refer to the sections on adrenocorticosteroids or nonsteroidal antiinflammatory analgesic agents as appropriate.

Antibacterial Agents
Common adverse reactions

Adverse reactions vary from drug subclass to drug subclass.

Pharmacology

Special considerations

Aminoglycosides (i.e., amikacin, gentamicin, tobramycin)
- Headache
- **Vertigo**
- **Ataxia**
- Nephrotoxicity
- Elevated liver function tests
- Ocular itching, burning with ophthalmic preparations
- **Blood dyscrasias (leukopenia, granulocytopenia)**

Cephalosporins (i.e., cefaclor, cefuroxime, cephalexin, cephradine)
- Headache
- Nausea
- Vomiting
- Diarrhea
- Dyspepsia
- Decreased appetite
- Altered taste sensation
- **Elevated liver function tests**
- **Blood dyscrasias (neutropenia, thrombocytopenia)**
- Rash

Macrolides (i.e., azithromycin, clarithromycin, erythromycin)
- Headache
- Abdominal pain
- **Angioedema**
- Dyspepsia
- Altered taste sensation
- **Pseudomembranous colitis**
- **Cholestatic jaundice**
- Rash

penicillin derivatives (i.e., amoxicillin, ampicillin, mezlocillin, piperacillin)
- Headache
- Dizziness
- Fatigue
- Gastrointestinal upset
- Jaundice
- Hepatitis
- Nephropathy
- **Reversible blood dyscrasias (agranulocytosis, neutropenia, thrombocytopenia)**
- Rash

quinolones (i.e., ciprofloxacin, levofloxacin, ofloxacin)
- Headache
- **Propensity for Achilles tendon inflammation and/or rupture**
- Photosensitivity
- Dyspepsia
- Altered taste sensation
- Rash

sulfa derivatives (i.e., sulfamethoxazole, sulfamethoxazole/trimethoprim)
- Stevens-Johnson syndrome
- Lupuslike symptoms
- Gastrointestinal upset
- Interstitial nephritis
- Hepatitis
- **Blood dyscrasias (agranulocytosis, thrombocytopenia)**
- Rash

tetracycline derivatives (i.e., doxycycline, tetracycline)
- Photosensitivity
- Dyspepsia
- Enterocolitis
- Jaundice
- **Elevated liver function tests**
- **Blood dyscrasias (aplastic anemia, hemolytic anemia, thrombocytopenia)**
- Rash

Anticholinergic Agents
Common adverse reactions
- Altered mental status (depression, hallucinations, nervousness)
- Lethargy
- Pupil constriction
- Blurred vision
- Dry mouth
- Tachycardia
- Nausea
- Vomiting
- Constipation
- Urinary retention

Special considerations
Systemic side effects are avoided with local (i.e., nasal) administration.

Anticoagulant Agents
Common adverse reactions
- Abdominal pain
- Vasculitis
- Asthenia
- Excessive bleeding (hemoptysis to gastrointestinal bleeding)
- Jaundice
- Elevated liver function tests
- Bruising
- Dermatitis
- Urticaria
- Alopecia
- Necrosis

Anticonvulsant Agents
Common adverse reactions
- Altered mental status (irritability, restlessness)
- Lethargy
- Headache
- Dizziness
- Ataxia

Special considerations
carbamazepine
- **Stevens-Johnson syndrome**
- Arthralgia
- Hypotension or hypertension
- Nausea
- **Jaundice**
- **Hepatitis**
- **Elevated liver function tests**
- **Aplastic anemia**
- Rash

felbamate
- Vomiting
- **Acute hepatic failure**
- **Aplastic anemia**

lamotrigine
- Cervical pain
- Arthralgia
- Hot flashes
- Visual disturbances (blurred vision, diplopia)
- **Arrhythmias**
- Pharyngitis
- Cough
- Rhinitis
- Myasthenia
- Nausea
- Vomiting
- Constipation or diarrhea
- Rash

phenytoin
- Dysphagia
- Gingival hyperplasia
- Nystagmus
- Epigastric pain
- Nausea
- Vomiting
- Constipation
- Anorexia

- **Jaundice**
- **Elevated liver function tests**
- **Blood dyscrasias (agranulocytosis, granulocytopenia)**
- Systemic lupus erythematous

valproic acid
- **Stevens-Johnson syndrome**
- **Fanconi's syndrome**
- Back pain
- Muscle weakness
- **Jaundice**
- Elevated liver function tests
- **Acute pancreatitis**
- **Blood dyscrasias (anemia, thrombocytopenia)**
- Rash

Antidepressant Agents
Common adverse reactions

- Lethargy
- Altered mental status (anxiety, nervousness)
- Nausea
- Constipation or diarrhea
- Sexual dysfunction (ejaculatory dysfunction, impotence)
- **Blood dyscrasias (agranulocytosis, leukopenia, thrombocytopenia)**
- Rash

Special considerations

Serotonin syndrome may occur as patients discontinue one antidepressant agent and start another.

fluoxetine
- Headache
- Fatigue
- Muscle weakness
- Tremor
- Anorexia

paroxetine
- Insomnia
- Dry mouth
- Asthenia

sertraline
- Tremor

tricyclic antidepressant agents (i.e., amitriptyline, nortriptyline)
- Altered mental status (disorientation, memory impairment)
- Arrhythmias
- Orthostatic hypotension
- Fatigue
- Tremor

Antidiarrheal Agents
Common adverse reactions

- Lethargy
- Epigastric pain
- Abdominal cramping
- Dizziness
- Vomiting

Special considerations
loperamide
- Dry mouth
- Fatigue
- Rash

diphenoxylate
- Altered mental status (depression, euphoria)
- Headache
- Paresthesias
- Urticaria
- Pruritus

Antiemetic Agents
Common adverse reactions

- Lethargy
- Dizziness

Special considerations
dolasteron
- Headache
- Tachycardia
- Diarrhea

granisetron
- Headache
- Hypertension
- Asthenia
- Diarrhea or constipation

metoclopramide
- Altered mental status (depression, mania, restlessness)
- Gastrointestinal upset
- Extrapyramidal reactions (i.e., bradykinesia, facial spasms, torticollis)
- Fatigue

prochlorperazine
- Agitation
- Extrapyramidal reactions (i.e., bradykinesia, facial spasms, torticollis)
- Hypotension
- Fatigue
- Jaundice
- **Blood dyscrasias (agranulocytosis, leukopenia)**

promethazine
- **Extrapyramidal reactions (i.e., bradykinesia, facial spasms, torticollis)**
- Anticholinergic reactions (i.e., blurred vision, dizziness, dry mouth, excitation, euphoria, lethargy, nervousness)
- Seizures
- Jaundice
- **Blood dyscrasias (agranulocytosis, leukopenia)**
- Rash

Antifungal Agents
Common adverse reactions
Adverse reactions vary from drug subclass to drug subclass.

Special considerations
amphotericin B
- Transient fever
- Transient chills
- Hearing loss
- **Tinnitus**
- **Arrhythmias**
- Hypotension
- **Bronchospasm**
- **Shock**
- **Anaphylaxis**
- Malaise
- Nephrotoxicity
- **Acute liver failure**
- Diarrhea

A premedication regimen including acetaminophen, hydrocortisone, and intravenous hydration may limit adverse reactions to amphotericin B.

clotrimazole
- Topical administration:
  - Stinging
  - Skin irritation
  - Erythema
- Oral administration:
  - Nausea
  - Vomiting
  - Elevated liver function tests

fluconazole
- Headache
- Abdominal pain
- Nausea
- Vomiting
- Diarrhea
- **Elevated liver function tests**
- **Exfoliative dermatitis**
- Rash

itraconazole
- Fever
- Headache
- Dizziness
- Fatigue
- Dyspepsia
- **Jaundice**
- **Elevated liver function tests**
- **Hepatitis**
- Rash

ketoconazole
- Abdominal pain
- **Anaphylaxis**
- Nausea
- Vomiting
- **Elevated liver function tests**
- Urticaria
- Pruritus
- Local skin reactions to topical application

terbinafine
- Headache
- Altered taste sensation
- Gastrointestinal upset
- **Elevated liver function tests**
- Urticaria
- Pruritus
- Rash

Antiglaucoma Agents
Common adverse reactions
- Local eye irritation (burning, stinging)
- Visual disturbances (blurring, myopia)

Special considerations
dorzolamide
- Bitter taste sensation
- Photophobia
- Ocular dryness
- Punctate keratitis

latanoprost
- Photophobia
- Increased pigmentation of iris
- Rash

pilocarpine
- Headache
- Ciliary spasm
- **Retinal detachment**
- **Lens opacity**

timolol
- Headache
- Systemic beta-blocker effects (i.e., bradycardia, hypotension)
- **Conjunctivitis**
- **Keratitis**
- **Diplopia**

Antigout Agents
Common adverse reactions

- Headache
- Gastrointestinal upset

Special considerations

allopurinol
- Fever
- **Stevens-Johnson syndrome**
- Lethargy
- **Renal impairment**
- **Jaundice**
- **Elevated liver function tests**
- **Hepatic necrosis**
- **Acute gout episodes**
- Exfoliative dermatitis
- **Toxic epidermal necrolysis**
- Rash

colchicine
- **Alopecia**
- Myopathy
- Peripheral neuropathy
- Almost certain to cause nausea, vomiting, and diarrhea during drug initiation for acute gout
- **Hematuria**
- **Paralytic ileus**
- Stomatitis
- **Bladder spasm**
- Anorexia
- **Sexual dysfunction (azoospermia, oligospermia)**
- **Blood dyscrasias (agranulocytosis, aplastic anemia, leukopenia, thrombocytopenia)**
- Rash

probenecid
- Gingival pain
- Dizziness
- Urinary frequency
- Uric acid kidney stones
- Pruritus
- Hematuria
- **Blood dyscrasias (aplastic anemia, hemolytic anemia, leukopenia)**

- Flushing
- Dermatitis

Antihistamines
Common adverse reactions

- Lethargy
- Dry mouth
- Dizziness
- Arrhythmias
- Fatigue
- Dyspepsia
- Anticholinergic effects (i.e., blurred vision, dizziness, dry mouth, excitation, lethargy, nervousness)
- **Blood dyscrasias (leukopenia, thrombocytopenia)**

Special considerations

Nonsedating antihistamines (i.e., astemizole, cetirizine, fexofenadine, loratidine) may have relatively lower incidence of central nervous system effects compared with other antihistamines.

Antihypertensive Agents
Common adverse reactions

Adverse effects vary from drug subclass to drug subclass.

Special considerations

Angiotensin converting enzyme (ACE) inhibitors (i.e., captopril, fosinopril, quinapril, ramipril)
- Headache
- Dizziness
- Orthostatic hypotension
- **Angioneurotic edema**
- Cough
- Dyspepsia
- Hyperkalemia

Alpha-adrenergic blockers (i.e., doxazosin, terazosin)
- Somnolence
- Dizziness
- Syncope
- **Tinnitus**
- Orthostatic hypotension
- Edema
- Fatigue
- Ataxia
- Sexual dysfunction (decreased libido, impotence)

Beta-blockers (i.e., atenolol, labetalol, metoprolol, propranolol)
- Insomnia
- **Lethargy**

- Altered mental status (depression, **psychosis**)
- Dizziness
- Bradycardia
- Hypotension
- Peripheral edema
- Cold extremities
- **Bronchospasm**
- Fatigue
- Diarrhea
- Impotence
- Rash

Calcium channel blockers
- Dihydropyridine (i.e., amlodipine, nicardipine, nifedipine)
  - Headache
  - Dizziness
  - Increased frequency of angina
  - Arrhythmias
  - Hypotension
  - Fatigue
  - Muscle weakness
  - Muscle cramping
  - Nausea
  - **Constipation or diarrhea**
  - Rash
- verapamil
  - Headache
  - Dizziness
  - Heart block
  - Bradycardia
  - Edema
  - Fatigue
  - Nausea
  - Constipation
  - Rash
  - **Flushing**

Central alpha-adrenergic agonists (clonidine)
- Altered mental status (agitation, confusion, dementia, hallucinations)
- Lethargy, sedation
- Insomnia
- Headache
- Myalgia
- Dizziness
- Dry mouth
- **Arrhythmias**
- **Bradycardia or tachycardia**
- Orthostatic hypotension
- Muscle weakness

- Nausea
- Constipation
- Rash

Vasodilators (i.e., hydralazine)
- Headache
- Angina
- Tachycardia
- Orthostatic hypotension
- **Edema**
- **Peripheral neuritis**
- Nausea
- Vomiting
- Diarrhea or constipation
- **Blood dyscrasias (agranulocytosis, thrombocytosis)**
- Nasal congestion
- Ocular tearing
- Rash
- Flushing

Antiinflammatory Agents
Common adverse reactions

Refer to the section on nonsteroidal antiinflammatory analgesic agents or adreno-corticosteroids as appropriate.

Antimigraine Agents
Common adverse reactions

dihydroergotamine
- Somnolence
- Dizziness
- Vasoconstrictive effects (paresthesias of extremities)
- Rhinitis
- Pharyngitis
- **Muscle weakness**
- Gastrointestinal upset
- **Nausea**
- **Vomiting**

ergotamine
- **Bradycardia or tachycardia**
- **Muscle weakness**
- Paresthesias
- Nausea
- Vomiting

Selective serotonin agonists (i.e., sumatriptan, zolmitriptan)
- Altered mental status (agitation, anxiety)
- Lethargy
- Headache
- Lightheadedness

- Dizziness
- Angina
- **Arrhythmias**
- **Hypertension**
- Fatigue
- **Paresthesias**
- **Asthenia**
- **Seizures**
- Diaphoresis
- Flushing

Antineoplastic Agents
Common adverse reactions

- Nausea
- Vomiting
- Gastrointestinal upset
- Dysuria
- Nephrotoxicity
- Cystitis
- Elevated liver function tests
- Blood dyscrasias (thrombocytopenia, leukopenia)
- Alopecia
- Rash

Special considerations

chlorambucil
- **Pulmonary fibrosis**

cyclophosphamide
- **Pulmonary fibrosis**

doxorubicin
- Myocardial toxicity

melphalan
- **Bronchopulmonary dysplasia**
- **Pulmonary fibrosis**

Antiosteoporosis Agents
Common adverse reactions

Adverse drug reactions vary from drug subclass to drug subclass.

Special considerations

Biphosphonates (i.e., alendronate, etidronate, tiludronate)
- Headache
- Arthralgia
- Myalgia
- Abdominal pain
- **Esophagitis**
- **Esophageal oral erosion**

- Acid regurgitation
- Gastrointestinal upset
- Nausea
- Dyspepsia
- Diarrhea
- Electrolyte imbalances (hypophosphatemia, hypomagnesemia)
- Minimized adverse drug reactions if dose taken with a full glass of water before first meal of the day (refer to specific drug information for exact time parameters)
- Avoidance of supine or reclining positions for at least 30 minutes after dosing decreases incidence of esophageal irritation
- etidronate—lower incidence of gastrointestinal reactions with etidronate than other biphosphonates

calcitonin
- Abdominal pain
- Rhinitis
- **Bronchospasm**
- **Anaphylactic shock**
- Nausea
- Vomiting
- Diarrhea
- Anorexia
- Rash
- Local skin reaction (i.e., injection site, nasal mucosa)
- Flushing

AntiParkinson's Agents
Common adverse reactions

Adverse drug reactions vary from drug subclass to drug subclass.

Special considerations

Anticholinergic agents (i.e., benztropine, trihexyphenidyl)
- Altered mental status (confusion, excitement, hallucinations)
- Lethargy
- Nausea
- Vomiting
- Constipation

dopamine agonists (i.e., amantadine, bromocriptine, pergolide)
- Somnolence or insomnia
- Altered mental status (confusion, hallucinations, irritability)
- Anticholinergic effects (i.e., anxiety, blurred vision, dizziness, dry mouth, euphoria, excitation, lethargy, nervousness)
- Orthostatic hypotension
- Dyskinesia
- Nausea
- Vomiting
- Diarrhea
- Dyspepsia

dopamine precursors (levodopa, levodopa/carbidopa)
- Altered mental status (anxiety, confusion)
- Headache
- Eyelid spasm
- Dizziness
- Arrhythmias
- Hypotension
- **Hypertension**
- Dystonias
- On-off phenomenon
- **Nausea**
- **Vomiting**
- Constipation or diarrhea
- Dyspepsia
- Monamine oxidase inhibitors (selegiline)
- Altered mental status (anxiety, apathy, confusion, depression, hallucinations, psychosis)
- Insomnia
- Headache
- Lightheadedness
- Dizziness
- Vertigo
- Syncope
- Dry mouth
- Nausea

Antipyretic Agents
Common adverse reactions
Adverse drug reactions vary from drug subclass to drug subclass.

Special considerations
acetaminophen
- **Angioedema**
- **Anaphylactoid reaction**
- Urticaria
- **Blood dyscrasias (thrombocytopenia, purpura)**
- Rash

See the section on nonsteroidal antiinflammatory analgesic agents or adrenocorticosteroids as appropriate.

Antipsychotic Agents
Common adverse reactions
- Lethargy
- Dizziness
- Hypotension
- Orthostatic hypotension
- Extrapyramidal reactions (i.e., bradykinesia, facial spasms, torticollis)
- **Neuroleptic malignant syndrome**

Pharmacology

- Lowered seizure threshold
- Tardive dyskinesia
- Gastrointestinal upset
- **Blood dyscrasias (agranulocytosis, thrombocytopenia)**
- Rash

Special considerations

clozapine—higher incidence of severe agranulocytosis than other antipsychotic agents

Antirhinitis Agents
Common adverse reactions

- Headache
- Nasal burning, stinging
- Nasal dryness
- Nasal congestion
- Epistaxis
- Nausea

Antiulcer Agents
Common adverse reactions

Adverse drug reactions vary from drug subclass to drug subclass.

Special considerations

carafate
- **Nausea**
- **Vomiting**
- **Diarrhea or constipation**
- **Gastrointestinal upset**

Histamine blockers (i.e., cimetidine, famotidine, ranitidine)
- Headache
- Dizziness
- Nausea
- Vomiting
- Diarrhea or constipation
- **Blood dyscrasias (anemia, granulocytopenia)**
- Pruritus
- Rash
- Cimetidine—higher incidence of adverse drug reactions compared with other histamine blockers

Proton pump inhibitors (lansoprozole, omeprazole)
- Altered mental status (confusion, agitation, hallucinations)
- Headache
- Dizziness
- Abdominal pain
- Nausea
- Vomiting
- Diarrhea or constipation
- **Erythema multiforme**

- **Toxic epidermal necrolysis**
- **Rash**

Antiviral Agents
Common adverse reactions

- Headache
- Abdominal pain
- Nausea
- Vomiting
- Diarrhea
- Rash

Special considerations

ganciclovir
- **Peripheral neuropathy**
- **Paresthesias**
- Blood dyscrasias (anemia, granulocytopenia, thrombocytopenia)
- Elevated liver function tests
- Pruritus

indinavir
- Insomnia
- Fatigue
- Nephrolithiasis
- Renal failure
- Elevated liver function tests
- Hepatitis
- Glucose intolerance to hyperglycemia
- Dysgeusia
- **Blood dyscrasias (neutropenia, thrombocytopenia)**

lamivudine
- Dizziness
- Arthralgia
- Myalgia
- Lactic acidosis
- Malaise
- Peripheral neuropathy
- Hepatomegaly

ritonavir
- Somnolence or insomnia
- Dizziness
- Asthenia
- Paresthesias
- Dysgeusia
- Blood dyscrasias (anemia, leukopenia, lymphocytosis, thrombocytopenia)

saquinavir
- Depression
- Insomnia
- Arthralgia

- Myalgia
- Fatigue
- Muscle weakness
- Muscle cramping
- Pancreatitis
- Glucose intolerance to hyperglycemia

zalcitabine
- Peripheral neuropathy
- Pancreatitis
- Blood dyscrasias (anemia, leukopenia, lymphocytosis, thrombocytopenia)

zidovudine
- Insomnia
- Myalgia
- Myopathy
- Blood dyscrasias (anemia, granulocytopenia)

Anxiolytic Agents
Common adverse reactions

- Altered mental status (confusion, depression, disorientation, excitement, memory impairment, paradoxical anxiety)
- Somnolence
- Dizziness

Special considerations

Potential for abuse of anxiolytic agents

Benign Prostate Hypertrophy Agents
Common adverse reactions

Adverse reactions vary from drug subclass to drug subclass.

Special considerations

Alpha-blockers (doxazosin, tamsulosin, terazosin)
- Somnolence
- Dizziness
- Syncope
- Orthostatic hypotension
- Edema
- Fatigue
- Ataxia
- Tinnitus
- Impotence

finasteride
- Sexual dysfunction (decreased libido, impotence)

Bronchodilators
Common adverse reactions

Adverse drug reactions vary from drug subclass to drug subclass.

Special considerations

Anticholinergic agents (ipratropium)
- Dizziness
- Cough
- Arrhythmias
- Local skin reaction

Beta-adrenergic agonists (i.e., albuterol, salmeterol)
- Altered mental status (anxiety, giddiness, nervousness)
- Headache
- Dizziness
- Tachycardia
- Hypertension
- Cough
- Tremor
- Gastrointestinal upset

Adrenocorticosteroids (i.e., beclomethasone, triamcinolone)
- Hoarseness
- Dry mouth
- Bronchospasm
- Oral fungal infection
- Rash

Xanthine derivatives (theophylline)
- Altered mental status (confusion, irritability, restlessness)
- Headache
- Arrhythmias
- Nausea
- Rash

Cardiac Glycosides
Common adverse reactions
- Confusion
- Headache
- Dizziness
- Visual disturbances (altered color vision, blurred vision, "halos" around bright objects)
- Heart block
- Arrhythmias (ventricular tachycardia, ventricular premature contractions)
- Muscle weakness
- Nausea
- Vomiting
- Diarrhea
- Anorexia

Central Nervous System Stimulants
Common adverse reactions
- Altered mental status (hallucinations, mania, nervousness)
- Insomnia

- Headache
- Tachycardia
- **Hypertension**
- **Seizures**
- Anorexia
- **Blood dyscrasias (anemia, thrombocytopenia)**

Special considerations

Potential for abuse of central nervous system stimulants

Cold Preparations
Common adverse reactions

- Central nervous system depression (lethargy, sedation) or stimulation (excitement, **psychosis**)
- Headache
- Dizziness
- Tremor
- Gastrointestinal upset
- Rash

Special considerations

Adverse drug reactions vary depending on the specific drug combination.

Diuretics
Common adverse reactions

- Headache
- Photosensitivity
- Hypotension
- Hyperglycemia
- Dehydration
- Electrolyte imbalance
- Gastrointestinal upset
- Rash

Special considerations

furosemide
- Dizziness
- Vertigo
- Tinnitus
- **Paresthesias**

hydrochlorothiazide
- Adverse lipid values

spironolactone
- Confusion
- Lethargy
- **Gynecomastia**

- Impotence
- Menstrual cycle changes (ammenorrhea, irregular menstrual cycle length, postmenopausal bleeding)
- Hirsutism

Electrolytes and Fluids
Common adverse reactions

- Electrolyte imbalance
- Fluid overload
- Phlebitis
- Local irritation

Erectile Dysfunction Agents
Common adverse reactions

Adverse drug reactions vary from drug subclass to drug subclass.

Special considerations

alprostadil
- Dizziness
- Hypotension
- Urethral burning
- Minor urethral bleeding
- Penile, urethral, testicular pain
- Priapism

sildenafil
- Headache
- Dizziness
- Visual disturbances (photosensitivity, blurring, color alteration)
- Cardiac complications in patients with coronary artery disease
- Nasal congestion
- Diarrhea
- Dyspepsia
- Rash
- Flushing

Estrogens
Common adverse reactions

- **Depression**
- Migraines
- **Dizziness**
- **Hypertension**
- Edema
- Nausea
- Vomiting
- **Break through menstrual bleeding**
- Swollen, tender breasts

- **Alopecia**
- **Hirsutism**
- Increased libido
- Body weight fluctuation

Special considerations

Increased risk of estrogen-dependent carcinoma, gallbladder disease, thromboembolic disorders, and hepatic tumors with long-term use

Gastrointestinal Motility Agents
Common adverse reactions

- Headache
- Abdominal pain
- **Visual disturbances**
- Tachycardia
- Rhinitis
- **Infection**
- Nausea
- Vomiting
- Diarrhea or constipation
- Rash
- Pruritus

Hemorrheologic Agents
Common adverse reactions

- Headache
- Dizziness
- **Hypotension**
- Flu like symptoms
- **Blurred vision**
- Nausea
- Vomiting
- **Bloating**
- Dyspepsia

Special considerations

Dyspepsia—reduced if doses taken with meals

Hyperthyroid Agents
Common adverse reactions

- Lethargy
- Fever
- Vertigo
- **Arthralgia**
- **Myalgia**
- Lupuslike symptoms
- **Paresthesias**

- Nausea
- Vomiting
- Blood dyscrasias (agranulocytosis, **leukopenia, thrombocytopenia**)
- Rash
- Urticaria
- Pruritus

Hypoglycemic Agents
Common adverse reactions

- Hypoglycemia
- Epigastric fullness sensation
- Gastrointestinal upset
- Nausea
- Dyspepsia

Special considerations

acarbose
- Abdominal pain
- Flatulence

glimepiride
- Headache
- Dizziness
- Asthenia
- **Blood dyscrasias (thrombocytopenia, anemia, agranulocytosis)**
- Allergic skin reaction

glipizide
- Cholestatic jaundice
- **Blood dyscrasias (thrombocytopenia, anemia, agranulocytosis)**
- Allergic skin reaction

glyburide
- Cholestatic jaundice
- **Blood dyscrasias (thrombocytopenia, anemia, agranulocytosis)**
- Allergic skin reaction

insulin
- Hypokalemia
- Lipodystrophy
- Local or systemic allergy

metformin
- Lactic acidosis
- Bloating
- Unpleasant or metallic taste sensation

troglitazone
- Back pain
- Dizziness
- Asthenia
- **Liver dysfunction**

Pharmacology

Hypolipidemic Agents
Common adverse reactions

Adverse drug reactions vary from drug subclass to drug subclass.

Special considerations

Bile acid sequestrants (cholestyramine, colestipol)
- Hemorrhoid irritation
- Fecal impaction
- Decreased vitamin absorption
- Rash

gemfibrozil
- Somnolence
- Headache
- **Blurred vision**
- Abdominal pain
- Arthralgia
- Jaundice
- Elevated liver function tests
- Myopathy
- Dyspepsia
- Gall bladder disease
- Sexual dysfunction (impotence, decreased libido)

HMG CoA reductase inhibitors (i.e., atorvastatin, fluvastatin, lovastatin, pravastatin, simvastatin)
- Headache
- **Dizziness**
- Abdominal pain
- Myalgia
- Arthralgia
- **Myopathy**
- Nausea
- Diarrhea or constipation
- Dyspepsia
- Elevated liver function tests
- **Rhabdomyolysis**
- Rash

niacin
- **Syncope**
- **Tachycardia**
- Hypotension
- Paresthesias
- Glucose intolerance
- Gastrointestinal upset
- Peptic ulcers
- Jaundice
- Elevated liver function tests
- Flushing
- Dry skin

Hypothyroid Agents
Common adverse reactions

- Angina
- Heart failure
- Hyperthyroidism

Laxatives
Common adverse reactions

- Diarrhea
- Potential for dependence on laxatives

Special considerations

Bulk-forming agents (psyllium)
- Abdominal fullness
- Flatulence

Concentrated stimulants (i.e., casanthranol, senna)
- Abdominal cramping

Osmotic agents (lactulose, sorbitol)
- Abdominal cramping
- Flatulence
- Nausea
- Vomiting
- Electrolyte imbalance

Stool softeners (docusate)
- Bitter taste sensation
- Throat irritation
- Nausea
- Rash

Muscle Relaxants
Common adverse reactions

- Lethargy
- Dizziness
- Gastrointestinal upset

Special considerations

baclofen
- Confusion
- Headache
- **Arrhythmias**
- Hypotension
- Fatigue
- **Paresthesias**
- Nausea
- Constipation

carisoprodol
- Headache
- Tachycardia

- Orthostatic hypotension
- Angioedema
- Epigastric distress
- Dyspnea
- Rash

cyclobenzaprine

- **Altered mental status (confusion, nervousness)**
- **Headache**
- Blurred vision
- Dry mouth
- **Tachycardia**
- **Arrhythmias**
- **Hypotension**
- **Muscle weakness**
- Paresthesias
- Bloating

methocarbamol

- Headache
- Visual disturbances (blurred vision, nystagmus)
- Bradycardia
- Gastrointestinal upset
- Nausea
- Vomiting
- Allergic skin reactions
- Flushing

Potential for abuse of muscle relaxants, particularly of carisoprodol

Sedatives
Common adverse reactions

- Altered mental status (confusion, depression, disorientation, excitement, memory impairment, paradoxical anxiety)
- Somnolence
- Dizziness

Special considerations

- Potential for abuse of sedatives

Critical Drug Interaction Gudelines

Drug agent	Interacting with	May cause
Analgesic Agents*		
AntiAlzheimer's Agents		
tacrine	• theophylline	Increased bronchodilator effect
Antiarrhythmic Agents		
quinidine	• amiodarone	Increased quinidine blood level
Anticoagulant Agents		
warfarin	• carbamazepine	Decreased anticoagulant effect
	• phenobarbital	
	• primidone	
warfarin	• amiodarone	Increased anticoagulant effect
	• aspirin	
	• cimetidine	
	• erythromycin	
	• fenofibrate	
	• fluconazole	
	• itraconazole	
	• ketoconazole	
	• lovastatin	
	• all nonsteroidal antiinflammatory agents (ibuprofen, ketoprofen)	
	• salsalate	
	• sulfamethoxazole	
Anticonvulsant Agents		
carbamazepine	• erythromycin	Increased carbamazepine blood level
	• propoxyphene	
fosphenytoin	• cimetidine	Increased phenytoin blood level
phenytoin	• amiodarone	Increased phenytoin blood level
	• cimetidine	
Antidepressant Agents		
lithium	• All thiazide diuretics (i.e., hydrochlorothiazide)	Increased lithium blood level
lithium	• Caution with other diuretics	Possible increased lithium blood level
Antigout Agents		
probenecid	• salicylates (i.e., aspirin, salsalate)	Decreased antigout effect

*See Antiinflammatory Agents section.

Continued

Table—cont'd

Drug agent	Interacting with	May cause
Antihistamine Agents		
astemizole	• azithromycin • clarithromycin • erythromycin • fluconazole • fluvoxamine • indinavir • itraconazole • ketoconazole • nefazodone • quinine • ritonavir	Potentially fatal arrhythmias
Antihypertensive Agents		
All beta-blockers (i.e., acebutolol, atenolol, carvedilol, labetalol, metoprolol, propranolol)	• verapamil	Potentially fatal arrhythmias
clonidine	• Tricyclic antidepressants (i.e., amitriptyline, desipramine, imipramine, nortriptyline)	Decreased antihypertensive effect
verapamil	• All beta-blockers (i.e., acebutolol, atenolol, carvedilol, labetalol, metoprolol, propranolol)	Potentially fatal arrhythmias
Antimigraine Agents		
dihydroergotamine	• azithromycin • clarithromycin • erythromycin	Increased risk for ergotamine adverse reaction
ergotamine	• azithromycin • clarithromycin • erythromycin	Increased risk for ergotamine adverse reaction
AntiParkinson's Agents		
selegiline	• Central nervous system stimulants (i.e., dextroamphetamine, methylphenidate, phentermine) • ephedrine • meperidine • phenylpropanolamine	Induced hypertensive crisis

Table—cont'd

Drug agent	Interacting with	May cause
AntiParkinson's Agents—cont'd		
selegiline	• amitriptyline • desipramine • fluoxetine • imipramine • nortriptyline • paroxetine • sertraline	Precipitation of serotonin syndrome
Antipsychotic Agents		
clomipramine	• clonidine	Decreased antihypertensive effect
lithium	• All thiazide diuretics (i.e., hydrochlorothiazide)	Increased lithium blood level
lithium	• Caution with other diuretics	Possible increased lithium blood level
Bronchodilators		
theophylline	• azithromycin • clarithromycin • cimetidine • ciprofloxacin • erythromycin • levofloxacin • ofloxacin • tacrine	Increased theophylline blood level
theophylline	• carbamazepine • phenobarbital • phenytoin	Decreased theophylline blood level
Cardiac Glycosides		
digoxin	• amiodarone • azithromycin • clarithromycin • erythromycin • verapamil	Increased digoxin blood level
Erectile Dysfunction Agents		
sildenafil	• nitroglycerin	Increased vasodilation
Estrogens		
Oral contraceptives	• carbamazepine	Decreased efficacy of hormonal birth control

Continued

Table—cont'd

Drug agent	Interacting with	May cause
Gastrointestinal Motility Agents		
cisapride	• azithromycin • clarithromycin • erythromycin • fluconazole • indinavir • itraconazole • ketoconazole	Potentially fatal arrhythmias
Hypolipidemic Agents		
gemfibrozil	• atorvastatin • fluvastatin • lovastatin • pravastatin • simvastatin	Increased risk of myopathy
niacin	• atorvastatin • fluvastatin • lovastatin • pravastatin • simvastatin	Increased risk of myopathy
Hypoglycemic Agents		
Hypoglycemic agents	• All beta-blockers (i.e., acebutolol, atenolol, carvedilol, labetalol, metoprolol, propranolol)	Hypoglycemia masked by pharmacologic effect of beta-blockers

Medication Guidelines for Drug Classes Affecting Rehabilitation

Adrenocorticosteroids

Dosing considerations

There are no onset, peak effect, or duration of action guidelines that affect rehabilitation if patients follow their prescribed medication regimens because most adrenocorticosteroids have a cumulative effect on chronic pain and inflammation.

Precautions

Pain symptoms may be masked.

Analgesic Agents

Dosing considerations

Narcotic analgesic agents (i.e., codeine, hydromorphone, meperidine, morphine, oxycodone, propoxyphene)

Onset of action
- Intravenous administration—≤5 minutes
- Intramuscular administration—10 to 30 minutes
- Oral administration—15 to 60 minutes

Peak effect
- propoxyphene—2 hours
- All other narcotic analgesic agents—30 to 60 minutes

Duration of action
- 4 hours (2 to 6 hours range)

Timing of rehabilitation—60 minutes after medication administration

Nonsteroidal antiinflammatory analgesic agents (i.e., diclofenac, etodolac, ibuprofen, nabumetone, piroxicam)

Onset of action
- Variable

Peak effect
- nabumetone—3 to 6 hours
- piroxicam—3 to 6 hours
- All other nonsteroidal antiinflammatory analgesic agents—1 to 2 hours

Duration of action
- nabumetone—24 hours
- piroxicam—24 hours
- All other nonsteroidal antiinflammatory analgesic agents—4 to 12 hours

Timing of rehabilitation—2 hours after medication administration

Precautions

Pain symptoms may be masked.
Narcotic analgesic agents cause central nervous system depression; therefore their use may adversely affect neurological findings (i.e., alertness, orientation).

Antianginal Agents
Dosing considerations

Onset of action
- isosorbide:
  - Chewable tablet—3 minutes
  - Oral tablet—45 to 60 minutes
  - Sustained release tablet—30 minutes
- nitroglycerin:
  - Sublingual—1 to 5 minutes
  - Paste—15 to 60 minutes
  - Patch—40 to 60 minutes

Peak effect—variable

Duration of action
- isosorbide:
  - Chewable tablet—30 minutes to 2 hours
  - Oral tablet—4 to 6 hours
  - Sustained release tablet—6 to 12 hours

- nitroglycerin:
  - Sublingual—1 to 2 hours
  - Paste—2 to 12 hours
  - Patch—18 to 24 hours

Timing of rehabilitation

With patients on scheduled regimens of isosorbide or nitroglycerin (versus "as needed" use for angina), therapists should consider the mode of administration for the timing of rehabilitation.

- Oral administration—60 minutes after administration
- Paste administration—60 minutes after administration
- Patch administration—either
  - Patch on at breakfast and off at bedtime—any waking hour
  - Patch on at bedtime and off at lunch—any waking hour before lunch

Precautions

Patients on scheduled nitrate regimens must have a nitrate-free period every 24 hours to prevent accommodation to nitrates.

Antiarrhythmic Agents
Dosing considerations

There are no onset, peak effect, or duration of action guidelines that affect rehabilitation if patients follow their prescribed medication regimens because the effects of antiarrhythmic agents are continuous and cumulative.

Precautions

These agents do not mask the occurrence of arrhythmias, but rather, limit arrhythmias as they occur. As a result, blood pressure and heart rate must be closely monitored to assess cardiac status arrhythmias.

Antigout Agents
Dosing considerations

There are no onset, peak effect, or duration of action guidelines that affect rehabilitation if patients follow their prescribed medication regimens because most antigout agents have a cumulative effect for chronic gout conditions.

For episodes of acute gouty arthritis, pain and edema usually diminish within 12 hours of intervention. Complete remission usually occurs within 48 to 72 hours.

Therapists may choose to reschedule rehabilitation until acute gouty attacks subside, particularly if affected joints are involved with the therapy program.

Precautions

indomethacin—may mask pain

Antihypertensive Agents
Dosing considerations

There are no onset, peak effect, or duration of action guidelines that affect rehabilitation if patients follow their prescribed medication regimens because the effects of antihypertensive agents are continuous and cumulative.

Precautions

Beta-blockers (i.e., atenolol, labetalol, metoprolol) and calcium channel blockers (verapamil) decrease the heart rate. Although heart rate monitoring reveals important arrhythmias, therapists should not monitor exercise tolerance and performance based solely on heart rate changes.

Patients with bronchial asthma, allergic bronchospasm, or severe chronic obstructive pulmonary disease taking beta-blockers are at an increased risk for bronchospasm. Therapists must closely monitor these patients for signs and symptoms of potentially fatal bronchospasm episodes.

AntiParkinson's Agents
Dosing considerations

The onset, peak effect, and duration of action guidelines vary by subclass and by patient and cannot be generalized.

Precautions

Patients experiencing changes in their usual response to antiParkinson's agents (i.e., early "wearing off," delayed onset of medication effects) may require a change in medication (i.e., sustained release), dosing (i.e., more frequent dosing), or medication administration (i.e., crushed tablet and dissolved in water for faster absorption).

Bronchodilators
Dosing considerations

Inhaled bronchodilators
- Onset of action—<1 to 2 minutes
- Peak effect—30 minutes to 2 hours
- Duration of action:
  - salmeterol—12 hours
  - Other bronchodilators—4 to 6 hours

Timing of rehabilitation
- 60 to 90 minutes after administration

Cardiac Glycosides
Dosing considerations

There are no onset, peak effect, or duration of action guidelines that affect rehabilitation if patients follow their prescribed medication regimens because the effects of cardiac glycosides are continuous and cumulative.

Precautions

Cardiac glycosides decrease the rate of ventricular contraction. Although heart rate monitoring reveals important arrhythmias, therapists should not monitor exercise tolerance and performance based solely on heart rate changes.

Hypoglycemic Agents
Dosing considerations

There are no onset, peak effect, or duration of action guidelines that affect rehabilitation if patients follow their prescribed medication and diet regimens.

Precautions

Hypoglycemia results if patients overmedicate or fail to follow their prescribed diet (i.e., skip meals).

Hyperglycemia results if patients undermedicate (i.e., miss doses, take incorrect doses) or fail to follow their prescribed diet (i.e., overeat).

Muscle Relaxants

Dosing considerations

- Onset of action—30 to 60 minutes
- Peak effect—unknown
- Duration of action—6 to 12 hours
- Timing of rehabilitation—60 minutes after medication administration

Precautions

Pain symptoms may be masked.

Muscle relaxants cause central nervous system depression; therefore their use may adversely affect neurological findings (i.e., alertness, orientation).

Therapeutic Medication Level Guidelines

Drug	Therapeutic concentration	Potentially toxic concentration
Antiarrhythmic Agents		
digoxin	Trough 0.5-2 ng/ml	Trough >2 ng/ml
procainamide	Trough 4-10 mcg/ml	>10 mcg/ml
quinidine	Trough 2-5 mcg/ml	Trough >10 mcg/ml
Antibacterial Agents		
amikacin	Peak 20-35 mcg/ml	Peak >35 mcg/ml
	Trough <8 mcg/ml	Trough >8 mcg/ml
gentamicin	Peak 4-10 mcg/ml	Peak >12 mcg/ml
	Trough 5-10 mcg/ml	Trough >2 mcg/ml
tobramycin	Peak 4-10 mcg/ml	Peak >12 mcg/ml
	Trough 5-10 mcg/ml	Trough >2 mcg/ml
vancomycin	Peak 30-40 mcg/ml	Peak >80 mcg/ml
	Trough 5-10 mcg/ml	Trough >13 mcg/ml
Anticonvulsant Agents		
carbamazepine	Trough 4-12 mcg/ml	Trough >12 mcg/ml
phenobarbital	Trough 15-40 mcg/ml	Trough >40 mcg/ml
phenytoin	Trough 10-20 mcg/ml	Trough >20 mcg/ml
primidone	Trough 5-12 mcg/ml	Trough >12 mcg/ml
valproic acid	Trough 50-100 mcg/ml	Trough >150 mcg/ml
Antidepressant Agents		
amitriptyline plus nortriptyline	Trough 120-250 ng/ml	Trough >500 ng/ml
desipramine	Trough 125-160 ng/ml	Trough >300 ng/ml
lithium	Trough 12 hours after dose 0.6-1.2 mEq/ml	Trough 12 hours after dose >3 mEq/ml
nortriptyline	Trough 50-140 ng/ml	Trough >500 ng/ml
Bronchodilators		
theophylline	Trough 10-20 mcg/ml	Trough >20 mcg/ml

Drug	INR* therapeutic range	Potentially toxic range
Anticoagulant Agents		
warfarin	Low intensity 2.0-3.0	>3.0
	High intensity 2.5-3.5	>3.5

*INR, International normalized ratio; standardized ratio for quantifying blood coagulation.

REFERENCES

Dipiro JT and others, eds: *Pharmacotherapy: a pathophysiological approach,* Stamford, Conn, 1997, Appleton & Lange.

Gilman AG and others, eds: *The pharmacological basis of therapeutics,* Elmsford, NY, 1990, Pergamon Press.

Kastrup EK, ed: *Facts and comparisons loose-leaf drug information service,* St Louis, 1998, Facts and Comparisons.

Lacy C and others: *Drug information handbook,* Hudson, Oh, 1995, Lexi-Comp.

McEvoy GK, ed: *American hospital formulary service 1998 drug information,* Bethesda, Md, 1998, The American Society of Health-System Pharmacists.

Murphy JL: *Monthly prescribing reference,* New York, 1998, Prescribing Reference.

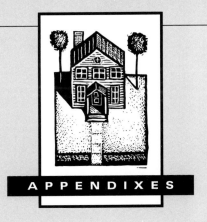

APPENDIXES

A. HIM-11 Coverage of Services

The Health Insurance Manual-11 (HIM-11) contains the federal rules and regulations concerning home health services for Medicare beneficiaries. It describes all facets of home care from billing procedures and beneficiary eligibility criteria to covered services and start of care procedures. Therapists must be aware of these rules to ensure proper reimbursement of home health services. This appendix contains the following HIM-11 excerpts pertinent to the provision of therapy services in the home:

The Health Care Financing Administration revised the Coverage of Services subsection of the HIM-11 in April of 1996. All Medicare-certified agencies possess a copy of the HIM-11. Consult the agency HIM-11 to stay abreast of recent changes or revisions to this manual.

COVERAGE OF SERVICES

<u>Covered and Noncovered Home Health Services</u>

203.   CONDITIONS TO BE MET FOR COVERAGE OF HOME HEALTH SERVICES

Home health agency (HHA) services are covered by Medicare when the following criteria are met:

- The person to whom the services are provided is an eligible Medicare beneficiary.

- The HHA that is providing the services to the beneficiary has in effect a valid agreement to participate in the Medicare program.

- The beneficiary qualifies for coverage of home health services as described in §204.

- The services for which payment is claimed are covered as described in §§205 and 206.

- Medicare is the appropriate payer.

- The services for which payment is claimed are not otherwise excluded from payment.

203.1 <u>Reasonable and Necessary Services</u>.—

A. <u>Background</u>.—In enacting the Medicare program, Congress recognized that the physician would play an important role in determining utilization of services. The law requires that payment may be made only if a physician certifies the need for services and establishes a plan of care. The Secretary is responsible for ensuring that the claimed services are covered by Medicare, including determining whether they are "reasonable and necessary."

B. <u>Determination of Coverage</u>.—The intermediary's decision on whether care is reasonable and necessary is based on information reflected in the home health plan of care (HCFA 485), in supplementary forms (e.g., HCFA 486 or an HHA's internal form), and the medical record concerning the unique medical condition of the individual patient. A coverage denial is not made solely on the basis of the reviewer's general inferences about patients with similar diagnoses or on data related to utilization generally, but is based upon objective clinical evidence regarding the patient's individual need for care. Additional information from the medical record must be requested when medical information needed to support a decision is not clearly present. The following examples illustrate this statement.

Examples of cases in which development of the case is needed:

EXAMPLE 1: A plan of care provides for daily skilled nursing visits for care of a pressure sore, but the description of the pressure sore and the dressing that is on the form causes the reviewer to question why daily skilled care is needed. The intermediary would not reduce the number of visits but would either request additional information to support the need for daily care or would request the nursing notes to determine if the patient required daily skilled care.

EXAMPLE 2: A patient with a diagnosis of congestive heart failure (CHF) has been hospitalized for 5 days. Posthospital skilled nursing care is ordered 3 × wk × 60 days for skilled observation, teaching of diet medication compliance and signs and symptoms of the disease. The documentation on the HCFA 485 and supplementary form shows that the patient has had CHF for 10 years with an exacerbation requiring recent hospitalization. The medications are not shown as changed or new. The clinical findings are contradictory. There is a possibility that this patient requires skilled observation and teaching although the documentation does not give a clear picture of the patient's needs. Therefore, the case would be developed further to determine if the criteria for coverage were met.

Examples of cases that would be denied without further development:

EXAMPLE 3: A plan of care provides for vitamin B-12 injections 1 × mo × 60 days for a patient who has been discharged from the hospital following a recent hip fracture. The patient has generalized weakness, but there is no diagnosis or clinical symptoms shown to support Medicare coverage of skilled nursing care for B-12 injections. The claim would be denied without further development.

EXAMPLE 4: A patient has a primary diagnosis of back sprain that resulted in a 7-day hospitalization. The patient also has a secondary diagnosis of emphysema with an onset 2 years prior to the start of care. Following the hospitalization, the physician ordered skilled nursing 2 × wk × 4 weeks for skilled observation of vital signs and response to medication and aide services 2 × wk × 4 weeks for personal care. The documentation on the HCFA 485 and supplementary form shows that the patient is up as tolerated, able to walk 10 feet without resting, and able to perform ADLs. Clinical facts show normal vital signs with no reference to emphysema. The patient is on colcace 100 mg BID. The documentation clearly does not support the medical necessity for skilled nursing care and the claim for the services would be denied without development.

Examples of cases in which payment may be made without further development:

EXAMPLE 5: A patient with a diagnosis of CHF has been hospitalized for five days. Post-hospital skilled nursing care is ordered 3 × wk × 60 days for skilled observation, teaching of a new diet regimen, compliance with multiple new medications, and signs and symptoms of the disease state. The documentation on the HCFA 485 and supplementary form shows the patient has had an acute exacerbation of a pre-existing CHF condition that required the recent acute hospitalization. The patient is discharged from the hospital with a medication regimen changed from previous medications. The HCFA forms documenting the clinical evidence of the recent acute exacerbation of the patient's cardiac condition combined with changed medications support the physician's order for care. Payment may be made without further development.

EXAMPLE 6: A plan of care provides for physical therapy treatments 3 × wk × 45 days for a patient who has been discharged from the hospital following a recent hip fracture. The patient was discharged using a walker 7 days before the start of home care. The HCFA 485 and supplementary form show that the patient was discharged from the hospital with restricted mobility in ambulation, transfers, and climbing of stairs. The patient had an unsafe gait indicating a need for gait training and had not been instructed in stair climbing and a home exercise program. The goal of the physical therapy was to increase strength, range of motion and to progress from walker to cane with safe gait. Information on the relevant HCFA forms also indicates that the patient had a previous functional capacity of full ambulation, mobility, and self care. The claim may be paid without further development, since there are no objective clinical factors in the medical evidence to contradict the order of the patient's treating physician.

203.2 <u>Impact of Other Available Caregivers and Other Available Coverage on Medicare Coverage of Home Health Services</u>.—Where the Medicare criteria for coverage of home health services are met, patients are entitled by law to coverage of reasonable and necessary home health services. Therefore, a patient is entitled to have the costs of reasonable and necessary services reimbursed by Medicare without regard to whether there is someone available to furnish the services. However, where a family member or other person is or will be providing services that adequately meet the patient's needs, it would not be reasonable and necessary for HHA personnel to furnish such services. Ordinarily it can be presumed that there is no able and willing person to provide the services being rendered by the HHA unless the patient or family indicates otherwise and objects to the provision of the services by the HHA, or the HHA has first hand knowledge to the contrary.

EXAMPLE: A patient, who lives with an adult daughter and otherwise qualifies for Medicare coverage of home health services, requires the assistance of a home health aide for bathing and assistance with an exercise program to improve endurance. The daughter is unwilling to bathe her elderly father and assist with the exercise program. Home health aide services to provide these services would be reasonable and necessary.

Similarly, a patient is entitled to have the costs of reasonable and necessary home health services reimbursed by Medicare even if the patient would qualify for institutional care (e.g., hospital care or skilled nursing facility care).

EXAMPLE: A patient who is discharged from a hospital with a diagnosis of osteomyelitis and requires continuation of the IV antibiotic therapy that was begun in the hospital was found to meet the criteria for Medicare coverage of skilled nursing facility services. If the patient also meets the qualifying criteria for coverage of home health services, payment may be made for the reasonable and necessary home health services the patient needs, notwithstanding the availability of coverage in a skilled nursing facility.

Medicare payment should be made for reasonable and necessary home health services where the patient is also receiving supplemental services that do not meet Medicare's definition of skilled nursing care or home health aide services.

EXAMPLE: A patient who needs skilled nursing care on an intermittent basis also hires a licensed practical (vocational) nurse to provide nighttime assistance while family members sleep. The care provided by the nurse, as respite to the family members, does not require the skills of a licensed nurse as defined in §205.1 and, therefore, has no impact on the patient's eligibility for Medicare payment of home health services even though another third party insurer may pay for that nursing care.

203.3 <u>Use of Utilization Screens and "Rules of Thumb"</u>.—Medicare recognizes that determinations of whether home health services are reasonable and necessary must be based on an assessment of each patient's individual care needs. Therefore, denial of services based on numerical utilization screens, diagnostic screens, diagnosis or specific treatment norms is not appropriate.

204. CONDITIONS THE PATIENT MUST MEET TO QUALIFY FOR COVERAGE OF HOME HEALTH SERVICES

To qualify for Medicare coverage of any home health services, the patient must meet each of the criteria described in this section. Patients who meet each of these criteria are eligible to have payment made on their behalf for the services discussed in §§205 and 206.

204.1 Confined to the Home.—

    A. Patient Confined to the Home.—In order for a patient to be eligible to receive covered home health services under both Part A and Part B, the law requires that a physician certify in all cases that the patient is confined to his/her home. (See §240.1.) An individual does not have to be bedridden to be considered as confined to the home. However, the condition of these patients should be such that there exists a normal inability to leave home and, consequently, leaving home would require a considerable and taxing effort. If the patient does in fact leave the home, the patient may nevertheless be considered homebound if the absences from the home are infrequent or for periods of relatively short duration, or are attributable to the need to receive medical treatment. Absences attributable to the need to receive medical treatment include attendance at adult day centers to receive medical care, ongoing receipt of outpatient kidney dialysis, and the receipt of outpatient chemotherapy or radiation therapy. It is expected that in most instances, absences from the home that occur will be for the purpose of receiving medical treatment. However, occasional absences from the home for nonmedical purposes, e.g., an occasional trip to the barber, a walk around the block or a drive, would not necessitate a finding that the patient is not homebound if the absences are undertaken on an infrequent basis or are of relatively short duration and do not indicate that the patient has the capacity to obtain the health care provided outside rather than in the home.

Generally speaking, a patient will be considered to be homebound if he/she has a condition due to an illness or injury that restricts his/her ability to leave his/her place of residence except with the aid of supportive devices such as crutches, canes, wheelchairs, and walkers, the use of special transportation, or the assistance of another person or if leaving home is medically contraindicated. Some examples of homebound patients that illustrate the factors used to determine whether a homebound condition exists would be: (1) a patient paralyzed from a stroke who is confined to a wheelchair or requires the aid of crutches in order to walk; (2) a patient who is blind or senile and requires the assistance of another person to leave his/her residence; (3) a patient who has lost the use of his/her upper extremities and, therefore, is unable to open doors, use handrails on stairways, etc., and requires the assistance of another individual to leave his/her residence; (4) a patient who has just returned from a hospital stay involving surgery suffering from resultant weakness and pain and, therefore, his/her actions may be restricted by his/her physician to certain specified and limited activities such as getting out of bed only for a specified period of time, walking stairs only once a day, etc.; (5) a patient with arteriosclerotic heart disease of such severity that he/she must avoid all stress and physical activity; and (6) a patient with a psychiatric problem if the illness is manifested in part by a refusal to leave home or is of such a nature that it would not be considered safe to leave home unattended, even if he/she has no physical limitations.

The aged person who does not often travel from home because of feebleness and insecurity brought on by advanced age would not be considered confined to the home for purposes of receiving home health services unless he/she meets one of the above conditions. A patient who requires skilled care must also be determined to be confined to the home in order for home health services to be covered.

Although a patient must be confined to the home to be eligible for covered home health services, some services cannot be provided at the patient's residence because equipment is required that cannot be made available there. If the services required by a patient involve the use of such equipment, the HHA may make arrangements with a hospital, skilled nursing facility, or a rehabilitation center to provide these services on an outpatient basis. (See §§200.2 and 206.5.) However, even in these situations, for the services to be covered as home health services, the patient must be considered confined to his/her home; and to receive such outpatient services a homebound patient will generally require the use of supportive devices, special transportation, or the assistance of another person to travel to the appropriate facility.

If a question is raised as to whether a patient is confined to the home, the HHA will be asked to furnish the intermediary with the information necessary to establish that the patient is homebound as defined above.

      B. Patient's Place of Residence.—A patient's residence is wherever he/she makes his/her home. This may be his/her own dwelling, an apartment, a relative's home, a home for the aged, or some other type of institution. However, an institution may not be considered a patient's home if the institution meets the requirements of §§1861(e)(1) or 1819(a)(1) of the Act. Included in this group are hospitals and skilled nursing facilities, as well as most nursing facilities under Medicaid.

Thus, if a patient is in an institution or distinct part of an institution identified above, the patient is not entitled to have payment made for home health services under either Part A or Part B since these institutions may not be considered his/her residence. When a patient remains in a participating SNF following his/her discharge from active care, the facility may not be considered his/her residence for purposes of home health coverage.

204.2 <u>Services Are Provided Under a Plan of Care Established and Approved by a Physician.</u>—

      A. <u>Content of the Plan of Care.</u>—The plan of care must contain all pertinent diagnoses, including the patient's mental status, the types of services, supplies, and equipment required, the frequency of visits to be made, prognosis, rehabilitation potential, functional limitations, activities permitted, nutritional requirements, all medications and treatments, safety measures to protect against injury, instructions for timely discharge or referral, and any additional items the HHA or physician choose to include.

NOTE: This manual uses the term "plan of care" to refer to the medical treatment plan established by the treating physician with the assistance of the home health care nurse. Although HCFA previously used the term "plan of treatment," the Omnibus Budget Reconciliation Act of 1987 replaced that term with "plan of care" without a change in definition. HCFA anticipates that a discipline-oriented plan of care will be established, where appropriate, by an HHA nurse regarding nursing and home health aide services and by skilled therapists regarding specific therapy treatment. These plans of care may be incorporated in the physician's plan of care or separately prepared.

      B. <u>Specificity of Orders.</u>—The orders on the plan of care must specify the type of services to be provided to the patient, both with respect to the professional who will provide them and the nature of the individual services, as well as the frequency of the services.

EXAMPLE: SN × 7/wk × 1 wk; 3/wk × 4 wk; 2/wk × 3 wk, (skilled nursing visits 7 times per week for 1 week; three times per week for 4 weeks; and two times per week for 3 weeks) for skilled observation and evaluation of the surgical site, for teaching sterile dressing changes and to perform sterile dressing changes. The sterile change consists of . . . (detail of procedure).

Orders for care may indicate a specific range in the frequency of visits to ensure that the most appropriate level of service is provided to home health patients. When a range of visits is ordered, the upper limit of the range is considered the specific frequency.

EXAMPLE: SN × 2-4/wk × 4 wk; 1-2/wk × 4 wk for skilled observation and evaluation of the surgical site. . . .

Orders for services to be furnished "as needed" or "PRN" must be accompanied by a description of the patient's medical signs and symptoms that would occasion a visit and a specific limit on the number of those visits to be made under the order before an additional physician order would have to be obtained.

        C. Who Signs the Plan of Care.—The physician who signs the plan of care must be qualified to sign the physician certification as described in 42 CFR 424.22.

        D. Timeliness of Signature.—The plan of care must be signed before the bill is submitted to the intermediary for payment.

        E. Use of Oral (Verbal) Orders.—When services are furnished based on a physician's oral order, the orders may be accepted and put in writing by personnel authorized to do so by applicable State and Federal laws and regulations, as well as by the HHA's internal policies. The orders must be signed and dated with the date of receipt by the registered nurse or qualified therapist (i.e., physical therapist, speech-language pathologist, occupational therapist, or medical social worker) responsible for furnishing or supervising the ordered services. The orders may be signed by the supervising registered nurse or qualified therapist after the services have been rendered, as long as HHA personnel who receive the oral orders notify that nurse or therapist before the service is rendered. Thus, the rendering of a service that is based on an oral order would not be delayed pending signature of the supervising nurse or therapist. Oral orders must be countersigned and dated by the physician before the HHA bills for the care in the same way as the plan of care.

        (1) Services that are provided from the beginning of the certification period and before the physician signs the plan of care are considered to be provided under a plan of care established and approved by the physician where there is an oral order for the care prior to rendering the services which is documented in the medical record and where the services are included in a signed plan of care.

EXAMPLE: The HHA acquires an oral order for venipuncture for a patient to be performed on August 1. The HHA provides the venipuncture on August 1 and evaluates the patient's need for continued care. The physician signs the plan of care for the venipuncture on August 15. Since the HHA had acquired an oral order prior to the delivery of services, the visit is considered to be provided under a plan of care established and approved by the physician.

        (2) Services that are provided in the subsequent certification period are considered to be provided under the subsequent plan of care where there is an oral order before the services provided in the subsequent period are furnished and the order is reflected in the medical record. However, services that are provided after the expiration of a plan of care, but before the acquisition of an oral order or a signed plan of care, cannot be considered to be provided under a plan of care.

EXAMPLE 1: The patient is under a plan of care in which the physician orders venipuncture every 2 weeks. The last day covered by the initial plan of care is July 31. The patient's next venipuncture is scheduled for August 5th and the physician signs the plan of care for the new period on August 1st. The venipuncture on August 5th was provided under a plan of care established and approved by the physician.

EXAMPLE 2: The patient is under a plan of care in which the physician orders venipuncture every 2 weeks. The last day covered by the plan of care is July 31. The patient's next venipuncture is scheduled for August 5th and the physician does not sign the plan of care until August 6th. The HHA acquires an oral order for the venipuncture before the August 5th visit, and therefore the visit is considered to be provided under a plan of care established and approved by the physician.

EXAMPLE 3: The patient is under a plan of care in which the physician orders venipuncture every 2 weeks. The last day covered by the plan of care is July 31. The patient's next venipuncture is scheduled for August 5th and the physician does not sign the plan of care until August 6th. The HHA *does not* acquire an oral order for the venipuncture before the August 5th visit, and therefore the visit cannot be considered to be provided under a plan of care established and approved by the physician. The prior plan of care expired and neither an oral order nor a signed plan of care was in effect on the date of the service. The visit is not covered.

(3) Any increase in the frequency of services or addition of new services during a certification period must be authorized by a physician by way of a written or oral order prior to the provision of the increased or additional services.

F. Frequency of Review of the Plan of Care.—The plan of care must be reviewed and signed by the physician who established the plan of care, in consultation with HHA professional personnel, at least every 62 days. Each review of a patient's plan of care must contain the signature of the physician and the date of review.

G. Facsimile Signatures.—The plan of care or oral order may be transmitted by facsimile machine. The HHA is not required to have the original signature on file. However, the HHA is responsible for obtaining original signatures if an issue surfaces that would require verification of an original signature.

H. Alternative Signatures.—HHAs that maintain patient records by computer rather than hard copy may use electronic signatures. However, all such entries must be appropriately authenticated and dated. Authentication must include signatures, written initials, or computer secure entry by a unique identifier of a primary author who has reviewed and approved the entry. The HHA must have safeguards to prevent unauthorized access to the records and a process for reconstruction of the records in the event of a system breakdown.

I. Termination of the Plan of Care.—The plan of care is considered to be terminated if the patient does not receive at least one covered skilled nursing, physical therapy, speech-language pathology service, or occupational therapy visit in a 62-day period unless the physician documents that the interval without such care is appropriate to the treatment of the patient's illness or injury.

204.3 Under the Care of a Physician.—The patient must be under the care of a physician who is qualified to sign the physician certification and plan of care in accordance with 42 CFR 424.22.

A patient is expected to be under the care of the physician who signs the plan of care and the physician certification. It is expected, but not required for coverage, that the physician who signs the plan of care will see the patient, but there is no specified interval of time within which the patient must be seen.

204.4 <u>Needs Skilled Nursing Care on an Intermittent Basis or Physical Therapy or Speech-Language Pathology Services or Has Continued Need for Occupational Therapy</u>.—The patient must need one of the following types of skilled services:

- Skilled nursing care that:

    —Is reasonable and necessary as defined in §§205.1A and B, and
    —Is needed on an "intermittent" basis as defined in §205.1C, or

- Physical therapy as defined in §§205.2A and B, or

- Speech-language pathology services as defined in §§205.2A and C, or

- A continuing need for occupational therapy as defined in §§205.2A and D.

The patient has a continued need for occupational therapy when:

- The services that the patient requires meet the definition of "occupational therapy" services of §§205.2A and D, and

- The patient's eligibility for home health services has been established by virtue of a prior need for skilled nursing care, speech-language pathology services, or physical therapy in the current or prior certification period.

EXAMPLE: A patient who is recovering from a cerebral vascular accident has an initial plan of care that called for physical therapy, speech-language pathology services, and home health aide services. In the next certification period, the physician orders only occupational therapy and home health aide services because the patient no longer needs the skills of a physical therapist or a speech-language pathologist, but needs the services provided by the occupational therapist. The patient's need for occupational therapy qualifies him or her for home health services, including home health aide services (presuming that all other qualifying criteria are met).

204.5 <u>Physician Certification</u>.—The HHA must be acting upon a physician certification that is part of the plan of care (HCFA-485) and meets the requirements of this section for HHA services to be covered.

    A. <u>Content of the Physician Certification</u>.—The physician must certify that:

      1. The home health services are or were needed because the patient is or was confined to the home as defined in §204.1;

      2. The patient needs or needed skilled nursing services on an intermittent basis, physical therapy, or speech-language pathology services, or continues or continued to need occupational therapy after the need for skilled nursing care, physical therapy, or speech-language pathology services ceased;

      3. A plan of care has been established and is periodically reviewed by a physician; and

      4. The services are or were furnished while the patient is or was under the care of a physician.

   B. <u>Periodic Recertification.</u>—The physician certification may cover a period less than but not greater than 62 days (2 months).

   C. <u>Who May Sign the Certification.</u>—The physician who signs the certification must be permitted to do so by 42 CFR 424.22.

205.   COVERAGE OF SERVICES WHICH ESTABLISH HOME HEALTH ELIGIBILITY

For any home health services to be covered by Medicare, the patient must meet the qualifying criteria as specified in §204, including having a need for skilled nursing care on an intermittent basis, physical therapy, speech-language pathology services, or a continuing need for occupational therapy as defined in this section.

205.2 <u>Skilled Therapy Services.</u>—

   A. <u>General Principles Governing Reasonable and Necessary Physical Therapy, Speech-Language Pathology Services, and Occupational Therapy.</u>—

   1. The service of a physical, speech-language pathologist or occupational therapist is a skilled therapy service if the inherent complexity of the service is such that it can be performed safely and/or effectively only by or under the general supervision of a skilled therapist. To be covered, the skilled services must also be reasonable and necessary to the treatment of the patient's illness or injury or to the restoration of maintenance of function affected by the patient's illness or injury. It is necessary to determine whether individual therapy services are skilled and whether, in view of the patient's overall condition, skilled management of the services provided is needed although many or all of the specific services needed to treat the illness or injury do not require the skills of a therapist.

   2. The development, implementation management and evaluation of a patient care plan based on the physician's orders constitute skilled therapy services when, because of the patient's condition, those activities require the involvement of a skilled therapist to meet the patient's needs, promote recovery and ensure medical safety. Where the skills of a therapist are needed to manage and periodically reevaluate the appropriateness of a maintenance program because of an identified danger to the patient, such services would be covered even if the skills of a therapist are not needed to carry out the activities performed as part of the maintenance program.

   3. While a patient's particular medical condition is a valid factor in deciding if skilled therapy services are needed, the diagnosis or prognosis should never be the sole factor in deciding that a service is or is not skilled. The key issue is whether the skills of a therapist are needed to treat the illness or injury, or whether the services can be carried out by nonskilled personnel.

   4. A service that is ordinarily considered nonskilled could be considered a skilled therapy service in cases in which there is clear documentation that, because of special medical complications, skilled rehabilitation personnel are required to perform or supervise the service or to observe the patient. However, the importance of a particular service to a patient or the frequency with which it must be performed does not, by itself, make a nonskilled service into a skilled service.

   5. The skilled therapy services must be reasonable and necessary to the treatment of the patient's illness or injury within the context of the patient's unique medical condition. To be considered reasonable and necessary for the treatment of the illness or injury:

a. The services must be consistent with the nature and severity of the illness or injury, the patient's particular medical needs, including the requirement that the amount, frequency and duration of the services must be reasonable;

b. The services must be considered, under accepted standards of medical practice, to be specific safe, and effective treatment for the patient's condition; and

c. The services must be provided with the expectation, based on the assessment made by the physician of the patient's rehabilitation potential, that:

—The condition of the patient will improve materially in a reasonable and generally predictable period of time; or

—The services are necessary to the establishment of a safe and effective maintenance program

Services involving activities for the general welfare of any patient, e.g., general exercises to promote overall fitness or flexibility and activities to provide diversion or general motivation, do not constitute skilled therapy. Those services can be performed by nonskilled individuals without the supervision of a therapist.

d. Services of skilled therapists for the purpose of teaching the patient, family or caregivers necessary techniques, exercises or precautions are covered to the extent that they are reasonable and necessary to treat illness or injury. However, visits made by skilled therapists to a patient's home solely to train other HHA staff (e.g., home health aides) are not billable as visits since the HHA is responsible for ensuring that its staff is properly trained to perform any service it furnishes. The cost of a skilled therapist's visit for the purpose of training HHA staff is an administrative cost to the agency.

EXAMPLE: A patient with a diagnosis of multiple sclerosis has recently been discharged from the hospital following an exacerbation of her condition that has left her wheelchair bound and, for the first time without any expectation of achieving ambulation again. The physician has ordered physical therapy to select the proper wheelchair for her long term use, to teach safe use of the wheelchair and safe transfer techniques to the patient and family. Physical therapy would be reasonable and necessary to evaluate the patient's overall needs, to make the selection of the proper wheelchair and to teach the patient and family safe use of the wheelchair and proper transfer techniques.

e. The amount, frequency, and duration of the services must be reasonable.

B. Application of the Principles to Physical Therapy Services.—The following discussion of skilled physical therapy services applies the principles in §205.2A to specific physical therapy services about which questions are most frequently raised.

1. Assessment.—The skills of a physical therapist to assess a patient's rehabilitation needs and potential or to develop and/or implement a physical therapy program are covered when they are reasonable and necessary because of the patient's condition. Skilled rehabilitation services concurrent with the management of a patient's care plan include objective tests and measurements such as, but not limited to, range of motion strength, balance coordination, endurance, or functional ability.

2. <u>Therapeutic Exercises</u>.—Therapeutic exercises which must be performed by or under the supervision of the qualified physical therapist to ensure the safety of the patient and effectiveness of the treatment, due either to the type of exercise employed or to the condition of the patient, constitute skilled physical therapy.

3. <u>Gait Training</u>.—Gait evaluation and training furnished to a patient whose ability to walk has been impaired by neurological, muscular or skeletal abnormality require the skills of a qualified physical therapist and constitute skilled physical therapy and are considered reasonable and necessary if training can be expected to improve materially the patient's ability to walk.

Gait evaluation and training that is furnished to a patient whose ability to walk has been impaired by a condition other than a neurological, muscular or skeletal abnormality would nevertheless be covered where physical therapy is reasonable and necessary to restore the lost function.

EXAMPLE 1: A physician has ordered gait evaluation and training for a patient whose gait has been materially impaired by scar tissue resulting from burns. Physical therapy services to evaluate the patient's gait, establish a gait training program, and provide the skilled services necessary to implement the program would be covered.

EXAMPLE 2: A patient who has had a total hip replacement is ambulatory but demonstrates weakness and is unable to climb stairs safely. Physical therapy would be reasonable and necessary to teach the patient to safely climb and descend stairs.

Repetitive exercises to improve gait, or to maintain strength and endurance and assistive walking are appropriately provided by nonskilled persons and ordinarily do not require the skills of a physical therapist. Where such services are performed by a physical therapist as part of the initial design and establishment of a safe and effective maintenance program, the services would, to the extent that they are reasonable and necessary, be covered.

EXAMPLE: A patient who has received gait training has reached his maximum restoration potential and the physical therapist is teaching the patient and family how to perform safely the activities that are a part of a maintenance program. The visits by the physical therapist to demonstrate and teach the activities (which by themselves do not require the skills of a therapist) would be covered since they are needed to establish the program.

4. <u>Range of Motion</u>.—Only a qualified physical therapist may perform range of motion tests and, therefore, such tests are skilled physical therapy.

Range of motion exercises constitute skilled physical therapy only if they are part of an active treatment for a specific disease state, illness, or injury, that has resulted in a loss or restriction of mobility (as evidenced by physical therapy notes showing the degree of motion lost and the degree to be restored). Range of motion exercises unrelated to the restoration of a specific loss of function often may be provided safely and effectively by nonskilled individuals. Passive exercises to maintain range of motion in paralyzed extremities that can be carried out by nonskilled persons do not constitute skilled physical therapy.

However, as indicated in §205.2A4, where there is clear documentation that, because of special medical complications (e.g., susceptible to pathological bone fractures), the skills of a therapist are needed to provide services that ordinarily do not need the skills of a therapist, then the services would be covered.

5. <u>Maintenance Therapy</u>.—Where repetitive services that are required to maintain function involve the use of complex and sophisticated procedures, the judgement and skill of a physical therapist might be required for the safe and effective rendition of such services. If the judgement and skill of a physical therapist is required to treat the illness or injury safely and effectively, the services would be covered as physical therapy services.

EXAMPLE: Where there is an unhealed, unstable fracture that requires regular exercise to maintain function until the fracture heals, the skills of a physical therapist would be needed to ensure that the fractured extremity is maintained in proper position and alignment during maintenance range of motion exercises.

Establishment of a maintenance program is a skilled physical therapy service where the specialized knowledge and judgement of a qualified physical therapist is required for the program to be safely carried out and the treatment aims of the physician achieved.

EXAMPLE: A Parkinson's patient or a patient with rheumatoid arthritis who has not been under a restorative physical therapy program may require the services of a physical therapist to determine what type of exercises are required to maintain his/her present level of function. The initial evaluation of the patient's needs, the designing of a maintenance program appropriate to the capacity and tolerance of the patient and the treatment objectives of the physician, the instruction of the patient, family or caregivers to carry out the program safely and effectively and such reevaluations as may be required by the patient's condition, would constitute skilled physical therapy.

While a patient is under a restorative physical therapy program, the physical therapist should regularly reevaluate his condition and adjust any exercise program the patient is expected to carry out himself or with the aid of supportive personnel to maintain the function being restored. Consequently, by the time it is determined that no further restoration is possible (i.e., by the end of the last restorative session) the physical therapist will already have designed the maintenance program required and instructed the patient or caregivers in carrying out the program.

6. <u>Ultrasound, Shortwave, and Microwave Diathermy Treatments</u>.—These treatments must always be performed by or under the supervision of a qualified physical therapist and are skilled therapy.

7. <u>Hot Packs, Infra-Red Treatments, Paraffin Baths and Whirlpool Baths</u>.—Heat treatments and baths of this type ordinarily do not require the skills of a qualified physical therapist. However, the skills, knowledge and judgment of a qualified physical therapist might be required in the giving of such treatments or baths in a particular case, e.g., where the patient's condition is complicated by circulatory deficiency, areas of desensitization, open wounds, fractures or other complications.

C. <u>Application of the General Principles to Speech-Language Pathology Services</u>.—Speech-language pathology services are those services necessary for the diagnosis and treatment of speech and language disorders that result in communication disabilities and for the diagnosis and treatment of swallowing disorders (dysphagia), regardless of the presence of a communication disability. The following discussion of skilled speech-language pathology services applies the principles to specific speech-language pathology services about which questions are most frequently raised.

1. The skills of a speech-language pathologist are required for the assessment of a patient's rehabilitation needs (including the causal factors and the severity of the speech and language disorders), and rehabilitation potential. Reevaluation would only be considered reasonable and necessary if the patient exhibited a change in functional speech or motivation, clearing of confusion or the remission of some other medical condition that previously contraindicated speech-language pathology services. Where a patient is undergoing restorative speech-language pathology services, routine reevaluations are considered to be a part of the therapy and could not be billed as a separate visit.

2. The services of a speech-language pathologist would be covered if they are needed as a result of an illness or injury and are directed towards specific speech/voice production.

3. Speech-language pathology would be covered where the service can only be provided by a speech-language pathologist and where it is reasonably expected that the service will materially improve the patient's ability to independently carry out any one or combination of communicative activities of daily living in a manner that is measurably at a higher level of attainment than that prior to the initiation of the services.

4. The services of a speech-language pathologist to establish a hierarchy of speech-voice-language communication tasks and cueing that directs a patient toward speech-language communication goals in the plan of care would be covered speech-language pathology services.

5. The services of a speech-language pathologist to train the patient, family, or other caregivers to augment the speech-language communication, treatment or to establish an effective maintenance program would be covered speech-language pathology services.

6. The services of a speech-language pathologist to assist patients with aphasia in rehabilitation of speech and language skills are covered when needed by a patient.

7. The services of a speech-language pathologist to assist patients with voice disorders to develop proper control of the vocal and respiratory systems for correct voice production are covered when needed by a patient.

D. Application of the General Principles to Occupational Therapy.—The following discussion of skilled occupational therapy services applies the principles to specific occupational therapy services about which questions are most frequently raised.

1. Assessment.—The skills of an occupational therapist to assess and reassess a patient's rehabilitation needs and potential or to develop and/or implement an occupational therapy program are covered when they are reasonable and necessary because of the patient's condition.

2. Planning, Implementing and Supervision of Therapeutic Programs.—The planning, implementing and supervision of therapeutic programs including, but not limited to those listed below, are skilled occupational therapy services, and if reasonable and necessary to the treatment of the patient's illness or injury would be covered.

a. Selecting and teaching task oriented therapeutic activities designed to restore physical function.

EXAMPLE: Use of woodworking activities on an inclined table to restore shoulder, elbow and wrist range of motion lost as a result of burns.

b. Planning, implementing and supervising therapeutic tasks and activities designed to restore sensory-integrative function.

EXAMPLE: Providing motor and tactile activities to increase sensory output and improve response for a stroke patient with functional loss resulting in a distorted body image.

c. Planning, implementing and supervising of individualized therapeutic activity programs as part of an overall "active treatment" program for a patient with a diagnosed psychiatric illness.

EXAMPLE: Use of sewing activities which require following a pattern to reduce confusion and restore reality orientation in a schizophrenic patient.

d. Teaching compensatory techniques to improve the level of independence in the activities of daily living.

EXAMPLE 1: Teaching a patient who has lost use of an arm how to pare potatoes and chop vegetables with one hand.

EXAMPLE 2: Teaching a stroke patient new techniques to enable him to perform feeding, dressing, and other activities of daily living as independently as possible.

e. The designing, fabricating, and fitting of orthotic and self-help devices.

EXAMPLE 1: Construction of a device that would enable a patient to hold a utensil and feed himself independently.

EXAMPLE 2: Construction of a hand splint for a patient with rheumatoid arthritis to maintain the hand in a functional position.

f. Vocational and prevocational assessment and training that is directed toward the restoration of function in the activities of daily living lost due to illness or injury would be covered. Where vocational or prevocational assessment and training is related solely to specific employment opportunities, work skills or work settings, such services would not be covered because they would not be directed toward the treatment of an illness or injury.

3. <u>Illustration of Covered Services.</u>—

EXAMPLE 1: A physician orders occupational therapy for a patient who is recovering from a fractured hip and who needs to be taught compensatory and safety techniques with regard to lower extremity dressing, hygiene, toileting and bathing. The occupational therapist will establish goals for the patient's rehabilitation (to be approved by the physician), and will undertake the teaching of the techniques necessary for the patient to reach the goals. Occupational therapy services would be covered at a duration and intensity appropriate to the severity of the impairment and the patient's response to treatment.

EXAMPLE 2: A physician has ordered occupational therapy for a patient who is recovering from a CVA. The patient has decreased range of motion, strength and sensation in both the upper and lower extremities on the right side and has perceptual and cognitive deficits resulting from the CVA. The patient's condition has resulted in decreased function in activities of daily living (specifically bathing, dressing, grooming, hygiene and toileting). The loss of function requires assistive devices to enable the patient to compensate for the loss of function and to maximize safety and independence. The patient also needs equipment such as himi-slings to prevent shoulder subluxation and a hand splint to prevent joint contracture and deformity in the right hand. The services of an occupational therapist would be necessary to assess the patient's needs, develop goals (to be approved by the physician), manufacture or adapt the needed equipment to the patient's use, teach compensatory techniques, strengthen the patient as necessary to permit use of compensatory techniques, and provide activities that are directed towards meeting the goals governing increased perceptual and cognitive function. Occupational therapy services would be covered at a duration and intensity appropriate to the severity of the impairment and the patient's response to treatment.

206. COVERAGE OF OTHER HOME HEALTH SERVICES

206.1 Skilled Nursing Care, Physical Therapy, Speech-Language Pathology Services, and Occupational Therapy.—Where the patient meets the qualifying criteria in §204, Medicare covers skilled nursing services that meet the requirements of §§205.1A and B and §206.7, physical therapy that meets the requirements of §§205.2A and B, speech-language pathology services that meet the requirements of §§205.2A and C, and occupational therapy that meets the requirements of §§205.2A and D.

Home health coverage is not available for services furnished to a qualified patient who is no longer in need of one of the qualifying skilled services specified in §205. Therefore, dependent services furnished after the final qualifying skilled service are not covered, except when the dependent service was followed by a qualifying skilled service as a result of the unexpected inpatient admission or death of the patient or due to some other unanticipated event.

206.2 Home Health Aide Services.—For home health aide services to be covered, the patient must meet the qualifying criteria as specified in §204; the services provided by the home health aide must be part-time or intermittent as discussed in §206.7; the services must meet the definition of home health aide services of this section; and the services must be reasonable and necessary to the treatment of the patient's illness or injury.

The reason for the visits by the home health aide must be to provide hands-on personal care to the patient or services that are needed to maintain the patient's health or to facilitate treatment of the patient's illness or injury.

The physician's order should indicate the frequency of the home health aide services required by the patient. These services may include but are not limited to:

a. Personal Care.—Personal care means:

- Bathing, dressing, grooming, caring for hair, nail and oral hygiene that are needed to facilitate treatment or prevent deterioration of the patient's health, changing the bed linens of an incontinent patient, shaving, deodorant application, skin care with lotions and/or powder, foot care, and ear care.

- Feeding, assistance with elimination (including enemas unless the skills of a licensed nurse are required due to the patient's condition), routine catheter care and routine colostomy care, assistance with ambulation, changing position in bed, assistance with transfers.

EXAMPLE 1: A physician has ordered home health aide visits to assist the patient in personal care because the patient is recovering from a stroke and continues to have significant right side weakness that causes him to be unable to bathe, dress or perform hair and oral care. The plan of care established by the HHA nurse sets forth the specific tasks with which the patient needs assistance. Home health aide visits at an appropriate frequency would be reasonable and necessary to assist in these tasks.

EXAMPLE 2: A physician ordered four home health aide visits per week for personal care for a multiple sclerosis patient who is unable to perform these functions because of increasing debilitation. The home health aide gave the patient a bath twice per week and washed hair on the other two visits each week. Only two visits are reasonable and necessary since the services could have been provided in the course of two visits.

EXAMPLE 3: A physician ordered seven home health aide visits per week for personal care for a bed-bound, incontinent patient. All visits are reasonable and necessary because the patient has extensive personal care needs.

EXAMPLE 4: A patient with a well-established colostomy forgets to change the bag regularly and has difficulty changing the bag. Home health aide services at an appropriate frequency to change the bag would be considered reasonable and necessary to the treatment of the illness or injury.

    b. Simple dressing changes that do not require the skills of a licensed nurse.

EXAMPLE: A patient who is confined to the bed has developed a small reddened area on the buttocks. The physician has ordered home health aide visits for more frequent repositioning, bathing and the application of a topical ointment and a gauze 4 × 4. Home health aide visits at an appropriate frequency would be reasonable and necessary.

    c. Assistance with medications that are ordinarily self-administered and do not require the skills of a licensed nurse to be provided safely and effectively.

NOTE: Prefilling of insulin syringes is ordinarily performed by the diabetic as part of the self-administration of the insulin and, unlike the injection of the insulin, does not require the skill of a licensed nurse to be performed properly. Therefore, if the prefilling of insulin syringes is performed by HHA staff, it is considered to be a home health aide service. However, where State law precludes the provision of this service by other than a licensed nurse or physician, Medicare will make payment for this service, when covered, as though it were a skilled nursing service. Where the patient needs only prefilling of insulin syringes and does not need skilled nursing care on an intermittent basis, physical therapy or speech-language pathology services or have a continuing need for occupational therapy, then Medicare cannot cover any home health services to the patient (even if State law requires that the insulin syringes be filled by a licensed nurse).

    d. Assistance with activities that are directly supportive of skilled therapy services but do not require the skills of a therapist to be safely and effectively performed such as routine maintenance exercises, and repetitive practice of functional communication skills to support speech-language pathology services.

    e. Routine care of prosthetic and orthotic devices.

When a home health aide visits a patient to provide a health related service as discussed above, the home health aide may also perform some incidental services that do not meet the definition of a home health aide service (e.g., light cleaning, preparation of a meal, taking out the trash, shopping). However, the purpose of a home health aide visit may not be to provide these incidental services since they are not health related services, but rather are necessary household tasks that must be performed by anyone to maintain a home.

EXAMPLE 1: A home health aide visits a recovering stroke patient whose right side weakness and poor endurance cause her to be able to leave the bed and chair only with extreme difficulty. The physician has ordered physical therapy and speech-language pathology services for the patient and has ordered home health aide services three or four times per week for personal care, assistance with ambulation as mobility increases, and assistance with repetitive speech exercises as her impaired speech improves. The home health aide also provides incidental household services such as preparation of meals, light cleaning and taking out the trash. The patient lives with an elderly frail sister who is disabled and cannot perform either the personal care or the incidental tasks. The home health aide visits at a frequency appropriate to the performance of the health related services would be covered, notwithstanding the incidental provision of noncovered services (i.e., the household services) in the course of the visits.

EXAMPLE 2: A physician orders home health aide visits three times per week. The only services provided are light housecleaning, meal preparation and trash removal. The home health aide visits cannot be covered, notwithstanding their importance to the patient, because the services provided do not meet Medicare's definition of "home health aide services."

206.3 <u>Medical Social Services</u>.—Medical social services that are provided by a qualified medical social worker or a social work assistant under the supervision of a qualified medical social worker may be covered as home health services where the patient meets the qualifying criteria specified in §204, and:

- The services of these professionals are necessary to resolve social or emotional problems that are or are expected to be an impediment to the effective treatment of the patient's medical condition or his or her rate of recovery; and

- The plan of care indicates how the services that are required necessitate the skills of a qualified social worker or a social work assistant under the supervision of a qualified medical social worker to be performed safely and effectively.

Where both of these requirements for coverage are met, services of these professionals that may be covered include, but are not limited to:

- Assessment of the social and emotional factors related to the patient's illness, need for care, response to treatment and adjustment to care;

- Assessment of the relationship of the patient's medical and nursing requirements to the patient's home situation, financial resources and availability of community resources;

- Appropriate action to obtain available community resources to assist in resolving the patient's problem. (Note: Medicare does not cover the services of a medical social worker to complete or assist in the completion of an application for Medicaid because Federal regulations require the State to provide assistance in completing the application to anyone who chooses to apply for Medicaid.);

- Counseling services which are required by the patient; and

- Medical social services furnished to the patient's family member or caregiver on a short-term basis when the HHA can demonstrate that a brief intervention (that is, two or three visits) by a medical social worker is necessary to remove a clear and direct impediment to the effective treatment of the patient's medical condition or to his or her rate of recovery. To be considered "clear and direct," the behavior or actions of the family member or caregiver must plainly obstruct, contravene, or prevent the patient's medical treatment or rate of recovery. Medical social services to address general problems that do not clearly and directly impede treatment or recovery as well as long-term social services furnished to family members, such as ongoing alcohol counseling, are not covered.

NOTE: Participating in the development of the plan of care, preparing clinical and progress notes, participating in discharge planning and inservice programs, and acting as a consultant to other agency personnel are appropriate administrative costs to the HHA.

EXAMPLE 1: The physician has ordered a medical social worker assessment of a diabetic patient who has recently become insulin dependent and is not yet stabilized. The nurse, who is providing skilled observation and evaluation to try to restabilize the patient, notices during her visits that supplies left in the home for the patient's use appear to be frequently missing and that the patient is not compliant with the regimen and refuses to discuss the matter. The assessment by a medical social worker would be reasonable and necessary to determine if there are underlying social or emotional problems that are impeding the patient's treatment.

EXAMPLE 2: A physician has ordered an assessment by a medical social worker for a multiple sclerosis patient who is unable to move anything but her head and has an indwelling catheter. The patient has experienced recurring urinary tract infections and multiple infected ulcers. The physician ordered medical social services after the HHA indicated to him that the home was not well cared for, the patient appeared to be neglected much of the time, and the relationship between the patient and family was very poor. The physician and HHA were concerned that social problems created by family caregivers were impeding the treatment of the recurring infections and ulcers. The assessment and follow-up for counseling both the patient and the family by a medical social worker would be reasonable and necessary.

EXAMPLE 3: A physician is aware that a patient with arteriosclerosis and hypertension is not taking medications as ordered and is not adhering to dietary restrictions because he is unable to afford the medication and is unable to cook. The physician orders several visits by a medical social worker to assist in resolving these problems. The visits by the medical social worker to review the patient's financial status, discuss options, and make appropriate contacts with social services agencies or other community resources to arrange for medications and meals would be a reasonable and necessary medical social service.

EXAMPLE 4: A physician has ordered counseling by a medical social worker for a patient with cirrhosis of the liver who has recently been discharged from a 28-day inpatient alcohol treatment program to her home that she shares with an alcoholic and neglectful adult child. The physician has ordered counseling several times a week to assist the patient in remaining free of alcohol and in dealing with the adult child. These services would be covered until the patient's social situation ceased to impact on her recovery and/or treatment.

EXAMPLE 5:   A physician has ordered medical social services for a patient who is worried about her financial arrangements and payment for medical care. The services ordered are to arrange Medicaid if possible and resolve unpaid medical bills. There is no evidence that the patient's concerns are adversely impacting recovery or treatment of her illness or injury. Medical social services cannot be covered.

EXAMPLE 6:   A physician has ordered medical social services for a patient of extremely limited income who has incurred large unpaid hospital and other medical bills following a significant illness. The patient's recovery is adversely affected because the patient is not maintaining a proper therapeutic diet, and cannot leave home to acquire the medication necessary to treat his/her illness. The medical social worker reviews the patient's financial status, arranges meal service to resolve the dietary problem, arranges for home delivered medications, gathers the information necessary for application to Medicaid to acquire coverage for the medications the patient needs, files the application on behalf of the patient, and follows up repeatedly with the Medicaid State agency.

The medical social services that are necessary to review the financial status of the patient, arrange for meal service, arrange for the medications to be delivered to the home, and arrange for the Medicaid State agency to assist the patient with the application for Medicaid are covered. The services related to the assistance in filing the application for Medicaid and the followup on the application are not covered since they are provided by the State agency free of charge, and hence the patient has no obligation to pay for such assistance.

EXAMPLE 7:   A physician has ordered medical social services for an insulin dependent diabetic whose blood sugar is elevated because she has run out of syringes and missed her insulin dose for two days. Upon making the assessment visit, the medical social worker learns that the patient's daughter, who is also an insulin dependent diabetic, has come to live with the patient because she is out of work. The daughter is now financially dependent on the patient for all of her financial needs and has been using the patient's insulin syringes. The social worker assesses the patient's financial resources and determines that they are adequate to support the patient and meet her own medical needs, but are not sufficient to support the daughter. She also counsels the daughter and helps her access community resources. These visits would be covered but only to the extent that the services are necessary to prevent interference with the patient's treatment plan.

EXAMPLE 8:   An Alzheimer's patient is being cared for by his wife. The nurse learns that the wife has not been giving the patient his medication correctly and seems distracted and forgetful about various aspects of the patient's care. In a conversation with the nurse, the wife relates that she is feeling depressed and overwhelmed by the patient's illness. The nurse contacts the patient's physician who orders a social work evaluation. In her assessment visit, the social worker learns that the patient's wife is so distraught over her situation that she cannot provide adequate care to the patient and is interfering with the patient's treatment program. While there, the social worker counsels the wife and assists her with referrals to a support group and her private physician for evaluation of her depression.

EXAMPLE 9:   The parent of a dependent disabled child has been discharged from the hospital following a hip replacement. Although arrangements for care of the disabled child during the hospitalization were made, the child has returned to the home. During a visit to the patient, the nurse observes that the patient is transferring the child from bed to a wheelchair. In an effort to avoid impeding the patient's recovery, the nurse contacts the patient's physician to order a visit by a social worker to mobilize family members or otherwise arrange for temporary care of the disabled child.

B. <u>Physical Therapy</u>.—These codes represent all services to be performed by the physical therapist. If services are provided by a nurse, they are included under A7. The following is a further explanation of each service:

- <u>B1. Evaluation</u>—Visit(s) made to determine patient's condition, physical therapy plans and rehabilitation potential. Also to evaluate home environment to eliminate structural barriers and improve safety to increase functional independence (ramps, adaptive wheelchair, bathroom aides).

- <u>B2. Therapeutic Exercise</u>—Exercises designed to restore function. Specific exercise techniques (e.g., Proprioceptive Neuromuscular Facilitation (PNF), Rood, Brunstrom, Codman's, William's) should be specified in the plan of care. The exercise technique should be listed in the medical record specific to the patient's condition. Also, manual therapy techniques which include soft tissue and joint mobilization to reduce joint deformity and increase functional range of motion.

- <u>B3. Transfer Training</u>—Evaluate and instruct safe transfers (bed, bath, toilet, sofa, chair, commode) using appropriate body mechanics, and equipment (sliding board, Hoyer lift, trapeze, bath bench, wheelchair). Instruct patient, family, and caregivers in appropriate transfer techniques.

- <u>B4. Establish or Upgrade Home Program</u>—To improve the patient's functional level by instruction to patient and other responsible individuals in exercise which may be used in adjunct to PT programs.

- <u>B5. Gait Training</u>—Includes gait evaluation and ambulation training of a patient whose ability to walk has been impaired. Gait training is the selection and instruction in use of various assistive devices (orthotic appliances, crutches, walker, cane, etc.).

- <u>B6. Pulmonary Physical Therapy</u>—Includes breathing exercises, postural drainage, etc., designed for patients with acute or severe pulmonary dysfunction.

- <u>B7. Ultra Sound</u>—Mechanism to produce heat or micro-massage in deep tissues for conditions in which relief of pain, increase in circulation, and increase in local metabolic activity are desirable.

- <u>B8. Electro Therapy</u>—Includes treatment for neuromuscular dysfunction and pain through use of electrotherapeutic devices (electromuscular stimulation, TENS, Functional Electrical Stimulation (FES), biofeedback, high voltage galvanic stimulation (HVGS) etc.).

- <u>B9. Prosthetic Training</u>—Includes stump conditioning (shrinking, shaping, etc.), range of motion, muscle strengthening and gait training with or without the prosthesis and appropriate assistive devices.

- <u>B10. Fabrication Temporary Devices</u>—Includes fabrication of temporary prostheses, braces, splints, and slings.

- B11. Muscle Reeducation—Includes therapy designed to restore function due to illness, disease or surgery affecting neuromuscular function.

- B12. Management and Evaluation of a Patient Care Plan—The complexity of necessary unskilled services require skilled management by a qualified physical therapist to ensure that these services achieve their purpose, and to promote the beneficiary's recovery and medical safety.

- B13. through B14. Reserved.

- B15. Other (Spec. Under Orders)—Include all PT services not identified above. Identify specific therapy services under physician's orders (HCFA-485 Item 21).

C. Speech Therapy (ST).—These codes represent all services to be performed by the speech therapist. Following is a further explanation of each.

- C1. Evaluation—Visit made to determine the type, severity and prognosis of a communication disorder, whether speech therapy is reasonable and necessary and to establish the goals, treatment plan, and estimated frequency and duration of treatment.

- C2. Voice Disorders Treatments—Procedures and treatment for patients with an absence or impairment of voice caused by neurologic impairment, structural abnormality, or surgical procedures affecting the muscles of voice production.

- C3. Speech Articulation Disorders Treatments—Procedures and treatment for patients with impaired intelligibility (clarity) of speech—usually referred to as anarthria or dysarthria and/or impaired ability to initiate, inhibit, and/or sequence speech sound muscle movements—usually referred to as apraxia/dyspraxia.

- C4. Dysphagia Treatments—Includes procedures designed to facilitate and restore a functional swallow.

- C5. Language Disorders Treatments—Includes procedures and treatment for patients with receptive and/or expressive aphasia/dysphasia, impaired reading comprehension, written language expression, and/or arithmetical processes.

- C6. Aural Rehabilitation—Procedures and treatment for patients with communication problems related to impaired hearing acuity.

- C7. Reserved.

- C8. Nonoral Communications—Includes any procedures designed to establish a nonoral or augmentive communication system.

- C9. Other (Spec. Under Orders)—Speech therapy services not included above. Specify service to be rendered under physician's orders (HCFA-485 Item 21).

    D. <u>Occupational Therapy</u>.—These codes represent all services to be rendered by the occupational therapist. Following is a further explanation:

- <u>D1. Evaluation</u>—Visit made to determine occupational therapy needs of the patient at the home. Includes physical and psychosocial testing, establishment of plan of treatment, rehabilitation goals, and evaluating the home environment for accessibility and safety and recommending modifications.

- <u>D2. Independent Living/Daily Living Skills (ADL training)</u>—Refers to the skills and performance of physical, cognitive and psychological/emotional self care, work, and play/leisure activities to a level of independence appropriate to age, life-space, and disability.

- <u>D3. Muscle Re-education</u>—Includes therapy designed to restore function lost due to disease or surgical intervention.

- <u>D4. Reserved</u>.

- <u>D5. Perceptual Motor Training</u>—Refers to enhancing skills necessary to interpret sensory information so that the individual can interact normally with the environment. Training designed to enhance perceptual motor function usually involves activities which stimulate visual and kinesthetic channels to increase awareness of the body and its movement.

- <u>D6. Fine Motor Coordination</u>—Refers to the skills and the performance in fine motor and dexterity activities.

- <u>D7. Neurodevelopmental Treatment</u>—Refers to enhancing the skills and the performance of movement through eliciting and/or inhibiting stereotyped, patterned, and/or involuntary responses which are coordinated at subcortical and cortical levels.

- <u>D8. Sensory Treatment</u>—Refers to enhancing the skills and performance in perceiving and differentiating external and internal stimuli such as tactile awareness, stereognosis, kinesthesia, proprioceptive awareness, ocular control, vestibular awareness, auditory awareness, gustatory awareness, and olfactory awareness necessary to increase function.

- <u>D9. Orthotics/Splinting</u>—Refers to the provision of dynamic and static splints, braces, and slings for relieving pain, maintaining joint alignment, protecting joint integrity, improving function, and/or decreasing deformity.

- <u>D10. Adaptive Equipment (fabrication and training)</u>—Refers to the provision of special devices that increase independent functions.

- <u>D11. Other</u>—Occupational therapy services not quantified above.

B. HIM-11 Durable Medical Equipment

As experts at assessing the need for durable medical equipment and instructing in its proper use, home care therapists must be aware of the federal rules concerning reimbursement for durable medical equipment. This appendix contains §220 Rental and Purchase of Durable Medical Equipment, which defines durable medical equipment, describes what makes equipment reasonable and necessary, and outlines billing issues such as rent versus purchase of equipment.

The Health Care Financing Administration revised the Rental and Purchase of Durable Medical Equipment subsection of the HIM-11 in September of 1987. All Medicare-certified agencies possess a copy of the HIM-11. Consult the agency HIM-11 to stay abreast of recent changes or revisions to this manual.

RENTAL AND PURCHASE OF DURABLE MEDICAL EQUIPMENT

A participating provider of service may be reimbursed under Part B on a reasonable cost basis for durable medical equipment which it rents or sells to a beneficiary for use in his home if the following three requirements are met:

- The equipment meets the definition of durable medical equipment (§220.1); and

- The equipment is necessary and reasonable for the treatment of the patient's illness or injury or to improve the functioning of his malformed body member (§220.2); and

- The equipment is used in the patient's home (§220.3).

Payment may also be made under this provision for repairs, maintenance, and delivery of equipment as well as for expendable and nonreusable items essential to the effective use of the equipment subject to the conditions in §220.4.

220.1 <u>Definition of Durable Medical Equipment</u>.—For purposes of coverage under Part B, durable medical equipment is equipment which (1) can withstand repeated use, and (2) is primarily and customarily used to serve a medical purpose, and (3) generally is not useful to a person in the absence of illness or injury, and (4) is appropriate for use in the home. All requirements of the definition must be met before an item can be considered to be durable medical equipment.

A. <u>Durability</u>.—An item is considered durable if it can withstand repeated use; i.e., the type of item which could normally be rented. Medical supplies of an expendable nature such as incontinent pads, lambs wool pads, catheters, ace bandages, elastic stockings, surgical face masks, irrigating kits, sheets, and bags are not considered "durable" within the meaning of the definition. There are other items which, although durable in nature, may fall into other coverage categories such as braces, prosthetic devices, artificial arms, legs, and eyes.

B. <u>Medical Equipment</u>.—Medical equipment is equipment which is primarily and customarily used for medical purposes and is not generally useful in the absence of illness or injury. In most instances, no development will be needed to determine whether a specific item of equipment is medical in nature. However, some cases will require development to determine whether the item constitutes medical equipment. This development would include the advice of local medical organizations (providers, medical schools, medical societies) and specialists in the field of physical medicine, and rehabilitation. If the equipment is new on the market, it may be necessary, prior to seeking professional advice, to obtain information from the supplier or manufacturer explaining the design, purpose, effectiveness, and method of using the equipment in the home as well as the results of any tests or clinical studies that have been conducted.

1. <u>Equipment Presumptively Medical</u>.—Items such as hospital beds, wheelchairs, hemodialysis equipment, iron lungs, respirators, intermittent positive pressure breathing machines, medical regulators, oxygen tents, crutches, canes, trapeze bars, walkers, inhalators, nebulizers, commodes, suction machines, and traction equipment presumptively constitute medical equipment. (Although hemodialysis equipment is a prosthetic device, it also meets the definition of durable medical equipment, and reimbursement for the rental or purchase of such equipment for use in the beneficiary's home will be made only under the provisions for payment applicable to durable medical equipment.)

2. <u>Equipment Presumptively Nonmedical</u>.—Equipment which is primarily and customarily used for a nonmedical purpose may not be considered "medical" equipment for which payment can be made under the medical insurance program. This is true even though the item has some remote medically related use. For example, in the case of a cardiac patient, an air conditioner might possibly be used to lower room temperature to reduce fluid loss in the patient and to restore an environment conducive to maintenance of the proper fluid balance. Nevertheless, because the primary and customary use of an air conditioner is a nonmedical one, the air conditioner <u>cannot</u> be deemed to be medical equipment for which payment can be made.

Other devices and equipment used for environmental control or to enhance the environmental setting in which the beneficiary is placed are not considered covered durable medical equipment. These include, for example, roomheaters, humidifiers, dehumidifiers, and electric air cleaners. Equipment which basically serves comfort or convenience functions or is primarily for the convenience of a person caring for the patient, such as elevators, stairway elevators, posture chairs, and cushion lift chairs do not constitute medical equipment. Similarly, physical fitness equipment, e.g., an exercycle; first-aid or precautionary-type equipment, e.g., preset portable oxygen units; self-help devices, e.g., safety grab bars; and training equipment, e.g., speech teaching machines and braille training texts, are considered nonmedical in nature.

3. <u>Special Exception Items</u>.—Specified items of equipment may be covered under certain conditions even though they do not meet the definition of durable medical equipment because they are not primarily and customarily used to serve a medical purpose and/or are generally useful in the absence of illness or injury. These items would be covered when it is clearly established that they serve a therapeutic purpose in an individual case and would include:

a. Gel pads and pressure and water mattresses (which generally serve a preventive purpose) when prescribed for a patient who has bed sores or there is medical evidence indicating that he is highly susceptible to such ulceration; and

b. Heat lamps for a medical rather than a soothing or cosmetic purpose, e.g., where the need for heat therapy has been established.

In establishing medical necessity for these items (see §220.2), the evidence must show that the item is included in the physician's course of treatment and a physician is supervising its use.

<u>NOTE</u>: The above items represent special exceptions and no extension of coverage to other items should be inferred.

220.2 <u>Necessary and Reasonable</u>.—Although an item may be classified as durable medical equipment, it may not be covered in every instance. Coverage in a particular case is subject to the requirement that the equipment be necessary and reasonable for treatment of an illness or injury, or to improve the functioning of a malformed body member. These considerations will bar payment for equipment which cannot reasonably be expected to perform a therapeutic function in an individual case or will permit only partial payment when the type of equipment furnished substantially exceeds that required for the treatment of the illness or injury involved.

A. <u>Necessity for the Equipment</u>.—Equipment is necessary when it can be expected to make a meaningful contribution to the treatment of the patient's illness or injury or to the improvement of his malformed body member. In most cases the physician's prescription for the equipment will be sufficient to establish that the equipment serves this purpose.

B. <u>Reasonableness of the Equipment</u>.—Even though an item of durable medical equipment may serve a useful medical purpose, the intermediary will also consider to what extent, if any, it would be reasonable for the Medicare program to pay for the item prescribed. The following considerations will enter into the intermediary's determination of reasonableness:

1. Would the expense of the item to the program be clearly disproportionate to the therapeutic benefits which could ordinarily be derived from use of the equipment?

2. Is the item substantially more costly than a medically appropriate and realistically feasible alternative pattern of care?

3. Does the item serve essentially the same purpose as equipment already available to the beneficiary?

The following example points up the applicability of these reasonableness guidelines:

<u>EXAMPLE:</u> The median price of standard whirlpool bath equipment is about $600 plus plumbing expenses necessary to install it in the patient's home. Program coverage of such equipment in the patient's home should be limited to those cases where it is prescribed for conditions where the whirlpool bath can be expected to provide a substantial therapeutic benefit justifying its cost. For example, bursitis or chronic osteoarthritis would not generally justify Medicare payment for whirlpool bath equipment in the home since it would not be reasonable to expect that a whirlpool bath would be significantly more beneficial than a normal warm bath. Moreover, where the patient is not homebound, payment for this item in the patient's home should be restricted to the cost of providing the service elsewhere, e.g., an outpatient department of a participating hospital, if that alternative is less costly.

C. <u>Payment Consistent With What Is Necessary and Reasonable</u>.—Where a claim is filed for equipment containing features of an aesthetic nature or features of a medical nature which are not required by the patient's condition or where there exists a reasonably feasible and medically appropriate alternative pattern of care which is less costly than the equipment furnished, the amount payable is based on the reasonable costs for the equipment or alternative treatment which meets the patient's medical needs.

The provider may not charge the beneficiary for features not medically required by his condition and which cannot be considered in determining the provider's allowable costs <u>unless</u> the beneficiary or his representative has specifically requested the excessive or deluxe item or services with knowledge of the amount he is to be charged.

220.3 <u>Definition of Beneficiary's Home</u>.—For purposes of rental and purchase of durable medical equipment, a beneficiary's home may be his own dwelling, an apartment, a relative's home, a home for the aged, or some other type of institution. However, an institution may not be considered a beneficiary's home if it:

A. Meets at least the basic requirement in the definition of a hospital (§112.1), i.e., it is primarily engaged in providing by or under the supervision of physicians, to inpatients, diagnostic and therapeutic services for medical diagnosis, treatment, and care of injured, disabled, and sick persons, or rehabilitation services for the rehabilitation of injured, disabled, or sick persons; or

B. Meets at least the basic requirement in the definition of a skilled nursing facility (§112.2), i.e., it is primarily engaged in providing to inpatients skilled nursing care and related services for patients who require medical or nursing care, or rehabilitation services for the rehabilitation of injured, disabled, or sick persons.

Thus, if an individual is a patient in an institution or distinct part of an institution which provides the services described in A or B above, he is not entitled to have payment made for rental or purchase of durable medical equipment since such an institution may not be considered his home.

When the beneficiary is at home for part of a month and is in an institution which cannot qualify as his home for a part of the same month, payment may be made for the entire month. However, where the provider charges for only part of a month in such a case payment will be made on a prorated basis.

220.4 Repairs, Maintenance, Replacement, and Delivery.—Under the circumstances specified below, payment may be made for repair, maintenance, and replacement of medically required durable medical equipment which the beneficiary owns or is purchasing, including equipment which had been in use before the user enrolled in Part B of the program. Since renters of equipment usually recover from the rental charge the expenses they incur with respect to maintaining in working order the equipment they rent out, separately itemized charges for repair, maintenance, and replacement of rented equipment are not covered.

A. Repairs.—Repairs to equipment which a beneficiary is purchasing or already owns are covered when necessary to make the equipment serviceable. If the expense for repairs exceeds the estimated expense of purchasing or renting another item of equipment for the remaining period of medical need, no payment can be made for the amount of the excess. Claims for repairs which suggest malicious damage or culpable neglect should be reported to the intermediary.

B. Maintenance.—Routine periodic servicing, such as testing, cleaning, regulating, and checking of the beneficiary's equipment is not covered. Such routine maintenance is generally expected to be done by the owner rather than by a retailer or some other person who would charge the beneficiary. Normally, purchasers of durable medical equipment are given operating manuals which describe the type of servicing an owner may perform to properly maintain the equipment. Thus, hiring a third party to do such work would be for the convenience of the beneficiary and would not be covered.

However, more extensive maintenance which, based on the manufacturers' recommendations, is to be performed by authorized technicians, would be covered as repairs. This might include, for example, breaking down sealed components and performing tests which require specialized testing equipment not available to the beneficiary.

C. Replacement.—Replacement of equipment which the beneficiary owns or is purchasing is covered in cases of loss or irreparable damage or wear and when required because of a change in the patient's condition. Expenses for replacement required because of loss or irreparable damage may be reimbursed without a physician's order when in the judgment of the intermediary the equipment as originally ordered, considering the age of the order, would still fill the patient's medical needs. However, claims involving replacement equipment necessitated because of wear or a change in the patient's condition should be supported by a current physician's order.

Cases suggesting malicious damage, culpable neglect, or wrongful disposition of equipment should be reported to the intermediary.

D. Delivery.—Reasonable costs for delivery of durable medical equipment whether rented or purchased are covered if the provider customarily makes separate charges for delivery and this is a common practice among the other local providers.

220.5 <u>Coverage of Supplies and Accessories</u>.—Reimbursement may be made for supplies, e.g., oxygen, only when essential to the effective use of medically necessary durable medical equipment. Medications which may be used in connection with durable medical equipment are generally not covered.

Medications fall within the drug restriction and are, therefore, not covered under Part B except for those which cannot be self-administered and are provided as incident to a physician's professional services. This exception would apply to tumor chemotherapy agents such as methotrexate, 5-fluorouracil, and FUDR when used in conjunction with an infusion pump which is considered to be durable medical equipment. Such drugs and related services in charging or recharging the pump are covered only when furnished by a physician or by a technician under circumstances which satisfy the requirements for coverage of the services of auxiliary personnel rendered "incident to" a physician's service (i.e., provided under his personal supervision with the charges for such services included in the physician's bill).

Reimbursement may be made for replacement of essential accessories such as hoses, tubes, mouth pieces, etc., for necessary durable medical equipment, only if the beneficiary owns or is purchasing the equipment.

220.6 <u>Miscellaneous Issues Included in the Coverage of Equipment</u>.—Payment can be made for the purchase of durable medical equipment even though rental payments may have been made for prior months. This could occur where, because of a change in his condition, the beneficiary feels that it would be to his advantage to purchase the equipment rather than to continue to rent it. When such a situation occurs, the provider may deduct all or part of the rentals paid from the purchase price of the equipment.

A beneficiary may sell or otherwise dispose of equipment for which he has no further use, for example, because of recovery from the illness or injury which gave rise to the need for the equipment. (There is no authority for the program to repossess the equipment.) If after such disposal there is again medical need for similar equipment, payment can be made for the rental or purchase of that equipment.

However, where an arrangement is motivated solely by a desire to create artificial expenses to be met by the program and to realize a profit thereby, such expenses would not be covered under the program. The resolution of questions involving the disposition and subsequent acquisition of durable medical equipment must be made on a case-by-case basis.

Cases where it appears that there has been an attempt to create an artificial expense and realize a profit thereby should be reported to the intermediary.

When payments stop because the beneficiary's condition has changed and the equipment is no longer medically necessary, he is responsible for the remaining noncovered charges. Similarly, when payments stop because the beneficiary dies, his estate is responsible for the remaining noncovered charges.

220.7 <u>Payment for Durable Medical Equipment</u>.—

    A. <u>The Decision to Rent or Purchase</u>.—A beneficiary may elect to rent an item of equipment rather than purchase it even though it may appear that purchase would be more economical for the program. However, the intermediary will determine the method of payment to be used by the program in making reimbursement for equipment that is purchased. In both rental and purchase on a periodic payment basis, the monthly amount payable to the provider is converted to estimated costs by using the established outpatient cost reimbursement rate.

1. <u>Rental Payments</u>.—Where a provider rents durable medical equipment to a beneficiary, the provider will be reimbursed 80 percent of the reasonable cost of making the equipment available less any unmet deductible. Where the provider <u>rents</u> the equipment to the patient, it submits an SSA-1483 for each month's rental charge. The patient is responsible to the provider for any unmet deductible and the monthly coinsurance.

2. <u>Purchase of Equipment</u>.—Where the provider sells the equipment to the patient, it submits one SSA-1483 to the intermediary showing the purchase price. The intermediary prepares an SSA-1483 for each month it makes payment showing the amount of the periodic payment for that month. The provider may either bill the patient once for his deductible and coinsurance liability or submit a bill to him each month. When equipment is purchased, the intermediary determines in accordance with the following guidelines whether program payment is to be made in a lump sum or in periodic payments.

    a. <u>Lump-Sum Payment for Inexpensive Equipment</u>.—Payment for inexpensive equipment will be made in a lump sum subject to the deductible and coinsurance when it is determined to be less costly or more practical to do so. <u>Inexpensive equipment</u> is normally any item of durable medical equipment for which the reasonable charge is $50 or less.

    b. <u>Periodic Payment</u>.—Where payment is not made in a lump sum, benefits will be paid in monthly installments equivalent to the payment that would have been made had the equipment been rented. However, periodic payments may be made only for the established period of medical necessity for the item or until the total program payments to the provider equal 80 percent of the estimated cost of the item, whichever comes first. The periodic payments are subject to the deductible and coinsurance provisions. While periodic payments will be made on a monthly basis, a single payment can be made for periodic payments which have accrued.

B. <u>When Expenses are Incurred</u>.—The first month's expense for rental of durable medical equipment is deemed incurred as of the date of delivery of the equipment for purposes of crediting the SMI deductible and for reimbursement. Expenses for subsequent months are incurred as of the same day of the month as the date of delivery. Where equipment is purchased, the periodic monthly benefits will be payable on the same basis. Providers may submit claims as of the date the expenses are incurred and the date of delivery should be specified on the bill.

EXAMPLE: In August 1973, Mr. Thomas, a paraplegic, signed an agreement with an HHA to purchase a wheelchair for $200 to use in his home. The wheelchair was delivered to him on September 8, 1973, and the HHA submitted a bill. The intermediary determined the reasonable rental charge was $20 a month. Since Mr. Thomas did not have any other covered Part B expenses during the year, periodic payments for September 1973, October 1973, and November 1973, were withheld to satisfy the deductible. The first payment became payable on December 8, 1973. Since $40 of the deductible was met in the last quarter of 1973, payment for January 1974 was withheld to satisfy the remaining deductible of $20 for 1974. Periodic payments resumed February 8, 1974.

C. <u>Determining Months for Which Periodic Payments May be Made for Purchased Equipment</u>.—No payment may be made for any month throughout which the patient is in an institution which does not qualify as his home. Where equipment is purchased by a patient for use in his home and he is subsequently admitted to a hospital or SNF which does not meet the definition of the patient's home (§220.3), payments should be suspended. Upon return of the patient to his home, payments should resume without loss of monthly installments because of the institutionalization. Assuming the deductible is met, payments would continue as long as the equipment is medically necessary or until 80 percent of the reasonable purchase price has been reimbursed, whichever occurs first. The following example illustrates the application of this policy.

<u>EXAMPLE</u>: Mrs. Jones, who had already met her deductible, purchased a wheelchair on February 1, which she used in her home until her admission to the hospital on April 15. She was discharged from the hospital to her home on June 15 and continued to need the wheelchair. The reasonable charge for the wheelchair was $150 and the reasonable rental charge was $15 per month. The intermediary scheduled 10 monthly payments of $12 each (80 percent of $15) and paid for February, March, and April. Since Mrs. Jones was hospitalized for the entire month of May, the fourth installment was suspended. This installment became the June payment, and payments continued through December rather than November, as originally scheduled.

D. <u>Durable Medical Equipment Purchased Before Beneficiary's Coverage Begins</u>.—The dates on which periodic payments for a covered purchased item are due and allocation of the installments for deductible purposes are determined under the rules in B above. However, in determining whether a purchased item is covered, the entire expense of the item is considered to have been incurred on the date the equipment was delivered to an individual. Accordingly, where a purchased item of durable medical equipment was delivered to an individual before his coverage period began, the entire expense of the item (whether it was paid for in its entirety at the time of purchase or on a deferred or installment basis), would be excluded from coverage since payment cannot be made for any expense incurred before an individual's coverage period began.

C. Therapy Abbreviation List

Abbreviations provide a medical shorthand to streamline documentation time. To facilitate communication, home care therapists must use universally accepted abbreviations that allow peers and other disciplines to interpret and understand therapy documentation correctly. This appendix lists common therapy abbreviations and symbols for home care documentation.*

ā	Before, prior to	bid	Twice a day
A	Assessment	biw	Twice a week
Ⓐ	Assist, assistive	BKA	Below knee amputation
AAROM	Active assistive range of motion	BM	Bowel movement
AB	Abduction	BP	Blood pressure
AC	Acromioclavicular	bpm	Beats per minute
ac	Before meals	BR	Bedrest
ACLF	Adult congregate living facility	BS	Breath sounds
ADD	Adduction	BSC	Bedside commode
ADL	Activities of daily living	BSDB	Bedside drainage bag
AEA	Above elbow amputation	BUH	Built-up handles
afib	Atrial fibrillation	c̄	With
AFO	Ankle foot orthosis	C	Centigrade
AIDS	Acquired immunodeficiency syndrome	C1-C7	Cervical vertebrae 1-7
AIIS	Anterior inferior iliac spine	CA	Cancer, carcinoma
AKA	Above knee amputation	CABG	Coronary artery bypass graft
ALF	Assisted living facility	CAD	Coronary artery disease
ALS	Amyotrophic lateral sclerosis	CAT	Computerized axial tomography
am, AM	Morning	cc	Chief complaint
amb	Ambulate	CF	Cystic fibrosis
AMA	Against medical advice	CHAP	Community Health Accreditation Program
AP	Anterior-posterior	CHF	Congestive heart failure
ARF	Acute renal failure	CHI	Closed head injury
AROM	Active range of motion	cm	Centimeter
ASAP	As soon as possible	CNA	Certified nursing assistant
ASCVD	Arteriosclerotic cardiovascular disease	CNS	Central nervous system
ASHD	Arteriosclerotic heart disease	c/o	Complains of
ASIS	Anterior superior iliac spine	comp	Compression
ausc	Auscultation	cont	Continue
AVN	Avascular necrosis	COPD	Chronic obstructive pulmonary disease
B	Bilateral	COPS	Conditions of participation
BADL	Basic activities of daily living	COTA	Certified occupational therapist assistant
BEA	Below elbow amputation	CP	Cerebral palsy, cold pack

*Appendix C modified from Anemaet WK, Moffa-Trotter ME: *The user friendly home care handbook,* Washington, DC, 1997, LEARN.

CPM	Continuous passive motion
CPR	Cardiopulmonary resuscitation
CR	Closed reduction
CRF	Chronic renal failure
CRRN	Certified rehabilitation registered nurse
CVA	Cerebrovascular accident
DC	Discharge
dept	Department
DIP	Distal interphalangeal joint
dist	Distraction
DJD	Degenerative joint disease
DM	Diabetes mellitus
DME	Durable medical equipment
DNR	Do not resuscitate
DOB	Date of birth
DOE	Dyspnea on exertion
DS	Dressing stick
DSD	Dry sterile dressing
DTR	Deep tendon reflex
DVT	Deep vein thrombosis
Dx	Diagnosis
ECF	Extended care facility
ECG	Electrocardiogram
EEG	Electroencephalogram
EENT	Ears, eyes, nose, throat
e.g.	For example
EMG	Electromyogram
EPS	Extrapyramidal symptoms
ER	Emergency room, external rotation
etc	Et cetera
ETOH	Alcohol
eval	Evaluation
ex	Exercise
ext	Extension
F	Fahrenheit, fair
FI	Fiscal intermediary
flex	Flexion
ft	Feet
f/u	Follow-up
FWB	Full weightbearing
FWW	Front-wheeled walker
Fx	Fracture
G	Good
GI	Gastrointestinal
GS	Gluteal set
gt	Gait
GU	Genitourinary
HA	Headache
HCFA	Health Care Financing Administration
HCVD	Hypertensive cardiovascular disease
hemi	Hemiplegia, hemiplegic

HEP	Home exercise program
HHA	Home health aide, home health agency
HIV	Human immunodeficiency virus
HNP	Herniated nucleous pulposus
h/o	History of
H$_2$O	Water
HOB	Head of bed
HOH	Hard of hearing
hosp	Hospital
HP	Hot pack
HR	Heart rate
hr	Hour
HS	Heel strike, heel slide, hamstring set, hemi sling
HTN	Hypertension
Hx	History
①	Independent
IADL	Instrumental activities of daily living
ICF	Intermediate care facility
ICU	Intensive care unit
IDDM	Insulin-dependent diabetes mellitus
i.e.	That is
in	Inch
IR	Internal rotation
IV	Intravenous
JCAHO	Joint Commission on the Accreditation of Healthcare Organizations
jt	Joint
KAFO	Knee ankle foot orthosis
L	Left
L1-L5	Lumbar vertebrae 1-5
lat	Lateral
lb	Pound
LBP	Low back pain
LE	Lower extremity
LOB	Loss of balance
lpm	Liters per minute
LPN	Licensed practical nurse
LS	Lumbosacral
Lsh	Long-handled shoehorn
Lsp	Long-handled sponge
LT	Lap tray
LTG	Long-term goal
LTM	Long-term memory
LVN	Licensed vocational nurse
m	Meter
max	Maximal, maximum
MCP	Metacarpophalangeal
MD	Medical doctor
med	Medial, medication, medicine
mets	Metastases

MH	Moist heat	p/o	Postop
MI	Myocardial infarction	PO	By mouth
min	Minimal, minimum, minute	POC	Plan of care
MMT	Manual muscle test	POD	Postoperative day
mo	Month	polio	Poliomyelitis
mob	Mobilization	POT	Plan of treatment
mod	Moderate	PRE	Progressive resistive exercise
MRE	Manual resistive exercise	pre-op	Preoperative
MRI	Magnetic resonance imaging	prn	As needed, as required
MRSA	Methacillin resistant staph areus	PROM	Passive range of motion
MS	Multiple sclerosis, mental status	PSIS	Posterior superior iliac spine
MSS	Medical social services	pt	Patient
MVA	Motor vehicle accident	PT	Physical therapy, physical therapist
NA	Not applicable	PTA	Physical therapist assistant
NC	Nasal cannula	PUD	Peptic ulcer disease
NDT	Neurodevelopmental treatment	PUW	Pick-up walker
neg	Negative	PVD	Peripheral vascular disease
NG	Nasogastric	PWB	Partial weight bearing
NH	Nursing home	$\bar{q}$	Each, every
NIDDM	Noninsulin–dependent diabetes mellitus	qd	Daily
NKA	No known allergies	qh	Every hour
no	Number	qid	Four times a day
noc	At night	qn	Every night
NPO	Nothing by mouth	qod	Every other day
NT	Not tested	QS	Quad set
N/V	Nausea and vomiting	qt	Quart
NWB	Non–weight bearing	quad	Quadriceps
O	Objective	R	Right, repetition
O_2	Oxygen	RA	Rheumatoid arthritis
OA	Osteoarthritis	re	Regarding
OBS	Organic brain syndrome	rehab	Rehabilitation
OOB	Out of bed	resp	Respiration, respiratory
OP	Osteoporosis	RHHI	Regional home health intermediary
OR	Operating room	RN	Registered nurse
ORIF	Open reduction internal fixation	r/o	Rule out
OSHA	Occupational Safety and Health Association	ROM	Range of motion
		RR	Respiration rate
OT	Occupational therapist, occupational therapy	RROM	Resistive range of motion
		RT	Respiratory therapist
oz	Ounce	Rx	Prescription
P	Poor, plan	S	Subjective, supervision
$\bar{p}$	After	$\bar{s}$	Without
PA	Physician's assistant	S1-S5	Sacral vertebrae 1-5
PA	Posterior-anterior	SA	Sock aide
pc	After meals	SAQ	Short arc quad
per	By, through	SBQC	Small base quad cane
PLB	Pursed-lip breathing	SC	Straight cane, sternoclavicular
PLF	Prior level of function	SDH	Subdural hematoma
pm, PM	Evening	sec	Second
PMHx	Past medical history	SI	Sacroiliac
PNF	Proprioceptive neuromuscular facilitation	SLP	Speech-language pathologist

SLR	Straight leg raise		**TPN**	Total parenteral nutrition
SNF	Skilled nursing facility		**TPR**	Temperature, pulse, respiration
SOB	Shortness of breath		**TSA**	Total shoulder arthroplasty
s/p	Status post		**TSR**	Total shoulder replacement
SP	Stand pivot		**TTWB**	Toe touch weight bearing
SPC	Single point cane		**Tx**	Treatment, traction
s/s	Signs and symptoms of		**UE**	Upper extremity
STAT	At once		**UMN**	Upper motor neuron
STG	Short-term goal		**URI**	Upper respiratory infection
STM	Short-term memory, soft tissue mobilization		**US**	Ultrasound
Sx	Surgery		**UTI**	Urinary tract infection
T	Trace		**VA**	Veteran's Administration
T1-T12	Thoracic vertebrae 1-12		**VO**	Verbal order
TB	Tuberculosis		**VS**	Vital signs
TBI	Traumatic brain injury		**WB**	Weight bearing
TENS	Transcutaneous electrical nerve stimulation		**WBAT**	Weight bearing as tolerated
TDWB	Toe down weight bearing		**WBQC**	Wide base quad cane
THA	Total hip arthroplasty		**WC**	Wheelchair
ther ex	Therapeutic exercise		**W/cm²**	Watts per square centimeter
THR	Total hip replacement		**WFL**	Within functional limits
TIA	Transient ischemic attack		**wk**	Week
tid	Three times a day		**WNL**	Within normal limits
tiw	Three times a week		**wt**	Weight
TKA	Total knee arthroplasty		**X**	Times
TKE	Terminal knee extension		**yd**	Yard
TKR	Total knee replacement		**YO**	Year old
TMJ	Temperomandibular joint		**yr**	Year
TP	Tender point			

SYMBOLS

1°	Primary		↑	Increased, more, elevated
2°	Secondary, secondary to		↓	Decreased, less, lower
?	Questionable, suspected		→	To
~	Approximately		←	From
=	Equal		↔	To and from
<	Less than		**#**	Number
>	Greater than		**@**	At, about
≤	Less than or equal to		**/**	Extension
≥	Greater than or equal to		✓	Flexion
°	Degree		**–**	Minus, negative
△	Change		**+**	Plus, and, positive

D. Common ICD-9-CM Therapy Diagnoses List

Therapy diagnoses are the disorders or deficits that therapists treat. All home care patients receiving therapy services must have therapy diagnoses. This appendix lists the more common therapy diagnoses treated by therapists in home health care. All diagnoses are coded using the International Classification of Diseases, Ninth Revision, Clinical Modification (ICD-9-CM), which provides a universal method for diagnosis classification and identification. This publication is frequently revised; home care therapists must confirm correct coding at least annually to stay abreast of changes.

ICD-9-CM Code	Therapy Diagnosis	ICD-9-CM Code	Therapy Diagnosis
042	Human immunodeficiency virus disease	337	Disorders of the autonomic nervous system
045	Acute poliomyelitis		*337.2 Reflex sympathetic dystrophy*
138	Late effects of acute poliomyelitis	340	Multiple sclerosis
250	Diabetes mellitus	344	Other paralytic syndromes
	250.6 Diabetes with neurological manifestations		*344.0 Quadriplegia and quadriparesis*
			344.1 Paraplegia
332	Parkinson's disease		*344.2 Diplegia of upper limbs*
	332.0 Paralysis agitans		*344.3 Monoplegia of lower limb*
	332.1 Secondary Parkinsonism		*344.4 Monoplegia of upper limb*
333	Other extrapyramidal disease and abnormal movement disorders	357	Inflammatory and toxic neuropathy
	333.0 Other degenerative diseases of the basal ganglia		*357.0 Acute infective polyneuritis*
			357.2 Polyneuropathy in diabetes
334	Spinocerebellar disease	432	Other and unspecified intracranial hemorrhage
	334.0 Friedreich's ataxia		*432.1 Subdural hemorrhage*
	334.1 Primary cerebellar degeneration		*432.9 Unspecified intracranial hemorrhage*
	334.3 Other cerebellar ataxia	434	Occlusion of cerebral arteries
335	Anterior horn cell disease		*434.0 Cerebral thrombosis*
	335.1 Spinal muscular atrophy		*434.1 Cerebral embolism*
	335.2 Motor neuron disease	435	Transient cerebral ischemia
	335.20 Amyotrophic lateral sclerosis	436	Acute, but ill-defined, cerebrovascular disease
	335.21 Progressive muscular atrophy		
	335.24 Primary lateral sclerosis		

ICD-9-CM Code	Therapy Diagnosis
438	Late effects of cerebrovascular disease
	438.2 Hemiplegia/hemiparesis
	438.3 Monoplegia of upper limb
	438.4 Monoplegia of lower limb
481	Pneumococcal pneumonia
482	Other bacterial pneumonia
491	Chronic bronchitis
	491.2 Obstructive chronic bronchitis
492	Emphysema
710	Diffuse diseases of connective tissue
	710.0 Systemic lupus erythematosus
	710.1 Systemic sclerosis
714	Rheumatoid arthritis and other inflammatory polyarthropathies
	714.0 Rheumatoid arthritis
715	Osteoarthritis and allied disorders
716	Other and unspecified arthropathies
718	Other derangement of joint
	718.4 Contracture of joint
	718.5 Ankylosis of joint
719	Other and unspecified disorders of joint
	719.7 Difficulty in walking
720	Ankylosing spondylitis and other inflammatory spondylopathies
	720.0 Ankylosing spondylitis
721	Spondylosis and allied disorders
	721.1 Cervical spondylosis with myelopathy
	721.4 Thoracic or lumber spondylosis with myelopathy
722	Intervertebral disc disorders
	722.4 Degeneration of cervical intervertebral disc
	722.5 Degeneration of thoracic or lumbar intervertebral disc
	722.7 Intervertebral disc disorder with myelopathy
	722.8 Postlaminectomy syndrome
723	Other disorders of cervical region
	723.0 Spinal stenosis in cervical region
724	Other and unspecified disorders of back
	724.0 Spinal stenosis, other than cervical

ICD-9-CM Code	Therapy Diagnosis
725	Polymyalgia rheumatica
726	Peripheral enthesopathies and allied syndromes
	726.0 Adhesive capsulitis of shoulder
	726.1 Rotator cuff syndrome of shoulder and allied disorders
	726.2 Other affections of shoulder region, not elsewhere classified
	726.5 Enthesopathy of hip region
	726.6 Enthesopathy of knee
728	Disorders of muscle, ligament, and fascia
	728.2 Muscular wasting and disuse atrophy, not elsewhere classified
730	Osteomyelitis, periostitis, and other infections involving bone
733	Other disorders of bone and cartilage
	733.0 Osteoporosis
	733.1 Pathologic bone fracture
	733.13 Pathologic fracture of vertebrae
737	Curvature of spine
	737.1 Kyphosis (acquired)
	737.2 Lordosis (acquired)
	737.3 Kyphoscoliosis and scoliosis
	737.4 Curvature of spine associated with other conditions
781	Symptoms involving nervous and musculoskeletal systems
	781.2 Abnormality of gait
805	Fracture of vertebral column without mention of spinal cord injury
807	Fracture of rib(s), strenum, larynx, and trachea
812	Fracture of humerus
820	Fracture of neck of femur
821	Fracture of other and unspecified parts of femur
822	Fracture of patella
823	Fracture of tibia and fibula
824	Fracture of ankle
831	Dislocation of shoulder
835	Dislocation of hip

E. Home Care Resources List

Home care resources provide information on a variety of diagnoses and disorders. They also assist therapists in directing patients and caregivers to specific support systems and databases relevant to specific patient conditions. This appendix lists resource centers for the following:

Resources on Aging
Resources on AIDS
Resources on Alcoholism
Resources on Arthritis
Resources on Bladder Incontinence
Resources on Brain Injury
Resources on Cancer
Resources on Dementia
Resources on Diabetes
Resources on Gastrointestinal Disorders
Resources on Hearing
Resources on Heart Disease
Resources on Influenza and Pneumonia Vaccines
Resources on Kidney Disorders
Resources on Leisure Activities
Resources on Lung Disease
Resources on Mental Disorders
Resources on Multiple Sclerosis
Resources on Osteoporosis
Resources on Parkinson's Disease
Resources on Personal and Emergency Response Systems
Resources on Speech and Communication Disorders
Resources on Stroke
Resources on Vision

RESOURCES ON AGING

The American Association of Homes and Services for the Aging Publications
Department 519
Washington, DC 20061-5119
1-800-508-9442

The American Association of Retired Persons
601 E Street NW
Washington, DC 20049
1-202-434-2277

Children of Aging Parents
1609 Woodbure Road, Suite 302A
Levittown, PA 19057
1-800-227-7294

The Coalition on Family Caregiving
2008 Dempster
Evanston, IL 60202
1-708-733-1400

National Association of Area Agencies on Aging
1112 16th Street NW, Suite 100
Washington, DC 20036
1-202-296-8130

National Association of State Units on Aging
2033 K Street NW, Suite 304
Washington, DC 20006
1-202-898-2578

The National Council on Aging
409 3rd Street SW, Suite 200
Washington, DC 20024
1-202-479-1200

National Council of Senior Citizens
1331 F Street
Washington, DC 20004
1-301-578-8800

The National Family Caregivers Association
9621 E Bexhill Drive
Kensington, MD 20895
1-800-896-3650

National Institute on Aging Information
The Age Page
PO Box 8057
Gaithersburg, MD 20898-8057
1-301-496-4000

Respite Care
825 Green Bay Road, Suite 112
Willamette, IL 60091
1-847-256-1705

RESOURCES ON AIDS

The Access Project
611 Broadway, Suite 613
New York, NY 10012-2608
1-800-734-7104

The AIDS Directory
LRP Publications, Department 440
747 Dresher Road, Suite 500
PO Box 980
Horsham, PA 19044-0980
1-800-341-7874 extension 310

American Foundation for AIDS
733 3rd Avenue, 12th Floor Research
New York, NY 10017
1-212-682-7440

Centers for Disease Control in Atlanta
MMWR Office
1600 Clifton Road, NE
Atlanta, GA 30333
1-800-342-2437 HIV Hotline

National Association of People with AIDS
1413 K Street NW, 7th Floor
Washington, DC 20005
1-202-898-0414

RESOURCES ON ALCOHOLISM

Alcoholics Anonymous
PO Box 459, Grand Central Station
New York, NY 10163
1-212-870-3400

National Clearinghouse for Alcohol Information
PO Box 2345
Rockville, MD 20852
1-301-468-2600

National Council on Alcoholism
12 West 21 Street
New Seventh Floor
New York, NY 10010
1-212-206-6770

RESOURCES ON ARTHRITIS

Arthritis Foundation
1330 W Peachtree Street
Atlanta, GA 30309
1-800-283-7800

National Institute of Arthritis and Musculoskeletal and Skin Diseases
1 AMS Circle
Bethesda, MD 20892-3675
1-301-495-4484

RESOURCES ON BLADDER INCONTINENCE

Alliance for Aging Research
2021 K Street NW, Suite 305
Washington, DC 20006
1-800-497-0360

Continence Restored
407 Strawberry Hill Avenue
Stanford, CT 06902
1-914-285-1470

National Association for Continence
PO Box 8310
Spartanburg, SC 29305
1-800-252-3337

Simon Foundation for Continence
Box 835
Wilmette, IL 60091
1-800-237-4666

RESOURCES ON BRAIN INJURY

The National Brain Injury Foundation
1-202-296-6443

RESOURCES ON CANCER

American Cancer Society
1-800-227-2345
1-404-320-3333
1-404-329-7616

The American Institute for Cancer Research
1759 R Street NW
Washington, DC 20069
1-800-843-8114

Cancer Fund of America
2901 Breezewood Lane
Knoxville, TN 37921-1099
1-423-938-5281

Cancer Information Service
Fred Hutchinson Cancer Research Center
1124 Columbia Street, MP-1700
Seattle, WA 98104
1-206-667-4675

ENCORE Plus-National YWCA
1-202-628-3636

Hospicelink
1-800-331-1620

Medic Alert Foundation
2323 Colorado Avenue
PO Box 1009
Turlock, CA 95380-1009
1-800-432-5378

National Alliance of Breast Cancer Organizations
9 East 37th Street, 10th Floor
New York, NY 10016
1-800-719-9154

National Cancer Institute
31 Center Drive, MSC 2580
Building 31, Room 10A16
Bethesda, MD 20892-2580
1-800-422-6237

National Hospice Organization
1901 N Moore Street, Suite 901
Arlington, VA 22209
1-703-243-5900

National Lymphedema Network
2211 Post Street, Suite 404
San Francisco, CA 94115-3427
1-800-541-3259

Y-ME
National Organization for Breast Cancer Information and Support
1-800-221-2141

RESOURCES ON DEMENTIA

Alzheimer's Association
919 N Michigan, Suite 1000
Chicago, IL 60611-1676
1-800-621-0379

Alzheimer's Disease Education and Referral Center (ADEAR)
PO Box 8250
Silver Spring, MD 20907-8250
1-800-438-4380

Alzheimer's Family Support Groups
USF Suncoast Gerontology Center
MDC Box 50
12901 Bruce B Downs Boulevard
Tampa, FL 33612
1-813-974-4355

Greater Ann Arbor Alzheimer's Association
PO Box 1713, Department N89
Ann Arbor, MI 48106
1-313-741-8200
ID Bracelets for $1

National Institute on Aging
NIA Information Office
9000 Rockville Pike
Building 31, Room 5C27
Bethesda, MD 20892
1-301-496-4000

United States Department of Health and Human Resources
Administration on Aging
HEW N Building
330 Independence Avenue SW
Washington, DC 20201
1-202-619-0724

RESOURCES ON DIABETES

American Diabetes Association
National Center
1660 Duke Street
PO Box 25757
Alexandria, VA 22314
1-800-232-3472

Diabetes Self-Care
3601 Thirlane Road NW, Suite 4
Roanoke, VA 24019
1-800-972-2323

HCF Research Foundation
PO Box 22124
Lexington, KY 40522
1-606-276-3119

Joslin Diabetes Center
1 Joslin Place
Boston, MA 02215
1-617-732-2400

National Diabetes Information Clearinghouse
1 Information Way
Bethesda, MD 20892-3560
1-301-654-3327

RESOURCES ON GASTROINTESTINAL DISORDERS

American Liver Foundation
1425 Pompton Avenue
Cedar Grove, NJ 07009
1-800-223-0179

National Foundation for Ileitis and Colitis
386 Park Avenue South, 17th Floor
New York, NY 10016
1-212-685-3440

United Ostomy Association
36 Executive Park, Suite 120
Irvine, CA 92614
1-800-826-0826

RESOURCES ON HEARING

American Speech-Language-Hearing Association
10801 Rockville Pike
Rockville, MD 20852
1-800-638-8255

Better Hearing Institute
PO Box 1840
Washington, DC 20013
1-888-482-4327
1-800-327-9355 (TTY)

HARC Mercantile Ltd
PO Box 3055
Kalamazoo, MI 49003-3055
1-800-445-9968

National Association of the Deaf
814 Thayer Avenue
Silver Spring, MD 20910
1-301-587-1788

National Information Center on Deafness
Gallaudet University
800 Florida Avenue NE
Washington, DC 20002
1-202-651-5051 Voice
1-202-651-5052 Voice and TTY

Office of Scientific and Health Reports
National Institute of Neurological Disorders and
    Stroke
Building 31, Room 8A06
Bethesda, MD 20892
1-301-496-5751

Self Help for Hard of Hearing People
7910 Woodmont Avenue, Suite 1200
Bethesda, MD 20814
1-301-657-2248
1-301-657-2249 TTY

RESOURCES ON HEART DISEASE

American Heart Association
7272 Greenville Avenue
Dallas, TX 75231
1-800-242-8721

National Heart, Lung, and Blood Institute
Information Center, Publications
PO Box 30105
Bethesda, MD 20824-0105
1-301-251-1222

National Heart, Lung, and Blood Institute
National Institute of Health
9000 Rockville Pike
Building 31, Room 4A21
Bethesda, MD 20892
1-301-496-4236

RESOURCES ON INFLUENZA AND PNEUMONIA VACCINES

American Lung Association
6160 Central Avenue
St. Petersburg, FL 33707
1-800-586-4872

Centers for Disease Control
National Center for Prevention Services
Division of Immunization
Atlanta, GA 30333
1-404-639-3747

National Institute on Aging
PO Box 8057
Gaithersburg, MD 20898-8057
1-800-222-2225

The National Institute of Allergy and Infectious Diseases
National Institutes of Health, Box AP
Building 31, Room 7A32
Bethesda, MD 20205
1-301-496-4000

RESOURCES ON KIDNEY DISORDERS

American Association of Kidney Patients
100 S Ashley Drive, Suite 280
Tampa, FL 33602
1-813-223-7099

National Kidney Foundation
30 East 33rd Street
New York, NY 10016
1-800-622-9010

United Network for Organ Sharing
1100 Boulders Parkway, Suite 500
Richmond, VA 23225-8770
1-800-243-6667

Polycystic Kidney Research Foundation
4901 Main, Suite 320
Kansas City, MO 64112
1-816-931-2600

RESOURCES ON LEISURE ACTIVITIES

Access to Recreation
PO Box 5072-430
Thousand Oaks, CA 91359
1-800-634-4351

Adventures in Cassettes
5353 Nathan Lane North
Plymouth, MN 55442
1-800-328-0108

Brookstone Hard-To-Find-Tools
1655 Bassford Drive
Mexico, MO 65265
1-800-846-3000

The Disability Bookshop Catalog
Twin Peaks Press
PO Box 129
Vancouver, WA 98666
1-360-694-2462

Eldergames
1331 H Street NW
Washington, DC 20005
1-800-637-2604

Geriatric Resources
PO Box 1509
Goldenrod, FL 33733
1-800-359-0390

S&S Worldwide
PO Box 513
Colchester, CT 06415
1-800-243-9232

Wireless: Minnesota Public Radio
PO Box 64422
St. Paul, MN 55164-0422
1-800-669-5959

RESOURCES ON LUNG DISEASE

American Association of Respiratory Care
11030 Ables Lane
Dallas, TX 75229
1-214-243-2272

American Lung Association
6160 Central Avenue
St. Petersburg, FL 33707
1-800-586-4872

RESOURCES ON MENTAL DISORDERS

The National Alliance for the Mentally Ill
200 N Glieb Road, Suite 1015
Arlington, VA 22203-3754
1-800-950-6264

National Mental Health Association
1021 Prince Street
Alexandria, VA 22314
1-800-969-6642

Reach c/o The Mental Health Association of MN
2021 E Hennepin Avenue, Suite 412
Minneapolis, MN 55413
1-612-331-6840

RESOURCES ON MULTIPLE SCLEROSIS

National Multiple Sclerosis Society
205 E 42nd Street
New York, NY 10017-5706
1-800-624-8236

RESOURCES ON OSTEOPOROSIS

National Institute on Aging
Information Center
PO Box 8057
Gaithersburg, MD 20898-8057
1-800-222-2225

National Osteoporosis Foundation
1150 17th Street NW, Suite 500
Washington, DC 20036-4603
202-223-2226

RESOURCES ON PARKINSON'S DISEASE

The American Parkinson Disease Association
1250 Highland Boulevard, Suite 4B
Staten Island, NY 10305
1-800-223-2732

National Institute of Neurological Disorders and
   Stroke: National Institute of Health
9000 Wisconsin Avenue
Bethesda, MD 20890
1-301-496-9746

Parkinson's Disease Foundation
Columbia University Med Research Building
710 W 168 Street, 3rd Floor
New York, NY 10032
1-212-923-4700

Parkinson's Disease Update
Medical Publishing Company
PO Box 450
Huntingdon Valley, PA 19006
1-800-947-6658

Parkinson Support Group of America
11376 Cherry Hill Road, Apt 204
Beltsville, MD 20705
1-301-937-1545

United Parkinson Foundation
833 W Washington Boulevard
Chicago, IL 60607
1-312-733-1893

RESOURCES ON PERSONAL AND EMERGENCY RESPONSE SYSTEMS

American Medical Alert Corporation
3265 Lawson Boulevard
Oceanside, NY 11572
1-516-536-5850

Life Alert Emergency Response
15301 Ventura Boulevard, Suite 3500
Sherman Oaks, CA 91403
1-800-367-8351

Lifeline Systems
1 Arsenal Marketplace
Watertown, MA 02172
1-800-543-3546

MedicAlert
2323 Colorado Avenue
PO Box 1009
Turlock, CA 95381-1009
1-800-432-5378

RESOURCES ON SPEECH AND COMMUNICATION DISORDERS

American Speech-Language-Hearing Association
10801 Rockville Pike
Rockville, MD 20852
1-800-638-8255

AT&T National Special Needs Center
5 Woodhollow
Parsippany, NJ 07054
1-800-233-1222

Crestwood Communication Aid Company
6625 N Sidney Place
Milwaukee, WI 53209-3259
1-414-352-5678

Don Johnson Developmental Equipment
1000 North Rand Road, Building 115
Wauconda, IL 60084
1-800-999-4660

Imaginart Communication Products
307 Arizona Street
Bisbee, AZ 85603
1-800-828-1376

Innocomp
26210 Emery Road, Suite 302
Warrensville Heights, OH 44128
1-800-382-8622

Luminaud
8688 Tyler Boulevard
Mentor, OH 44060-4348
1-216-255-9082

Mayer Johnson Company
PO Box 1579
Solana Beach, CA 92075-1579
1-619-550-0084

The National Easter Seal Society, Inc.
230 W Monroe, Suite 1800
Chicago, IL 60606
1-800-221-6827

National Institute of Neurological and Communicative Disorders and Stroke
National Institute of Health
Bethesda, MA 20892
1-301-496-9746

Sentient Systems Technology
2100 Wharton Boulevard, Suite 360
Pittsburgh, PA 15203
1-800-344-1778

Words +
40015 Sierra Highway, Building 145
South Palmdale, CA 93550
1-805-266-8500

RESOURCES ON STROKE

National Institute of Neurological and Communicative Disorders and Stroke
National Institute of Health
Bethesda, MA 20892
1-301-496-9746

National Stroke Association
8480 E Orchard Road, Suite 1000
Englewood, CO 80111-5015
1-303-649-9299

Office of Scientific and Health Reports
National Institute of Neurological Disorders and Stroke, Building 31, Room 8A06
Bethesda, MD 20892
1-301-496-5751

RESOURCES ON VISION

American Academy of Ophthalmology
PO Box 7424
San Francisco, CA 94210
1-800-222-3937

American Council of the Blind
1155 15th Street NW, Suite 720
Washington, DC 20005
1-800-424-8666

American Foundation for the Blind
National Headquarters
15 West 16th Street
New York, NY 10011
1-800-232-5463

American Optometric Association
Communication Division
243 North Lindbergh Boulevard
St. Louis, MO 63141
1-314-991-4100

Better Vision Institute
1800 N Kent Street, Suite 904
Rosslen, VA 27209
1-800-424-8422

Jewish Guild for the Blind
15 West 65th Street
New York, NY 10023
1-212-769-6237

The Lighthouse Low Vision Catalog
3620 Northern Boulevard
Long Island, NY 11101
1-800-453-4923

Lighthouse National Center for Vision & Aging
111 E 59th
New York, NY 10022
1-800-334-5497

National Eye Institute
31 Center Drive, MSC 2510
Building 31, Room 6A32
Bethesda, MD 20892-2510
1-301-496-5248

National Library Service for the Blind and Physically Handicapped: Library of Congress
1291 Taylor Street NW
Washington, DC 20542
1-800-424-8567

National Society to Prevent Blindness
160 E 56th Street
New York, NY 10022
1-800-331-2020

Sun Sounds Radio Service
3124 E Roosevelt
Phoenix, AZ 85008
1-602-231-0500

TeleSensory Corporation
455 N Bernardo Avenue
Mountain View, CA 94043
1-800-227-8418

Vision Foundation
818 Mount Auburn Street
Watertown, MA 02172
1-617-926-4232

Modified from Anemaet WK, Moffa-Trotter ME: *The user friendly home care handbook,* Washington, DC, 1997, LEARN.

F. Home Care Journals and Publications List

One of the keys to success in any practice setting is staying informed on current policy, research, and clinical practice guidelines. This appendix provides home care therapists with access to a variety of journals, newsletters, and publications devoted to the home health arena.

The American Journal of Hospice and Palliative Care
470 Boston Post Road
Weston, MA 02193
1-800-869-2700

CCH Home Care Front
4025 W Patterson Avenue
Chicago, IL 60646-6085
1-800-835-5224

CCH Home Care Provider's Guide
4025 W Patterson Avenue
Chicago, IL 60646-6085
1-800-835-5224

Healthward
Dependicare Home Health
1815 Gardner Road
Broadview, IL 60513

Homecare Direction
Beacon Health Corporation
1001 W Glen Oaks Lane, Suite 104
Mequon, WI 53092
1-414-241-3765

Homecare Quality Management
American Health Consultants
PO Box 71266
Chicago, IL 60691-9986
1-800-688-2421

Home Care Accreditation Alert
11300 Rockville Pike, Suite 1100
Rockville, MD 20852
1-800-929-4824 extension 223

Home Care Automation
11300 Rockville Pike, Suite 1100
Rockville, MD 20852
1-800-929-4824

Home Care Case Management
American Health Consultants
PO Box 71266
Chicago, IL 60691-9986
1-800-688-2421

Homecare Clinical Advisor
Beacon Health Corporation
12308 N Corporate Parkway, Suite 100
Mequon, WI 53092
1-800-553-2041

Homecare Education Management
American Health Consultants
PO Box 71266
Chicago, IL 60691-9986
1-800-688-2421

Home Health Business Report
American Health Consultants
PO Box 71266
Chicago, IL 60691-9986
1-800-688-2421

699

Home Health Care Management and Practice
Aspen Publishers
Professional Sales Department
200 Orchard Ridge Drive
Gaithersburg, MD 20878
1-800-638-8437

Home Health Digest
Aspen Publishers
7201 McKinney Circle
Frederick, MD 21701
1-800-234-1660

Home Health Focus
Mosby Yearbook
11830 Westline Industrial Drive
St. Louis, MO 63146
1-800-453-4351

Home Health Line
11300 Rockville Pike, #1100
Rockville, MD 20852-3030
1-800-929-4824

Home Health Resource Library
American Health Consultants
PO Box 740060
Atlanta, GA 30374-9823
1-800-688-2421

The Hospice Journal
The Hawthorne Press
10 Alice Street
Bingingham, NY 13904
1-800-342-9678

Hospital Home Health
American Health Consultants
PO Box 71266
Chicago, IL 60691-9986
1-800-688-2421

National Association for Home Care
519 C Street NE
Washington, DC 20002-5809
1-202-547-7424

Success in Home Care
11300 Rockville Pike, Suite 1100
Rockville, MD 20852-3032
1-301-287-2223

Modified from Anemaet WK, Moffa-Trotter ME: *Home care reality seminar handout,* Chevy Chase, Md, 1998, GREAT SEMINARS.

Index